Evidence-based
Neurology:
Management of
Neurological Disorders

Evidence-based Neurology: Management of Neurological Disorders

EDITED BY

Livia Candelise
Cochrane Neurological Network
Ospedale Maggiore Policlinico
University of Milan
Milan, Italy

WITH

Richard Hughes
King's College London School of Medicine at Guy's
King's College and St Thomas' Hospitals
London, UK

Alessandro Liberati
Università di Modena e Reggio Emilia
Modena, Italy

Bernard M.J. Uitdehaag
VU University Medical Center
Amsterdam, The Netherlands

Charles Warlow
University of Edinburgh
Western General Hospital
Edinburgh, UK

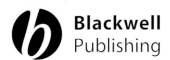
Blackwell Publishing

BMJ|Books

© 2007 by Blackwell Publishing
BMJ Books is an imprint of the BMJ Publishing Group Limited, used under licence
Blackwell Publishing, Inc., 350 Main Street, Malden, MA 02148-5020, USA
Blackwell Publishing Ltd, 9600 Garsington Road, Oxford OX4 2DQ, UK
Blackwell Publishing Asia Pty Ltd, 550 Swanston Street, Carlton, Victoria 3053, Australia

First published 2007
2   2008

Library of Congress Cataloging-in-Publication Data

Evidence-based neurology : management of neurological disorders / edited by
Livia Candelise ... [et al.].
    p. ; cm.
  "BMJ Books."
  Includes bibliographical references and index.
  ISBN 978-0-7279-1811-6 (hardback : alk. paper)
 1. Nervous system—Diseases. 2. Neurology. 3. Evidence-based medicine.
 I. Candelise, Livia. [DNLM: 1. Nervous System Diseases—therapy. 2. Evidence-Based
Medicine. WL 140 E93 2007]

RC346.E972 2007
616.8—dc22

                        2006038415

ISBN: 978-0-7279-18116

A catalogue record for this title is available from the British Library

Set in 9/12pt Meridian by Charon Tec Ltd (A Macmillan Company),
Chennai, India, www.charontec.com
Printed and bound in Singapore by COS Printers Pte Ltd

Commissioning Editor: Mary Banks
Editorial Assistant: Victoria Pittman
Development Editors: Vicki Donald, Simone Dudziak
Production Controller: Rachel Edwards

For further information on Blackwell Publishing, visit our website:
http://www.blackwellpublishing.com

The publisher's policy is to use permanent paper from mills that operate a sustainable
forestry policy, and which has been manufactured from pulp processed using acid-free
and elementary chlorine-free practices. Furthermore, the publisher ensures that the text
paper and cover board used have met acceptable environmental accreditation standards.

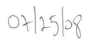
07/25/08

Contents

Contributors

Miguel F. Arango, MD

Assistant Professor
Department of Anesthesia and Perioperative Medicine
London Health Sciences Centre (University Campus)
London, Canada

Nadine Attal, MD, PhD

Neurologist and Pain Specialist
INSERM U 792 & Centre d'Evaluation et de Traitement de la Douleur
Hôpital Ambroise Paré
Boulogne-Billancourt, France

Thomas Benke, MD

Klinik für Neurologie
Medizinische Universität Innsbruck
Innsbruck, Austria

Michel Billiard, MD

Professor of Neurology
School of Medicine
Gui de Chauliac Hospital
Montpellier, France

Jeremy D.P. Bland

Consultant in Clinical Neurophysiology
Department of Clinical Neurophysiology
Kent and Canterbury Hospital
Canterbury, UK

Thomas Brandt, MD, FRCP

Professor and Chairman
Department of Neurology
Ludwig-Maximilians-University
Munich, Germany

Jorge G. Burneo, MD, MSPH

Assistant Professor of Neurology
Co-director, UWO Evidence-Based Neurology Group
University of Western Ontario
London, Canada

Livia Candelise

Professor of Neurology
Cochrane Neurological Network
Department of Neurological Sciences
Ospedale Maggiore Policlinico
University of Milan
Milan, Italy

Stefano F. Cappa, MD

Professor of Neuropsychology
Department of Psychology
Università Vita-Salute San Raffaele
Milan, Italy

Richard J. Caselli, MD

Professor of Neurology
Chairman, Department of Neurology
Mayo Clinic College of Medicine
Mayo Clinic Arizona
Scottsdale, USA

Stephanie Clarke

Professor of Neuropsychology
Centre Hospitalier Universitaire Vaudois
Head of the Division of Neuropsychology
Faculty of Biology and Medicine
University of Lausanne
Lausanne, Switzerland

Christian Daniel Cnyrim

Resident, Department of Neurology
University Hospital 'Grosshadern'
University of Munich
Munich, Germany

Miguel Coelho, MD

Neurologist, Neurological Clinical Research Unit
Institute of Molecular Medicine
Centro de Estudos Egas Moniz
Faculdade de Medicina de Lisboa
Lisbon, Portugal

Giorgio Cruccu

Professor of Neurology
Department of Neurological Sciences
La Sapienza University
Rome, Italy

Bart M. Demaerschalk, MD, MSc, FRCPC

Assistant Professor of Neurology
Division of Cerebrovascular Diseases and Critical Care Neurology
Mayo Clinic Arizona
Scottsdale, USA

George Ebers, MD, MA, FRCPC, FMedSci, FRCP
Action Research Professor of Neurology
Department of Clinical Neurology
University of Oxford
Radcliffe Infirmary
Oxford, UK

Eva L. Feldman, MD, PhD
Russell N. DeJong Professor of Neurology
University of Michigan
Ann Arbor, USA

Joaquim Ferreira, MD
Neurologist, Neurological Clinical Research Unit
Institute of Molecular Medicine
Centro de Estudos Egas Moniz
Faculdade de Medicina de Lisboa
Lisbon, Portugal

Graziella Filippini, MD
Director, Unit of Neuroepidemiology
National Neurological Institute 'Carlo Besta'
Milan, Italy

Paul Garner, MD, FFPHM
International Health Group
Liverpool School of Tropical Medicine
Liverpool, UK

Jan van Gijn, MD, FRCP, FRCPEdin
Professor and Chairman
Department of Neurology
University Medical Centre
Utrecht, The Netherlands

Gord Gubitz, MD, FRCPC, FRCPEdin
Assistant Professor of Neurology
Division of Neurology
Halifax Infirmary
Halifax, Canada

Robin Grant
Consultant Neurologist, Honorary Senior Lecturer
Department of Clinical Neurosciences
Western General Hospital
Edinburgh, UK

Michael G. Hart
Department of Clinical Neurosciences
Western General Hospital
Edinburgh, UK

Caroline M. van Heugten, PhD
Neuropsychologist
Senior Researcher in Cognitive Rehabilitation
Institute for Rehabilitation Research Hoensbroek
Institute of Brain and Behaviour
University of Maastricht
Hoensbroek, The Netherlands

Richard Hughes, MD, FRCP, FMedSci
Professor of Neurology
Department of Clinical Neuroscience
King's College London School of Medicine at Guy's
King's College and St Thomas' Hospitals
London, UK

Anu Jacob, MD, MRCP, DM
Consultant Neurologist
The Walton Centre for Neurology and Neurosurgery
Liverpool, UK

Paula Kersten, BSc, MSc, PhD
Senior Lecturer, School of Health Professions and Rehabilitation
   Sciences
University of Southampton
Southampton, UK

Alessandro Liberati
Professor of Clinical Epidemiology and Biostatics
Department of Hematology and Oncology
Università di Modena e Reggio Emilia
Modena, Italy

Anne MacGregor, MB, BS, MFFP, DIPM
Director of Clinical Research
The City of London Migraine Clinic
London, UK

Anthony Marson
Senior Lecturer and Honorary Consultant
The Division of Neurological Science
University of Liverpool
Liverpool, UK

Harry McNaughton, PhD
Programme Director, Rehabilitation Research
Medical Research Institute of New Zealand
Wellington, New Zealand

Kathryn McPherson, RN, RM, BA (Hons), PhD
Professor of Rehabilitation (Laura Fergusson Chair)
Division of Rehabilitation and Occupation Studies
Auckland University of Technology
Auckland, New Zealand

Douglas Mitchell, MD, FRCP
Director, Preston MND Care and Research Centre
Royal Preston Hospital
Preston, UK

Lorenzo P. Moja
Researcher
Centro Cochrane Italiano
Istituto Mario Negri
Milan, Italy

Ivan Moschetti, MD

Researcher
Centro Cochrane Italiano
Istituto Mario Negri
Milan, Italy

Fiona Norwood, PhD, MRCP

Consultant Neurologist
King's Neuroscience Centre
King's College Hospital
London, UK

Corina Puppo, MD

Assistant Professor
Intensive Care Unit
Hospital de Clínicas
Universidad de la República
Montevideo, Uruguay

Sridharan Ramaratnam

Senior Consultant Neurologist
Apollo Hospitals
Chennai, India

Gabriel J.E. Rinkel, MD

Professor of Neurology
Department of Neurology
University Medical Centre
Utrecht, The Netherlands

Bruno Rossi

Professor of Physical Medicine and Rehabilitation
Director, Academic Unit of Neurorehabilitation
Department of Neuroscience
University of Pisa
Pisa, Italy

Michael R. Rose, MD, FRCP

Consultant and Honorary Senior Lecturer in Neurology
Department of Neurology
King's College Hospital
London, UK

Peter M. Rothwell, MD, PhD, FRCP

Professor of Clinical Neurology
University Department of Clinical Neurology
Radcliffe Infirmary
Oxford, UK

Cristina Sampaio, MD, PhD

Professor, Laboratório de Farmacologia Clinica e Terapêutica
Faculdade de Medicina de Lisboa
Lisbon, Portugal

David T. Shakespeare, MSc, MRCP

Consultant in Rehabilitation Medicine
Preston Neuro-Rehabilitation Unit
Preston, UK

Tom Solomon, BA, BM, BCh, MRCP, DCH, DTMH, PhD

MRC Senior Clinical Fellow, Senior Lecturer in Neurology
Medical Microbiology and Tropical Medicine
University of Liverpool
Liverpool, UK

Brigitte Stemmer, MD, PhD

Professor, Canada Research Chair in Neuroscience and
  Neuropragmatics
Centre de recherche, IUGM
University of Montreal
Montreal, Canada

Michael Strupp, MD

Professor of Neurology and Clinical Neurophysiology
University of Munich
University Hospital 'Grosshadern'
Munich, Germany

Rod Taylor, MSc, PhD

Reader in Health Services Research
Peninsula Medical School
Exeter, UK

Lynne Turner-Stokes, DM, FRCP

Director, Regional Rehabilitation Unit
Northwick Park and Herbert Dunhill Chair of Rehabilitation
King's College London
London, UK

Bernard M.J. Uitdehaag, MD, PhD

Associate Professor of Neurology and Epidemiology
Department of Neurology and Department of Clinical
Epidemiology and Biostatistics
VU University Medical Centre
Amsterdam, The Netherlands

Walter Videtta, MD

Neurocritical Care, ICU
Hospital Nacional 'Prof. A. Posadas'
De Buenos Aires, Argentina

Charles Warlow

Professor of Medical Neurology
Department of Clinical Neurosciences
University of Edinburgh
Western General Hospital
Edinburgh, UK

Samuel Wiebe, MD, MSc, FRCPC

Professor and Head, Division of Neurology
Foothills Medical Centre
Calgary, Canada

Bryan K. Woodruff, MD

Instructor in Neurology
Mayo Clinic College of Medicine
Mayo Clinic Arizona
Scottsdale, USA

Preface

A carefully selected group of collaborators contributed to this book on evidence-based neurology, which aims to answer more than 100 clinical questions about treatment and management of neurological disorders. Participating authors, all of whom have clinical experience in specific neurological disorders, used a standard approach to search and summarize the results of existing scientific evidence in an attempt to provide readers with a straightforward text.

Thus we hope that this volume will be a useful tool for all general neurologists, from the oldest to the youngest, in their everyday clinical practice.

We aim to offer a product that:
- summarizes the most recent and important findings on treatments for neurological patients;
- provides answers to at least one treatment uncertainty;
- measures the benefit and, when applicable, the risk of harm inherent in specific neurological interventions.

We do not pretend to have provided complete coverage of the neurological field, because some important topics were not included. We also do not pretend to be completely evidence based, because some important clinical questions do not have an evidence-based answer. We selected a set of topics on the basis of practical judgement, and we systematically searched the literature that contained answers. We hope that the reader will not be disappointed that the whole of neurological treatment is not covered, or that the information provided for each topic is not 100% comprehensive.

Nowadays regulatory agencies such as the FDA and EMEA play a role in guiding clinical practice. Guidelines and practice parameters, more and more frequently, produce internationally and locally applicable clinical rules. Of course clinicians must be able to obtain these guidelines and know how to use them in their practice. However, sometimes they also need to refer back to primary studies and to weigh their personal experience against specific clinical research, taking into account both the design and results of that research. They need to know the characteristics of the patients included in the studies, which modalities were used to give the intervention being evaluated, which drugs and dosages were used, and they need a complete list of the outcome measures evaluated and the side effects reported by the original papers. Furthermore, they need to understand to what degree these studies are in line with their knowledge of the physio-pathology and of the natural history of the disease. This volume provides some of this information. It is intended to fill the gap between guidelines and primary studies as well as between primary and secondary scientific medical literature.

Book structure

This book has three sections and 24 chapters. Part 1 includes four introductory chapters on methodological issues related to evidence-based neurology (EBN). Part 2 (8 chapters) covers some routine interventions for symptoms common to several neurological diseases. Part 3 (12 chapters) covers a range of common or important illnesses and conditions.

We followed the Cochrane Collaboration guidelines for search strategies (Cochrane Reviewers' Handbook 4.2.2; Chapter 5: Locating and selecting studies for reviews) unless otherwise specified in each chapter. We used different types of studies to present the best possible summary of the evidence, joining a number of different sources using the usual hierarchical order proposed by the evidence-based movement. We preferred systematic reviews (Cochrane and non-Cochrane) as first choices. Randomized clinical trials (RCTs) were considered the gold standard. Other types of studies were only used if clinical questions could be better answered with non-randomized studies. We tried to select articles and studies of good methodological quality and to provide a critical appraisal of those of lower levels of quality.

We graded evidence in few cases because we didn't want to provide guidelines or recommendations. When we used a grading system we followed the European Federation of Neurological Societies (EFNS) grading system (*European Journal of Neurology* 2004; **11**: 577–81).

The selection of chapter titles and topics was done in collaboration with the editors and the authors of each chapter. We tried to identify important and common clinical conditions seen in neurological wards and outpatient clinics.

Each chapter starts with a brief definition of the clinical condition/s, together with its/their incidence and natural history. A clear formulation of a real-world scenario or question usually follows. The questions are structured using the standard three elements of patient, intervention, and outcome. The section covering critical review of the evidence for each question is mostly devoted to the presentation of the findings. The results are as quantitative as possible. Quantifying the expected benefit/harm for any intervention, rather than coming up with a single yes-or-no answer provides useful elements for deciding whether the expected benefit outweighs the potential harm. It also gives insight into the probability for a patient to gain or lose if treated with the intervention. Tables summarizing the quantitative, and, when this was not possible, the qualitative, results are included in each chapter. For each comparison, the tables list the number of patients, the risk in the control group, the relative risk (RR), and the absolute risk reduction (ARR). The weighted mean difference (WMD) is used for continuous outcome variables. A qualitative description of the results is provided when quantitative data are not available from the primary studies. Some chapters include the implications that the findings could have on clinical practice and on organization of health care, as well as an insight into the questions that have no answers and for which further evidence is required for better informed decisions.

Within this general framework among chapters, differences remain due to an intrinsic non-homogeneity of the primary reference studies, and also to the different cultural backgrounds of the internationally represented authors. This could be a limitation of the volume, or indeed a strength, making it more lively and nearer to real clinical needs. We hope that with future updating, which will of course be necessary (most of our references do not supersede 2006), we will be able to improve the format and the homogeneity of the chapters.

Finally, a few people deserve special acknowledgement for their contribution to this book. Debbie Jordan was responsible for all communications. She served as a valuable liaison between the publisher, editors and authors. Rodrigo Salinas contributed to the initial concept, helping to outline the chapter titles and topics. Mary Banks at Blackwell Publishing provided capable and consistent support throughout the project. I would like to express my sincere appreciation for this work.

Livia Candelise

PART 1
Introduction

CHAPTER 1

Evidence-based medicine: its contributions in the way we search, appraise and apply scientific information to patient care

Alessandro Liberati, Lorenzo P. Moja, Ivan Moschetti

Terms of reference

Reflections and elaborations about how evidence-based medicine (EBM) has been, and will increasingly be, able to influence clinical practice and the teaching of medicine abound, and it is very hard to try to say something original that is not already available [1]. This book, as Livia Candelise states in her introduction, is an attempt to summarize and compile examples of the contributions that a systematic approach to the search, identification and critical appraisal of scientific information can bring as an added value to the appropriate care of a patient with neurological problems/diseases. It is, therefore, very likely that this book will be read and used mostly by clinicians that – with different level of appreciation of the EBM approach – will seek information useful for their daily practice. The benefits, however, of putting together an account of what we know and do not know about the best ways to diagnose and treat neurological diseases are that one can see how far we are from being able to properly address patients problems and, more importantly, whether the ways in which the many uncertainties that still surround the care of patients with neurological disorders are being addressed in a proper way.

In short, the purposes of this chapter are:

(a) To revisit what EBM is and is not in the light of the strong positive, as well as negative, feelings that its appearance has brought about.

(b) To discuss the fact that the term 'evidence' itself is not so simple as it is sometimes portrayed, and try to see the extent to which this is at the heart of the controversial feelings about EBM.

(c) To summarize what the steps recommended by an 'EBM approach' are and exemplify the different ways in which users can take advantage of it.

In the concluding part of this chapter an attempt to reflect of who are the 'enemies' of EBM and how EBM itself has raised our awareness of the challenges that are ahead of us in terms of clinical practice, clinical research and health care policies will be attempted.

The EBM movement has provoked strong restatements from within the clinical world about the essence of the patient–clinician relationship and the balance between scientific approach and personal experience.

Some commentators saw the movement partly as an attempt by clinicians to keep control of decision making in the face of governments set on increasing intervention in the previously relative autonomous professions. Health policies worldwide, however, reveal the growth of mechanisms aimed at establishing parameters for acceptable clinical practice and a range of apparatus for monitoring and enforcing these parameters. On another track, some critics have questioned the movement's sometimes exclusive focus on one particular research design (i.e. the randomized controlled trial, RCT) as unnecessarily narrow and reinforcing the cultural and political values of particular research groups. Also embedded in this phenomenon is a staging of the confrontation between science and progress on one hand and myth and reaction on the other.

Whether the current debate addresses the real issues or is rather confounded by extraneous factors is the main 'file rouge' that the reader will recognize within this chapter. Our personal conviction is that in the current debate there is a mixture of epistemological confusion about the proper definition of 'proof' and 'evidence', resistances to cultural and professional changes from within the medical profession, misplaced criticisms from EBM scepticists and, to some extent, over-enthusiasm and reductionism from those that fail to recognize EBM's practical and methodological limitations.

What is EBM and what it is not?

The term EBM, as we use it nowadays, was introduced in 1992 by the same group of people that, years before, started the discipline called 'Clinical Epidemiology' (CE) [2]. CE stemmed essentially from the idea of adapting and expanding epidemiological methods to medical and health care decision making; CE was in fact defined as 'the discipline dealing with the study of the occurrence of medical decisions in relation to its determinants' [3].

CE has been very successful in illustrating new ways of teaching medicine and training health professionals and positioned itself around the notion of 'critical appraisal skills' as yet another essential ability that – in addition to the interpersonal, diagnostic and prognostic ones – a good doctor should master. An important CE's by-product was the documentation that much of the available evidence on diagnosis, prognosis and treatment of diseases was of poor methodological quality and quite often of dubious transferability to everyday clinical practice.

This led to a strong call for improving the scientific basis of clinical practice that was seen as too often dominated by practices of unproven effectiveness. This was the background for the 1992 *Journal of American Medical Association* (*JAMA*) article that first used the term 'Evidence-Based Medicine' [2].

In essence, proponents of EBM said that 'all medical actions of diagnosis, prognosis and therapy should rely on solid quantitative evidence based on the best of clinical epidemiological research'. Also they stated that 'we should be cautious about actions that are only based on experience or extrapolation from basic science'. Indeed this is not a new concept as recent research into the history of medicine has documented [4]. Vandenbroucke recently discussed the well-rooted historical precedents for the CE and EBM movements in the history of methodological research in medicine quoting, among others, Alexandre Louis who led in 1830 in France an initiative called 'Medicine d'Observation' [4]. Finding, not surprisingly, strong resistance from his fellows' environment, Louis stated that 'physicians should not rely on speculation and theory about causes of disease, nor on single experiences, but they should make large series of observations and derive numerical summaries from which real truth about the actual treatment of patients will emerge'.

Parallels and differences between now and then are worth noting here. In the early 1800s proponents of 'Medicine d'Observation' were reacting against a kind of medicine that derived its theories from many things that we would consider 'nonsense' by today scientific standards. Today EBM acts in the context of a very different environment where modern medical basic science has a solid experimental background. We now know that 'Medicine d'Observation' shortly after its appearance failed. A strong reaction from the medical profession together with the absence of contextual conditions account for this unfavourable outcome. Will EBM experience a different outcome as it leaves in a more scientifically oriented medical world? In many ways a similarly strong negative reaction has emerged today against EBM. No doubts that one of the reasons of such a negative

reaction against EBM has been the fact that it was labelled as a 'shift in medical paradigm' [2,4]. Such a definition would imply that EBM means scientific medicine and that all medicine practised before it was unscientific. This is not only simplistic but, to any closer scrutiny, profoundly wrong. The difference between the pre- and post-EBM era is not that before it people did not use the evidence. Rather, the real failure was the lack of a framework and set of rules to use the evidence in a systematic and explicit fashion.

Seen in this way the current fight around EBM and its nature could be advanced by moving the discussion from principles into a more pragmatic perspective where the attention is centred on a 'better use of evidence in medicine'. This would have the distinct advantage of indicating that it is the way and the rules according to which we use and interpret evidence that needs to be changed.

In contrast with the traditional wisdom of clinical practice, stressing the need for a 'better use of evidence in medicine' would indicate that that intuition and unsystematic clinical experience as well as pathophysiological rationale are insufficient ground for clinical decision making. On the contrary, modern practice of medicine finds its way on formal rules aimed at interpreting the results of clinical research effectively; these rules must complement medical training and common sense of clinicians whose uncontrolled dominance is no longer ethically and scientifically acceptable.

Struggling for a better use of evidence in medicine has also other important advantages. It challenges the paternalistic and authoritarian nature of much medical practice and helps understanding that – even when based on scientific methods – there is a selective and structural imbalance in the nature of the evidence that is available. This is skewed and biased towards therapeutic versus preventative interventions and towards simple pharmacological versus complex behavioural/social care. Acquiring critical appraisal skills – one of the most important tenets of the EBM movement – is the necessary (though not sufficient) best immunization against ignoring that there is a structural imbalance in the research agenda. An imbalance that should be overcome in order to make fully available the sort of evidence that is needed to provide effective and comprehensive health care to all patients [5].

The many faces of evidence (proof, causality and uncertainty) and their implications for clinical decision

Having set this background it should be clear that some definition of 'proof' is also needed to distinguish between scientific medicine and charlatanism. Pathophysiology – that is the reference to a mechanism to support the introduction of a new drug – is a criterion that has failed several times in the past: for example, the widespread practice of phlebotomy in 18th century medicine had some 'pathophysiological' basis, but no effectiveness at all. To define what we accept as a proof is clearly a problem of transparency of medical practice.

Our thesis is that, unfortunately, the 'evidence/lack of evidence balance' is not a black/white one for several reasons:
(a) For many clinical practices, even if we have well-conducted RCTs, all we can achieve is a 'weight-of-evidence' overall evaluation, because we face conflicting results from RCTs.
(b) In other instances RCTs are not available simply because they have not been conducted, and we only have access to observational investigations.
(c) The quality of the RCT is poor, so that a meta-analysis is not easily interpretable.
(d) RCT cannot be easily conducted for practical or ethical reasons.
Of course, we also have clear instances in which systematic reviews and meta-analyses contribute in an unequivocal way to the adoption or banning of a treatment.

In addition, we need to integrate the scientific evidence with the patient's preferences, with economic constraints, with the health care organization, with ethical obligations … This kind of integration is the object of clinical guidelines, in which ideally evidence is a necessary but insufficient component.

The model we can use comes from a different field, causality, and has been suggested by the philosopher John Mackie. Mackie claims that causality cannot be reduced to single necessary and sufficient causes, but rather should be described in terms of elements that he calls INUS (Insufficient Non-redundant component of an Unnecessary Sufficient complex). In his example, why did the house burn? The causal complex is formed by the association of fire in the fireplace, a strong wind, a defect in the alarm system and the fact that the house is wooden. If we analyse each component, none of them is a single sufficient cause, but only their conjunction gives origin to an overall sufficient complex. However, the complex is not necessary, because the house could burn in many different ways (e.g. because I put it deliberately on fire). According to Mackie, although none of the elements are sufficient, at least one is necessary (non-redundant), that is in its absence the complex would be ineffective (in the example: eliminating the fire in the fireplace would make the whole complex ineffective). Let us try to apply this same reasoning to medical decision. The physician has to integrate several elements into a decisional complex. Consider, for example, the prescription of interferon in patients with a diagnosis of relapsing–remitting multiple sclerosis (MS). According to the systematic review in the Cochrane Library, there are only seven trials including approximately 1200 patients with reliable information only on short-term follow-up (i.e. up to 2 years; example in the Appendix). The evidence overall suggests some advantage associated with interferon but results are hampered by the high proportion of drop-outs and the type of outcome measures

chosen. Should the neurologist decide to prescribe interferon? Instead of being an exception, the example is the rule. In other words, we often face 'grey' areas and the practicing neurologist might decide that, based on the Cochrane Review, the weight of evidence is quite strong or can reason exactly in the opposite way considering the relatively short follow-up, the questionable methodological quality of the studies and the important side effects. In other words, the weight of the empirical evidence can determine the ultimate therapeutic choice depending on the array of factors that, in the face of the same empirical evidence, a practitioner will consider.

Having said that it is important to perceive correctly one important feature of Mackie's definition of INUS, that is that at least one component is necessary (non-redundant). This component is evidence and without evidence there will never be good and justifiable clinical decision.

If we accept that evidence is a necessary component, still how to weigh the evidence depends on the definition of effectiveness one adopts. Effectiveness, like disease, is a 'fuzzy' concept. Concepts are almost never sharp, that is defined on the basis of a single property, but they tend to be fuzzy. In particular, the concept of effectiveness cannot be defined on the basis of a singular property (reducing mortality, disability, etc.), but of several properties that are partially overlapping in the actual instances: for some people effectiveness is mainly subjective, for others it is mainly objective, and no single definition is the right one. In summary, we have to face that effectiveness is a 'fuzzy' concept. This means that we cannot use the results of clinical trials (or of their synthesis in the form of systematic reviews or meta-analyses) as the only source of information and decisions about care: the work of the physician consists just in integrating different kinds of knowledge, although evidence is a necessary component.

Different modes of developing and using EBM skills and their ability to bring about evidence-based practice

The rapid spread of EBM has arisen from two main awareness:
1 The need for valid information about diagnosis, prognosis, therapy and prevention.
2 The inadequacy of traditional sources for this information because they are out of date (textbooks), frequently wrong (experts), ineffective (didactic continuing medical education), or too overwhelming in their volume and too variable in their validity for practical clinical use (medical journals).
Until recently, coping with these problems was impossible for full-time clinicians. However, developments in the 'technology of EBM' have permitted a change in this situation:
• The development of strategies for efficiently tracking down and appraising evidence (for its validity and relevance).
• The creation of systematic reviews of the effects of health care (see the Cochrane Collaboration).

• The creation of evidence-based journals of secondary publication and of evidence-based summary services such as clinical evidence.

• The creation of information systems for bringing the foregoing to us in a timely fashion.

The essence of the EBM approach to patients care comprises four steps [6]:

• *Step 1*: Transforming the need for information (about prevention, diagnosis, prognosis, therapy, causation, etc.) into an answerable question.

• *Step 2*: Locating the best evidence with which to answer that question.

• *Step 3*: Critically appraising the evidence for its validity (closeness to the truth), impact (size of the effect) and applicability (usefulness in our clinical practice).

• *Step 4*: Integrating the critical appraisal with our clinical expertise and with the patients characteristics, values and circumstances.

Depending on her/his different needs each health professional will use all or part of the above steps in different modes.

First is the 'doer' mode, in which all the four steps above are carried out.

Second is the 'user' mode, where searches are restricted to evidence resources that have already undergone critical appraisal by others such as evidence summaries.

Third is the 'replicator' mode, where the decisions of respected opinion leaders are followed.

All three of these modes involve the integration of evidence (from whatever source) with patient's unique characteristics, values and circumstances, but they vary in the execution of the other steps.

An intuitively appealing way to achieve such evidence-based practice is to generalize EBM teaching and training so that all clinicians become able to independently find, appraise and apply the best evidence. This strategy, however, has limitations as attaining all the necessary skills requires favourable personal attitude(s) and predisposition(s), intensive study and frequent, time-consuming, application. It is neither realistic nor feasible to expect and pretend that all practitioners will get to this advanced level of EBM skills. It has been repeatedly shown that practitioners welcome the availability of evidence-based summaries generated by others and evidence-based practice guidelines or protocols as long as they see them as helping tools and not compulsory obligations for their practice [6].

Thus, producing more comprehensive and more easily accessible pre-appraised resources is a second strategy for ensuring evidence-based care. The availability of evidence-based resources and recommendations will, however, still be insufficient to produce consistent evidence-based care. Habit, local practice patterns and product marketing may often be stronger determinants of practice. Studies have shown that traditional continuing education has little effect on combating these forces and shaping doctors' behaviour [7]. On the other hand, approaches that do change targeted clinical behaviours include one-to-one conversations with an expert, computerized alerts and reminders, preceptorships, advice from opinion leaders, and targeted audit and feedback. Other effective strategies include restricted drug formularies, financial incentives and institutional guidelines. Application of these strategies, which do not demand even a rudimentary ability to use the original medical literature and instead focus on behaviour change, thus constitute the pivotal strategy for achieving evidence-based care [7]. Therefore, educators, managers and policy makers should be aware that the widespread availability of comprehensive pre-appraised evidence-based summaries and the implementation of strategies known to change clinicians' behaviour will both be necessary to ensure high levels of evidence-based health care.

Internal and external enemies of EBM

But the difficulties that hamper a prudent and systematic use of evidence come not only from its imperfect and limited nature and from the medical establishment's resistance to change. There are also 'internal enemies' (which we will call the 'enthusiasts' here) who seem to have limited understanding of EBM's structural limitations and are dominated by unduly (optimistic) expectations of its sufficiency to guide medical practice. We mention below some of the relevant problems that should be kept in mind before blaming EBM as the sole culprit of its limitations.

First is the bias in the research agenda and the lack of mechanisms to prioritize it with respect to health needs. The increasing commercial influences in health care have produced a structural distortion in the setting of the research agenda and we see today a systematic bias in research priorities with a lot of (often redundant) data on pharmacological treatments and a dearth of information on potentially very relevant non-pharmacological interventions. Only recently this is starting to attract attention but this is still far from what would be needed to bring about the necessary changes [8]. Health services, on the other hand, have not traditionally been interested in investing in research and with some noticeable recent exceptions (see the UK R&D programme as well as part of the NIH research programme in the US) this is still the case. Consumers' input into research agenda is far from systematic and often the role of patients' charities ends up with lobbying for a particular disease or health problem rather than for the advocacy of an open and transparent prioritization [5].

The lack of independence of medical information and the 'pollution' caused by the commercial interference in it is another key factor. The imbalance between commercial and independent information is so striking that it may be naive to imagine that EBM alone can maintain its credibility without structural and cultural investments. When relevant information is not properly disseminated and implemented it is as if it would not exist. The recent example of the pharmacological treatment of hypertension is a case in point here: very expensive drugs have been for many years marketed without good evidence of their superiority to the equally effective and much less expensive old diuretics and only thanks to a publicly funded large scale trial [9] we now know that millions of dollars have been probably wasted without substantial benefits for patients. But lack of independence and monopoly of scientific information manifests itself also in the increasing medicalization of common problems and in the making of 'new diseases' as a way to make the health care market bigger and more profitable [10]. In this scenario as far as people identify as 'evidence-based' procedures and interventions for which studies exist and as 'non-evidence-based' areas where studies could exists but have not been carried out because there is no commercial interest in running them, EBM is at high risk of being used a fashionable yet misleading key word [11].

The 'paternalism' inherent in the idea that experts 'know it better' and that they are thus entitled to make decisions on behalf of their patients is a third important enemy. Paternalism has many components all of which are dangerous and should be recognized. One component comes from the idea that the increasing complexity of modern medicine requires increasing specialization. More and more medicine is fragmented into sub-specialities where people have a very deep knowledge into an increasingly narrow spectrum of problems. This technical knowledge leads to an overemphasis of the yield of a particular intervention where benefits are much too overrated with respect to risks [12]. Linked to this is the inherent conflict of interest that unavoidably links the social and professional prestige of those that are experts in a given field to the success of the intervention/technology of which they are champions. Like for the bias of the research agenda there are signs of increasing awareness that conflicts of interest are a threat to an equitable and effective practice of medicine but still much less than it should be [13]. And, again, a narrow technical view of EBM could be insufficient and perhaps even misleading in this respect.

Lack of awareness of the above-mentioned problems is – we believe – a great danger to EBM. Assuming that all relevant 'information needs' can be derived from published studies, that all practice skills can be derived from being updated with the medical literature, that methodological rigor is the only dimension that matters – even divorced from clinical and epidemiological relevance – and that health policies should be dictated (rather than more humbly 'informed') by evidence of effectiveness alone, are all internal threats that should be seriously considered and challenged.

What have we learned from EBM?

Having discussed EBM's epistemological, structural and practical limitations it is also fair to reflect on what it has

helped us to understand as of the major problems and limitations of today's clinical practice and health policies. Given the space constraints of this chapter we will summarize in short statements what we believe are issues that should inform an health care policy agenda that takes seriously some of the challenges that are ahead of us, if we care for effective and equitable systems of delivering health care. The list is tentative and incomplete and would hopefully be instrumental to stimulate a discussion on EBM's benefit/harm balance thus far.

Clinical practice

• There are not organized mechanisms and efforts to transfer and disseminate information on interventions that work from research to clinical practice; these efforts should become an integral part of the functioning of a good health care system.
• Medical practice is fraught with ineffective interventions and long delays before effective care enters clinical practice. Special attention should be given to in continuing medical education activities.
• Doctors and health professionals are not, by themselves alone, able to critically appraise the results of clinical research; consequently they can be (easily) misguided by unintentionally or intentionally wrong messages. Teaching critical appraisal skills should be an essential part of medical education.
• Clinical practice should (and can) be informed by results of systematic reviews of the best available information; knowledge of a given field based on just the few better known studies is dangerous because it ignores 'publication bias' and false negative results, etc. Medical education should stress the idea that knowledge is a 'cumulative' rather then a 'discrete' process and appropriate information tools should be made available to all health professionals [14].

Clinical research

• The quality of medical research is often poor and urgent improvements are needed. Poor quality has to do both with failure to apply appropriate designs and methodologies as well as paying attention to the search for relevant outcomes and for interventions that are generalizable outside the research settings.
• There are not explicit and transparent mechanisms for prioritizing research. Health care systems have almost exclusively delegated the responsibility to pharmaceutical companies and the commercial sector in general. Public and independent support to research is an urgent need [5].
• Conflicts of interest and lack of independence of investigators represent an increasing threat to the credibility of research [15,16].
• Patients' participation can be instrumental both in improving relevance and applicability of clinical research and in facilitating shared decision making. There is some evidence that, if properly involved, at the level of planning and identifying priorities, patients and consumers can provide valuable

inputs for research [17]. However, this is a process that requires a governance effort in order to avoid that increasing fragmentation is included in the prioritization process [18].

Health care policies
• Evidence should 'inform' but may be often inadequate to 'guide' decision making at the policy level. The sort of evidence that is usually produced by traditional clinical research is too narrow and lacks important elements that are otherwise crucial in policy making [19].
• Resources are often wasted by not acting against the use of ineffective interventions or by implementing effective interventions with ineffective strategies. A better link between efforts to improve quality at the micro level is needed.
• Health care system should assume more responsibility in knowledge production and should themselves promote research into areas that are likely not to attract resources due to limited commercial return [5].

Conclusions

There is no doubt that EBM does not, and cannot, answer all the epistemological and practical questions surrounding the practice of medicine. On the contrary, it is important that expectations from EBM are appropriate in order to prevent conceptual and practical mistakes. EBM provides methodological tools and a cultural framework. Methodologically it is useful to understand how we can produce valid and relevant information about the effectiveness of medical care. Culturally, its anti-authoritarian spirit is important to increase the participation of different stakeholders and to increase the opportunity for a multidisciplinary approach to health care problems.

It is clear that, thus far, the potential of EBM has not been fully exploited and that too narrow views of it have created avoidable confrontations with those that may be concerned that an 'EBM-dominated view' can do more harm than good. As efforts by methodologists have chiefly focused on how to design, conduct and interpret studies aimed at assessing efficacy/effectiveness of drugs, EBM is today mostly 'evidence-based therapy' with robust tools (i.e. RCTs) especially for assessing the worth of relatively simple interventions. The fact that we currently have limited ability to reliably assess complex interventions, preventative care in general as well as diagnosis or prognosis, should be seen not only as the results of the greater intrinsic complexity of these areas, but also as the consequence of the lower intellectual investments. A reflection, in turn, of the more limited commercial interests is at stake here.

It is our view that – despite the many limitations we have highlighted in this chapter – EBM has, at least in some areas of medicine, resulted in better clinical research and greater awareness of health professionals, health administrators and policy makers. A lot remains to be done in order to create a better understanding of the nature of proof, evidence and uncertainty; a more balanced research agenda; more coherent

mechanisms to improve quality of care; more substantial cultural efforts to empower patients and consumers. But we should be ready to recognize that most of this goes beyond what EBM can do alone and depends, more broadly, on health policy and politics with capital 'P'.

References

1 Strauss SE, Richardson SW, Glasziou P, Haynes RB. *Evidence Based Medicine: How to Practice and Teach EBM*. Elsevier, Churchill Livingstone, London and Philadelphia, 2005.

2 Evidence-Based Medicine Working Group. Evidence based medicine: a new approach to the teaching of medicine. *JAMA* 1992; **268**: 2420–5.

3 Spitzer WO. Clinical epidemiology. *J. Chronic Dis.* 1986; **39**(6): 412–5.

4 Vandenbroucke IP. Evidence based medicine and 'Medicine d'Observation'. *J. Clin. Epidemiol.* 1996; **49**: 1335–8.

5 Liberati A. Consumer participation in research and health care. *BMJ* 1997; **315**: 499.

6 Guyatt G, Deborah CD, Haynes B. Evidence based medicine has come a long way. *BMJ* 2004; **329**: 990–1.

7 Grol R, Grimshaw J. From best evidence to best practice: effective implementation of change in patients' care. *Lancet* 2003; **362**: 1225–30.

8 Garattini S, Liberati A. Bias by omitted research. *BMJ* 2000; **321**: 845–6.

9 Appel L. The verdict from the ALLHAT: thiazide diuretics are the preferred initial therapy for hypertension. *JAMA* 2002; **288**: 3039–41.

10 Freemantle N, Hill S. Medicalisation, limits to medicine or never enough money to go around. *BMJ* 2002; **4**: 864–5.

11 Charlton B. The rise and fall of EBM. *Quart. J. Med.* 1998; **91**: 371–4.

12 Sackett DL. The arrogance of preventive medicine. *Can. Med. Assoc. J.* 2002; **167**(4): 363–4.

13 Bekelman JE, Li Y, et al. Scope and impact of financial conflicts of interests in biomedical research. *JAMA* 2003; **289**: 454–65.

14 The Cochrane Library, Issue 4, 2005. http://www3.interscience. wiley.com/cgi-bin/mrwhome/106568753/HOME

15 Korn D. Conflicts of interest in biomedical research. *JAMA* 2000; **284**(17): 2234–6.

16 Angell M. Is academic medicine for sale? *N. Eng. J. Med.* 2000; **342**(20): 1516–18.

17 Rice GPA, Incorvaia B, Munari L, Ebers G, Polman C, D'Amico R, Filippini G. Interferon in relapsing–remitting multiple sclerosis. *Cochrane Database Syst. Rev.* 2001; 4: CD002002. DOI: 10.1002/14651858.CD002002.

18 Hanley B. Involvement works: the 2nd report of the Standing Committee on Consumer Involvement in NHS research. *NHS Executive* 2000 (available at www.conres.co.uk).

19 Maynard A. Evidence based medicine: an incomplete method to inform treatment choice. *Lancet* 1997; **349**: 126–8.

Appendix

The Appendix shows summaries from the Cochrane Library [14]. We have chosen four examples that can be considered typical of a few categories that have been mentioned above. In the first example, the evidence is rather sparse (only 453 patients) and results are conflicting, with a non-statistically significant trial showing protection and one significant trial showing an excess of deaths in the corticosteroid arm. The second example is more complex, since the information available was not enough to evaluate the efficacy of treatment. If all missing data (drop-outs) are attributed to disease progression (worst-case scenario) then treatment is associated with a slight adverse effect. Lack of data of good quality is the main problem in this example.

The third example shows how useful a systematic review and meta-analysis can be. Individual trials were equivocal, but the overall consideration of their results showed and that anticoagulants do more harm than benefit in acute ischaemic stroke. On the opposite, the fourth example (Warfarin in atrial fibrillation, AF) is paradigmatic of a situation in which a systematic review and meta-analysis clearly reveals – more than single trials – that the benefits are considerable and the treatment should be transferred into practice.

1 *Corticosteroids in ischaemic stroke*: Seven trials involving 453 people were included. Details of trial quality that may relate to bias were not available from most trials. No difference was shown in the odds of death within 1 year (odds ratio (OR) 1.08, 95% confidence interval (CI) 0.68–1.72). Treatment did not appear to improve functional outcome in survivors. Six trials reported neurological impairment but pooling the data was impossible because no common scale or time interval was used. The results were inconsistent among individual trials. The only adverse effects reported were small numbers of gastrointestinal bleeds, infections and deterioration of hyperglycaemia across both groups.

2 *Interferon and MS*: Although 1215 patients from seven trials were included in this review, only 919 (76%) contributed to the results concerning exacerbations and progression of the disease at 2 years. Specifically, interferon significantly reduced the occurrence of exacerbations (relative risk (RR) = 0.80, 95% CI 0.73, 0.88, $P < 0.001$) and progression of the disease (RR = 0.69, 95% CI 0.55, 0.87, $P = 0.002$) 2 years after randomization. However, the correct assignment of drop-outs was essential to the demonstration of efficacy, most conspicuously concerning the effect of the drug on disease progression. If interferon-treated patients who dropped out were deemed to have progressed (worst-case scenario) the significance of these effects was lost (RR = 1.31, CI 0.60, 2.89, $P = 0.5$). The evolution in magnetic resonance imaging (MRI) technology in the decade in which these trials were performed and different reporting of data among trials made it impossible to perform a quantitative analysis of the MRI results. Both clinical and laboratory side effects reported in the trials were more frequent in treated patients than in controls. No information was available regarding side effects and adverse events after 2 years of follow-up. The impact of interferon treatment (and its side effects) on the quality of life of patients was not reported in any trial included in this review. Reviewers' conclusions: The efficacy of interferon on exacerbations and disease progression in patients with relapsing–remitting MS was modest after 1 and 2 years of treatment. It was not possible to conduct a quantitative analysis beyond 2 years. Longer follow-up and more uniform reporting of clinical and MRI outcomes among these trials might have allowed for a more convincing conclusion.

3 *Anticoagulants in ischaemic stroke*: Twenty-one trials involving 23,427 patients were included. The quality of the trials varied considerably. The anticoagulants tested were standard unfractionated heparin, low-molecular-weight heparins, heparinoids, oral anticoagulants and thrombin inhibitors. Based on eight trials (22,450 patients) there was no evidence that anticoagulant therapy reduced the odds of death from all causes (OR 1.05, 95% CI 0.98–1.12). Similarly, based on five trials (21,846 patients), there was no evidence that anticoagulants reduced the odds of being dead or dependent at the end of follow-up (OR 0.99, 95% CI 0.94–1.05). Although anticoagulant therapy was associated with about 9 fewer recurrent ischaemic strokes per 1000 patients treated, it was also associated with a similar sized 9 per 1000 increase in symptomatic intracranial haemorrhages. Similarly, anticoagulants avoided about 4 pulmonary emboli per 1000, but this benefit was offset by an extra 9 major extracranial haemorrhages per 1000.

Sensitivity analyses did not identify a particular type of anticoagulant regimen or patient characteristic associated with net benefit.

4 *Warfarin in patients with AF*: Fourteen articles were included in this review. Warfarin was more efficacious than placebo for primary stroke prevention (aggregate OR of stroke = 0.30 (95% CI 0.19, 0.48)), with moderate evidence of more major bleeding (OR = 1.90 (95% CI 0.89, 4.04)). Aspirin was inconclusively more efficacious than placebo for stroke prevention (OR = 0.68 (95% CI 0.29, 1.57)), with inconclusive evidence regarding more major bleeds (OR = 0.81 (95% CI 0.37, 1.78)). For primary prevention, assuming a baseline risk of 45 strokes per 1000 patient-years, warfarin could prevent 30 strokes at the expense of only six additional major bleeds. Aspirin could prevent 17 strokes, without increasing major haemorrhage. In direct comparison, there was moderate evidence for fewer strokes among patients on warfarin than on aspirin (aggregate OR = 0.64 (95% CI 0.43, 0.96)), with only suggestive evidence for more major haemorrhage (OR = 1.58 (95% CI 0.76, 3.27)). However, in younger patients, with a mean age of 65 years, the absolute reduction in stroke rate with warfarin compared to aspirin was low (5.5 per 1000 person-years) compared to an older group (15 per 1000 person-years). Low-dose warfarin or low-dose warfarin with aspirin was less efficacious for stroke prevention than adjusted-dose warfarin. Reviewers' conclusions: The evidence strongly supports warfarin in AF for patients at average or greater risk of stroke, although clearly there is a risk of haemorrhage. Although not definitively supported by the evidence, aspirin may prove to be useful for stroke prevention in subgroups with a low risk of stroke, with less risk of haemorrhage than with warfarin. Further studies are needed of low-molecular-weight heparin and aspirin in lower-risk patients.

CHAPTER 2

What to do when there is no evidence

Charles Warlow

In every day practice busy neurologists have to make decisions about therapeutic interventions which are not supported by randomized controlled trials (RCTs) or meta-analyses of RCTs. Either no RCTs have been done at all, or those that have been done are unconvincing – even when put together in a meta-analysis; perhaps the sample size was too small for reasonable precision, or there was some problem with bias. Under these all too familiar circumstances one cannot decide what to do for the best on the basis of what has come to be known as 'evidence-based medicine' (EBM). And yet there is no avoiding the fact that decisions have to be made when managing individual patients, there always are options, even if one option is to do nothing. For example, wait and see versus spinal cord decompression for cervical spondylotic myelopathy, thymectomy or not for myasthenia gravis, sodium valproate or carbamezipine for partial epilepsy in an elderly patient, levodopa or a dopaminergic agonist in early Parkinson's disease, admit a subarachnoid haemorrhage patient to a neurology rather than to a neurosurgery ward, and so on. While many would argue that RCTs are not the only source of evidence in making therapeutic intervention decisions, most agree that RCTs generally provide the best evidence – if they are available and properly carried out. So what should we do when there is no adequate evidence, at least from RCTs?

Do not succumb to EBMitis

There has never been an RCT to support the use of parachutes to prevent death after jumping out of aeroplanes – and I am sure there never will be. The only entry in the Cochrane Library on 'parachute' is in a review on the treatment of sprained ankles, a well-known complication of parachute jumping but hardly serious enough to withdraw parachutes from general use [1]. Like parachutes, some interventions are so obviously useful on the basis of pathophysiology, experience, common sense, and wisdom that RCTs really are unnecessary; penicillin for meningococcal meningitis and evacuation of extradural haematoma spring to mind. These treatments may not be 'evidence-based' in the sense of having adequate support from RCTs (there are none) but they work, they are widely

used and everyone is comfortable with them. But naturally even these interventions could be improved on and so maybe an RCT would be necessary to compare a new with the current intervention (an improved type of parachute versus the standard parachute, a likely better antibiotic versus penicillin). Of course one does have to guard against extremes of therapeutic optimism that lead to the epidemic of tonsillectomies in the first half of the 20th century [2] and the zeal bordering on madness that drove Aloysius Cotton to remove one or more potentially infected organs as a treatment for insanity [3]. Interventions such as penicillin for meningococcal meningitis would be included in a book on treatment of neurological disorders by a wise clinician, but not in a hard-core book on evidence-based neurology where authors would have succumbed to EBMitis, the disease which afflicts clinicians, authors, managers, and policy makers which makes them refuse to accept, support, use or fund any therapeutic intervention without RCT-based support – a very dangerous disease indeed (particularly for pilots who have their parachutes withdrawn for lack of RCTs of efficacy, notwithstanding the availability of other forms of evidence that parachutes work, and for patients with an extradural haematoma denied neurosurgical intervention). EBMitis may not matter when considering the myriad of what sometimes appear to be rather trivial therapeutic interventions which do not have any RCT support and yet are widely accepted and used – some may work, others may not. But this is probably of no great concern unless there is a significant opportunity cost in carrying on with them in which case RCTs would have to be done to prevent non-evidence-based treatments which do actually work from being withdrawn. Possible examples include turning unconscious patients every 4 h to prevent pressure areas, pain relief with non-steroidal anti-inflammatory drugs for polymyositis, resting for a few weeks after subarachnoid haemorrhage, and setting up a support group for patients with the Guillain–Barre syndrome. In the middle ground are interventions with very clear adverse effects which nonetheless seem to be effective and which are used by many people despite the lack of good RCT evidence: for example pyridostigmine for myasthenia gravis, amantadine for fatigue in multiple sclerosis, a check angiogram a few months after coiling an intracranial aneurysm.

Are you absolutely sure there is no evidence?

Having avoided the temptation to do absolutely nothing unless there is a formal RCT showing that any benefit outweighs the risks (in other words EBMitis), it is important to make sure there really is no evidence to support or refute a particular course of action. There have been some remarkable examples of treatments still being tested long after it was obvious they worked, either because the trialists were unaware of previous evidence or just ignored it; for example the use of aprotinin to reduce blood loss during cardiac surgery [4].

The obvious place to look for evidence is in the Cochrane Library (http://www.nelh.nhs.uk/cochrane.asp), both for reviews and – if necessary – for individual RCTs. Indeed, the Cochrane Library is now so comprehensive that it is probably not worth looking much further, although a quick PubMed or Medline search would be wise, and also asking an expert in the condition if one is easily available. Of course there are excellent non-Cochrane Systematic Reviews but these are still likely to be referenced in the Cochrane Library, or in the reference list of a relevant review or RCT in the library.

Can you generalize from what evidence there is?

Very often there is formal evidence but not quite in the relevant area for an individual patient. For example, although it is clear from the Antithrombotic Trialists' Collaboration (ATT) that long term aspirin reduces the risk of major vascular events in those at high risk, there were very few patients over the age of 90 in the trials [5]. It is conceivable that for them the harms might outweigh the benefits. So what to do in this group? Clearly one has to use judgement with an individual patient about whether to generalize the overall result of the ATT and give aspirin, or not (or if there is an ongoing RCT going in this older group of patients randomization would be an alternative – see below). So, in a very spry 95-year old with a mild ischaemic stroke, aspirin might well be sensible, while in a not so spry patient with a history of duodenal ulceration and a tendency to fall and bang their head, aspirin would not be such a good idea. But can one generalize even further and support the widespread use of aspirin to prevent clot formation and embolism from coils which have just been inserted into ruptured intracranial aneurysms? Here one would be relying much more on pathophysiology (see below) because there really are no relevant RCTs to help make the decision; although aspirin might prevent platelets adhering to the naked coils, it may also interfere with endothelialization of the coil surface adjacent to the flowing blood. It is difficult to know what best to do under the circumstances.

Of course those with severe EBMitis, who only see the world in black and white and insist that all decisions have to follow strict guidelines based on RCTs, would have great trouble generalizing from one sort of patient in an RCT to a slightly different sort in real life. Clinical judgement would not be high on their list of desirable attributes (many with EBMitis are not clinically qualified anyway).

Can you use non-randomized evidence from good observational studies?

Yes, but with great care, and generally as a second best to a good RCT if one is possible (which it may not be). Even the best observational studies comparing groups of patients treated one way versus another during the same time period but not in the context of a formal RCT, using the same outcomes and adjusting for all known confounding factors, can come up with the wrong answer – usually because it is impossible to adjust for prognostic variables which are not known about, or are not measurable, and which may be unevenly distributed between the treated and untreated patients. Even adjusting for confounders that are known about is not an exact science, particularly when the confounding variable is not measured accurately. Hormone replacement therapy (HRT) for post-menopausal women is a spectacular example of observational epidemiology getting it wrong. The observational epidemiology suggested protection from strokes, the eventual randomized trials showed the opposite [6]. This saga does make one wonder about the other widely used hormonal treatment in healthy women, oral contraceptives which have not been, and cannot be, tested in RCTs. Is the risk of stroke derived from observational epidemiology smaller or larger than we think, or maybe there is no risk at all? Of more relevance to neurologists, there is some evidence from non-randomized data from the medical groups in the randomized trials of carotid surgery that the usual positive relationship between increasing blood pressure and stroke risk is inverted when there is severe bilateral carotid disease (Figure 2.1). This makes pathophysiological sense and fits with anecdotal experience that lowering blood pressure in these patients may lead to a stroke within a few days. So is this enough to recommend leaving the blood pressure alone, at least until the severe carotid disease is relieved? Perhaps – it certainly sends out a message to be very cautious about blood pressure lowering if one is tempted to intervene.

What about relying on pathophysiology?

The first two thirds of the 20th century was the golden age for exploiting pathophysiology to understand disease, and from that understanding to designing treatments – many were hugely successful such as drugs to lower the blood pressure, dilate the bronchi, stop the stomach producing acid, and put dopamine back into the brain. But still the question must always remain, do the theoretical benefits based on pathophysiology outweigh the expected – and unexpected – harms? Does lowering the blood pressure really reduce the

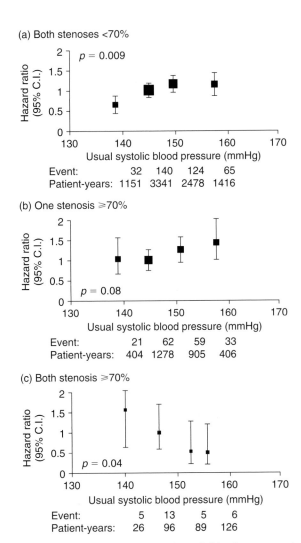

Figure 2.1 Relationships between usual systolic blood pressure and stroke risk in the patients randomized to medical care only from the North American Symptomatic Carotid Endarterectomy Trial (NASCET) and European Carotid Surgery Trial (ECST) of carotid endarterectomy, stratified according to severity of carotid disease. Hazard ratios are derived from a Cox model and adjusted for age, sex and previous ischaemic heart disease and stratified by study. From Rothwell et al. [7] with permission.

risk of stroke (yes from the subsequent RCTs), are the expected harms less than the benefits (yes, provided problems such as symptomatic postural hypotension are avoided), and are the unexpected harms less than the benefits (no in the case of practolol, the beta blocker which was withdrawn because of pulmonary fibrosis). But relying on our necessarily incomplete understanding of pathophysiology can, and often does, lead to more harm than good. When beta blockers were introduced in the 1960s they were known to be negatively inotropic and were therefore considered a contraindication if there was any chance of heart failure. Several decades later, on the basis of RCTs, they are now a treatment for heart failure [8]. So even convincing pathophysiology has ideally to

be put to the test in RCTs – does what *ought* to work really work, and are the harms less than the benefits?

Is there such a thing as clinical wisdom?

I think so, and I hope so, otherwise medicine would become no more than plugging patients into some computer which would dictate therapeutic interventions – like 'painting by numbers'. Maybe this is the holy grail of those with EBMitis, but it will not occur in our lifetime. Patients are too different from each other in their genes, environment, diseases, reactions to their diseases, desires and acceptance of risk. Decisions still have to be made, with or without evidence – riluzole may or may not be a reasonably evidence-based treatment for motor neurone disease [9] but do seriously disabled patients really want to prolong their lives by a couple of months on average? Radiotherapy may give a malignant glioma patient a few more months of life along with treatment-induced fatigue [10], but he or she may prefer to get away for a final cruise rather than return every week for 6 weeks to hospital for treatment. On the other hand, something simply because that is what is usually done may be not such a bad idea, at least for a properly informed patient. But the doctor must keep an open mind and a serious sense of curiosity and scepticism, at least until an RCT can be organized. For treatments for fairly stable symptoms, another option is an n-of-1 trial in an individual patient so that at least for that particular individual one can work out whether something works or not – for example various pain killers for migraine, one anti-epileptic drug rather than another. Even if RCTs have given information that on average one intervention is better than another, patients are different from each other and if there is the opportunity to try manipulating different interventions in an individual, or different doses of the same intervention, then it seems silly not to take it. Of course, the symptoms have to be stable, reasonably easy to measure, and it is best to use a placebo where possible but all this can be expensive and difficult to organize [11].

Join a clinical trial

Ideally when confronted by genuine uncertainty clinicians and patients should join together to do the appropriate RCTs. Decision-making then becomes easy; when there is no formal evidence and you and the patient are uncertain which treatment option to take, ask the patient to join the trial. But so often this is not an option because:

• The disease is deemed to be too rare for a trial (e.g. Wilson's disease) although I am not sure this really is a valid excuse.

• The trial may have to be so long that it is thought impossible, although again that may not be a valid excuse (e.g. drugs to modify the course of multiple sclerosis); one reliable answer every 5–10 years would be better than a stream of unreliable answers based on short follow-up and surrogate outcomes every 1–2 years.

• The nearest collaborating centre in the trial is too far away.

• A trial is not being done because of difficulty with ethics, for example obtaining consent from unconscious patients.

• The intervention may seem to be too 'trivial' for an RCT (e.g. turning unconscious patients) or so new it is still evolving (e.g. middle cerebral artery clot extraction).

• Intransigent innovators or clinicians with much to gain financially or academically may impede trials (e.g. endarterectomy for carotid stenosis in the 1980s, stenting nowadays).

• Lack of incentives for busy clinicians to be involved in trials.

• Lack of regulation which allows surgical innovations and devices to enter routine practice on the basis of 'evidence' which is far inferior to the RCTs required for new drugs.

• Lack of funding which is always in short supply, but it must be cost-effective to have reliable answers to therapeutic questions (it would help, therefore, if funding for routine treatments and funding for RCTs came from the same source).

How hard to push for an RCT must depend on factors such as:

• How much harm to patients would arise if no trial was done and a new intervention was allowed into clinical practice without proper evaluation (a lot of harm potentially if carotid stenting is allowed to replace carotid endarterectom which is, an undoubtedly effective intervention, without good evidence of equivalence).

• How costly the new treatment is (so RCTs of the interferons in multiple sclerosis were absolutely necessary).

• The opportunity cost of doing a trial of one intervention and so not being able to evaluate another (which tends to occur when industry dominates a field leaving non-drug interventions un-evaluated).

Remain humble, do not succumb to therapeutic nihilism or the company dinner

I believe it is best to start from the position that something *may* work rather than it *must* work, but at the same time not to become hopelessly nihilistic in the expectation that nothing ever works in practice. While it is true that many interventions have turned out not to work (vitamins and cancer prevention, neuroprotection for acute ischaemic stroke) or to

work rather trivially (beta interferon for multiple sclerosis), there have been huge successes – coils rather than clips for ruptured intracranial aneurysms, statins to prevent strokes, triptans for migraine. On the other hand, over optimism fuelled by too many drug company dinners is equally damaging. Well-informed uncertainty is a legitimate professional position, but it must not lead to paralysis of action in individual cases, even if the action is 'do nothing'.

References

1 Handoll HHG, Rowe BH, Quinn KM, de Bie R. Interventions for preventing ankle ligament injuries. *Cochrane Database Syst. Rev.* 2001; 3: CD000018. DOI: 10.1002/14651858.CD000018.

2 American Child Health Association. *Physical Defects*, Chapter 8. School Health Influence on Tonsillectomy, 1934.

3 Scull A. *Madhouse: A Tragic Tale of Megalomania and Modern Medicine*, Yale University Press, 2005.

4 Fergusson D, Glass KC, Hutton B, Shapiro S. Randomised controlled trials of aprotinin in cardiac surgery: could clinical equipoise have stopped the bleeding? *Clin. Trial.* 2005; **2**: 218–32.

5 Antithrombotic Trialists' Collaboration. Collaborative meta-analysis of randomised trials of antiplatelet therapy for prevention of death, myocardial infarction, and stroke in high risk patients. *BMJ* 2002; **324**: 71–86.

6 Bath, PMW, Gray, LJ. Association between hormone replacement therapy and subsequent stroke: a meta-analysis. *BMJ* 2005; **330**: 342–6.

7 Rothwell PM, Howard SC, Spence JD. for the Carotid Endarterectomy Trialists' Collaboration. Relationship between blood pressure and stroke risk in patients with symptomatic carotid occlusive disease. *Stroke* 2003; **34**: 2583.

8 McMurray JJV. Heart failure. *Lancet* 2005; **365**: 1877–89.

9 Miller RG, Mitchell JD, Lyon M, Moore DH. Riluzole for amyotrophic lateral sclerosis (ALS)/motor neuron disease (MND). *Cochrane Database Syst. Rev.* 2002; 2: CD001447. DOI: 10.1002/14651858.CD001447.

10 Brada M. HGG – how effective is radiotherapy? In: Chris W, ed., *Evidence-Based Oncology*. Blackwell BMJ Books, Oxford, 2003: pp. 568–70.

11 Hankey GJ, Todd AA, Yap PL, Warlow CP. An 'n of 1' trial of intravenous immunoglobulin treatment for chronic inflammatory demyelinating polyneuropathy. *J. Neurol. Neurosurg. Psychiatr.* 1994; **57**: 1137.

CHAPTER 3

Outcome and adverse effect measures in neurology

Jorge G. Burneo, Samuel Wiebe

Measuring outcomes

What is a good outcome measure?
Defining primary and secondary outcomes

Outcomes in clinical neurosciences research should be directly relevant to the question being addressed, and susceptible to the effects of the intervention under investigation. Although several outcomes are usually measured in any study, investigators must define a priori which outcome is their primary target, and which are secondary. The distinction is important because the sample size, significance level, and power of the study to find a difference when there is one, are all based on one primary outcome measure. All other outcomes are 'secondary' because the study may or may not be powered to formally test their significance. Hence, secondary outcome measures may be useful to generate hypotheses and they may lend support to notions, but may not necessarily prove the effect of an intervention. If readers of a medical paper are unable to readily identify a primary outcome measure, they should use caution in interpreting the results. Primary and secondary outcomes are critical to the validity of a study, and analysis strategies for these variables should be pre-specified. Completeness and accuracy of primary outcome data collection is paramount; incomplete data can seriously affect the study validity [1]. Examples of typical primary outcomes in neurosciences include ⩾50% seizure reduction, stroke or vascular death, and relapse of multiple sclerosis. Note that these outcomes should have direct clinical relevance. When the latter is in question (e.g. ⩾50% seizure reduction), the clinical usefulness of the study is equally questionable, regardless of its statistical significance.

An equally important aspect of defining outcomes pertains to the applicability of study results. All outcome assessment entails a specific method of measurement, a time frame within which it is measured, and a notion of reliability and validity of the measurement. An explicit description of these elements is necessary for clinicians to judge the relevance and applicability of research results to the care of individual patients. For example, most clinical trials of interventions in chronic neurological conditions use short-term outcomes. Other trials assess outcomes for interventions that have a highly restricted application or patient population. These factors determine the applicability of the results in clinical practice.

Standardizing outcome measures

Measuring outcomes in a consistent (e.g. standardized) manner in all study participants and at all time points, is necessary to avoid error and bias, and to ensure reproducibility [2]). In addition to decreasing the 'noise' inherent in any measurement process, rigorous adherence to standardized outcome measurement is necessary to obtain valid (i.e. believable) results.

Numerical results from standardized measures (e.g. scores of rating scales) have many advantages over qualitative assessments (e.g. adjectives like 'improved significantly'), unless the latter are clearly defined, preferably with an external reference value. Numerical indices allow more detailed and precise reporting than qualitative assessments, lend themselves to statistical analysis, and are easier to communicate. Although developing valid standardized measures is labour intensive, they are usually more informative and efficient than subjective evaluations. Even when seemingly simple outcomes are assessed (e.g. stroke versus no stroke, MS attack versus no attack, etc.), it is essential to standardize the definition of what constitutes an event.

Useful outcome measures must be valid, reliable, and responsive to change. Validity refers to the ability to measure the specific domains we are interested in; for example, pain, activity limitation (disability), or quality of life (QOL). Reliability pertains to obtaining the same result when applied to similar patients by different outcome assessors or at different points in time. Responsiveness ensures that small but clinically important changes are captured. This is particularly relevant when assessing the effect of interventions or change over time in individual patients. Unresponsive measures, even if valid and reliable, are futile for assessing the effect of interventions or the effect of time. Clinicians faced with evidence about an intervention must be satisfied that the measures used by researchers have been demonstrated to have satisfactory responsiveness.

Using surrogate outcomes, advantages, and pitfalls

A surrogate outcome measure can be conceptualized as a laboratory, physiologic, or sub-clinical measurement used as a substitute to measuring outcomes that are directly related to how patients feel and function, or related to their survival [3,4]. Examples include using infarct size on brain CT in lieu of clinical stroke severity, carotid plaque changes in lieu of stroke occurrence, and MS lesion burden on MRI in lieu of disability. Surrogate outcomes may provide important background information about the potential usefulness of an intervention, which can then be tested formally in clinical trials. They also lend themselves more readily to blinded assessment. In stroke, for example, an independent radiologist who is unaware of treatment and clinical outcome could determine the size of an infarct, a surrogate outcome that is easier to blind and may be related to clinical outcome.

However, clinicians must use surrogate markers cautiously because they cannot reliably predict the outcome for which they have been substituted. Although surrogate outcomes may be more reliable if they are causally and consistently associated with the clinically important outcome, widespread adoption of interventions based on surrogate outcomes can be seriously misleading [5]. Classic examples include the use of Xylocaine in acute myocardial infarction, which prevents the surrogate outcome of arrhythmias but increases the risk of death; and clofibrate, which improves the surrogate outcome of hypercholesterolemia but increases overall mortality.

Statistical versus clinical significance

Although assessing statistical significance is straightforward, the same is not true about clinical significance. Both concepts are important in evaluating the usefulness and safety of interventions. Statistical significance provides us with some level of confidence (95% for a P value of 0.05) that the results are not due to chance or error, regardless of their clinical significance. On the other hand, clinical significance can be defined in terms of the minimum clinically important difference. That is, the minimum change that patients or clinicians consider sufficient to justify an intervention, in the absence of adverse events [6]. In the context of clinical interventions, assessing clinical significance must also account for the differences between experimental and control groups [7].

In contrast to the universally accepted statistical significance threshold ($P < 0.05$), the magnitude of change required for clinical significance varies depending on the disease under consideration and the outcome measure used (see below). Other factors such as cost are also relevant and may influence the relationship between the magnitude of change in the clinical outcome and its clinical significance. Perhaps in an attempt to clarify the concept, some commentators suggest that clinical significance is reached when the results lead to a change in clinical behaviour or improvement in the patients' QOL [7].

Clearly, statistical and clinical significance are related. With the exception of interventions for which historical incontrovertible clinical evidence of benefit exists (e.g. insulin for diabetes), statistically non-significant findings are inconclusive and not widely adopted, unless no other therapies exist. Similarly, statistically significant results that do not reach the threshold for clinical significance are rarely worth implementing. Whereas statistically significance is directly related to sample size and can be enhanced by increasing the number of study subjects, clinical significance is not. Consider the evidence for donepezil (Aricept) in slowing the progression of dementia. A Cochrane meta-analysis revealed a statistically significant mean improvement of 2.9 points at 24 weeks in the primary outcome measure, the ADAS-cog scale, using 10 mg of donepezil. However, the ADAS-cog's score ranges from 0 to 70 and one must wonder whether a change that is less than 5% of the total range has any clinical significance (www.uwo.ca/cns/ebn). A similar observation can be made about vagus nerve stimulation for medically refractory seizures. A meta-analysis of randomized trials (www.uwo.ca/cns/ebn) demonstrated a mean improvement of 16% in seizure frequency at 3 months. Although this was statistically significant, its clinical significance is difficult to ascertain because of the small effect size and the brief duration of follow-up.

How are outcome measures applied in clinical research?

Avoiding measurement bias

Bias may be conceptualized as any process at any stage of research or inference which results in systematically over- or underestimating the effect of an intervention. Bias differs from random error in that the latter does not have a consistent direction, for example, does not consistently over or under-estimate outcomes. Sackett has compiled a comprehensive catalogue of the different kinds of biases that threaten the validity of clinical research at various levels of implementation [8]. In studies of interventions and randomized trials, bias occurs when outcome assessors (clinicians, researchers, or patients themselves) are not blinded to the type of intervention received and their knowledge influences their assessment. Consequently, interpreter-dependent measures (e.g. clinical assessment and tests requiring clinical interpretation) are more prone to bias than physiologic- or interpreter-independent measures (e.g. standardized laboratory or biochemical indicators).

Another important source of bias in interventional studies is the imbalance between patients and controls of known or unknown variables that affect outcome, that is, confounders. Imbalance in confounders may predetermine the results and is a serious threat to the validity of the results. The universal approach to balancing confounders among experimental and control groups is randomization. In this process, each patient has an equal chance of receiving experimental or control interventions. Ideally, randomization results in experimental and control patients that are similar in every respect but the intervention under investigation. However, imbalances may still occur with randomization, especially if the sample size is small. In this situation, post hoc adjustments may be used in data analyses for variables that are known, but this does not correct for unknown confounders.

Placebos and blinding

Correctly conducted, blinded, randomized controlled trials (RCTs) provide the most valid estimates of treatment effects, and account for phenomena such as regression to the mean (the tendency of extreme measures to become less extreme on repeated assessment), the effects associated with being a research participant (Hawthorne effect), [9] and the effects of receiving an apparently therapeutic intervention (the placebo effect) [10]. Blinded outcome assessment is often accomplished through the use of placebos whose appearance is similar or identical to the experimental intervention. Although the use of placebos in pharmacological interventions is relatively simple, the same is not true about surgical interventions, procedures, and devices. The ethical and emotional issues surrounding sham procedures, and especially sham surgery, are enormous. In the neurosciences, even minimally invasive interventions, such as non-penetrating skull burr holes in surgical trials for movement disorders, aroused intense controversy, and vehement expression of polarized views [11]. Viable alternatives to this methodological impasse include the adjudication of outcomes by independent, blinded assessors, and the use of interpreter-independent, clinically relevant primary outcome measures.

Whose viewpoint should outcome measures reflect?

Every clinical outcome measure requiring judgement or interpretation captures the viewpoint of the assessor (e.g. the clinician, researcher, observer, or patient). This is important because there is empirical evidence that patients, clinicians, and families assess the same outcomes in different ways [12–14]. As the clinical community moves towards patient-centered care, and as the practice of medicine moves towards a model of best-agency and away from paternalism, the importance of the patients' viewpoint is increasingly recognized. Patients' self-rated outcome measures, especially if valid and standardized, provide the viewpoint of the most important stakeholder in clinical practice, that is, the patient. In addition, these measures allow the assessment of minimum clinically important differences. As a general principle, the viewpoint captured by outcome measures should be that of the recipient of the intervention. Therefore, if interventions are geared towards families, societal groups, or clinicians, the corresponding viewpoints should be obtained.

Applying outcome measures in clinical practice

Dichotomous outcomes
Relative versus absolute measures

The relative risk (RR) and the relative risk reduction (RRR) express the impact of treatment on dichotomous (e.g. yes–no) outcomes. The RR is simply the ratio of two proportions and it provides the ratio of the event risk in the treatment or experimental group versus that in the control group (Table 3.1). The RRR is an estimate of the proportion of baseline or control group risk that is removed by the intervention (Table 3.1). A third relative measure of treatment effect is the odds ratio (OR), which is the ratio of two odds, for example, the odds of experimental patients having the target outcome and the odds of control patients having the target outcome (Table 3.1).

The most commonly used absolute measure is the absolute risk difference (ARD). The ARD tells us what proportion of patients is spared the adverse outcome if they receive the treatment under study, rather than the control treatment or placebo, and is obtained by subtracting the proportion of patients with the target event in the control group from that in the treatment or experimental group (Table 3.1). The ARD is more useful clinically because one can easily derive the number needed to treat (NNT) [15,16]. This represents the number of patients that need to be treated over a certain period of time to prevent one adverse or target event, and is obtained by taking the reciprocal of the ARD expressed as a proportion; that is 1/ARD. A negative number, denotes that the experimental intervention is harmful because it increases the risk of an adverse event. The resulting number is referred to as the number needed to harm (NNH) [16] (Table 3.1).

The main disadvantage of relative measures (RRR) is that they do not account for the baseline risk. For example,

Table 3.1 Definition of commonly used measures of therapeutic efficacy

Treatment	Adverse event	
	Present	Absent
Yes	a	b
No (control)	c	d
Control event rate	CER	$= c/c + d$
Experimental event rate	EER	$= a/a + b$
Relative risk	RR	$=$ EER/CER
Relative risk reduction	RRR	$= 1 - $ RR
Absolute risk difference	ARD	$=$ CER $-$ EER
Control odds	CO	$= c/d$
Experimental odds	EO	$= a/b$
Odds ratio	OR	$=$ EO/CO or ad/bc
Number needed to treat	NNT	$= 1/$ARD

reducing the risk of seizure recurrence from 90% with medical therapy to 40% with temporal lobe surgery yields an RRR of 56% and an NNT of 2. If the risk of seizure recurrence were decreased from 9% with medical therapy to 4% with surgical therapy, this would yield an identical RRR of 56%, but the NNT would be 20 (10 times higher!).

Calculating NNTs from OR, RR, or RRR

When NNTs are not provided by researchers, one can calculate them from the probability of an event in the treatment group (experimental event rate = EER) and the probability of an event in the control group (control event rate = CER). If the CER and either the RR or RRR are provided, the NNT can be calculated with the following formulas [16,17]:

$$\text{if the RR} < 1 \text{ then NNT} = \frac{1}{(1 - \text{RR}) \times \text{CER}}$$

$$\text{if the RR} > 1 \text{ then NNT} = \frac{1}{(\text{RR} - 1) \times \text{CER}}$$

If the CER and OR are provided, the NNT can be calculated using the following formulas:

$$\text{if the OR} < 1 \text{ then NNT} = \frac{1 - [\text{CER} \times (1 - \text{OR})]}{[(1 - \text{CER}) \times \text{CER} \times (1 - \text{OR})]}$$

$$\text{if the OR} > 1 \text{ then NNT} = \frac{1 + \text{CER} \times (\text{OR} - 1)}{[\text{CER} \times (\text{OR} - 1) \times (1 - \text{CER})]}$$

Numerous freely accessible OR and NNT web calculators are available. For example see http://www.uwo.ca/cns/ebn/ebntools.xls.

Continuous outcomes
How can we interpret and use grouped outcome measures, for example means and medians?

Because dichotomous outcomes (e.g. occurrence of seizures versus not) can yield ARDs and NNTs, they lend themselves to clinical interpretation and application of research results at the bedside. However, many clinically relevant outcomes are expressed numerically as a continuum (e.g. pain, disability, cognitive function, symptom severity, QOL) and reported as the group's mean or median, with some measure of variability (e.g. standard deviation or standard error). How are clinicians to interpret these reports? Typically, studies exploring the impact of treatments on continuous measures compare the means in treatment and control groups and assess whether the differences are statistically significant. However, the clinical importance of grouped or mean changes is difficult to interpret, regardless of their statistical significance. This is because aggregate or grouped data (means, medians) convey no information about the number of individuals in a group who experience clinically important change. For example, when the mean change for the group is not statistically significant or when it is lower than a pre-specified minimum threshold, clinicians may erroneously conclude that the treatment has no important effects for the group. In reality, this conveys no information about the proportion of individuals in that group who experienced clinically significant improvement or worsening. Conversely, large mean changes can be misconstrued as a group overall's improvement, when in reality this can be accounted for by a small number of individuals experiencing large changes, while the majority of the group remains unchanged [18]. Clinical interpretation of continuous outcomes requires a notion of what constitute clinically important, small, medium, and large changes in individual patients, a concept alluded to earlier. Assessing clinically important change in individual patients is increasingly recognized as a prerequisite for judging the impact of interventions on outcomes measured along a continuum. If clinicians know how many patients improved, worsened, or did not change, they can obtain ARD and NNTs or NNHs, using the simple methods outlined earlier. These measures are much more meaningful than a mean with an attached P value, regardless of its statistical significance [19].

In the absence of a notion of what constitutes a minimum clinically important difference for a specific outcome measure, clinicians can resort to the 'half-standard deviation' rule. There is evidence that in many circumstances, the minimum important difference can be approximated by one half (0.5) of the standard deviation of the score of the instrument assessing the outcome of interest (e.g. pain, QOL, life satisfaction, disability, etc.) [20]. The standard deviation for an instrument or scale can usually be obtained from the reports of an instrument's measurement properties, or from studies reporting the instrument's finding in populations similar to the patients in whom one is applying the measure.

A simple, useful method to obtain NNTs from parallel (not cross-over) RCTs using a continuous outcome measure has been suggested by Guyatt et al. [18] and is illustrated below. If the outcome is categorized according to the minimum clinically important difference into three groups (improved, unchanged, and worsened), we obtain the following table:

Control	Treatment		
	% Improved (x)	% Unchanged (y)	% Worsened (z)
% Improved (d)	dx	dy	dz
% Unchanged (e)	ex	ey	ez
% Worsened (f)	fx	fy	fz

(From Bussiere M, Wiebe S, *Can. J. Neurol. Sci.* 2005; **32**: 420–3, with permission.)

Each cell is the product of multiplying the proportions in the corresponding headings. For example, cell *dx* is obtained by multiplying proportion (*d*) by proportion (*x*). Patients along the diagonal (clear cells) are unchanged. To obtain the NNT we add up the cells of those who improved (gray cells, $ex + fx + fy$), subtract the cells of those who deteriorated (dark cells, $dy + dz + ez$), and divide 1 by the result. A spreadsheet that calculates this NNT is available at http://www.uwo.ca/cns/ebn/ebntools.xls (click on the tab labeled 'NNT-3 category').

Quality of life

Health related QOL entails aspects of well-being and health as they impact on a person's life, as rated by patients themselves and encompassing a number of areas or domains, including psychosocial and physical function, general health, specific symptoms, and limitations imposed by health problems [21]. QOL is particularly germane to neurological disorders because of their chronicity and because of the risk–benefit trade-offs incurred in their treatment (e.g. brain tumour resection at the risk of loss of function). Moreover, although no models currently exist to incorporate QOL information into routine clinical care [22], evidence is accumulating for its role in neurological disorders. For example, Gilliam et al. demonstrated in an RCT that patients with epilepsy randomized to QOL measurement had a higher rate of detection and treatment of drug of adverse effects than those in whom QOL was not measured [23]. Similarly, Wagner et al. showed that 63% of clinicians gained new information and 14% changed management based on QOL assessment using the generic instrument SF-36 in the routine care of patients with epilepsy [24]. Although QOL assessment is still in its infancy and is often discounted as subjective or soft, increasingly, studies are including QOL measures in their outcomes or even as primary outcomes, in recognition of the importance of patient-centred outcome assessment. A large number of QOL tools have been developed in the last decade. These can be categorized as generic or non-targeted (e.g. SF-36, Sickness Impact Profile, EQ-5D, etc.), or specific (targeted) tools. The latter can be specific to a condition, a population or a symptom. The choice of QOL tool to assess outcomes should be determined by the question being asked, the characteristics of the tool (ease of administration, validity, reliability, and responsiveness), and whether comparisons with other conditions are important. If the latter is important, generic tools allow for comparisons across conditions and populations. On the other hand, there is empirical evidence that disease-specific or targeted QOL instruments are more responsive to change than generic or non-targeted measures [25].

Measuring adverse effects

What types of studies do we need?

Adverse effects of interventions are as important as their efficacy; however, their assessment is less well developed for a number of reasons. One of the most important barriers is study design. Currently, study designs used to demonstrate efficacy follow the criteria of regulatory agencies upon which market licenses are granted. These studies are too short, too small, and completely inadequate to assess harm. Because interventions that reach the licensing trial stage typically have a relatively low rate of severe adverse events, their assessment requires prospective cohort studies with large numbers of patients observed for prolonged period of time and evaluated in a systematic manner. For instance, 30,000 patient-years would be needed to have 95% confidence to detect an adverse event that occurs once in every 10,000 patient-years [26]. On the other hand, clinicians must also be wary about inferring causality based on single or small reports of adverse events in the absence of robust data. Contribution to central adverse event registers, and a watchful, informed clinical practice style are preferable responses. The lack of robust evidence for causality of adverse events has resulted in unwarranted and prolonged withdrawal from use of important interventions (e.g. digoxin and metformin). Exceptionally, the adverse event rate is sufficiently high to allow astute clinicians to establish a causal association, for example 30% risk of irreversible visual field constriction with vigabatrin.

Funding studies geared at assessing adverse effects is largely non-existent. Case–control and pharmacosurveillance studies are the surrogate method whereby clinicians can gain understanding about adverse effects. However, although these studies provide a notion of the occurrence of adverse effects, the true incidence, and more importantly, the causal association with putative interventions are very difficult to establish. Another problem in the assessment of adverse effects relates to the method used to probe for their occurrence. Adverse effects spontaneously reported by patients can potentially underestimate, and less frequently overestimate their frequency. To overcome this problem, some studies use questionnaires or checklists with standard terminology and content. However, these questionnaires may miss adverse events that were not probed, and the prompting induced by a list of symptoms may lead to over-reporting. Also, clinical trials of new interventions usually exclude pregnant women, those with inadequate contraception methods, and paediatric populations, further contributing to the scarcity of data in these groups of patients.

Five study designs have been used in the literature to assess harm, that is, RCTs, cohort studies, case–control studies, case series, and case reports. Each has strengths and weaknesses. A defining feature of the first three is the assembly of one or more comparison groups. The last two are typically retrospective, lack comparison groups, and should be used for hypothesis generation rather than to claim an association. The appropriateness of any study depends on the exposure and outcome of interest. Hence, carefully conducted RCTs are useful for frequent adverse events that occur early after the intervention, for example, harm related to epilepsy surgery. However, case–control studies are the preferred vehicle for rare or late adverse effects.

Applying information about adverse effects in clinical practice

Likelihood of being helped versus harmed (LHH). The NNH is a simple measure that tells us how many patients need to receive an intervention for one patient to experience an adverse effect. The larger the NNH the safer or better tolerated the intervention. A more meaningful measure that incorporates information about benefit and harm is the LHH, which expresses the 'pros' (benefits) and 'cons' (harm) of a treatment in a single value. In its simplest expression the LHH is simply the ratio of the NNH and the NNT: LHH = NNH/NNT. An LHH > 1 means that the expected benefits outweigh the possible harm, an LHH < 1 means that the possible harm outweighs the expected benefits.

One problem with the crude LHH is that it implies equal severity weights for the adverse event and for the beneficial effect. For example, according to a meta-analysis of thrombolysis for acute ischemic stroke, [27] the NNT to reduce death or dependency is 7, and the NNH for fatal intracranial haemorrhage is 40. Hence, LHH = (40/7) = 6. Because both outcomes are fairly similar in severity (both include a risk of death), one may say that IV tPA is 6 times more likely to help than to harm this select group of patients. The same is not true for symptomatic intracranial haemorrhage, whose NNH is 14, hence LHH = (14/2) = 2. Because death/dependency is a more severe outcome than symptomatic haemorrhage, we cannot meaningfully use this crude LHH. In this case, clinicians and patients may give each outcome a different severity weight. For example, if symptomatic haemorrhage were judged to be one tenth (0.1) as severe as death/dependency, the adjusted LHH would be [(NNH/weight)/(NNT)]; thus, [(14/0.1)/7] = 20. Therefore, a milder adverse effect results in a larger LHH, indicating a more effective and safe procedure, for example, intravenous tPA is 20 times more likely to help than to harm patients when considering this particular adverse effect.

Illustrating outcomes measures with an example: Epilepsy

An example of the complexity of outcome assessment in neurology is found in epilepsy. Clinical trials in epilepsy present a wide range of challenges. Four main types of outcome measures are used in clinical trials of epilepsy, for example, seizure frequency, seizure severity, adverse effects, and QOL. Seizure frequency is the most commonly used. Although superficially simple, measuring this outcome is not straightforward. First, few studies have explored the validity of seizure diaries, the standard method of capturing this outcome. Second, there is no consensus about the optimum specific

seizure measure. Most pharmaceutical trials focus on some measure of improvement in seizure frequency (e.g. $\geq 50\%$), for which no notion of a minimum clinically important change exists, as opposed to seizure freedom, which is always clinically meaningful. Third, comparing mean seizure counts is an alternative; however, the clinical interpretation of group means and medians is problematic (see above).

Finally, the overall objective of any intervention in epilepsy is to improve the patients' QOL. Numerous scales have been designed to assess QOL in epilepsy, their reliability, validity, and responsiveness have been established [28], and thresholds that constitute minimum clinically important change in individual instruments have been reported [19]. Yet, because of regulatory and licensing requirements, few studies emphasize or adequately assess the impact of interventions on QOL.

Interpreting outcomes in epilepsy surgery

Clinicians at the University of Western Ontario wished to know if they should refer a patient with temporal-lobe epilepsy (TLE) for surgery. After searching the literature for the best evidence, they came across a study that compared surgery and medical treatment in patients with TLE [29].

The study was a RCT that assessed the safety and efficacy of temporal lobe surgery as compared to medical treatment. The primary outcome was freedom from seizures. Secondary outcomes were frequency and severity of seizures, QOL, disability, and death. Clinicians calculated the CER (medical therapy), EER (surgical therapy), ARD, NNTs, and their respective confidence intervals using a simple, 2 × 2 table, and produced a critically appraised topic (Appendix) (http://www.uwo.ca/clinns/ebn).

References

1 Biller J, Bogousslavsky J. *Clinical Trials in Neurologic Practice.* Butterworth-Heinemann, Woburn, MA, 2001.

2 Nunnally JCJ. *Introduction to Psychological Measurement.* McGraw-Hill, New York, 1970.

3 Temple RJ. A regulatory authority's opinion about surrogate endpoints. In: Nimmo WS & Tucker GT, eds., *Clinical Measurement in Drug Evaluation*, John Wiley & Sons, New York, 1995.

4 Bucher H, Guyatt G, Cook DJ, Holbrook A, McAlister F. Therapy and applying the results: surrogate outcomes. In: Guyatt G & Rennie D, eds., *Users' Guides to the Medical Literature.* American Medical Association, Chicago, 2002: pp. 393–413.

5 Valori RM. Outcome measures. In: McGovern DPB, Summerskill WSM, Valori RM, Levi M & McManus RJ, eds., *Evidence-Based Medicine in General Practice.* BIOS, Oxford, 2001.

6 Jaeschke R, Singer J, Guyatt GH. Measurement of health status. Ascertaining the minimal clinically important difference. *Contr. Clin. Trials* 1989; **10**(4): 407–15.

7 Sackett DL, Haynes RB, Guyatt GH, Tugwell P. *Clinical Epidemiology*, 2nd edn. Little Brown, London, 1991.

8 Sackett DL. Bias in analytic research. *J. Chronic Dis.* 1979; **32**(1–2): 51–63.

9 Parsons HM. What happened at Hawthorne? *Science* 1974; **183**: 922–32.

10 Burneo JG, Montori VM, Faught E. Magnitude of the placebo effect in randomized trials of antiepileptic agents. *Epilepsy Behav.* 2002; **3**(6): 532–4.

11 Macklin R. The ethical problems with sham surgery in clinical research. *N. Engl. J. Med.* 1999; **34**(13): 992–6.

12 Eiser C, Morse R. Can parents rate their child's health-related quality of life? Results of a systematic review. *Qual. Life Res.* 2001; **10**(4): 347–57.

13 Gordon K, MacSween J, Dooley J, Camfield C, Camfield P, Smith B. Families are content to discontinue antiepileptic drugs at different risks than their physicians. *Epilepsia* 1996; **37**(6): 557–62.

14 Rothwell PM, McDowell Z, Wong CK, Dorman PJ. Doctors and patients don't agree: cross sectional study of patients' and doctors' perceptions and assessments of disability in multiple sclerosis. *BMJ* 1997; **314**(7094): 1580–3.

15 Laupacis A, Sackett DL, Roberts RS. An assessment of clinically useful measures of the consequences of treatment. *N. Engl. J. Med.* 1988; **318**(26): 1728–33.

16 Bussiere M, Wiebe S. Measuring the benefit of therapies for neurological disorders. *Can. J. Neurol. Sci.* 2005; **32**: 419–24.

17 Sackett DL, Strauss SE, Richardson WS, Rosenberg W, Haynes B. *Evidence-Based Medicine. How to Practice and Teach EBM*, 2nd edn. Churchill Livingstone, London, 2000.

18 Guyatt GH, Juniper EF, Walter SD, Griffith LE, Goldstein RS. Interpreting treatment effects in randomised trials. *BMJ* 1998; **316**(7132): 690–3.

19 Wiebe S, Matijevic S, Eliasziw M, Derry PA. Clinically important change in quality of life in epilepsy. *J. Neurol. Neurosurg. Psychiatr.* 2002; **73**(2): 116–20.

20 Norman GR, Sloan JA, Wyrwich KW. Interpretation of changes in health-related quality of life: the remarkable universality of half a standard deviation. *Med. Care* 2003; **41**(5): 582–92.

21 Guyatt GH, Feeny DH, Patrick DL. Measuring health-related quality of life. *Ann. Intern. Med.* 1993; **118**(8): 622–9.

22 Greenhalgh J, Long AF, Flynn R. The use of patient reported outcome measures in routine clinical practice: lack of impact or lack of theory? *Soc. Sci. Med.* 2005; **60**(4): 833–43.

23 Gilliam FG, Fessler AJ, Baker G, Vahle V, Carter J, Attarian H. Systematic screening allows reduction of adverse antiepileptic drug effects: a randomized trial. *Neurology* 2004; **62**(1): 23–7.

24 Wagner AK, Ehrenberg BL, Tran TA, Bungay KM, Cynn DJ, Rogers WH. Patient-based health status measurement in clinical practice: a study of its impact on epilepsy patients' care. *Qual. Life Res.* 1997; **6**(4): 329–41.

25 Wiebe S, Guyatt G, Weaver B, Matijevic S, Sidwell C. Comparative responsiveness of generic and specific quality-of-life instruments. *J. Clin. Epidemiol.* 2003; **56**(1): 52–60.

26 Walker MC, Sander JW, Shorvon SD. Epilepsy: ethics, outcome variables and clinical scales. In: Guiloff RJ, ed., *Clinical Trials in Neurology*, Springer-Verlag, London, 2001.

27 Thrombolysis for acute ischaemic stroke (Cochrane Review). The Cochrane Library, 2003. (Accessed on July 23rd, 2006).

28 Cramer JA. Principles of health-related quality of life: assessment in clinical trials. *Epilepsia* 2002; **43**(9): 1084–95.

29 Wiebe S, Blume WT, Girvin JP, Eliasziw M. A randomized, controlled trial of surgery for temporal-lobe epilepsy. *N. Engl. J. Med.* 2001; **345**(5): 311–8.

Appendix

In patients with TLE, surgery was superior to medical therapy at 1 year. The NNT was 3 to render patients free from all seizures, and to render them free of seizures impairing awareness.

Clinical Problem: The patient is a 36-year-old male with long-standing history of medically refractory TLE and mesial temporal sclerosis on MRI.

Clinical Question: What is the efficacy and safety of temporal lobe surgery in patients with TLE?

Search Strategy: PubMed: Search 'TLE' and 'surgery', All Fields, Limit to RCT, Human. Yielded eight citations. The article chosen was cited first.

Clinical bottom lines:
1 With temporal lobe surgery, the NNT for freedom from all seizures at 1 year was 3 (95% CI 2, 5), while it was 2 (95% CI 1.5, 3) for freedom from seizures impairing awareness.
2 The proportion of patients that remained free of seizures impairing awareness at 1 year was 58% in the surgical group and 8% in the medical group ($P < 0.001$).
3 The proportion of patients that remained free of all seizures was 38% in the surgical group and 3% the medical group ($P < 0.001$).
4 The QOL was better among the patients in the surgical group than among those in the medical group ($P < 0.001$), and it improved over time in both groups ($P < 0.003$).
5 Temporal lobe surgery was safe in patients with TLE (see data interpretation below).

The evidence:
This parallel group RCT assessed the safety and efficacy of temporal lobe surgery as compared to optimum medical treatment at 1 year in 80 patients with TLE. Optimal medical therapy and primary outcomes were assessed by blinded epileptologists. Analysis was by intention to treat. The primary outcome was freedom from seizures that impair awareness. Secondary outcomes were frequency and severity of seizures, QOL, disability, and death.

Data and interpretation:

1 Freedom of seizures impairing awareness at 1 year

	Seizure free	Seizures	Total
Surgery	23	17	40
Medical therapy	3	37	40
Total	26	54	

CER = 0.08, EER = 0.58, ARR = 0.5, NNT = 2 (95% CI 1.5, 3).

2 Freedom of all seizures at 1 year

	Seizure free	Seizures	Total
Surgery	15	25	40
Medical therapy	1	39	40
Total	16	64	

CER = 0.025, EER = 0.375, ARR = 0.35, NNT = 3 (95% CI 2, 5).

3 Risk and harm

	ARI (%)	NNH (1/ARI)	95% CI (ARI)
Surgery			
Total risks (surgical complications)	11	9	
Thalamic infarct	2.5	40	0.06, 13
Wound infection	2.5	40	0.06, 13
Decreased verbal memory	5	20	
Asymptomatic superior quadrantanopsia	61	1.5	
Medical therapy			
Death	2.5	40	0.06, 13

ARI: absolute risk increase; NNH: number needed to harm.

Comments about the evidence:

1 Although two blinded epileptologists assessed the patient's seizure diaries, one wonders whether patients may have had seizures that impaired awareness and thus were not recorded. However, this is the only feasible manner of measuring seizure outcome, and is standard for all medical or surgical epilepsy trials.

2 No clear description was given specifically about how adverse events were collected.

3 The long-term outcome of surgery was not addressed by this RCT. However, long-term outcomes are unlikely to be derived from RCTs, which are typically of limited duration.

4

CHAPTER 4

Systematic reviews of diagnostic research

Bernard M.J. Uitdehaag, Peter M. Rothwell

Introduction

Obtaining an accurate diagnosis is essential in clinical practice. Almost all clinical actions are in one way or the other related to the diagnosis. When confronted with a patient with a medical problem, the first effort goes – either implicitly or explicitly – into making a diagnosis. This should translate into an expected prognosis and guide further action, either immediate therapeutic intervention or further diagnostic testing. An accurate diagnosis is crucial in choosing the right therapy and, vice versa, it is often only possible to properly evaluate the results of any treatment within the context of a certain diagnosis.

Despite the pivotal role of diagnosis in clinical practice, it has been the focus of much less research than has the development and evaluation of treatments. As in football, scoring the goal draws more attention than giving the assist. Consequently the methodological development of therapeutic research is more advanced. Randomized controlled trials (RCTs) are now widespread and standardized approaches to evaluating the quality of these trials have been developed. Moreover, given that sometimes the omissions are not in the execution of research but in the reporting of the findings, guidelines have been developed to improve the reporting of RCTs and thus facilitating the assessment of the validity of the results [1]. This so-called CONSORT statement is now accepted and applied by the major medical journals.

Progress is now being made in the field of diagnostic testing, such as the STARD initiative [2]. Like the CONSORT, STARD is intended to improve the quality of reporting of studies to the advantage of clinicians, reviewers and others. However, since this is a relatively recent development, most published studies on diagnostic tests that are included in present reviews may suffer from a lack of information on key elements of design, conduct and analysis [3].

Importance of diagnostic research

One of the main problems facing research into diagnosis is the fact that the field of diagnostic test development is often exceedingly dynamic. With progressing technical abilities new diagnostic procedures are introduced at a high rate, frequently without careful clinical evaluation. Indeed, the speed of development of new tests (e.g. in the field of molecular genetics or radiology) can undermine careful evaluation of their diagnostic properties. However, the importance of rigorous diagnostic research should not be underestimated. The lack of reliable information on the accuracy of new diagnostic tests or procedures can result in incorrect diagnoses, unnecessary procedures, avoidable burden for patients and increased health care costs. It is also important to realize that this is not only applicable to new diagnostic tests, but also to diagnostic procedures that have been used in clinical practice for many decades (and still are used) despite never having been properly analysed with respect to their diagnostic features.

Introduction and application of diagnostic test procedures must be based on adequate clinical evaluation. Clinicians must therefore be familiar with concepts such as sensitivity and specificity, pre- and post-test odds, likelihood ratios, pre- and post-test probabilities and diagnostic-odds ratios. Moreover, they should be aware of strengths and limitations of these concepts since this is critical for the judgement on the potential relevance of any test in daily practice.

The design of diagnostic research depends to a great extent on the objective of the test. Some tests focus on identifying a disorder whereas others focus on prognosis or decisions concerning therapy. For each of these questions different designs may be appropriate. So far, no standards for the evaluation of diagnostics are formulated as a requirement for acceptance [4].

Importance of systematic reviews of diagnostic research

There are at least three situations in which systematic reviews of diagnostic research should be advocated. First, if there are many publications on a specific topic there is, of course, a need for efficiently integrating this existing information. All parties involved in decision making – health care providers, researchers and policy makers – often have access to large numbers of publications, but it may be hard to properly weight all this information. Systematic reviews and meta-analysis may help, where possible, to amalgamate all information and to draw well-balanced and more reliable conclusions. Second, if there are few publications on a specific topic a detailed literature search and systematic review is equally important in order not to miss what previous work has been done. Finally, if there are insufficient publications on a specific topic, systematic reviews are essential to convincingly document this lack of information and thereby influence the research agenda.

Construction of diagnostic reviews

There are five key elements in systematic reviews in general and these are also present in diagnostic reviews [5]. These elements mark the steps that should be taken by the authors in chronologic order and as a rule are present in the manuscript in the same sequence.

All systematic diagnostic reviews must start with the *formulation of a review question*. This question should be sufficiently detailed to be of help in the next steps of the review. This means that the question not only includes the test and its objective, which – as indicated earlier [4] – can vary but which must specify the patient population and the setting. In addition, the reference test 'gold standard' and outcomes should be included in the question. This results in a focussed question that is on the one hand helpful for the review process and on the other hand enables the reader to judge whether the review is addressing the issue he or she is interested in.

Based on this focussed question a *comprehensive search of the literature and selection of primary studies* must be performed. The search for primary studies must be thorough in order not to miss studies. This is an important element in the review that should be described in detail. Details about the search strategy, including the databases that were explored, the reference lists that were scanned and the experts that were contacted, should be described in order to allow the reader to see whether the strategy was sufficient to be reasonably comprehensive and to minimize bias in study selection. After all potentially relevant studies are identified, the process by which studies were selected and excluded must be explained and justified.

The *critical appraisal of the quality of included studies and the extraction of data* from these studies forms the next step in the process and the subsequent part of the paper. The quality criteria to be evaluated include study design, patient sample (e.g. recruitment, setting and characteristics), reference diagnosis, execution of the experimental test and the completeness of the report [6]. It will often be necessary to contact the authors of the original papers to ask for additional information. Lack of information in the publication on some aspects of the study related to quality does not necessarily imply a reduced quality in the execution of the study. Implementation of the STARD initiative [2] will eventually improve the reporting of diagnostic studies, but systematic reviews will often

continue to need to include older studies. Results from the quality assessment must be included in the review. If studies fail to reach a certain standard of quality they can either be excluded from the review or analyses of the results can be stratified by (aspects of) study quality. This decision should be clearly indicated in the report. From all included studies data concerning diagnostic accuracy should be extracted. This can be done in parallel with quality assessment.

The next phase is the *synthesis and summary of study results*. After collecting all available relevant data from the included studies these data should be analysed and, if possible and meaningful, pooled. Although statistical techniques are available to combine outcome measures, the resulting summary estimate is not always useful. For example, there may be substantial variability in results of the included studies, in which case, identification and description of the sources of this heterogeneity is more informative than reporting a single pooled measure of accuracy. When reading this section of a review, attention must be paid both to the decision to perform a meta-analysis or not and to the choice of the applied methods.

In certain circumstances, it can be helpful to obtain the individual patient data from studies in order to better understand apparent differences in findings or to stratify analyses by important covariates. For example, despite concerted attempts to review and draw conclusions from the published literature comparing non-invasive tests for imaging carotid stenosis with the Gold Standard of arterial angiography, there was significant heterogeneity of test accuracy for virtually all non-invasive modalities and it was not possible to perform any key subgroup analyses (e.g. accuracy in symptomatic versus asymptomatic arteries) or determine the effect of using several non-invasive tests together [7–11]. These difficulties forced researchers to resort to pooled analyses of individual patient data [12].

Finally, *interpretation of the results* must result in a balanced discussion about the strengths and limitations of the review. The implications for clinical practice should be expounded and in addition suggestions for further research may be included.

Critical issues in diagnostic reviews

There are several critical issues in diagnostic research in general and more specifically in diagnostic reviews [13]. Some of the most important issues will be briefly addressed here. They match the key elements described in the previous section.

If performed adequately, the answer one can get from a diagnostic review is determined by the question from which the review started. If for instance one is interested to find out whether a new test can replace an existing test, a review should contain studies in which both tests are compared [6]. Combined data from studies in which both tests are evaluated independently from each other may be less informative and more difficult to interpret.

For the validity of a systematic review it is crucial that all available data that are relevant for the research question is identified. Therefore, a comprehensive and systematic search of the literature is needed. Search strategies to identify studies of diagnostic test in specific databases have been developed [14,15] but these cannot guide the search in the so-called 'grey literature' [16]. The use of a methodological filter can be helpful in reducing the search results, but should not lead to elimination of relevant studies. Their use in intervention studies may be advantageous, but it has been shown that the use of these filters in diagnostic reviews may lead to omission of many studies and consequently jeopardize the validity of the review and should thus be avoided [17].

Apart from being incomplete when searching the literature another threat for the validity of the review is publication bias. If studies with poor test performance results are not published the diagnostic accuracy of the test will be overestimated in the review [13]. Research on the underlying causes for publication bias and the impact on in diagnostic reviews is limited. In common with therapeutic reviews, funnel plots can be used to evaluate publication bias in diagnostic reviews [18], although careful consideration of the structure of the plot is needed [19].

After identifying all relevant studies, the methodological quality of all these studies should be assessed. Methodological shortcomings may affect estimates of the accuracy of a diagnostic test in either way [20]. However, only a small minority of diagnostic reviews take differences in quality into account [21]. Using a Delphi procedure an evidence based quality assessment tool (QUADAS) was developed for use in systematic reviews of diagnostic accuracy studies [22]. The QUADAS tool is a list of 14 questions focussing predominantly on several potential sources of bias (which may limit the validity of the study results). In addition, sources of variability (which may limit the generalizability of the results) and the quality of reporting are included. Clear instructions on how to score each item are available, but the use of an overall quality score is discouraged. An overall score implies the need for combining different aspects of quality and so far, there is no generally accepted method of weighting the individual quality items against one another. In addition, because of the frequently poor reporting of the primary study any scoring system will be hampered. But even if all elements are available, investigating the association between different quality aspects and diagnostic performance estimates may be preferred to using combined quality scores [23]. So far the empirical evidence about the size and the effect of these associations is limited [24].

In systematic reviews, the way in which estimates of diagnostic accuracy obtained from the individual studies are summarized is variable. Also the choice of outcome measure may differ from review to review. Based on their familiarity to clinicians, sensitivity and specificity are often reported as main outcomes. In addition, the advantage of these measures is that most diagnostic studies report these outcomes and alternative measures like likelihood ratios and diagnostic odds ratios can be derived from them [25]. It should be kept in mind that some diagnostic procedures result in a value on a continuous (e.g. serum level), discrete or ordinal scale. For the purpose of clinical decision making, often a cut-off level is chosen resulting in a dichotomous scale, from which sensitivity (the proportion of true positives in the diseased) and specificity (the proportion of true negatives in the non-diseased) are calculated. However, sensitivity and specificity depend on the chosen cut-off value, which may vary from study to study. Sensitivity and specificity are often inversely correlated within studies and should not be pooled separately over studies [26], but analysed in pairs. Test performance within studies is described by the receiver-operating characteristic (ROC) curve in which the sensitivity is plotted against 1-specificity. For combining results on several studies summary ROC (sROC) curves can be constructed in which the pairs of sensitivity and specificity of each study is plotted in the ROC space [27]. The sROC approach has become a standard method for meta-analysis in diagnostic reviews. The major advantage is that it makes it possible to handle problems with pooling of data. However, there are also clear limitations [28]. Apart from assumptions on the comparability of endpoints, threshold values and study quality, possibly the major limitation is the lack of understanding of the concept and interpretation of the sROC approach by clinicians. If results from diagnostic reviews cannot be applied in clinical practice, the effort is wasted.

Finally, the societal impact of diagnostic strategies is seldom addressed in diagnostic research [13] and it is therefore hardly possible to incorporate that aspect of (new) tests in reviews. Although many people recognize the potential importance of cost-effectiveness studies of diagnostic strategies, these studies are extremely complex. Diagnostic procedures are sometimes performed in isolation, sometimes in parallel with other tests and sometimes conditional depending on the results of others tests. In addition, both correct and incorrect diagnoses must be considered and treatments with their variable costs and success rate are part of the model.

Conclusion

Diagnostic research lags behind therapeutic research in many ways. Nevertheless, the diagnostic field may use all methodological knowledge that has been gathered in the therapeutic field to their own benefit. By doing that progress of diagnostic research may be more rapid compared to therapeutic research in the past.

Systematic reviews are invaluable tools in diagnostic research. They help to collect all available data, identify variability between studies, make reliable estimates of diagnostic characteristics of tests using a powerful approach and highlight areas where further research is necessary.

References

1 Moher D, Schulz KF, Altman DG. The CONSORT statement: revised recommendations for improving the quality of reports of parallel-group randomised trials. *Lancet* 2001; **357**: 1191–4.

2 Bossuyt PM, Reitsma JB, Bruns DE, Gatsonis CA, Glasziou PP, Irwig LM, Lijmer JG, Moher D, Rennie D, de Vet HC. Towards complete and accurate reporting of studies of diagnostic accuracy: the STARD initiative. *BMJ* 2003; **326**: 41–4.

3 Reid MC, Lachs MS, Feinstein AR. Use of methodological standards in diagnostic test research. Getting better but still not good. *JAMA* 1995; **274**: 645–51.

4 Knottnerus JA, van Weel C. Evaluation of diagnostic procedures. In: Knottnerus JA, ed *'The Evidence Base of Clinical Diagnosis'*, BMJ Books, London, 2002.

5 Madhukar P, McCulloch M, Enanoria W, Colford Jr JM. Systematic reviews of diagnostic test evaluations: what's behind the scenes? *Evid. Based Med.* 2004; **9**: 101–3.

6 Deeks JJ. Systematic reviews of evaluations of diagnostic and screening tests. *BMJ* 2001; **323**: 157–62.

7 Rothwell PM, Pendlebury ST, Wardlaw J, Warlow CP. A critical appraisal of the design and reporting of studies of imaging and measurement of carotid stenosis. *Stroke* 2000; **31**: 1444–50.

8 Blakeley DD, Oddone EZ, Hasselblad V, Simel DL, Matchar DB. Noninvasive carotid artery testing. A meta-analytic review. *Ann. Intern. Med.* 1995; **122**: 360–7.

9 Fisher CM, Appleberg M, Irwig L, Macaskill P. A systematic review of the accuracy of diagnosis of 70% carotid artery stenosis by duplex scanning. *J. Vascul. Invest.* 1998; **4**: 91–8.

10 Westwood ME, Kelly S, Berry E, Bamford JM, Gough MJ, Airey CM, et al. Use of magnetic resonance angiography to select candidates with recently symptomatic carotid stenosis for surgery: systematic review. *BMJ* 2002; **324**: 198.

11 Koelemay MJ, Nederkoorn PJ, Reitsma JB, Majoie CB. Systematic review of computed tomographic angiography for assessment of carotid artery disease. *Stroke* 2004; **35**: 2306–12.

12 Wardlaw JM, Chappell F, Stevenson M, DeNigris E, Thomas S, Gillard J, Berry E, Young G, Rothwell P, Roditi G, Gough M, Brennan A, Bamford J, Best J. Accurate, practical and cost-effective assessment of carotid stenosis in the UK. NHS Health Technology Assessment, 2005.

13 Tatsioni A, Zarin DA, Aronson N, Samson DJ, Flamm CR, Schmid C, Lau J. Challenges in systematic reviews of diagnostic technologies. *Ann. Intern. Med.* 2005; **142**: 1048–55.

14 Leeflang MM, Scholten RJ, Rutjes AW, Reitsma JB, Bossuyt PM. Use of methodological search filters to identify diagnostic accuracy studies can lead to the omission of relevant studies. *J. Clin. Epidemiol.* 2006; **59**: 234–40.

15 Wilczynski NL, Haynes RB, the Hedges Team. EMBASE search strategies for identifying methodologically sound diagnostic studies for use by clinicians and researchers. *BMC Med.* 2005; **3**: 7.

16 Haynes RB, Wilczynski NL. Optimal search strategies for retrieving scientifically strong studies of diagnosis from Medline: analytical survey. *BMJ* 2004; **328**: 1040–1042.

17 Alberani V, De Castro Pietrangeli P, Mazza AM. The use of grey literature in health sciences: a preliminary survey. *Bull. Med. Libr. Assoc.* 1990; **78**: 358–63.

18 Song F, Khan KS, Dinnes J, Sutton AJ. Asymmetric funnel plots and publication bias in meta-analyses of diagnostic accuracy. *Int. J. Epidemiol.* 2002; **31**: 88–95.

19 Deeks JJ, Macaskill P, Irwig L. The performance of tests of publication bias and other sample size effects in systematic reviews of diagnostic test accuracy was assessed. *J. Clin. Epidemiol.* 2005; **58**: 882–93.

20 Rutjes AW, Reitsma JB, Di Nisio M, Smidt N, van Rijn JC, Bossuyt PM. Evidence of bias and variation in diagnostic accuracy studies. *CMAJ* 2006; **174**: 469–76.

21 Whiting P, Rutjes AW, Dinnes J, Reitsma JB, Bossuyt PM, Kleijnen J. A systematic review finds that diagnostic reviews fail to incorporate quality despite available tools. *J. Clin. Epidemiol.* 2005; **58**: 1–12.

22 Whiting P, Rutjes AW, Reitsma JB, Bossuyt PM, Kleijnen J. The development of QUADAS: a tool for the quality assessment of studies of diagnostic accuracy included in systematic reviews. *BMC Med. Res. Methodol.* 2003; **3**: 25.

23 Whiting P, Harbord R, Kleijnen J. No role for quality scores in systematic reviews of diagnostic accuracy studies. *BMC Med. Res. Methodol.* 2005; **5**: 19.

24 Whiting P, Rutjes AW, Reitsma JB, Glas AS, Bossuyt PM, Kleijnen J. Sources of variation and bias in studies of diagnostic accuracy: a systematic review. *Ann. Intern. Med.* 2004; **140**: 189–202.

25 Reitsma JB, Glas AS, Rutjes AW, Scholten RJ, Bossuyt PM, Zwinderman AH. Bivariate analysis of sensitivity and specificity produces informative summary measures in diagnostic reviews. *J. Clin. Epidemiol.* 2005; **58**: 982–90.

26 Honest H, Khan KS. Reporting of measures of accuracy in systematic reviews of diagnostic literature. *BMC Med. Res. Methodol.* 2002; **2**: 4.

27 Moses LE, Shapiro D, Littenberg B. Combining independent studies of a diagnostic test into a summary ROC curve: data-analytic approaches and some additional considerations. *Stat. Med.* 1993; **12**: 1293–316.

28 Jones CM, Athanasiou T. Summary receiver operating characteristic curve analysis techniques in the evaluation of diagnostic tests. *Ann. Thorac. Surg.* 2005; **79**: 16–20.

PART 2

Neurological symptoms/problems

CHAPTER 5
Acute migraine attacks

Anne MacGregor

Background

Headache is the most common neurological condition in the world, with more than 90% of the population reporting headaches at some time in their lives [1]. Most headaches can be accounted for by two types of primary headache, as defined in the International Headache Society (IHS) classification of headache disorders – migraine and tension-type headache – and by one type of secondary headache, associated with the overuse of headache medication (medication-overuse headache) [2] (Table 5.1).

Migraine is more prevalent than diabetes, epilepsy and asthma combined, affecting more than 14% (7.6% of men and 18.3% of women) of the UK population – over 6 million people[3]. Migraine has been ranked by the World Health Organization (WHO) as 19th among all diseases worldwide causing disability (12th in women) [4]. WHO has also recognized the impact that headache has on public health [5]. Research shows that in the UK alone, an estimated 5.7 working days are lost per year for every working or student migraineur and each working day up to 90,000 people are absent from work or school as a result of migraine [3]. Prevalence of migraine varies with age, rising through early adult life and peaking during the most productive working years.

Despite all these facts, migraine is not seen as a public health problem; it is widely under diagnosed and under treated, in children and adults [6,7]. It has been estimated that in the UK and the USA around two-thirds of patients with migraine never consult their doctor, are not given a correct diagnosis and are treated (or treat themselves) with only over-the-counter medication [6]. Many patients would benefit from correct diagnosis and medical management (notably those with medication-overuse headache) or from treatment with more specific drugs (notably the triptans for migraine sufferers). Under-treatment – as well as causing unnecessary disability and suffering – is not economically cost-effective in terms of time lost from work and burden placed on the families of sufferers; more effective health care would alleviate much of the suffering and therefore reduce both the personal and financial costs of headache [8]. However, in many countries, headache is seen as a self-limiting and essentially unimportant condition, and therefore worthy of scant regard and scant resources. Recent advances in the treatment of headache, particularly of migraine, increase the possibilities of improving headache care [8].

Case scenario

A 43-year-old government officer has had recurring headaches since her early teens. She recalls that when they first started she had two or three attacks per year of severe headaches lasting part of day. She would feel sick and noticed that the headaches resolved once she vomited. At university, they became particularly bad and in her final year, she was having headaches most days. However, she managed to control them with painkillers. She sought medical advice and was told that she had chronic sinusitis. When she left university the pattern initially reverted to infrequent attacks but after she had children she experienced monthly attacks, with her periods. However, they would only last a day and would respond to painkillers. For the last couple of years the headaches have become more frequent and more severe. She now has two to three attacks per month of severe headache with nausea, each lasting 2–3 days. Her usual painkillers no longer help and she is losing time from work. Her doctor has suggested that she is 'stressed' and advised antidepressants. She was angered by this suggestion, as between attacks she feels completely well. She has asked to see you for a second opinion. She wants to know why no one has suggested a brain scan and why she cannot just have some stronger painkillers.

Framing answerable clinical questions

You are concerned that the increased frequency of headaches might suggest underlying pathology although, on the basis of 'common headaches occur commonly', the most likely diagnosis is a primary headache such as migraine. However, she has been diagnosed in the past with chronic sinusitis and, most recently, depression. Are these valid diagnoses?

You frame six specific questions to address.

1 In middle-aged people, what is the likelihood that recurrent headaches are migraine? [baseline risk]

2 In middle-aged people what is the utility of investigations and brain scans in the diagnosis of headache? [baseline risk]

Table 5.1 *The International Classification of Headache Disorders*, 2nd Edition (adapted from IHS [2] with permission).

Primary headaches

1. Migraine, *including*:
   - 1.1 Migraine without aura
   - 1.2 Migraine with aura
2. Tension-type headache, *including*:
   - 2.1 Infrequent episodic tension-type headache
   - 2.2 Frequent episodic tension-type headache
   - 2.3 Chronic tension-type headache
3. Cluster headache and other trigeminal autonomic cephalalgias, *including*:
   - 3.1 Cluster headache
4. Other primary headaches

Secondary headaches

5. Headache attributed to head and/or neck trauma, *including*:
   - 5.2 Chronic post-traumatic headache
6. Headache attributed to cranial or cervical vascular disorder, *including*:
   - 6.2.2 Headache attributed to subarachnoid haemorrhage
   - 6.4.1 Headache attributed to giant cell arteritis
7. Headache attributed to non-vascular intracranial disorder, *including*:
   - 7.1.1 Headache attributed to idiopathic intracranial hypertension
   - 7.4 Headache attributed to intracranial neoplasm
8. Headache attributed to a substance or its withdrawal, *including*:
   - 8.1.3 Carbon monoxide-induced headache
   - 8.1.4 Alcohol-induced headache
   - 8.2 Medication-overuse headache
   - 8.2.1 Ergotamine-overuse headache
   - 8.2.2 Triptan-overuse headache
   - 8.2.3 Analgesic-overuse headache
9. Headache attributed to infection, *including*:
   - 9.1 Headache attributed to intracranial infection
10. Headache attributed to disorder of homoeostasis
11. Headache or facial pain attributed to disorder of cranium, neck, eyes, ears, nose, sinuses, teeth, mouth or other facial or cranial structures, *including*:
    - 11.2.1 Cervicogenic headache
    - 11.3.1 Headache attributed to acute glaucoma
12. Headache attributed to psychiatric disorder

Neuralgias and other headaches

13. Cranial neuralgias, central and primary facial pain and other headaches, *including*:
    - 13.1 Trigeminal neuralgia
14. Other headache, cranial neuralgia, central or primary facial pain

---

3 For people with migraine, which non-specific acute treatments are effective in increasing the probability of response or pain-free at 2 h? [therapy]

4 For people with migraine, which specific acute treatments are effective in increasing the probability of response or pain-free at 2 h? How great are the adverse events? [therapy]

5 For people with migraine, which treatments for prophylaxis are effective at reducing the frequency of migraine by 50%? What are the likely adverse events? [therapy]

6. For people with migraine, what is the likelihood of attacks persisting life-long? [prognosis]

Critical review of the evidence

1. Diagnosis

In middle-aged people, what is the likelihood that the headaches are migraine?

Migraine is the commonest form of disabling headache presenting to doctors. Some studies suggest that the lifetime prevalence of migraine in women is as great as 25%, compared with only 8% in men [9]. Adults with migraine describe episodic attacks of moderate to severe headache lasting between part of a day and 3 days, with associated nausea, photo- and/or phono-phobia [2]. During attacks, activity is limited. Less commonly, attacks are preceded by a neurological aura, typically visual, lasting 5–60 min preceding and resolving before the onset of headache. Epidemiological studies confirm the clinical impression that migraine is a predominantly female disorder. Although migraine is equally common in both sexes before puberty, there is increased female prevalence following menarche [10]. This difference between the sexes becomes greater with increasing age, peaking during the early 40s and declining thereafter [11,12]. This sex difference during the reproductive years is generally considered to result from the additional trigger of the fluctuating hormones of the menstrual cycle, particularly during the perimenopause [13]. Attacks of migraine occur between once a week and once a year, with a median of one per month, and with complete freedom from symptoms between attacks [3].

Of the differential diagnosis of common headache, tension-type headache, although more prevalent, is less disabling and lacks the specific features or associated symptoms of migraine. It can occur daily. Medication-overuse headache is increasingly identified as a cause of daily or near-daily headache, estimated to affect 1 in 50 adults with a 5:1 female to male ratio [14]. It typically arises when symptomatic treatment for headache is taken more often than 2–3 days a week [2]. Medication overuse must always be managed because it can mask the diagnosis, causes illness and markedly reduces the effectiveness of all forms of headache treatment.

Sinusitis is a common mistaken diagnosis of primary headache. No headache, whether episodic or chronic, should be attributed to sinus disease in the absence of other symptoms suggestive of it. Depression is often comorbid with migraine and, if present, should be treated. However, there is little evidence to suggest that treating depression affects the outcome of migraine. Several prophylactic drugs used for migraine are antidepressant but they are effective on migraine at doses lower than the effective antidepressive doses.

2. CT scan

In middle-aged people what is the utility of investigations and brain scans in the diagnosis of headache?

In clinical practice, a primary concern is differentiation of primary headaches from secondary sinister headaches.

Table 5.2 Non-specific acute treatments for migraine.

Types of study (reference)	Intervention	Outcome	Number of patients (number of trials)	Control group risk	Absolute risk reduction	NNT (95% CI)
SR [20]	Tolfenamic acid 200 mg versus placebo	2 h response	84 (1)	29%	48%	2.1 (1.5–3.5)
SR [20]	Aspirin 900 mg plus metoclopramide 10 mg versus placebo	2 h response 2 h pain-free	749 (N/A) 753 (3)	25% 7%	32% 11%	3.2 (2.6–4.0) 8.6 (6.2–14)
SR [20]	Paracetamol 500 mg plus aspirin 500 mg plus caffeine 130 mg versus placebo	2 h response	1220 (3)	No data	No data	3.9 (3.2–4.9)
SR [20]	Paracetamol 1000 mg versus placebo	2 h response	289 (1)	39%	19%	5.2 (3.3–13)
RCT [19]	Aspirin 1000 mg versus placebo	2 h response 2 h pain-free	401 (1)	34% 6%	18% 14%	5.6 7.1
RCT [17]	Ibuprofen 200 mg versus 400 mg versus 600 mg versus placebo	2 h response 2 h pain-free	729 (1)	50% 13%	14–22% 12–16%	4.5–7.1 6.3–8.3
RCT [18]	Diclofenac 50 mg (tablet or sachet) versus placebo	2 h response 2 h pain-free	328 (1)	24% 12%	17.5–22% 7–13%	4.5–5.7 7 sachet (5.5–13.4) 15.8 tablet (8.6–96.2)

SR: systematic review; RCT: randomised controlled trial; NNT: number needed to treat; CI: confidence interval.

History is a crucial step in diagnosis of primary headaches, together with a normal neurological examination. A separate history is required for each type of headache reported, particularly noting the course and duration of each. Many specialists advocate the use of a symptom diary, which patients can use at home to establish a temporal pattern for their headache. A review of four studies of screening questions for migraine in patients with headache identified five predictors: pulsating, duration 4–72 h, unilateral, nausea and disabling [15]. If three predictors are present, the likelihood ratio for migraine is 3.5 (95% CI, 1.3–9.2), increasing to 24 (95% CI, 1.5–388) if four predictors are present.

Investigations, including neuroimaging, do not contribute to the diagnosis [16]. Imaging is necessary only if secondary headache is suspected because of undefined headache, atypical symptoms, persistent neurological or psychopathological abnormalities, or abnormal findings on neurologic examination [15].

3. Non-specific acute treatments

For people with migraine, which non-specific acute treatments are effective in increasing the probability of response or pain-free at 2 h?

Analgesics and non-steroidal anti-inflammatory drugs

Analgesics are the first-line acute treatment for migraine. Many analgesics have been shown in multiple trials to be more effective than placebo, including aspirin (500–1000 mg), diclofenac (50–100 mg), flubiprofen (100–300 mg), ibuprofen (400–2400 mg), naproxen (750–1250 mg), paracetamol (1000 mg), piroxicam (40 mg) and tolfenamic acid (200–400 mg) [17–21]. Several trials have examined the efficacy of a proprietary combination of paracetamol, aspirin and caffeine; each trial found that the combination analgesic was significantly more effective than placebo [20–21] (Table 5.2).

Antiemetics

Nausea and vomiting are usual symptoms of migraine. For some individuals these symptoms can be far more distressing and difficult to control than the headache itself. Several antiemetics are commonly used although clinical trial data are limited. The recognition that gastric stasis accompanies migraine led to trials with gastroprokinetic agents metoclopramide (10 mg po, im or iv), and domperidone (20–30 mg po or pr) which may have the additional advantage of enhancing the bioavailability of concomitant drugs given orally to treat migraine [22]. Chlorpromazine (25–50 mg im), metoclopramide (10 mg iv or im) and prochlorperazine (10 mg iv or im) have also been used as single-agent therapies in migraine with success [21].

4. Specific acute treatments

For people with migraine, which specific acute treatments are effective in increasing the probability of response or pain-free at 2 h? How great are the adverse events?

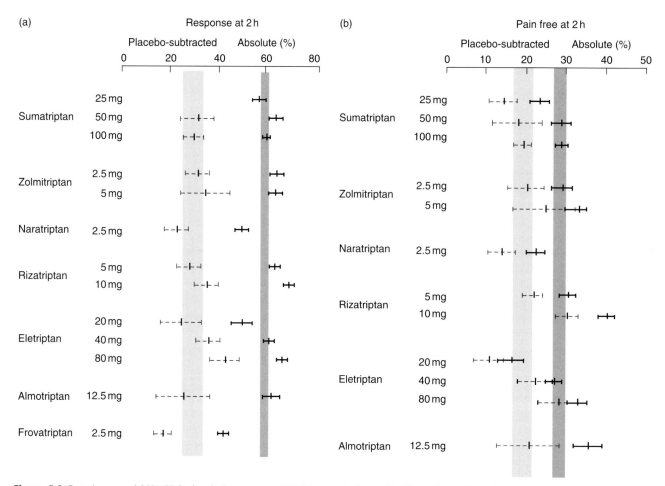

Figure 5.1 Data (mean and 95% CI) for headache response at 2 h (a) and pain free at 2 h (b) are shown for each triptan. Absolute and placebo subtracted outcomes are presented with the hatched region being the 95% CI envelope for sumatriptan 100 mg (adapted from Ferrari et al. [25] with permission).

Triptans

Sumatriptan, the first triptan to become available, was initially available in its subcutaneous form. At least 11 placebo-controlled trials have been consistent in showing that 6 mg of subcutaneous sumatriptan is better than placebo in providing headache relief at 1 h [23]. Sixteen trials have compared oral sumatriptan with placebo and findings are consistent in showing that oral sumatriptan is an effective drug for the treatment of a single acute attack of migraine. It is well tolerated, though minor adverse events are not uncommon [24]. Overall, the proportion of patients reporting relief with oral sumatriptan is lower than that with subcutaneous sumatriptan [25].

Six triptans have become available since sumatriptan appeared on the market: almotriptan, eletriptan, frovatriptan, naratriptan rizatriptan and zolmitriptan. Eletriptan and rizatriptan have been subject to Cochrane Reviews confirming efficacy [26,27]. A systematic review and meta-analysis that took data from 53 trials involving over 24,000 patients compared the oral triptans, using oral sumatriptan (at a dose of 100 mg) as the comparator [25]. All the triptans were found to be more effective than placebo at relieving the headache and other symptoms of migraine. The typical end-point was the headache response at 2 h (a positive response being defined as reduction of pain from moderate or severe at baseline to absent or mild by 2 h) (Figures 5.1 and 5.2).

More stringent parameters are pain-free at 2 h (reduction of pain from moderate or severe at baseline to absent by 2 h), sustained pain-free at 24 h (reduction of pain from moderate or severe at baseline to absent by 2 h, headache does not return and no other headache medication taken) and adverse event data are shown in Table 5.3.

A number of conclusions can be drawn about the efficacies of the various oral triptans:

• Fastest onset to effect is with subcutaneous sumatriptan.
• Eletriptan and rizatriptan are the most rapidly acting oral triptans, with effect seen from 30 min.
• Oral almotriptan, sumatriptan and zolmitriptan act within 45–60 min.

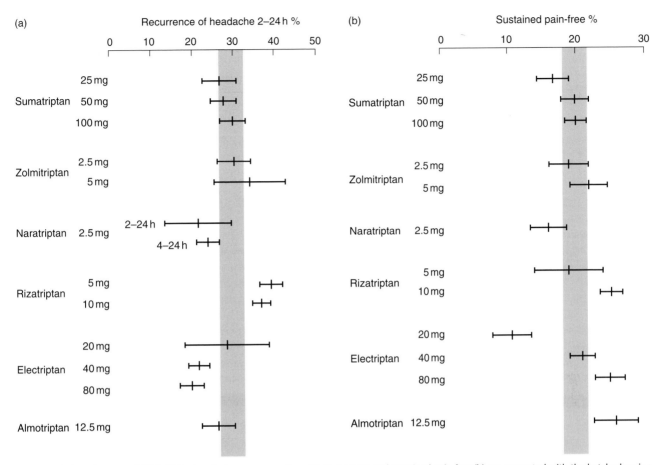

Figure 5.2 Data (mean and 95% CI) for headache recurrence from 2 h to 24 h (a) and sustained pain free (b) are presented with the hatched region being the 95% CI envelope for sumatriptan 100 mg. For naratriptan the recurrence rate is given for the time period 4–24 h post-dose (as presented in the original publications) and for 2–24 h post-dose (after recalculating the data) (adapted from Ferrari et al. [25] with permission).

- Frovatriptan and naratriptan are the slowest, taking up to 4 h before effect is seen.
- Intranasal zolmitriptan is faster acting than oral zolmitriptan.
- Pain-free rates at 2 h and sustained pain-free rates over 24 h are higher for almotriptan, eletriptan and rizatriptan than for sumatriptan.
- The highest likelihood of consistent success is with almotriptan, eletriptan and rizatriptan.
- The lowest rate of adverse events is with almotriptan, eletriptan and naratriptan.

Guidelines published suggest the following approach to symptomatic treatment of migraine, based on the available evidence and expert consensus [21,28]:

- Initial treatment with and NSAID ± a prokinetic anti-emetic is a reasonable choice for mild to moderate migraine.
- Initial treatment with any triptan is a reasonable choice when the headache is moderate to severe or when the migraine, whatever its severity, has failed to respond to non-specific medication in the past.

- Intranasal zolmitriptan or subcutaneous sumatriptan may be useful in patients with nausea and vomiting or when a rapid response is important.

A rational hierarchy of the use of triptans has been proposed (Table 5.4).

Triptans are more effective when taken while the headache is mild. They are ineffective if taken before the onset of headache, during premonitory symptoms or aura [29].

Relapse of headache, typically the day following initial treatment, is a significant problem in clinical practice, the rate being between 15–40%. The highest relapse rate is associated with subcutaneous sumatriptan and the lowest with naratriptan and frovatriptan. If migraine relapses after successful treatment, a second dose of triptan can be given. There is also some evidence that the combination of a triptan and an NSAID reduces the likelihood of relapse [30].

Contraindications to triptans include untreated arterial disease, Raynaud's disease, pregnancy, lactation and severe renal or liver failure.

Table 5.3 Meta-analysis of triptans: NNTs of 2-h pain-free and 24-h sustained pain-free and NNH (adapted from Ferrari et al. [25] with permission).

Intervention	Number of participants (number of trials)	Outcome	Absolute risk reduction/ increase (95% CI)	NNT or NNH (95% CI)	Ratio of NNH/NNT
Sumatriptan 100 mg versus placebo	2071 (9)	2 h pain-free	19.5 (17.3; 21.8)	5.1 (4.6–5.8)	1.5
		24 h sustained pain-free	20.0 (18.2; 21.3)	5.0 (4.7–5.5)	1.5
		Adverse events	13.2 (8.6; 17.8)	7.6 (5.6–11.6)	
Sumatriptan 50 mg versus placebo	583 (3)	2 h pain-free	18.0 (11.7; 24.3)	5.6 (4.1–8.5)	2.3
		24 h sustained pain-free	19.8 (17.8; 21.8)	5.1 (4.6–5.6)	2.5
		Adverse events	7.8 (2.6; 13.1)	12.8 (7.6–38)	
Zolmitriptan 2.5 mg versus placebo	1320 (3)	2 h pain-free	20.4 (15.6; 25.1)	4.9 (4.0–6.4)	1.3
		24 h sustained pain-free	19.0 (16.1; 21.8)	5.3 (4.6–6.2)	1.2
		Adverse events	15.9 (9.6; 22.1)	6.3 (4.5–10.4)	
Zolmitriptan 5 mg versus placebo	1596 (5)	2 h pain-free	25.2 (16.9; 33.5)	4.0 (3.0–5.9)	1
		24 h sustained pain-free	21.9 (19.3; 24.6)	4.6 (4.1–5.2)	0.9
		Adverse events	24.5 (15.5; 33.5)	4.1 (3.0–6.5)	
Rizatriptan 10 mg versus placebo	4437 (11)	2 h pain-free	30.4 (27.5; 33.2)	3.3 (3.0–3.6)	2.2
		24 h sustained pain-free	25.3 (23.7; 26.9)	3.9 (3.7–4.2)	1.9
		Adverse events	13.5 (10.6; 16.3)	7.4 (6.1–9.4)	
Eletriptan 40 mg versus placebo	2894 (7)	2 h pain-free	27.2 (25.2; 29.2)	3.7 (3.4–4.0)	3.7
		24 h sustained pain-free	20.9 (19.1; 22.7)	4.8 (4.4–5.2)	2.9
		Adverse events	7.3 (2.7; 11.8)	13.7 (8.5–37)	
Almotriptan 12.5 mg versus placebo	1074 (3)	2 h pain-free	21.0 (13.3; 28.7)	4.8 (3.5–7.5)	11.7
		24 h sustained pain-free	25.9 (22.7; 29.1)	3.9 (3.4–4.4)	14.3
		Adverse events	1.8 (−2.7; 6.2)	56 (16.1–no harm)	
Naratriptan 5 mg versus placebo	2023 (5)	2 h pain-free	14.1 (10.7; 17.5)	7.0 (5.7–9.3)	6.0
		24 h sustained pain-free	15.9 (13.4; 18.5)	6.3 (5.4–7.5)	6.7
		Adverse events	2.4 (−2.2; 7.0)	42 (14.2–no harm)	
Frovatriptan 2.5 mg versus placebo	2892 (5)	2 h pain-free			Approximately 10

NNT: number needed to treat; NNH: number needed to harm; CI: confidence interval.

Table 5.4 Proposed rational hierarchy for the use of triptans (adapted from Steiner et al. [28] with permission).

Use	Dose regimen
Appropriate for first use of a triptan	Almotriptan 12.5 mg, eletriptan 40 mg, sumatriptan 50 mg or zolmitriptan 2.5 mg orally
When greater efficacy is needed	Eletriptan 80 mg or rizatriptan 10 mg, sumatriptan 100 mg or zolmitriptan 5 mg orally or sumatriptan 20 mg nasal spray
When a rapid response is important above all	Sumatriptan 6 mg subcutaneously or zolmitriptan 5 mg intranasal
When nausea or vomiting precludes oral therapy	Sumatriptan 6 mg subcutaneously or zolmitriptan 5 mg intranasal
When side effects are troublesome with other triptans	Naratriptan 2.5 mg or almotriptan 12.5 mg orally or frovatriptan 2.5 mg
When headache relapse is a problem	Ergotamine tartrate 1–2 mg may be helpful

Ergot derivatives

The evidence for the efficacy of ergot derivatives in the symptomatic treatment of migraine is inconsistent, and their use is largely based on long-standing and wide clinical experience. A review of 18 trials found that oral ergotamine was more effective than placebo for some parameters in seven trials, but no better than placebo in three trials [31].

There are few studies on non-oral routes of ergotamine (rectal, sublingual, nasal, inhaled). Since oral bioavailability is poor, these other routes should, theoretically, be advantageous. An evidence-based expert consensus statement has produced recommendations for the use of ergotamine (Table 5.5).

Dihydroergotamine can be administered intramuscularly, intravenously, subcutaneously and intranasally but few trials have assessed its efficacy.

Ergot derivatives have been used less commonly since the triptans became available, but they still have a place in the

Table 5.5 Recommendations for the use of ergotamine (adapted from Tfelt-Hansen et al. [31] with permission).

Parameter	Recommendations	Comments
Which patients?	Patients requiring migraine-specific therapy	When a migraine-specific therapy is indicated, a triptan is a better choice than ergotamine for most patients.
	Patients established on ergotamine	Patients who are responding satisfactorily, have no contraindications and no signs of dose escalation, should not usually be switched to a triptan.
Special cases	Patients with very long attacks	Attacks lasting >48 h may be usefully treated with ergotamine
	Patients with frequent headache relapse	Headache relapse is probably less likely with ergotamine
Frequency of dosing	Once a week or six times a month	Ergotamine-induced headache and rebound headache are associated with frequent use. This can be limited by restricting ergotamine consumption and encouraging use of a preventative medication as headache becomes more frequent. May be modified to four consecutive doses for menstrual migraine
Dose per attack	Single dose (0.5–2 mg)	Should be given as a single dose as early as practicable in the attack at a dose that produces a response with as few side effects as possible. It is useful to test this dose for tolerability for nausea between attacks.
Preferred route	Rectal	Generally better used rectally, provided it is acceptable to the patient, because of improved absorption.

management of migraine, not least because there are some patients who do better with ergots than with triptans.

Contraindications to ergot derivatives include untreated arterial disease, Raynaud's disease, pregnancy, lactation and severe renal or liver failure. Toxicity and misuse potential are greater risks with ergotamine than with triptans so the frequency of intake should be restricted to a maximum of 10 days per month.

5. Prophylaxis

For people with migraine, which treatments for prophylaxis are effective at reducing the frequency of migraine by 50%? What are the likely adverse events?

Prophylactic drugs aim to reduce the frequency of migraine attacks, their duration or their severity. Agents used include beta-blockers, antidepressants, calcium-channel blockers, serotonin antagonists, anticonvulsants and NSAIDs. Overall, about one-third of patients who are treated with prophylactic agents can be expected to have a 50% reduction in the frequency of their headaches (Table 5.6).

A second or third prophylactic agent taken concomitantly may be needed in some cases.

Guidelines published by the American Academy of Neurology suggest the following indications for prophylactic treatment of migraine, based on the available evidence and expert consensus [32]:
• Recurrent migraine that, in the patient's opinion, significantly interferes with his or her daily routine in spite of acute treatment.
• Frequent headaches.
• Acute therapies cannot be used because of contraindications, failure, overuse or adverse effects.

• Cost considerations.
• Patient preference.
• The presence of uncommon migraine conditions that may predispose to permanent neurological sequelae, such as hemiplegic migraine, basilar migraine, migraine with prolonged aura or migrainous infarction.

The guidelines go on to give further consensus-based recommendations for selecting the most appropriate prophylactic medication:
• Start with medications that have the highest level of evidence-based efficacy.
• Start with the lowest dose that has been shown to be effective, and increase it slowly until clinical benefits are achieved for the patient in the absence of, or until limited by, adverse effects.
• Give each medication an adequate trial, which may mean 2–3 months in some cases.
• Consider reducing the dose or even discontinuing the medication if, after 3–6 months headaches are well controlled.
• Long-acting formulations may improve compliance.
• Establish that any agent chosen is not contraindicated in any coexisting illness.
• Choose an agent that may be beneficial in any coexisting illness, remembering that some conditions are more common in people with migraine (e.g. anxiety disorders, affective disorders, stroke, myocardial infarction, epilepsy, Raynaud's phenomenon).

Beta-blockers

There is extensive clinical experience of using beta-blockers in the prophylaxis of migraine, and multiple clinical trials have been shown to be 60–80% effective in producing a reduction of more than 50% in the frequency of attacks. Propranolol

Table 5.6 Prophylactic drugs with data on ⩾50% reduction in migraine attacks.

Intervention	Outcome	Number of participants (number of trials)	Control group risk (range)	Relative risk (95% CI)	Absolute risk increase (95% CI)	Comment
Propranolol (SR) Ref [33]	⩾50% reduction of migraine or headache index	688 (9)	30% (11–50)	1.9 (1.6–2.3)	28% (21; 35)	Parallel group and pooled crossover data (PROP CR) Main AEs: fatigue (<10%).
	Adverse effects	619 (6)	24% (4–65)	1.4 (1.2–1.8)	10% (3; 16)	
Topiramate (SR) Ref [20]	⩾50% reduction of migraine	822 (5)	22%	2.1 (1.7–2.6)	24%	21% on topiramate withdrew because of AE. Main AEs: paraesthesiae (50%), fatigue (15%), nausea (13%).
Sodium valproate (SR) Ref [20]	⩾50% reduction of migraine	349 (3)	18% (14–20)	2.6 (1.7–4.0)	28% (24; 34)	15% on sodium valproate withdrew because of AEs Main AEs: weight gain (>10%), somonolence (<10%), alopecia (<10%).
	Adverse effects	369 (3)	35%	1.5	17%	
Gabapentin (SR) Ref [35]	⩾50% reduction of migraine	87 (1)	16%	2.9 (1.23–6.74)	30% (12; 49)	Just one small trial. Main AEs: Dizziness (28%), somnolence (21%).
Flunarizine 5 mg versus 10 mg (RCT) Ref [37]	⩾50% reduction of migraine compared to run-in	783 (1)	No placebo control		46–53%	Propranolol 160 mg used as an active comparator with 48% responders. Main AEs: somnolence (20%), weight gain (11%).

SR: systematic review; RCT: randomised controlled trial; CI: confidence interval.

has been the most extensively studied, and there is consistent evidence for its effectiveness at daily doses of 120–240 mg [33]. Studies reporting on lower doses (80–160 mg) have reported mixed results [32]. Multiple trials of metoprolol versus placebo have also reported mixed results, although direct comparisons between metoprolol and propranolol have shown few significant differences, suggesting that metoprolol is an effective migraine prophylactic agent [33]. Similarly, timolol, atenolol and nadolol are also effective on the basis of direct comparisons with propranolol or placebo [33]. Beta-blockers with intrinsic sympathomimetic activity (acebutolol, alprenolol, oxprenolol and pindolol) seem not to be effective.

Antidepressants

The antidepressant most commonly used in the prophylaxis of migraine is amitriptyline, which also has the strongest evidence base for its use [32]. Amitriptyline may be particularly effective for patients with mixed migraine and tension-type headache. Selective serotonin reuptake inhibitors (SSRIs) have also been tried in migraine prophylaxis. Although there is some evidence to support the efficacy of fluoxetine (10–40 mg) a Cochrane Review suggests that other SSRIs are no better than placebo for preventing migraine [34].

Antiepileptic drugs/neuromodulators

Divalproex sodium and valproate and have been shown in at least five studies to be effective in the prophylaxis of migraine [35]. Daily doses of 500, 1000 and 1500 mg can all be effective; titration is required. The multiple daily dosing that is needed may be able to be avoided by using extended-release preparations. Topiramate, the most recently licenced migraine prophylactic, has proven effective at doses of 100 mg per day in three randomized placebo-controlled dose-ranging studies [36].

Evidence for the use of other antiepileptics such as gabapentin and lamotrigine is weak.

Calcium-channel blockers

The evidence is best for the use of flunarizine, which has been the subject of more than 25 trials. Eight trials comparing it with placebo have been conducted, and a meta-analysis of seven of these shows that flunarizine is more effective than placebo. Comparisons of flunarizine with either propranolol or metoprolol have shown no significant differences between the agents [32,37]. Trials for the use of other calcium-channel blockers have either given mixed results or are difficult to interpret [32]. For example, vera-pamil was found to be more effective than placebo in two trials, but both of these trials were small and had high drop-out rates; results of a third trial shown no significant differences for verapamil versus placebo but also for verapamil versus propranolol. Two trials comparing nifedipine with placebo found differences that were statistically insignificant, but clinically important effects could not be excluded. Difficult-to-interpret results were also reported in two trials comparing nifedipine with propranolol and in another trail comparing nifedipine with flunarizine. One placebo-controlled trial reported efficacy for nicardipine.

Methysergide and pizotifen
Methysergide and pizotifen are serotonin antagonists. Methysergide, a semisynthetic ergot alkaloid, was one of the first agents to be used and studied for migraine prophylaxis, and multiple trials have suggested that it is effective at reducing headache frequency [32]. However, its use is limited by adverse effects, including retroperitoneal, endocardial and retropleural fibrosis. These side effects occur in about one in 2500 patients and are usually associated with long-term, uninterrupted use. Risk can be reduced with a 1-month drug 'holiday' for every 6 months of treatment. Analysis of placebo-controlled trials of pizotifen suggests that it has a statistically significant clinical effect, and in comparison trials, no significant differences were demonstrated between pizotifen and methysergide, metoprolol, naproxen or flunarizine. However, the design of these trials has been questioned. Sedation and weight gain limit its use in clinical practice [32].

Herbs and vitamins
Often seen as 'non-drug' options, herbs and vitamins are popular therapeutic options for many people with migraine and are increasingly scrutinized in randomized placebo-controlled trials.

A Cochrane Review of five trials assessed the efficacy of oral feverfew (*Tanacetum parthenium*) compared with placebo. The results did not convincingly establish that feverfew is more effective than placebo for preventing migraine [38]. No major side effects were associated with feverfew.

Riboflavin (vitamin B2), in doses of 400 mg daily (more than 20 times the recommended daily intake) has been assessed against placebo in 55 patients with migraine in a randomized trial of 3 months duration. Using an intention-to-treat analysis, riboflavin was significantly superior to placebo in reducing attack frequency [39]. The proportion of patients who reported at least 50% fewer headache days was at 15% for placebo and 59% for riboflavin, a significant difference. There were no serious side effects.

Like riboflavin, Coenzyme Q10 (CoQ10) also improves energy metabolism and 3×100 mg/day has been compared with placebo in 42 migraine patients in a double-blind, randomized, trial [40]. The 50%-responder-rate for attack frequency was 14.4% for placebo and 47.6% for CoQ10, a significant difference. CoQ10 was well tolerated.

Magnesium has not been shown to be effective in two trials of migraine prevention [41,42].

A randomized double-blind placebo-controlled trial of a compound providing a daily dose of riboflavin 400 mg, magnesium 300 mg and feverfew 100 mg was compared against 25 mg riboflavin ('placebo') [43]. Of 49 patients who completed the 3-month trial there was no difference between active and 'placebo' groups reporting a 50% or greater reduction in migraines (42% and 44%, respectively) neither was there a difference in 50% or greater reduction in migraine days (33% and 40%). Compared to baseline, however, both groups showed a significant reduction in number of migraines, migraine days and migraine index.

Two randomized placebo-controlled trials of butterbur (*Petasites hybridus*) for migraine prophylaxis have suggested efficacy [44,45].

However, further large and rigorously conducted trials of herbs and vitamin treatments are needed before they can be recommended as an alternative to standard therapies.

Physical treatments
A number of physical treatments for migraine have been studied, including transcutaneous electrical nerve stimulation (TENS), occlusal adjustment, cervical manipulation and acupuncture. With the exception of acupuncture, there are few studies reported on these treatments. Of 17 trials comparing true and sham (placebo) acupuncture in migraine and tension-type headache patients, eight reported true acupuncture to be significantly superior; four reported a trend in favour of true acupuncture and in three trials there was no difference between the two interventions. Two trials were uninterpretable [46,47].

Behavioural therapy
Behavioural therapies that have been studied include relaxation training, biofeedback and cognitive behavioural therapy. A review of 70 prospective controlled trials of behavioural treatments for migraine showed that, compared with controls, all of these therapies are somewhat effective in preventing migraine [48].

6. Prognosis
For people with migraine, what is the likelihood of attacks persisting life-long?

In general, the prognosis of migraine is favourable. Studies consistently show that migraine peaks during the 40 s but usually remits in later life [49]. The reason for this decline in prevalence is unknown although it has been postulated that it could relate to a reduced vascular response with advancing years.

Conclusion

The prevalence of migraine in a middle-aged woman is around 25% and hence is the most likely diagnosis for recurrent episodic 'sick' headaches in an otherwise well person. Having established the diagnosis on history, in the absence of abnormal findings on physical examination, you are reassured by the evidence that there is no need to undertake any investigations to confirm this diagnosis.

Since the severity of your patient's attacks varies, there is good quality evidence to recommend a NSAID together with a prokinetic antiemetic. You also prescribe a triptan for attacks that do not respond to this and recommend that if a triptan is always required, it can be taken together with the NSAID to increase efficacy and reduce the likelihood of relapse. Given the frequency of the attacks you discuss prophylactic options and settle on a beta-blocker as being the most suitable first-line agent, as she does not wish to take an antidepressant. You assure her that the present increased frequency of attacks is in keeping with the expected pattern of migraine for her age and sex. Further, the natural history of migraine is such that migraine is likely to improve post-menopause.

Future research needs

The reliance on the history for diagnosing migraine is often a cause for uncertainty and there would be considerable benefit if a specific and sensitive test were available.

Although the majority of people with migraine recognize that a cure is unlikely, they would benefit from more effective symptomatic and prophylactic medication. It is likely that this will result from research into the pathophysiology of migraine. Despite considerable recent advances, much remains obscure. In particular, relapse of symptoms following effective treatment with triptans is a considerable clinical problem and can extend the total duration of attack.

Similarly, prophylaxis has limited efficacy and is often associated with unwanted side effects on days when the individual would otherwise by symptom-free.

Few studies have adequately compared behavioural and pharmacological treatments for migraine, or even the combination of such treatments.

Finally, there is the issue of more effective management of migraine and comorbid conditions such as depression.

References

1 Rasmussen BK. Epidemiology of headache. *Cephalalgia*. 1995; **15**(1): 45–68.

2 Headache Classification Subcommittee of the International Headache Society (IHS). *The International Classification of Headache Disorders*, 2nd edn. *Cephalalgia*. 2004; **24**(Suppl. 1): 1–160.

3 Steiner TJ, Scher AI, Stewart WF, Kolodner K, Liberman J, Lipton RB. The prevalence and disability burden of adult migraine in England and their relationships to age, gender and ethnicity. *Cephalalgia*. 2003; **23**(7): 519–27.

4 World Health Organization. *Mental Health: New Understanding*, WHO: New Hope, Geneva, 2001.

5 World Health Organization. Headache disorders and public health. Education and management implications. World Health Organization 2000 [www.migraines.org/new/pdfs/who.pdf].

6 Lipton RB, Scher AI, Steiner TJ, et al. Patterns of health care utilization for migraine in England and in the United States. *Neurology*. 2003; **60**(3): 441–8.

7 Bigal ME, Kolodner KB, Lafata JE, Leotta C, Lipton RB. Patterns of medical diagnosis and treatment of migraine and probable migraine in a health plan. *Cephalalgia*. 2006; **26**(1): 43–9.

8 Steiner TJ. Lifting the burden: the global campaign against headache. *Lancet Neurol*. 2004; **3**(4): 204–5.

9 Rasmussen BK, Jensen R, Schroll M, Olesen J. Epidemiology of headache in a general population – a prevalence study. *J. Clin. Epidemiol*. 1991; **44**(11): 1147–57.

10 Bille B. Migraine in school children. *Acta. Paed. Scand.* 1962; **51**(Suppl. 136): 1–151.

11 Scher A, Stewart W, Lipton R. Migraine and headache: a meta-analytic approach. In: Crombie I, ed. *Epidemiology of Pain*. IASP Press, Seattle, 1999.

12 Stewart WF, Lipton RB, Celentano DD, Reed ML. Prevalence of migraine headache in the United States. Relation to age, income, race, and other sociodemographic factors. *JAMA*. 1992; **267**(1): 64–9.

13 MacGregor EA, Frith A, Ellis J, Aspinall L, Hackshaw A. Incidence of migraine relative to menstrual cycle phases of rising and falling estrogen. *Neurology*. 2006; **67**. Published September 13, 2006 as doi:10.1212/01.wnl.0000233888. 18228.19

14 Diener HC, Limmroth V. Medication-overuse headache: a worldwide problem. *Lancet Neurol*. 2004; **3**(8): 475–83.

15 Detsky ME, McDonald DR, Baerlocker MO, Tomlinson GA, McCory DC, Booth CM. Does this patient with headache have a migraine or need neuroimaging? *JAMA*. 2006; **296**: 1274–83.

16 Practice parameter: the utility of neuroimaging in the evaluation of headache in patients with normal neurologic examinations (summary statement). Report of the Quality Standards Subcommittee of the American Academy of Neurology. *Neurology*. 1994; **44**(7): 1353–4.

17 Kellstein DE, Lipton RB, Geetha R, et al. Evaluation of a novel solubilized formulation of ibuprofen in the treatment of migraine headache: a randomized, double-blind, placebo-controlled, dose-ranging study. *Cephalalgia*. 2000; **20**(4): 233–43.

18 Diener HC, Montagna P, Gacs G, et al. Efficacy and tolerability of diclofenac potassium sachets in migraine: a randomized, double-blind, cross-over study in comparison with diclofenac potassium tablets and placebo. *Cephalalgia*. 2006; **26**(5): 537–47.

19 Lipton RB, Goldstein J, Baggish JS, Yataco AR, Sorrentino JV, Quiring JN. Aspirin is efficacious for the treatment of acute migraine. *Headache*. 2005; **45**(4): 283–92.

20 Bandolier. www.jr2.ox.ac.uk/bandolier/booth/booths/migraine. html Accessed: 5th October 2006.

21 US Headache Consortium. Evidence-based guidelines for migraine headache in the primary care setting: pharmacological management of acute attacks. Available at www.americanheadachesociety.org/professionalresources/USHeadacheConsortiumGuidelines.asp 2000: Accessed 10 September 2006.

22 Ross-Lee LM, Eadie MJ, Heazlewood V, Bochner F, Tyrer JH. Aspirin pharmacokinetics in migraine. The effect of metoclopramide. *Eur. J. Clin. Pharmacol.* 1983; **24**: 777–85.

23 Tfelt-Hansen P. Efficacy and adverse events of subcutaneous, oral, and intranasal sumatriptan used for migraine treatment: a systematic review based on number needed to treat. *Cephalalgia.* 1998; **18**(8): 532–8.

24 McCory DC, Gray RN. Oral sumatriptan for acute migraine. *Cochrane Database Syst. Rev.* 2003; 3: CD002915. DOI: 10.1002/14651858.CD002915.

25 Ferrari MD, Goadsby PJ, Roon KI, Lipton RB. Triptans (serotonin, 5-HT1B/1D agonists) in migraine: detailed results and methods of a meta-analysis of 53 trials. *Cephalalgia.* 2002; **22**(8): 633–58.

26 Smith LA, Oldman AD, McQuay HJ, Moore RA. Eletriptan for acute migraine. *Cochrane Database Syst. Rev.* 2000; 4: CD003224. DOI: 10.1002/14651858.CD003224.

27 Oldman AD, Smith LA, McQuay HJ, Moore RA. Rizatriptan for acute migraine. *Cochrane Database Syst. Rev.* 2000; 4: CD003221. DOI: 10.1002/14651858.CD003221.

28 Steiner TJS, MacGregor EA, Davies PT. Guidelines for all doctors in the management and diagnosis of Migraine and Tension-Type Headache 2nd ed, 2004. www.bash.org.uk Accessed 10 September 2006.

29 Bates D, Ashford E, Dawson R, et al. Subcutaneous sumatriptan during the migraine aura. Sumatriptan Aura Study Group. *Neurology.* 1994; **44**(9): 1587–92.

30 Smith TR, Sunshine A, Stark SR, Littlefield DE, Spruill SE, Alexander WJ. Sumatriptan and naproxen sodium for the acute treatment of migraine. *Headache.* 2005; **45**(8): 983–91.

31 Tfelt-Hansen P, Saxena PR, Dahlof C, et al. Ergotamine in the acute treatment of migraine: a review and European consensus. *Brain.* 2000; **123**(Pt 1): 9–18.

32 US Headache Consortium. Evidence-based guidelines for migraine headache in the primary care setting: pharmacological management for prevention of migraine. Available at www.americanheadachesociety.org/professionalresources/USHeadacheConsortiumGuidelines.asp 2000: Accessed 10 September 2006.

33 Linde K, Rossnagel K. Propranolol for migraine. *Cochrane Database Syst. Rev.* 2004; 2: CD003225. DOI: 10.1002/14651858.CD003225.pub2.

34 Moja PL, Cusi C, Sterzi RR, Canepari C. Selective serotonin re-uptake inhibitors (SSRIs) for preventing migraine and tension-type headaches. *Cochrane Database Syst. Rev.* 2005; 3: CD002919. DOI: 10.1002/14651858.CD002919.pub2.

35 Chronicle E, Mulleners W. Anticonvulsant drugs for migraine prophylaxis. *Cochrane Database Syst. Rev.* 2004; 3: CD003226. DOI: 10.1002/14651858.CD003226.pub2.

36 Bussone G, Usai S, D'Amico D. Topiramate in migraine prophylaxis: data from a pooled analysis and open-label extension study. *Neurol. Sci.* 2006; **27** (Suppl. 2): S159–63.

37 Diener HC, Matias-Guiu J, Hartung E, et al. Efficacy and tolerability in migraine prophylaxis of flunarizine in reduced doses: a comparison with propranolol 160 mg daily. *Cephalalgia.* 2002; **22**(3): 209–21.

38 Pittler MH, Ernst E. Feverfew for preventing migraine. *Cochrane Database Syst. Rev.* 2004; 1: CD002286. DOI: 10.1002/14651858.CD002286.pub2.

39 Schoenen J, Jacquy J, Lenaerts M. Effectiveness of high-dose riboflavin in migraine prophylaxis. A randomized controlled trial. *Neurology.* 1998; **50**(2): 466–70.

40 Sandor PS, Di Clemente L, Coppola G, et al. Efficacy of coenzyme Q10 in migraine prophylaxis: a randomized controlled trial. *Neurology.* 2005; **64**(4): 713–15.

41 Peikert A, Wilimzig C, Kohne-Volland R. Prophylaxis of migraine with oral magnesium: results from a prospective, multi-center, placebo-controlled and double-blind randomized study. *Cephalalgia.* 1996; **16**(4): 257–63.

42 Pfaffenrath V, Wessely P, Meyer C, et al. Magnesium in the prophylaxis of migraine – a double-blind placebo-controlled study. *Cephalalgia.* 1996; **16**(6): 436–40.

43 Maizels M, Blumenfeld A, Burchette R. A combination of riboflavin, magnesium, and feverfew for migraine prophylaxis: a randomized trial. *Headache.* 2004; **44**(9): 885–90.

44 Diener HC, Rahlfs VW, Danesch U. The first placebo-controlled trial of a special butterbur root extract for the prevention of migraine: reanalysis of efficacy criteria. *Eur. Neurol.* 2004; **51**(2): 89–97.

45 Lipton RB, Gobel H, Einhaupl KM, Wilks K, Mauskop A. Petasites hybridus root (butterbur) is an effective preventive treatment for migraine. *Neurology.* 2004; **63**(12): 2240–4.

46 Diener HC, Kronfeld K, Boewing G, et al. Efficacy of acupuncture for the prophylaxis of migraine: a multicentre randomised controlled clinical trial. *Lancet. Neurol.* 2006; **5**(4): 310–16.

47 Melchart D, Linde K, Berman B, et al. Acupuncture for idiopathic headache. *Cochrane Database Syst. Rev.* 2001; 1: CD001218. DOI: 10.1002/14651858.CD001218.

48 US Headache Consortium. Evidence-based guidelines for migraine headache: behavioral and physical treatments. Available at www.americanheadachesociety.org/professionalresources/USHeadacheConsortiumGuidelines.asp 2000:Accessed 10 September 2006.

49 Lipton RB, Stewart WF, Diamond S, Diamond ML, Reed M. Prevalence and burden of migraine in the United States: data from the American Migraine Study II. *Headache.* 2001; **41**(7): 646–57.

6 CHAPTER 6
Back and neck pain

Harry McNaughton

Background

Low back pain (LBP) is a very common problem with a lifetime prevalence of 60% or more. The rate at which neurologists are consulted by people with back pain varies across countries. In the US, people with back pain may represent around 10% of all patients seen by a neurologist but it is likely to be considerably less than this in countries with lower concentrations of neurologists per head of population.

Perhaps 90% of the LBP in the population can be described as 'non-specific' implying no underlying serious pathology. Attempts to improve diagnostic specificity in this large group have not been successful despite a multitude of diagnostic labels, often reflecting treatment strategies of the providers involved. Neurologists are most likely to see people with back pain and neurological symptoms and/or signs. 'Sciatica', now more commonly referred to in the back pain literature simply as 'leg pain', may complicate up to 5% of new cases of back pain which represents a considerable number of potential new consultations each year.

There is considerable variation in the published studies of the natural history of episodes of acute back pain. This variation reflects the population studied, length of follow-up and outcome instruments used. There is reasonable agreement among the studies that for people with a new episode of acute LBP, particularly if there are no preceding episodes, outcome is very favourable, with 'full recovery' rates of >80% by 4 weeks and about 5% who are still symptomatic by 3 months or so. However, a significant proportion of the population with a new episode of back pain will report recurrent symptoms over the subsequent 12 months. Persistent back pain appears to be more common as people age and with more episodes of acute back pain. The very favourable natural history for acute episodes of back pain probably explains why so many treatments for back pain appear effective both to patients and practitioners. In this setting, randomized controlled trials (RCTs) are necessary to separate true treatment effects. However, one of the problems with these trials is the need to include a fairly homogeneous population in the study, often excluding people with a significant history of previous back pain or prior treatment with one of the modalities being tested. This can limit the generalizability of these trials to ordinary clinical practice.

Very few investigations in the context of acute LBP have adequate sensitivity and specificity to make them useful. CT scans and MRI scans are over-sensitive in terms of abnormalities that may be interpreted as 'causing' the episode of back pain. Around one third of adults with no current or previous back symptoms will have evidence of bulging or herniated discs on MRI scan [1].

Framing clinical questions

1 For adults within 6 weeks of onset of acute back or neck pain, with or without radiation, what interventions improve recovery and reduce long-term chronicity? Specifically, what is the place of bed rest, non-steroidal anti-inflammatory drugs (NSAIDs), steroids and 'physical therapies' including manipulation?

2 For people with chronic back pain, do exercise-based interventions improve functional outcomes?

3 For people with back or neck pain, does surgery improve outcomes for any particular group and/or at any particular time?

Critical review of the evidence for each question

1. Bed rest for acute back pain episode

1 *For adults with an acute episode of low back or neck pain without radicular features, does prescription of bed rest lead to better outcomes compared to advice to continue normal activities?*

2 *For adults with an acute episode of LBP with sciatica, does prescription of bed rest lead to better outcomes compared to advice to continue normal activities?*

1 Bed rest has been a traditional treatment for back pain, and particularly back pain with leg pain (or 'sciatica'). A systematic review of RCTs of bed rest versus other treatments is available with the date of the most recent substantive amendment being May 2004 [2]. Eleven trials (1963 patients) were included in this updated Cochrane Review (Table 6.1). The authors report that there is high quality evidence from two trials that people with acute LBP who are advised to rest in bed have more pain (standardized mean difference (SMD) 0.22 (95% confidence interval (CI) 0.02, 0.41)) and less functional

Table 6.1 Bed rest compared to other treatments for people with back pain. Result of systematic review [2].

Patient	Intervention	Outcome (follow-up time)	Number of patients (number of trials)	Control group mean change from baseline (range)	SMD or WMD (95% CI)	Control group risk (range)	Relative risk (95% CI)	Absolute risk reduction	Comment
Acute LBP	Bed rest versus advice to stay active	Pain intensity (3–4 weeks)	400 (2)	12.9* (1.9–23.9)	0.22 (0.02–0.41)				Bed rest worse One study excluded by risk of bias
		Functional status (3–4 weeks)	400 (2)	8.1* (10.0–6.3)	0.29 (0.09–0.49)				Bed rest worst
Acute LBP with sciatica	Bed rest versus advice to stay active	Pain intensity (3–4 weeks)	346 (2)	38.6 (37.3–40.0)	0.03 (ns)				Bed rest better
		Functional status (3–4 weeks)	346 (2)	30.6 (20.1–41.2)	0.19 (ns)				Bed rest worse
Acute LBP with or without sciatica	Bed rest 2–3 days versus bed rest 7 days	Complete recovery (3 weeks)	189 (1)			62%	1.03 (0.63–1.28)	2% (ns)	2–3 days better
		Pain intensity	47 (1)	1.10	0.2 (ns)				2–3 days better

LBP: low back pain; SR: systematic review; SMD: standardised mean difference; WMD: weighted mean difference; CI: confidence interval; RCT: randomized controlled trial; ns: not statistically significant. *Different scales.

recovery (SMD 0.29 (95% CI 0.05, 0.45)) at both 3–4 weeks and 12 weeks of follow-up than those advised to stay active but that these differences are small.

2 For patients with sciatica, which in this review was defined by the presence of neurological deficit, there is moderate quality evidence from two trials of no difference in pain (SMD −0.03 (95% CI −0.24, 0.18)) or functional status (SMD 0.19 (95% CI −0.02, 0.41)) between bed rest and staying active. There is moderate quality evidence from two studies of little or no difference in pain intensity or functional status between 2 to 3 days and 7 days of bed rest. There is at least theoretical risk in prescribing bed rest, with evidence of rapid deconditioning of muscles with complete bed rest.

2. NSAIDs for acute back pain episode

1 *For adults with an acute episode of LBP with or without radicular features, does prescription of NSAIDs lead to better outcomes compared to placebo and/or other medications?*

2 *For adults with an acute episode of neck pain with or without radicular features, does prescription of NSAIDs lead to better outcomes compared to placebo and/or other medications?*

1 NSAIDs are commonly prescribed for acute LBP. Studies in general practice suggest that around 50% of patients are given a prescription for analgesics with most of these getting NSAIDs. A systematic review of the use of NSAIDs for LBP is available including 51 trials with 6057 patients. The most recent substantive update was in February 2000 [3]. The systematic review examined the effectiveness of NSAIDs versus placebo, versus paracetamol and versus other analgesics. Outcomes were generally pain (most often using visual analogue scores) and 'global improvement', all short term (generally 1 week). There was evidence from 11 RCTs including 1622 patients, comparing NSAIDs with placebo. Pooled results showed no difference for pain but significantly improved global improvement: relative risk (RR) 1.24 (95% CI 1.10, 1.41) and a significant reduction in other analgesic use: RR 1.29 (95% CI 1.05, 1.57) in the first week (Table 6.2). These trials included patients with acute LBP, with or without sciatica. When compared to paracetamol the results were conflicting. It was not possible to pool the results of the five trials. In trials comparing NSAIDs with other analgesics (not paracetamol), there was reasonable

Table 6.2 NSAIDs compared to various controls for people with back pain and neck pain.

Type of study (reference)	Patient	Intervention	Outcome (follow-up time)	Number of patients (number of trials)	Control group mean change from baseline (range)	SMD (95% CI)	Control group risk (range)	Relative risk (95% CI)	Absolute risk reduction (95% CI)	Comment
SR** [3]	Acute LBP with or without sciatica	NSAIDs versus placebo	Pain intensity (1 week)	452 (3)	20.3* (0.56 to 33.4)	0.53 (ns)				NSAID worst. Non statistical significant
			Global improvement (1 week)	535 (6)			63% (20–78)	1.24 (1.1–1.4)	13% (6–20)	NSAID better
	Mainly acute LBP with or without sciatica (some chronic)	NSAIDs versus paracetamol	Pain intensity short term	255 (5)	Unable to pool the results					Conflicting results
	Chronic mechanical neck pain	NSAIDs versus various (acupuncture, manipulation, sham physical therapy)	Pain intensity short term	198 (4)	Unable to pool the results					No benefit of NSAIDs over other treatments

LBP: low back pain; SR: systematic review; SMD: standardised mean difference; CI: confidence interval; RCT: randomized controlled trial; ns: not statistically significant. *Different scales; **The SR was recently withdrawn from the Cochrane Library.

evidence of no advantage for NSAIDs and in 'head-to-head' trials of different NSAIDs there was no consistent best performer.

2 There has also been a systematic review of trials of NSAID treatment in patients with chronic mechanical neck pain [4], defined by exclusion of a range of disorders including rheumatoid arthritis, presence of myelopathy, ankylosing spondylitis, spasmodic torticollis, fractures and dislocations but including 'whiplash'. NSAIDs were compared to various other treatments including acupuncture, manipulation and sham physical therapy. Four trials, including 198 patients were included with short-term pain as the endpoint. Overall, there was no evidence that NSAIDs were superior to the treatments to which they were compared, some of which were effectively 'placebo' treatments for neck pain.

There is a substantial literature on the risks of treatment with NSAIDs, particularly gastrointestinal side-effects. Any benefit in short-term reduction of symptoms in acute low back and neck pain needs to be balanced against that risk.

3. Epidural steroids for subacute back pain

1 *For adults with an episode of subacute LBP with sciatica, does the use of epidural steroid lead to better outcomes, including pain reduction and a reduced need for surgical intervention?*

2 *For adults with an episode of subacute neck pain with radicular symptoms, does the use of epidural steroid lead to better outcomes, including pain reduction and a reduced need for surgical intervention?*

Although the natural history of acute episodes of back and neck pain, with or without radicular symptoms is favourable, there will still be a considerable number of people that fail to fully recover by 6–12 weeks, so-called 'subacute' back or neck pain. For the clinician, the clinical options may include referral for consideration of surgery or continuation of conservative measures such as more physical therapy. Epidural steroid injections are commonly employed as an intermediate step between conservative management and surgery. To offset the risks and costs involved with this invasive procedure, it is necessary to have confidence that the treatment is superior to conservative management both for symptom relief and, preferably, leading to a reduced need for surgery.

1 There are a number of RCTs of epidural steroid injections in different back pain populations with different steroid preparations, with or without anaesthetic agent, with or without fluoroscopy or CT guidance, with different control groups, outcome measures and follow-up periods. There have been several systematic reviews between 1995 and 2005 generally including the same trials but coming to different conclusions about the overall efficacy of epidural steroids. One of the systematic reviews [5] which attempted to pool all available results concluded that epidural steroids were effective in reducing sciatica (pooled odds ratio 2.61 (95%CI 1.9–3.77)) for short-term pain relief and 1.87 (95%CI 1.3–2.68) for long-term pain relief). Most of the systematic reviews however, including those with the most rigorous searching, inclusion and analysis strategies, have concluded that the case for epidural steroid injections in patients with sciatica is unproven. In a Cochrane Review [6], the pooled RR for short-term benefit with epidural steroids was 0.93 (95%CI 0.79, 1.09) and long-term benefit RR 0.92 (95% CI 0.76, 1.11). Most of the trials employed pain (using a visual analogue scale (VAS)) as an endpoint although some included need for further surgery. A number of small RCTs have been published since these systematic reviews. Two high quality trials in particular compared outcomes for patients where epidural injections with steroid (and/or anaesthetic agent) were compared with injections with either saline or anaesthetic agent alone. In the trial with saline injection controls [7], there was evidence of short-term benefit for the intervention group (symptom control and patient satisfaction) but not longer-term benefit. In the trial with anaesthetic only injection controls [8], there was a reduction in the need for surgery in the intervention group. However, because of the small numbers in these trials, it is likely that a further systematic review including these trials will still reach a conclusion of 'conflicting results' from the available studies. As a guide to the size of any treatment effect from epidural steroids, one systematic review estimated that the number needed to treat for short-term benefit (i.e. less than 60 days) with 75% relief was around 7 and for 50% relief around 3. However, for longer-term improvement (3–12 months) the NNT for 50% pain relief was around 13 with wide confidence intervals (95%CI 6.6–314) [5]. These numbers are dependent on the most positive reading of the pooled results from the various trials and should be considered optimistic.

2 For neck pain with radicular symptoms, a systematic review of various injection therapies is available with the last substantive amendment made in December 2004 [4]. That review found only one trial comparing epidural steroid given with lignocaine and intramuscular steroid given with lignocaine in 50 subjects with chronic neck pain and radiation. There was a benefit for the epidural group for pain (SMD −1.46 (95%CI −2.16, −0.76)) and return to work (RR 0.49

(95%CI 0.29, 0.92)) at 4 weeks. That review also identified two RCTs comparing intramuscular lignocaine with placebo for people with chronic mechanical neck pain (166 subjects) with follow-up between 2 weeks and 3 months and favouring the intervention (SMD −1.36 (95%CI −1.93, −0.80)). Overall, the quality of this evidence is, at best, modest and should be applied clinically with considerable caution until further studies are available. Clearly there are risks associated with these treatments and the small numbers studied make it impossible to quantify the size of benefit (if any) with any certainty.

4. Manipulation for acute back pain episode

1 *For adults with an acute episode of LBP with or without radicular features, does prescription of manipulation lead to better outcomes compared to no manipulation and/or other treatments?*
2 *For adults with an acute episode of neck pain with or without radicular features, does prescription of manipulation lead to better outcomes compared to no manipulation and/or other treatments?*

Manipulation is often prescribed for acute and chronic back and neck pain. Manipulation is practised in different forms by the same and different practitioners including chiropractors, osteopaths, physical therapists and musculoskeletal medicine doctors. The related procedure – mobilization – is also frequently employed, the difference between the two procedures generally being one of extent, where most manipulation techniques aim to move the joint or segment beyond its passive range while mobilization techniques stay within the passive range of movement of a joint or segment. There are many RCTs of manipulation in its various forms undertaken by many different practitioners with varying levels of training. Chiropractic manipulation has been the most extensively studied. There are a number of systematic reviews of the RCTs along with several international guidelines which do not agree on the role of manipulation in the management of acute LBP.

1 The most recent systematic review is of high quality and attempts to quantify the clinical effect of manipulation for LBP [9]. In 29 RCTs with over 3000 patients, comparing manipulation to a range of 'inactive' treatments (such as sham manipulation or detuned electrical stimulators), there was a clear treatment effect from manipulation. This was quantified at around 10 mm (95%CI 2, 17) on a 100 mm VAS for pain where 0 is no pain and 100 mm is the worst pain imaginable. There was also a benefit of manipulation compared to 'inactive' treatments in terms of function: 2.8 points (95%CI −0.1, 5.6) on the Roland Disability Questionnaire (which has a range of 23 points). Endpoints were generally measured within weeks of treatment. However, when manipulation was compared to other 'active' treatments for back pain such as exercise treatments, no difference was found. In subanalyses, there was no change in the findings if only studies with patients with sciatica were included.

2 A systematic review with most recent substantive update in March 2002 is available [10] which considers the impact of manipulation and mobilization on various outcomes for acute, subacute and chronic neck pain, with and without radicular symptoms. Although 33 RCTs were included in the review, only one had more than 70 subjects. The authors concluded that there was evidence of no impact on pain and functional outcomes of either a single manipulation or 6–20 manipulations over a few weeks. They came to a similar conclusion about mobilization. They identified 15 trials of 'multi-modal therapy with an exercise focus' which generally meant manipulation and/or mobilization and an active exercise programme. Compared to waiting list controls, there were improvements for pain (pooled SMD −0.85 (95% CI −1.20 to −0.50)), function (generally measured using the Northwick Park Neck Pain Questionnaire) (pooled SMD −0.57 (95% CI −0.94 to −0.21)) and 'global perceived effect' (SMD −2.73 (95% CI −3.30 to −2.16)). Most of the trials included in this analysis involved subjects with chronic or subacute neck pain. The major reservation about the results is the use of waiting list controls and uncertainty about the 'active element' of the treatment given the evidence that manipulation and mobilization alone appear to be ineffective. It was not possible to make comment on the subgroup of subjects with radicular symptoms. Regarding the safety of cervical manipulation, estimates of between one significant adverse event per 3000 and one per 1,000,000 manipulations have been made with too little information available to narrow this discrepancy.

5. Exercise therapy for chronic back pain

For people with chronic back pain, do exercise-based interventions improve functional outcomes?

Exercise treatments are commonly prescribed for people with acute, subacute and chronic LBP. There is considerable heterogeneity in the many trials of exercise therapy with respect to the study population, the exercise intervention, control groups, follow-up times and outcome measures used. A high quality systematic review with the most substantive update in February 2005 is available [11] which included 61 RCTs (6390 participants). Most of these trials (43/61) were in subjects with chronic back pain.

For people with acute back pain, there was evidence of no benefit for exercise interventions from 11 trials (1192 subjects) for pain outcomes at different time points. For people with subacute back pain there was modest evidence of benefit in reducing work loss from two trials using a graded exercise programme but no evidence of benefit for pain and functional outcomes (usually using either the Oswestry disability index or Roland-Morris disability questionnaires) for subjects in eight trials when the results were combined. For people with chronic back pain there was strong evidence of benefit for exercise treatments compared to no treatment and to other

conservative treatments with regard to pain, especially for patients seeking care from health professionals (as opposed to community populations with back pain recruited specifically for study). The benefit on functional outcomes was small and unlikely to be clinically significant. Because of the wide variety of interventions in these trials it is difficult to draw conclusions about whether particular exercise regimens are better than others or what might constitute appropriate duration and intensity of treatment.

A further systematic review of physical conditioning programmes with a return to work focus [12], concluded that for patients with chronic LBP, physical conditioning programmes resulted in an average 45 days less work loss at 12 months follow-up (95% CI 87.6, 3.3) based on pooled results from two RCTs. However there was no significant difference if the outcome of 'off work' at 12 months was used.

6. Surgery

1 *For people with acute or subacute back pain with radicular features and radiographic evidence of an appropriate disc/other lesion, does a surgical procedure to remove, or modify, the disc/other structure lead to better pain and/or functional outcomes than non-surgical management? If effective, what is the ideal timing for surgery in terms of a preceding period of non-surgical management? What are the long-term risks of surgical treatment for back pain with radicular features?*
2 *For people with chronic back pain, with or without degenerative features on imaging of the lumbar spine, who fail to respond to conservative treatment, is spinal fusion more effective than best non-surgical therapy, particularly on outcomes at the level of activity limitation and participation?*

1 Surgery has been considered an option for people with back pain that does not recover with conservative treatment, particularly when sciatica is present. These four clinical questions relate to LBP. The same general questions apply also to neck pain although with somewhat less emphasis on disc lesions.

In an ideal world there would be systematic reviews based on multiple high-quality RCTs to consider these questions which come up reasonably often in clinical practice. Distressingly, there remains only a single RCT of surgery versus no surgery for sciatica with radiographic evidence of a disc lesion, published over 20 years ago. The reason for this paucity remains uncertain. There is clearly a large amount of clinical uncertainty, manifest by large variations in surgery rates among countries.

Taken at face value, the one RCT [13] provides modest support for surgery as an effective intervention. In that trial 126 subjects with sciatica, a radiologically proven disc lesion and *uncertainty* about the appropriateness of surgical intervention were randomized to surgery or no surgery groups and followed for up to 10 years. At 1 year, there was a statistically significant, but small, benefit for surgery with 'satisfaction' rates of 92% for the surgical group and 79% for the non-surgical group. By 4 years there was no difference between the two groups – satisfaction rates of 82% and 88%, respectively. This study has been criticized, primarily because of a high crossover rate from no surgery to surgery along with insensitive outcome measures. It should be pointed out that, of the original 280 patients that Weber assembled, 67 were assigned to surgery without randomization, because they 'had symptoms and signs that beyond doubt, required surgical therapy'. Some reviewers of the original study have taken this to mean that the results of this trial cannot be generalized to a population of newly presenting patients with sciatica where surgery is being contemplated as a treatment option. Equally it could be argued, as no randomized trial of newly presenting patients with sciatica, contemplating surgery, is available, that this is the best information we have. A new RCT of surgery versus prolonged conservative treatment for sciatica is planned in the Netherlands [14] aiming to recruit 300 patients within 12 weeks of a new episode of sciatica.

A systematic review of surgery for lumbar disc prolapse is available [15]. However, of the 27 RCTs included in that review, 16 tested chemonucleolysis. Ten trials compared different surgical techniques without a 'no surgery' group with the remaining trial being that of Weber, referred to above.

Problems of bias preclude the use of cohort studies to answer the clinical questions posed above.

Surgery for neck pain with radicular features is the subject of a systematic review [16]. The authors found one RCT (81 patients) comparing surgical decompression for cervical radiculopathy with physiotherapy or cervical collar immobilization. Three months after surgery, the surgical group had less pain (mean difference (MD) −14 (out of 100), 95% CI −27.84, −0.16) compared to the physiotherapy group. By 1 year after surgery there were no differences between the two groups (MD −9, 95% CI −23.39, 5.39). Results were similar when surgery was compared to cervical collar immobilization. There was also a significant short-term improvement in sensory loss in the surgery group compared to either control but this difference was no longer present after 1 year.

2 The effectiveness of surgery for back pain without radicular features has been the subject of a systematic review [17] with most recent substantive update in February 2005 but most of the RCTs were of different types of operation. Two recent RCTs with non-operative control groups were included. A further RCT with non-operative control group has been published since then. These three RCTs are considered below, making the point that each trial used different inclusion and exclusion criteria and the control population also varied.

One trial [18] randomized 294 subjects with chronic LBP of more than 2 years duration (median approximately 8 years) to one of three surgical groups for spinal fusion using different techniques or no surgery (physical therapy). Prior to entry to the study all subjects had to have completed a course of conservative therapy which failed to improve them, so

the control group effectively repeated this non-effective treatment. By 2 years follow-up the surgical group as a whole had better outcomes than the non-surgical group including pain, disability and depressive symptoms.

A further RCT [19] enrolled 349 subjects with more than 1 year's duration LBP considered candidates for spinal fusion to either surgery or an intensive rehabilitation programme including cognitive behavioural therapy. There were significant falls in disability scores in both groups by 2 years of follow-up. There was a much smaller difference between the groups which just reached statistical significance, favouring surgery.

A third trial [20] enrolled 64 patients with chronic LBP for more than 1 year and randomly assigned them to spinal fusion or cognitive intervention and exercises. By 1-year follow-up there were significant falls in disability scores in both groups. There was no significant difference between the groups on disability scores.

Taken together, these studies suggest that spinal fusion surgery is as effective as a combined programme of exercises and cognitive intervention for people with long-term (greater than 1 year) LBP but may be more effective than physical therapy alone for patients with chronic LBP >2 years duration. Evidence from the Swedish study [17] suggests that more complicated and higher risk surgical techniques are no better than the most straightforward technique of posterolateral fusion without internal fixation. The complication rate of surgery in these and other trials has been reported as between 6% and 31% depending on the technique used. Reintervention rates are between 6% and 22%.

Summary

We know that back pain and neck pain are common complaints and associated with considerable misery and cost, particularly when the problem becomes chronic. The reductionist model of medical thinking that has prevailed for the last 250 years ('every symptom has a cause, remove the cause and the symptoms disappear'), has largely failed in an attempt to find 'cures' for these problems which are almost ubiquitous in adult life and carry a generally favourable prognosis. The various systematic reviews of individual treatments suggest a small favourable treatment effect for 'active' therapies including advice to stay active, exercise and manipulation although the size of these effects is very small. The evidence for surgery as an effective option for back pain with or without radicular features is less than impressive considering the frequency with which it used, along with the known complications and costs involved. A recent *BMJ* editorial [21] referred to spinal fusion for chronic back pain as 'an experimental treatment'. There is clearly a place for more high-quality RCTs of surgery with non-surgical control groups *and* of non-surgical treatments for people with chronic LBP aiming to identify the best non-surgical treatment against which surgical interventions should be compared. At present, most support can be found for intensive multi-disciplinary bio-psycho-social rehabilitation programmes [22].

In the absence of compelling evidence for many of the commonly used interventions for people with back and neck pain, a reasonable approach for clinicians managing these patients is a combination of adequate assessment, reassurance in the absence of significant disease, encouraging activity and 'doing least harm' in the way of interventional therapy. In the long term, taking the medicine out of musculoskeletal pain complaints and encouraging clinicians and lay people to recognize them as part of our adult experience may lead to less overall misery.

References

1 Boden SD, Davis DO, Dina TS, Patronas NJ, Wiesel SW. Abnormal magnetic-resonance scans of the lumbar spine in asymptomatic subjects. A prospective investigation. *J. Bone Joint Surg. Am.* 1990; **72**: 403–8.

2 Hagen KB, Hilde G, Jamtvedt G, Winnem M. Bed rest for acute low-back pain and sciatica. *Cochrane Database Syst. Rev.* 2005; **3**.

3 van Tulder MW, Scholten RJPM, Koes BW, Deyo RA. Non-steroidal anti-inflammatory drugs for low-back pain. *Cochrane Database Syst. Rev.* 2005; **3**.

4 Peloso P, Gross A, Haines T, Trinh K, Goldsmith CH, Aker P. Medicinal and Injection therapies for mechanical neck disorders. *Cochrane Database Syst. Rev.* 2005; **3**.

5 Watts RW, Silagy CA. A meta-analysis on the efficacy of epidural corticosteroids in the treatment of sciatica. *Anaesth. Intens. Care* 1995; **23**: 564–9.

6 Nelemans PJ, de Bie RA, de Vet HCW, Sturmans F. Injection therapy for subacute and chronic benign low-back pain. *Cochrane Database Syst. Rev.* 2005; **3**.

7 Vad VB, Bhat AL, Lutz GE, Cammisa F. Transforaminal epidural steroid injections in lumbosacral radiculopathy: a prospective randomized study. *Spine* 2002; **27**: 11–16.

8 Riew KD, Yin Y, Gilula L, et al. The effect of nerve-root injections on the need for operative treatment of lumbar radicular pain. prospective, randomized, controlled, double-blind study. *J. Bone Joint Surg. Am.* 2000; **82-A**: 1589–93.

9 Assendelft WJJ, Morton SC, Yu Emily I, Suttorp MJ, Shekelle PG. Spinal manipulative therapy for low-back pain. *Cochrane Database Syst. Rev.* 2005; **3**.

10 Gross AR, Hoving JL, Haines TA, Goldsmith CH, Kay T, Aker P, Bronfort G. Manipulation and mobilisation for mechanical neck disorders. *Cochrane Database Syst. Rev.* 2005; **3**.

11 Hayden JA, Tulder van MW, Malmivaara A, Koes BW. Exercise therapy for treatment of non-specific low back pain. *Cochrane Database Syst. Rev.* 2005; **3**.

12 Schonstein E, Kenny DT, Keating J, Koes BW. Work conditioning, work hardening and functional restoration for workers with back and neck pain. *Cochrane Database Syst. Rev.* 2005; **3**.

13 Weber H. Lumbar disc herniation. A controlled, prospective study with ten years of observation. *Spine* 1983; **8**: 131–40.

14 Peul WC, van Houwelingen HC, van der Hout WB, et al. Prolonged conservative treatment or 'early' surgery in sciatica caused by a lumbar disc herniation: rationale and design of a randomized trial [ISRCT 26872154]. *BMC Musculoskeletal Disorders* 2005; **6**: 8. doi:10.1186/1471-2474-6-8.

15 Gibson JNA, Grant IC, Waddell, G. Surgery for lumbar disc prolapse. *Cochrane Database Syst. Rev.* 2005; **3**.

16 Fouyas, IP. Statham, PFX. Sandercock, PAG. Lynch, C. Surgery for cervical radiculomyelopathy. *Cochrane Database Syst. Rev.* 2005; **3**.

17 Gibson JNA, Waddell G. Surgery for degenerative lumbar spondylosis. *Cochrane Database Syst. Rev.* 2005; **3**.

18 Fritzell P, Hagg O, Wessberg P, Nordwall A. Swedish Lumbar Spine Study Group. 2001 Volvo Award Winner in Clinical Studies: Lumbar fusion versus nonsurgical treatment for chronic low back pain: a multicenter randomized controlled trial from the Swedish Lumbar Spine Study Group. *Spine* 2001; **26**: 2521–32.

19 Fairbank J. Frost H. Wilson-MacDonald J. Yu LM. Barker K. Collins R. *Spine* Stabilisation Trial Group. Randomised controlled trial to compare surgical stabilisation of the lumbar spine with an intensive rehabilitation programme for patients with chronic low back pain: the MRC spine stabilisation trial. *BMJ.* 2005; **330**: 1233–8.

20 Ivar Brox J. Sorensen R. Friis A. Nygaard O. Indahl A. Keller A. Ingebrigtsen T. Eriksen HR. Holm I. Koller AK. Riise R. Reikeras O. Randomized clinical trial of lumbar instrumented fusion and cognitive intervention and exercises in patients with chronic low back pain and disc degeneration. *Spine* 2003; **28**: 1913–21.

21 Koes BW. Surgery versus intensive rehabilitation programmes for chronic low back pain. *BMJ.* 2005; **330**: 1220–21.

22 Guzman J, Esmail R, Karjalainen K, et al. Multi-disciplinary bio-psycho-social rehabilitation for chronic low-back pain. *Cochrane Database Syst. Rev.* 2005; **3**.

7

CHAPTER 7

Neuropathic pain

Giorgio Cruccu, Nadine Attal, Rod Taylor

Introduction

Neuropathic pain has been defined as pain initiated, or caused by, a primary lesion or dysfunction of the nervous system [1]. Neuropathic pain can take a variety of forms and is a major disability in common neurological diseases, such as neuropathy, myelopathy, multiple sclerosis (MS), or stroke. It is estimated that 1.5% of the general population is affected by neuropathic pain. However, this figure is a crude estimate and there are few published data on the incidence and prevalence of the various forms and aetiologies of neuropathic pain [2,3].

The burden of neuropathic pain on patients and healthcare systems appears to be potentially large. A number of studies demonstrated that patients with neuropathic pain experience a poor health-related quality of life [4,5]. Furthermore, a recent analysis of US insurance claims data has shown annual healthcare charges three-fold higher for neuropathic patients than age and sex matched patients without a recent claim for neuropathic pain [6].

Despite the considerable increase in the number of randomized placebo-controlled trials in neuropathic pain over the last few years, the medical treatment of neuropathic pain is still far from satisfactory, with less than half of the patients achieving significant benefit with any pharmacological drug [3,7,8]. Randomized controlled trials (RCT) have generally been performed in patients categorized according to their aetiologies. Most RCTs have been conducted in postherpetic neuralgia (PHN) and painful polyneuropathy (PPN), whereas there are very few trials in other peripheral neuropathic pains – including trigeminal neuralgia – and central pain (CP), and no RCTs in painful radiculopathies [7,8].

Framing clinical questions

To avoid unclear and non-definite neuropathic pain conditions, and also taking in account commonality of neuropathic conditions and number of available RCTs, we decided to focus on painful polyneuropathies and PHN. In addition we included CPs, as they are well known to neurologists but differ in pain characteristics, mechanisms, and therapy.

These three conditions are representative of diseases affecting different portions of the nociceptive pathways: in distal–proximal order, painful polyneuropathies are distal axonopathies, PHN is a ganglionopathy, spinal cord injury (SCI) may damage the dorsal horn or spinothalamic tract, and post-stroke pain mostly affects the thalamo-cortical neurons.

PPN is a common neuropathic pain condition. Diabetic polyneuropathy is the most classical example with a reported prevalence of 54–1100 cases per 100 000 [9,10]. Patients usually present with spontaneous and stimulus-evoked pains with a distal and symmetrical distribution [11]. Although one or more of the pain symptoms characteristics of neuropathic conditions are seen in the majority of the patients, the most frequent single pain symptom is deep aching pain [11]. Diabetic and non-diabetic PPN are similar in symptomatology and with respect to treatment response [12].

PHN is a painful aftermath of shingles with a reported prevalence of 6.8–38.3 cases per 100 000 [13]. Patients with PHN often describe a constant generally burning pain and a paroxysmal pain with lancinating or shooting quality, and brush-induced allodynia is found in most cases. In an individual patient, any of these three components can be the most distressing feature of the pain [14]. The incidence of PHN (defined as pain persisting for more than 1 month after the herpes zoster skin rash) has been estimated to range 9–14% [15].

CP or central neuropathic pain is pain due to a lesion in the central nervous system (CNS). We were unable to locate an estimate of the incidence or prevalence of CP. CP can be a consequence of stroke (central post-stroke pain, CPSP), SCI, MS, but also other aetiologies [16]. Pain may be burning, shooting, aching, or pricking and is often accompanied by dysesthesia, hyperalgesia or allodynia, particularly to brush or cold [17,16].

Search methods, ranking criteria, and statistical analysis

Our search, adhering to the methods described in the book introduction, was based on the Cochrane Collaboration guidelines for search strategies and conducted up to January 2006. We sought Cochrane Systematic Reviews [18,19,20–22], other systematic reviews [3,7,8,23,24,25,26,27], and RCTs (randomized double-blind studies using chronic dosing and placebo and studying at least 10 patients). The grading of evidence followed the European Federation of Neurological Studies (EFNS) system [28]. As recommended by the EFNS guidelines on neuropathic pain assessment [29], we checked and duly commented upon the RCTs that assessed sleep, mood, and quality of life. But unless otherwise specified, we took as primary measure of benefit the number of responders (i.e. patients with at least 50% pain relief), and as primary measure of harm the number of patients that discontinued because of adverse events. Differences between active and control groups were evaluated with the Fisher's exact test, with calculation of 95% confidence intervals (CI).

In order to reflect the relative importance of both the quality of evidence and the relative efficacy/safety of treatments we developed two summary metrics for group of trials for each drug by indication:

'Reliability' that is a metric based on sample size and quality of the RCTs), where reliability = sample size (1–5 scale of patients with active treatment)* × quality score (as assessed by 1–5 Jadad scale)#. *Sample scale: in these analysis we extracted numerical data from 81 trials for a total of 4956 patients treated with active treatment; the sample size ranged from 11–878, with a non-normal distribution, median = 33, 25% percentile = 19, and 75% percentile = 72; hence we used a scale assigning 1 to trials with <19, 2 to those with 19–32, 3 to those with 33, 4 to those with 34–72, and 5 to those with >72 patients with active. #Quality scale: the Jadad scale is a commonly used method of scoring the quality of trials on the basis of the type of randomization, placebo, and blinding, but does not take into account the sample size [30]; total Reliability over several trials was calculated by summing the reliability calculated for each trial.

'Net Gain' that is a metric based on the relative benefit) and harm in a trial where Net Gain = (% patients with beneficial outcome with active minus % patients with beneficial outcome with control) minus (% patients with harmful outcome with active minus % patients with harmful outcome with control). For the purposes of this chapter, benefit was defined as the proportion of patients achieving a 50% or more pain relief while harm was defined as the proportion of patients dropping out due to adverse events. To prevent double taxing the drug-induced gain, the proportion of patients benefiting from therapy was calculated based on the population excluding those who dropped out due to adverse events. Net Gain for each drug class (or individual drug) was calculated by first pooling total data from all trials and then applying the formula. Net Gain is only reported in those circumstances where there was a statistically significant difference (P < 0.05) in the benefit outcome.

For each of the three pain conditions, a table reports the results for each drug or drug class, including absolute values of Reliability and Net Gain (Tables 7.1–7.3); Reliability and Net Gain values are then normalized to maximum and minimum values found in the given pain condition and plotted on diagrams of Reliability/Gain, where best drugs are located in the upper-right quadrant (Figures 7.1–7.3).

Critical review of the evidence for each question

1. Painful neuropathy

In patients with painful neuropathy, how do drug treatments affect the probability of reducing pain? What is the probability of adverse effects?

PPN is the neuropathic pain condition that has been most intensively studied in controlled trials (a total of 3567 patients in our analysis) (Table 7.1).

Tricyclic antidepressants

Eleven small cross-over, class-I or II RCTs, dating from 1984 to 2003, have established the efficacy of Tricyclic antidepressants (TCA) (amitriptyline, clomipramine, desipramine, imipramine, nortriptyline, and the tetracyclic maprotiline) in PPN [19,27]. TCA in PPN was significantly better than placebo (P < 0.0001), with a combined Reliability over 11 trials of 77 and Net Gain of 38%. The TCA most effective is nortriptyline 30 mg, scoring 84% gain; amitriptyline (probably the most used in clinical practice) provides on average a 41% Net Gain. There were only two head-to-head trials (both Class I). In one, clomipramine and desipramine were not significantly different [31]. In the other amitriptyline was slightly but significantly more effective than maprotiline [39]. The most common side effects of TCA are dry mouth, constipation, sweating, dizziness, disturbed vision, drowsiness, palpitation, orthostatic hypotension, sedation, and urinary hesitation. More selective TCAs such as nortriptyline are better tolerated than the non-selective TCA, with less anticholinergic effects and sedation [40]. A suspected association between TCA treatment and sudden cardiac death has raised concern. A recent epidemiological study found a slight increase in sudden cardiac death with TCA doses greater than 100 mg/day [41]. Therefore caution is recommended for older patients, particularly those with cardiovascular risk factors [3,27].

Serotonin–noradrenaline reuptake inhibitors

Venlafaxine 150–225 mg/day and duloxetine 60–120 mg/day [7,8,42] are significantly effective in PPN (P < 0.0001), with a combined Reliability of 128. The Net Gain, however, is comparatively low: 16%. Duloxetine has been shown to improve quality of life and sleep in a large, class-I RCT [43]. In a head-to-head comparison, venlafaxine was as efficacious as the TCA imipramine [44].

Serotonin–noradrenaline reuptake inhibitors (SNRI) are a better option than tricyclics in patients with cardiac disease [7]. The relative risk for withdrawal is not significantly different from placebo and there is no need for drug-level

Table 7.1 Treatments for painful polyneuropathies.

Drugs	Sample size (trials)	Benefit with active (range)	Benefit with control (range)	Relative Risk (95% CI)	Harm with active (range)	Harm with control (range)	Relative Risk (95% CI)	Reliability and Net Gain	
TCA	564 (11)	56.6% (37–89)	11.6% (0–24)	4.9 (3.4–7) P < 0.0001	8.9% (0–24)	2.1% (0–6)	4.3 (1.7–11) P = 0.0008	**77**	**38**
SNRI	1013 (4)	51.8% (27–63)	28.5% (7–35)	1.8 (1.4–2.1) P < 0.0001	11.2% (9–20)	4.0% (4–5.3)	2.8 (1.6–4.9) P < 0.0001	**128**	**16**
SSRI	162 (3)	43.2% (20–50)	28.4% (15–41)	1.5 (1–2.3) ns	5.4% (0–6)	2.2% (0–4)	2.5 (0.5–13) ns	**24**	–
PGB/GBP	797 (5)	50.3% (43–61)	20.7% (14–31)	2.4 (1.9–3) P < 0.0001	8.5% (6.5–11)	4.4% (2.9–6.7)	1.9 (1.1–3.4) P = 0.022	**101**	**26**
NaCB	282 (3)	60.1% (48–74)	20.8% (18–26)	2.9 (2.1–4.1) P < 0.0001	15.3% (0–28)	4.1% (0–8)	3.7 (1.5–8.9) P = 0.019	**32**	**22**
LTG	59 (1)	44.4%	17.9%	2.5 (1–6.1) P = 0.044	6.9%	6.7%	1.0 (0.2–6.9) ns	**10**	**26**
Topiramate	1092 (2)	45.7%	23.0%	1.99 (1.3–3) P < 0.0002	24.3%	8.3%	2.9 (1.5–5.7) P < 0.0005	**50**	**6**
Valproate	130 (2)	56.1% (26–83)	13.8% (10–18)	4.1 (2.1–8) P < 0.0001	4.6% (3–6)	1.5% (0–3)	3.0 (0.3–28) ns	**23**	**39**
Opioids	300 (3)	69.4% (41–80)	27.4% (10–37)	2.5 (1.8–3.5) P < 0.0001	15.2% (14–16)	4.7% (1.5–9)	3.2 (1.4–7.3) P = 0.0033	**80**	**32**
Mexiletine	158 (2)	72.7% (12–87)	59.6% (33–70)	1.2 (0.9–1.6) ns	9.1% (8–13)	8.5% (3–20)	1.1 (0.4–3.2) ns	**25**	–
NMDA	106 (3)	58% (47–68)	27.5% (0–37)	2.1 (1.3–3.5) P = 0.0025	1.8% (0–4.3)	0% (0–0)	1 ns	**13**	**29**
Capsaicin	439 (5)	59.5% (47–89)	45.9% (18–65)	1.3 (1.1–1.5) P = 0.0045	11.9% (7–13)	2.8% (0–4)	4.2 (1.6–11) P = 0.0017	**42**	**5**

Outcome measure of benefit: number of patients with at least 50% pain relief. Outcome measure of harm: number of drops out due to adverse events. In all instances control is placebo.

Reliability: a metric based on quality of evidence and sample size (see Methods).

Net Gain: a metric based on the relative benefit and harm in a trial where Net Gain = (% patients with benefit with active minus % patients with benefit with placebo) minus (% patients with harm with active minus % patients with harm with placebo); it only applies to treatments significantly different from placebo. *P*-value from Fisher's exact test.

TCA: tricyclic antidepressants (amitriptyline 75–90 mg, clomipramine 75 mg, desipramine 200 mg, imipramine 100–200 mg, nortriptyline 30 mg, and the tetracyclic maprotiline 75 mg). SNRI: serotonin–noradrenalin reuptake inhibitors (duloxetine 60–120 mg, venlafaxine 150–225 mg). SSRI: selective serotonin reuptake inhibitors (citalopram 40 mg, fluoxetine 40 mg, paroxetine 40 mg). PGB/GBP: presynaptic calcium-channel modulators (gabapentin (GBP) up to 3600 mg; pregabalin (PGB) 150–600 mg). NaCB: sodium-channel blocking antiepileptic drugs (carbamazepine (CBZ) 200–600 mg, oxcarbazepine (OXC) 600–1800 mg, phenytoin 300 mg).

LTG: lamotrigine, various-action antiepileptic drug (50–400 mg). Another study in 100 patients with mixed neuropathic pains found no difference between LTG 200 mg and placebo [31].

Topiramate: various-action antiepileptic drug (100–400 mg). Two high-quality, very ample sample size; one, resulting in topiramate = placebo, had no calculation of responders [32].

Valproate: various-action antiepileptic drug (1000–1500 mg). Opioids: predominantly acting on mu-opioid receptor (oxycodone 20–80 mg, tramadol 200–400 mg). Mexiletine: antiarrhythmic drug (225–675 mg).

NMDA: N-methyl-D-aspartate antagonists of the NMDA receptor (dextromethorphan 400 mg, memantine 55 mg). In two studies the outcome measure was not 50% pain relief and in one the control group had lorazepam instead of placebo [7,8,33]. Capsaicin, topical: 0.075% cream q.i.d.

monitoring. The most frequently observed adverse events with duloxetine are nausea, somnolence, dry mouth, increased sweating, loss of appetite, and weakness [43]. Although immediate release venlafaxine is associated with adverse CNS and somatic symptoms such as agitation, diarrhoea, increased liver enzymes, hypertension, and hyponatremia [45], the extended release formulation appears to be far more tolerable, the main side effects being gastrointestinal disturbances [44,46].

The optimal dosage of duloxetine is 60 mg/day: 120 mg/day is no better than 60 mg/day and 20 mg/day is ineffective (class I: 32,59). Only high doses of venlafaxine (150–225 mg/day) are effective [7].

Selective serotonin reuptake inhibitors

Paroxetine, fluoxetine, and citalopram have been evaluated in one small-sample class-II RCT each [7,8]. The combined Reliability is low: 24, the efficacy is not significantly different from placebo. It is worth mentioning, however, that paroxetine 40 mg/day was significantly better than placebo, with a Net Gain of 35%, in one 20-patient, cross-over RCT [47].

Presynaptic calcium-channel modulators (PGB/GBP)

Both pregabalin (PGB) 300–600 mg/day and gabapentin (GBP) 1800–3600 mg/day have good evidence for efficacy in PPN, with several high-quality RCTs [48,49,50,51]. These drugs relieve the pain of diabetic PPN consistently across trials, with a combined Reliability of 101 and Net Gain of 26%. Some of the initial PGB trials were flawed by exclusion of GBP non-responders, but two more recent class-I RCTs that did not profit from this kind of enriched enrolment still reported a similar efficacy [52,53]. The two drugs have never been compared head-to-head; an indirect comparison between placebo-controlled trials shows similar Net Gains for GBP and PGB. One head-to-head class-II study compared GBP (1800 mg/day) to amitriptyline (75 mg/day): because of an insufficient sample size, the relative efficacy and tolerability of these drugs could not be definitively assessed [54]. Significant improvement of health-related quality of life and sleep has been documented for GBP in one class-I RCT [48] and for PGB in three class-I RCTs [49,50,52]. The most common side effects of GBP and PGB include dizziness, somnolence, peripheral oedema, and dry mouth, with a similar frequency for both drugs. While GBP is widely accepted as highly tolerable even at high dosages (>2400 mg) [20,21], the reports on PGB change remarkably with the daily dose: with 150–300 mg there is almost no difference with placebo [49,53], while the withdrawal rate reaches 20% with 600 mg [52,55].

Sodium-channel blockers

Three small cross-over double-blind trials, published some 30 years ago, reported significant effects of phenytoin and carbamazepine (CBZ) in diabetic PPN, but their methods and reporting do not live up to current standards [7,8]. Oxcarbazepine (OXC) data were equivocal in PPN, with some unpublished or open-label trial evidence [56]. However, in a recent double-blind parallel-group placebo trial of 16-week duration, OXC (300–1800 mg/day) was moderately efficacious in diabetic PPN [57]. For the NaCB class, the mean Net Gain is good (22%), but the overall Reliability is very low: 32. One small class-II study reported similar efficacy of CBZ and nortriptyline–fluphenazine, but the small sample size ($n = 16$) might prevent disclosing a difference [58]. In general, NaCB drugs in PPN do not seem as efficacious as they are in trigeminal neuralgia. CBZ entails frequent adverse events, which include sedation, dizziness, gait abnormalities. Liver enzymes, blood cells, and platelets must be monitored for at least one year, because of possible toxic effects. Induction of microsomal enzyme systems may influence the metabolism of several drugs. In contrast to CBZ, OXC does not entail enzyme induction and there is little risk for crossed cutaneous allergy. In the first months of treatment, sodium levels must be monitored because OXC induces hyponatraemia, about 6% in the elderly [59]. As regards other side effects, although a better tolerance has been claimed with OXC

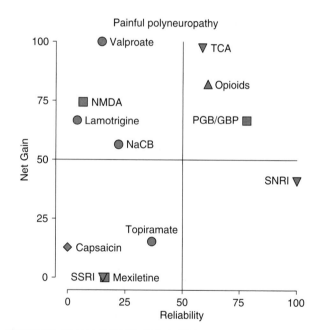

Figure 7.1 Diagram Reliability/Gain in PPN.

X-axis: Reliability of the evidence, based on quality and sample size of the available trials (see text). *Y*-axis: Net Gain of active over control both in terms of efficacy and tolerability (see text). Both measures are normalized to maximum and minimum value found in PPN. Drugs in the upper-right quadrant are most reliably efficacious and tolerable, those in the left half are provided with lower-level evidence, those in the lower half are less efficacious or less tolerable. For instance, valproate would be most effective but has poor evidence to support its effectiveness, Serotonin–noradrenaline reuptake inhibitors (SNRI) have top-level evidence but are, comparatively, moderately effective.

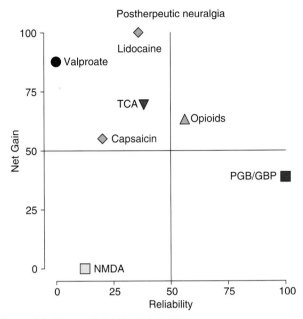

Figure 7.2 Diagram Reliability/Gain in PHN.
X-axis: Reliability of the evidence, based on quality and sample size of the available trials (see text). *Y*-axis: Net Gain of active over control both in terms of efficacy and tolerability (see text). Both measures are normalized to maximum and minimum value found in PHN. Drugs in the upper-right quadrant are most reliably efficacious and tolerable, those in the left half are provided with lower-level evidence, those in the lower half are less efficacious or less tolerable.

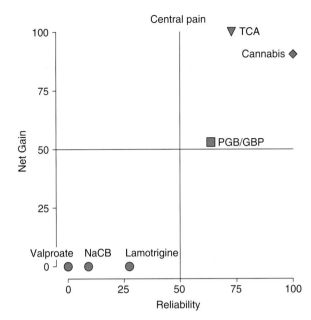

Figure 7.3 Diagram Reliability/Gain in CP.
X-axis: Reliability of the evidence, based on quality and sample size of the available trials (see text). *Y*-axis: Net Gain of active over control both in terms of efficacy and tolerability (see text). Both measures are normalized to maximum and minimum value found in CP. Drugs in the upper-right quadrant are most reliably efficacious and tolerable, those in the left half are provided with lower-level evidence, those in the lower half are less efficacious or less tolerable.

compared with CBZ [7,25], this notion lacks consistent evidence from class-I trials. In a recent trial in diabetic PPN, 27.5% of the OXC group discontinued treatment due to central or gastrointestinal side effects versus 8% with the placebo [57]. Both drugs should be initiated with low dosages and slowly increased up to efficacy or intolerable side effects. Effective dosages range from 200–1200 mg/day for CBZ and 600–1800 mg/day for OXC.

Lamotrigine

Lamotrigine (LTG) up to 400 mg/day, was studied in one high-quality, small sample-size RCT [60], but the difference in pain compared with placebo was only weakly significant ($P = 0.047$). Furthermore, LTG 200 mg/day was found to be equivalent to placebo (Net Gain 0%) in a class-I study in 100 patients with various peripheral neuropathic pains [31]. Side effects of LTG include dizziness, nausea, headache, and fatigue [7,8]. It may induce potentially severe allergic skin reactions. In a meta-analysis collecting data from 572 patients, 9% of patients were withdrawn because of major adverse events, most commonly rash (class I: 9). To minimize the occurrence of cutaneous rashes, a very slow dose titration is recommended: treatment should be initiated with 25 mg daily and increased by 25 mg every other week. The analgesic dosages of LTG range from 200–400 mg/ day.

Valproate

Data about valproate are controversial, because it gave good pain relief results in two class-II studies from the same group [61,62], whereas the drug was no better than placebo in a third, class-I study [63]. Hence its potential in PPN needs further evidence.

Topiramate

Topiramate 100–400 mg/day has been assessed in two class-I RCTs in over 1000 patients with diabetic PPN [32,64]. In one it was very weakly efficacious (Net Gain 6%) and in the other it did not prove better than placebo.

Opioids

Only two RCTs assessed a pure opioid (oxycodone) in PPN. Both were high-quality and demonstrated that controlled release (CR) oxycodone 20–80 mg/day is efficacious and tolerable [65,66], with a Net Gain of 44%. In these trials, however, patients previously receiving opioids were allowed to participate, which may enhance the proportion of opioid responders and reduce the incidence of side effects. Also tramadol 200–400 mg/day, a drug with both opioid and monoaminergic effects that is usually classified among the minor opioids, was significantly better than placebo in PPN in two class-I RCTs [67,68]. The Net Gain yielded by tramadol

(27%), however, is far lower than that of oxycodone. The combined Reliability is 80, the Net Gain 32%. The two largest, high-class, trials that demonstrated efficacy of CR oxycodone and tramadol [65,67] also found these drugs ineffective on quality of life and comorbidities. The most common side effects of opioids are constipation, sedation, and nausea. The risk of cognitive impairment has been reported to be negligible and the side effect profile good, particularly for oxycodone [65,66,69,70,71]. However, less than 20% of patients continue with opioids after 1 year, because of an unfavourable balance between side effects and efficacy [72]. Because of tolerability and tolerance problems in the long term, recent European recommendations indicate that opioids should be considered for chronic non-cancer pain as second line, if other reasonable therapies fail to provide adequate analgesia [7,73]. Tramadol has been reported to induce dizziness, dry mouth, nausea, constipation, and somnolence with significantly more dropouts compared to placebo [68,70,74]. There is an increased risk of seizures in patients with a history of epilepsy or receiving drugs which may reduce the seizure threshold. Serotonergic syndrome may occur if tramadol is used as an add-on treatment to other serotonergic medications (particularly selective serotonin reuptake inhibitors (SSRIs)).

Mexiletine

It is an antiarrhythmic drug, did not yield significant pain relief in four class I–II trials in PPN [7,8].

NMDA-antagonists

Memantine has not shown convincing efficacy in PPN, while pain relief was found for the weak N-methyl-D-aspartate (NMDA)-antagonist dextromethorphan in two small trials [8,33]. The combined Net Gain for this drug class is high (29%) but Reliability is low: 13.

Topical capsaicin

Across five class I–II studies [7,8] there is inconsistent evidence that capsaicin provides a clinically noticeable pain relief in PPN (the Net Gain is 5% only). Furthermore the intense burning sensation caused by this agent decreases compliance and may cause unblinding.

Combination therapy

The usefulness of combination therapy has been assessed in only two RCTs. The largest one, which also included patients with PHN, was a class-I study demonstrating synergistic effects of GBP–morphine combination, with better analgesia at lower doses of each drug than either as a single agent [75]. The other study, class II, showed the superiority of GBP–venlafaxine combination on pain, mood, and quality of life when compared with GBP plus placebo, but the sample was 11 patients only [51].

Practical recommendations

As summarized in Figure 7.1, three drug classes lie in the upper-right quadrant of higher Reliability of evidence and higher Net Gain over placebo, and should therefore be considered first line in PPN: Opioids, PGB/GBP, and TCA. The choice among these drugs is subject to several considerations that are non-quantitative but must be taken into account in clinical practice. For example, an elderly patient with cardiovascular risks factors should not take TCA. A patient with a severe limitation in quality of life should try first PGB (best evidence for quality of life and comorbidities) rather than opioids (evidence for ineffectiveness on quality of life). A patient with an overt depression will probably receive an additional therapeutic gain with antidepressants. In a patient with a particularly severe pain that cannot wait for slow titration times it is better to try PGB rather than GBP. In case of failure, because the mechanisms of action of these three drug classes are completely different, it is reasonable to try – unless contraindicated – all three.

Dosages of opioids should be titrated individually up to efficacy and according to side effects; effective doses for oxycodone range 20–80 mg/day. Tramadol should be initiated at low dosages, particularly in the elderly patient (25 mg once daily) and then titrated as tolerated; the effective dosages range 200–400 mg/day. Effective dosages range 1200–3600 mg/day for GBP and 150–600 mg/day for PGB. GBP needs slow individual titration with initial dosages of 300 mg/day (or less in elderly patients) while PGB can be titrated more rapidly and has a short onset of action (less than 1 week); whereas GBP should be administered t.i.d., PGB can be administered b.i.d. TCA should be initiated at low dosages (amitriptyline 10–25 mg in a single dose taken at bedtime) and then slowly titrated, as tolerated. Effective dosages are highly variable from one subject to another, the average dosage for amitriptyline being 75 mg/day, that for nortriptyline 30 mg/day. Whether TCA blood concentrations should be measured is still controversial [7,27].

2. Postherpetic neuralgia

In patients with PHN, how do drug treatments affect the probability of reducing pain? What is the probability of adverse effects?

TCA antidepressants

Amitriptyline (average dosages 65–100 mg/day), nortriptyline (average 89 mg), and desipramine (average 65–73 mg) are effective in PHN ($P < 0.0001$) on the basis of three class I–II RCTs with a combined Reliability of 40 and Net Gain of 34% (Table 7.2). In two small head-to-head, class-II trials, the tetracyclic maprotiline has been found slightly less effective than amitriptyline [76] and nortriptyline as effective as amitriptyline, but better tolerated [40]. There are no RCTs reporting the efficacy of SSRI or SNRI antidepressant in PHN. For contraindications, side effects, and suggested titration of TCA, see previous section on PPN.

Table 7.2 Treatments for postherpetic neuralgia.

Drugs	Sample size (trials)	Benefit with active (range)	Benefit with control (range)	Relative Risk (95% CI)	Harm with active (range)	Harm with control (range)	Relative Risk (95% CI)	Reliability and Net Gain	
TCA	133 (4)	51.3% (37–70)	10.2% (4–23)	5.0 (2.9–8.9) $P < 0.0001$	12.8% (1.2–24)	5.3% (0–17)	2.4 (1.0–5.6) $P = 0.037$	40	38
PGB/GBP	974 (4)	43.3% (31–72)	15.0% (11–21)	2.9 (2.2–3.8) $P < 0.0001$	17.9% (13–31)	8.4% (5–12)	2.1 (1.5–3.1) $P < 0.0001$	95	19
Valproate	45 (1)	56.5%	9.1%	6.5 (1.7–26) $P = 0.0011$	4.4%	0.0%	1.0 NS	6	43
Opioids	230 (3)	66.7% (45–77)	28.8% (7–56)	2.3 (1.8–3.1) $P < 0.0001$	10.0% (7.9–12)	3.3% (0–10.2)	3.1 (1.1–8.9) $P = 0.04$	56	31
NMDA	71 (4)	27.5% (12–38)	15.5% (12–23)	1.8 (0.8–3.7) NS	11.8% (0–25)	1.6% (0–8.4)	7.2 (0.9–56) $P = 0.35$	17	–
Capsaicin	175 (2)	70.8% (44–79)	26.5% (6–31)	2.7 (1.8–3.9) $P < 0.0001$	20.0% (0–24)	2.4% (0–3)	8.5 (2.0–35) $P = 0.0002$	24	27
Lidocaine	128 (4)	60.4% (33–78)	9.3% (9.1–9.4)	6.5 (2.8–15) $P < 0.0001$	1.8% (0–2)	0.0% (0–0)	1.0 NS	38	49

Outcome measure of benefit: number of patients with at least 50% pain relief. Outcome measure of harm: number of drops out due to adverse events. In all instances control is placebo.

Reliability: a metric based on quality of evidence and sample size (see Methods).

Net Gain: a metric based on the relative benefit and harm in a trial where Net Gain = (% patients with benefit with active minus % patients with benefit with placebo) minus (% patients with harm with active minus % patients with harm with placebo); it only applies to treatments significantly different from placebo. P-value from Fisher's exact test.

TCA: tricyclic antidepressants (amitriptyline 65–73 mg, desipramine 63–167 mg, nortriptyline 89 mg). PGB/GBP: presynaptic calcium-channel modulators (GBP 1200–3600 mg, PGB 150–600 mg). Valproate: various-action antiepileptic drug (1000 mg). Opioids: predominantly acting on mu-opioid receptor (oxycodone 20–60 mg, methadone 91 mg, tramadol 300–400 mg). NMDA: N-methyl-D-aspartate antagonists of the NMDA receptor (dextromethorphan 400–439 mg, memantine 20–35 mg). Capsaicin, topical: 0.075% cream q.i.d. Lidocaine, topical: 5% gel or patch. Several medium-quality trials, but only two with calculation of responders. The outcome measure is relief from allodynia, rather than overall pain intensity. A further trial [34] was negative on overall pain intensity.

Presynaptic calcium-channel modulators (PGB/GBP)

PGB 150–600 mg/day (class I: 21, 69) and GBP 1800–3600 mg/day (class I: 61,66) have consistently shown significant efficacy in PHN, with a combined Reliability of 95, though with the modest Net Gain of 19%. Both PGB and GBP improved mood, sleep, or other items of quality of life [55,77,78,79]. For side effects and suggested titration of GBP and PGB see previous section on PPN.

Opioids

Oxycodone, morphine, and methadone have shown efficacy in PHN in two class-I, cross-over RCTs [69,71]. One non-placebo-controlled study reported better efficacy of high versus low dosages of levorphanol in PHN patients (extracted from a larger group of patients with multiple-aetiology neuropathic pains) [70]. Tramadol 300–400 mg/day was shown

moderately effective on some measures of spontaneous pain intensity in PHN; in this class-I study, only patients with pain lasting for less than 1 year were included, thus several patients tended to recover spontaneously during the trial, which may account for the high rate of placebo response [74]. The combined Reliability for strong and mild opioids is 56, the Net Gain 31%. But there is an important within-class difference, oxycodone (20–60 mg) scoring 42.7% versus 21.4% of tramadol (300–400 mg).

In one trial comparing slow-release morphine (91 mg/day, range 15–225) and methadone (15 mg/day) with TCA and placebo, pain relief was significantly greater with morphine than with nortriptyline, whereas the analgesic efficacy of methadone was comparable to that of TCA [69]. There were significantly more withdrawals during the opioid treatment than during the TCA treatment, but cognitive deterioration was seen only with TCA.

Valproate

Valproate has been assessed in PHN by one class-II trial only, with a small sample size [80]: valproate 1000 mg/day gave very good results (Net Gain 43%), but the Reliability of evidence is very low: 6.

NMDA-antagonists

Dextromethorphan and memantine have been studied in two trials each (class I–II), all with very small sample size [8,33,81]. Neither in the individual trials nor in the pooled results was there is significant gain with the drugs over placebo.

Topical lidocaine

Repeated application of lidocaine patches (5%) has shown efficacy in PHN patients with allodynia in some class-II studies, all with short duration (up to 3 weeks) [34,82,83]. One cross-over study did not report baseline levels of pain and used an enriched enrolment (i.e. only patients with open-label clinical improvement with topical lidocaine were recruited) [82]. The combined Reliability is 38, the efficacy depends on whether ongoing pain or allodynia are considered. Whereas the efficacy on ongoing pain is still controversial [7], the effect on allodynia is excellent, with a Net Gain of 49%. The use of lidocaine patches is very safe with a very low systemic absorption and only local adverse effects (mild skin reactions) have been reported [34,82]. Up to four patches per day for a maximum of 12 h may be used to cover the painful area; titration is not necessary [7].

Capsaicin

Topical capsaicin 0.075% has been found effective, though to a small degree, in two class-I RCTs [2,84] with a combined Reliability of 24 and Net Gain of 27%. As already mentioned, there are no major adverse events with topical capsaicin, but the intense burning sensation caused by this agent decreases compliance and may cause unblinding.

Practical recommendations

The reliability/gain diagram for PHN shows one drug class alone in the upper-right quadrant: Opioids (Figure 7.2). Were we to rely on one 38-patient trial only, we might select among the opioid oxycodone, which has a very high Net Gain. However, oxycodone is a major opioid, thus raising the concern of tolerance in the long-term treatment necessary for this chronic benign condition [7,73]. Similarly, valproate has scored an excellent Net Gain, although in one 45-patient trial only. We would need at least one further RCT with oxycodone and one with valproate. Unlike PPN, in PHN TCA are located in the upper-left quadrant because of a weaker reliability of evidence, while PGB/GBP are in the lower-right quadrant because of weaker efficacy. Topical lidocaine has the highest Net Gain, considering its efficacy on allodynic pain rather than overall pain. For the moment, we would suggest to use lidocaine patches (up to four patches a day) in those patients having a small area of allodynia, and to try, for ongoing pain, oxycodone, TCA, or GBP/PGB, according to the same considerations that we made in the previous section on PPN.

3. Central pain

In patients with CP, how do drug treatments affect the probability of reducing pain? What is the probability of adverse effects?

In general, very few trials have been carried out in patients with CPs, including pain due to SCI, post-stroke pain, and pain associated to MS. We are aware of 12 trials, 8 of these reporting the number of responders and thus included in Table 7.3.

Tricyclic antidepressants

Amitriptyline has been assessed both in post-stroke and SCI pain. In 15 patients with post-stroke pain, amitriptyline 75 mg daily was superior to placebo (class I: 44). In a large class-I study of patients with SCI pain, amitriptyline (average dose 55 mg/day) was found to be ineffective, but the lack of effect might be due to inadequate assessment of neuropathic pain [85]. The overall Reliability was 20, the mean Net Gain 21%.

Presynaptic calcium-channel modulators (PGB/GBP)

In a class-II cross-over trial of 20 patients with SCI pain, GBP up to 3600 mg was significantly effective [36]. PGB (average dose 460 mg/day) was significantly efficacious in a large class-I parallel-group RCT in SCI [35]. Although the PGB/GBP efficacy in SCI pain has been established by these two high-quality studies, only the latter study with PGB reports the number of patients with >50% pain relief: the Reliability is 18; the Net Gain over placebo is low: 11%.

Sodium-channel blockers

We are aware of only one trial (class I) on CBZ 800 mg/day in post-stroke pain [86]; the difference with placebo was not significant. In the same study, CBZ was found to be less efficacious compared with amitriptyline.

Lamotrigine

LTG 200 mg/day was significantly better than placebo in a class-I study of 30 patients with post-stroke pain [37]. Unfortunately this study did not report number of responders. In patients with SCI pain, in contrast, LTG up to 400 mg/day was exactly equal to placebo, although an effect was observed in a post hoc analysis in patients with incomplete SCI [87].

Valproate

Valproate (up to 2400 mg/day for 3 weeks) did not differ from placebo in one class-II trial in SCI [88].

Table 7.3 Results in central pain.

Drugs	Sample size (trials)	Benefit with active (range)	Benefit with control (range)	Relative Risk (95% CI)	Harm with active (range)	Harm with control (range)	Relative Risk (95% CI)	Reliability and Net Gain	
Amitriptyline	99 (2)	34.6% (22–67)	5.8% (5–7)	6.0 (1.9–19) P = 0.0004	11.9% (0–16)	3.6% (0–5)	3.26 (0.7–15) NS	20	21
PGB	137 (1)	27.8%	8.6%	3.2 (1.3–8.3) P = 0.012	21.4%	13.4%	1.6 (0.7–3.4) NS	18	11
CBZ	15 (1)	38.5%	6.7%	5.77 (0.8–43) NS	6.7%	0.0%	1.0 NS	4	–
LTG	22 (1)	20.0%	21.0%	0.95 (0.3–3) NS	3.7%	7.1%	0.52 (0.05–5) NS	10	–
Valproate	20 (1)	30.0%	20.0%	1.5 (0.5–4.5) NS	0.0%	0.0%	1.0 NS	6	–
Cannabis	90 (2)	35.1% (27–46)	14.3% (13–17)	2.46 (1.2–5) P = 0.0158	1.8% (0–3)	0.0% (0–0)	1.0 NS	26	19

Outcome measure of benefit: number of patients with at least 50% pain relief. Outcome measure of harm: number of drops out due to adverse events. Unless otherwise specified control is placebo.

Reliability: a metric based on quality of evidence and sample size (see Methods).

Net Gain: a metric based on the relative benefit and harm in a trial where Net Gain = (% patients with benefit with active minus % patients with benefit with placebo) minus (% patients with harm with active minus % patients with harm with placebo); it only applies to treatments significantly different from placebo. P-value from Fisher's exact test.

Amitriptyline: tricyclic antidepressant (50–75 mg). One study in post-stroke pain and one in SCI. PGB: presynaptic calcium-channel modulator (150–600 mg) in SCI [35]. In another study in SCI, GBP up to 3600 mg was significantly better than placebo, but number of responders was not reported [36]. CBZ: carbamazepine, predominantly NaCB (800 mg) in post-stroke pain. LTG: lamotrigine, various-action antiepileptic drug (200–400 mg) in SCI. In another study in post-stroke pain, LTG 200 mg was better than placebo, but number of responders was not reported [37]. Valproate: various-action antiepileptic drug (1000 mg) in SCI. Cannabinoids: tetrahydrocannabinol (THC) 5–10 mg, delta-9-tetra-hydrocannabinol: cannabidiol (THC:CBD) via oromucosal spray, both in MS.

Opioids

There is one (class-I) RCT on opioids, in multiple-aetiology peripheral or CP: levorphanol at high dose (8.9 mg/day) was more effective than levorphanol at low dose (2.7 mg/day) in patients with CP, but there was no placebo group [70]. There was no difference in response between patients with SCI, MS, PHN, or PPN, but patients with brain lesions had more early dropouts due to side effects compared with the others.

Cannabinoids

Cannabinoids have recently been assessed in two class-I RCTs, both on pain associated to MS. In one trial in 24 patients, the oral cannabinoid tetrahydrocannabinol (THC) 5–10 mg/day for 3 weeks, was superior to placebo [89]. THC was effective on ongoing and paroxysmal pain, but not on mechanical allodynia. Cannabinoids delivered via an oromucosal spray (2.7 mg of THC, 2.5 mg of cannabidiol; mean number of sprays 9.6, range 2–25) have shown beneficial effects on pain and sleep in one parallel RCT in patients with

MS [90]; the patients included either had neuropathic or spasm-related pain and post hoc analyses indicated a trend towards better effects in patients with painful muscle spasms. The overall Reliability for cannabinoids is 26 and the mean Net Gain 19%.

Mexiletine

Mexiletine 450 mg/day was no better than placebo in a small cross-over trial involving 11 SCI patients [91]. Low doses and small number of patients might play a role for lack of efficacy.

Practical recommendations

Both reliability of evidence and efficacy are lower in central than peripheral neuropathic pains. Figure 7.3 shows the normalized values. So far, cannabinoids (in pain associated to MS), amitriptyline (in post-stroke pain), and PGB (in SCI pain) are the best choice. CBZ and valproate are no better than placebo. We must mention that both GBP and LTG have been found to be significantly efficacious in CP in two high-quality RCTs. However, these trials could not be compared with the other trials because the number of responders was not reported. Considering the small number of RCTs in CP and the generally small sample sizes, treatment of CP may be based on general principles for peripheral neuropathic pain treatment and for side effect profile. Currently, we suggest GBP, LTG, PGB or TCA as first choice for poststroke or SCI pain. The level of evidence is lower for opioids given the lack of placebo-controlled studies. For CP associated to MS, cannabinoids have high-level efficacy, but may raise safety concerns, thus we recommend initially a trial with other drugs found effective in other CP conditions.

References

1 Merskey H, Bogduk N. *Classification of Chronic Pain*, 2nd edition. IASP Press, Seattle, 1994.

2 Bernstein JE, Korman NJ, Bickers DR, et al. Topical capsaicin treatment of chronic postherpetic neuralgia. *J. Am. Acad. Dermatol.* 1989; **21**: 265–70.

3 Dworkin RH, Backonja M, Rowbotham MC, et al. Advances in neuropathic pain: diagnosis, mechanisms, and treatment recommendations. *Arch. Neurol.* 2003a; **60**: 1524–34.

4 Kosinski MR, Schein JR, Vallow SM et al. An observational study of health-related quality of life and pain outcomes in chronic low back pain patients treated with fentanyl transdermal system. *Curr. Med. Res. Opin.* 2005; **21**: 869–62.

5 Mayer-Rosberg K, Burckhardt CS, Huizar K et al. A comparison of the SF-36 and Nottingham Health Profile in patients with chronic neuropathic pain. *Eur. J. Pain* 2001; **5**: 391–403.

6 Berger A, Dukes EM, Oster G. Clinical characteristics and economics costs patients with painful neuropathic disorders. *J. Pain* 2004; **5**: 143–9.

7 Attal N, Cruccu G, Haanpaa M, et al. EFNS Guidelines on pharmacological treatment of neuropathic pain. *Eur. J. Neurol.* 2006; **13**: 1153–69.

8 Finnerup NB, Otto M, McQuay HJ, et al. Algorithm for neuropathic pain treatment: an evidence based proposal. *Pain* 2005; **118**: 289–305.

9 Bennett G. Neuropathic pain: new insights, new interventions. *Hosp. Pract.* 1998; **33**: 95–110.

10 McDonald BK, Cockerell OC, Sander JWAS, Shorvon SD. The incidence and lifetime prevalence of neurological disorders in a prospective community-based study in the UK. *Brain* 2000; **123**: 665–676.

11 Otto M, Bak S, Bach FW, et al. Pain phenomena and possible mechanisms in patients with painful polyneuropathy. *Pain* 2003; **101**: 87–92.

12 Sindrup SH, Jensen TS. Pharmacologic treatment of pain in polyneuropathy. *Neurology* 2000; **55**: 915–20.

13 Gudmundsson S, Helgason S, Sigurdsson JA. The clinical course of herpes zoster: a prospective study in primary care. *Eur. J. Gen. Practice,* 1996; **2**: 12–16.

14 Nurmikko T, Bowsher D. Somatosensory findings in postherpetic neuralgia. *J. Neurol. Neurosurg. Psychiatr.* 1990; **53**: 135–41.

15 Watson CP. The treatment of postherpetic neuralgia. *Neurology* 1995; **45**(Suppl. 8): S58–60.

16 Boivie J. Central pain. In: MacMahon, SB & Koltzenburg M, eds., *Wall and Melzack's Textbook of Pain.* Elsevier, Churchill Livlingstone, 2005: pp. 1057–75.

17 Attal N, Bouhassira D. Central neuropathic pain. In: Pappagallo M, ed., *The Neurological Basis of Pain.* McGraw Hill, New York, 2005: pp. 301–9.

18 Duhmke RM, Cornblath DD, Hollingshead JR. Tramadol for neuropathic pain. *Cochrane Database Syst. Rev.* 2004: CD003726.

19 Saarto T, Wiffen P. Antidepressants for neuropathic pain. *Cochrane Database Syst. Rev.* 2005; **20**: CD005454.

20 Wiffen P, Collins S, McQuay H, et al. Anticonvulsant drugs for acute and chronic pain. *Cochrane Database Syst. Rev.* 2005c; **20**: CD001133.

21 Wiffen P, McQuay H, Edwards J, et al. Gabapentin for acute and chronic pain. *Cochrane Database Syst. Rev.* 2005a; **20**: CD005452.

22 Wiffen P, McQuay H, Moore R. Carbamazepine for acute and chronic pain. *Cochrane Database Syst. Rev.* 2005b; **20**: CD005451.

23 Adriaensen H, Plaghki L, Mathieu C, et al. Critical review of oral drug treatments for diabetic neuropathic pain–clinical outcomes based on efficacy and safety data from placebo-controlled and direct comparative studies. *Diabetes Metab. Res. Rev.* 2005; **21**: 231–40.

24 Eisenberg E, McNicol ED, Carr DB. Efficacy and safety of opioid agonists in the treatment of neuropathic pain of nonmalignant origin: systematic review and meta-analysis of randomized controlled trials. *JAMA* 2005; **293**: 3043–52.

25 Jensen TS. Anticonvulsants in neuropathic pain: rationale and clinical evidence. *Eur. J. Pain* 2002; **6**(A): 61–8.

26 McQuay HJ. Neuropathic pain: evidence matters. *Eur. J. Pain* 2002; **6**(Suppl. A): 11–18.

27 Sindrup SH, Otto M, Finnerup NB, Jensen TS. Antidepressants in the treatment of neuropathic pain. *Basic Clin. Pharmacol. Toxicol.* 2005; **96**: 399–409.

28 Brainin M, Barnes M, Baron JC, et al. Guideline Standards Subcommittee of the EFNS Scientific Committee. Guidance for the preparation of neurological management guidelines by EFNS scientific task forces – revised recommendations. *Eur. J. Neurol.* 2004; **11**: 577–81.

29 Cruccu G, Anand P, Attal N, et al. EFNS guidelines on neuropathic pain assessment. *Eur. J. Neurol.* 2004; **11**: 153–62.

30 Jadad AR, Moore RA, Carroll D, et al. Assessing the quality of reports of randomized clinical trials: is blinding necessary? *Contr. Clin. Trial.* 1996; **17**: 1–12.

31 McCleane GJ. 200 mg daily of lamotrigine has no analgesic effect in neuropathic pain: a randomised, double-blind, placebo controlled trial. *Pain* 1999; **83**: 105–7.

32 Thienel U, Neto W, Schwabe SK, et al. Topiramate Diabetic Neuropathic Pain Study Group. Topiramate in painful diabetic polyneuropathy: findings from three double-blind placebo-controlled trials. *Acta. Neurol. Scand.* 2004; **110**: 221–31.

33 Sang CN, Booher S, Gilron I, et al. Dextromethorphan and memantine in painful diabetic neuropathy and postherpetic neuralgia. Efficacy and dose–response trials. *Anesthesiology* 2002; **96**: 1053–61.

34 Galer BS, Jensen MP, Ma T, et al. The lidocaine patch 5% effectively treats all neuropathic pain qualities: results of a randomized, double-blind, vehicle-controlled, 3-week efficacy study with use of the neuropathic pain scale. *Clin. J. Pain* 2002; **18**: 297–301.

35 Siddall PJ, Cousins MJ, Otte A, et al. Pregabalin in central neuropathic pain: a placebo controlled trial in spinal cord injury. *Neurology* 2006, in press.

36 Levendoglu F, Ogun CO, Ozerbil O, et al. Gabapentin is a first line drug for the treatment of neuropathic pain in spinal cord injury. *Spine* 2004; **29**: 743–51.

37 Vestergaard K, Andersen G, Gottrup H, et al. Lamotrigine for central poststroke pain: A randomized controlled trial. *Neurology* 2001; **56**: 184–90.

38 Sindrup SH, Gram LF, Skjold T, et al. Clomipramine vs desipramine vs placebo in the treatment of diabetic neuropathy symptoms. A double-blind cross-over study. *Br. J. Clin. Pharmacol.* 1990; **30**: 683–91.

39 Vrethem M, Boivie J, Arnqvist H, et al. A comparison a amitriptyline and maprotiline in the treatment of painful polyneuropathy in diabetics and nondiabetics. *Clin. J. Pain* 1997; **13**: 313–23.

40 Watson CP, Vernich L, Chipman M, et al. Nortriptyline versus amitriptyline in postherpetic neuralgia: a randomized trial. *Neurology* 1998; **51**: 1166–71.

41 Ray WA, Meredith S, Thapa PB, et al. Cyclic antidepressants and the risk of sudden cardiac death. *Clin. Pharmacol. Ther.* 2004; **75**: 234–41.

42 Raskin J, Pritchett YL, Wang F, et al. A double-blind, randomized multicenter trial comparing duloxetine with placebo in the management of diabetic peripheral neuropathic pain. *Pain Med.* 2005; **6**: 346–56.

43 Goldstein DJ, Lu Y, Detke MJ, et al. Duloxetine versus placebo in patients with painful diabetic neuropathy. *Pain* 2005; **116**: 109–18.

44 Sindrup SH, Bach FW, Madsen C, et al. Venlafaxine versus imipramine in painful polyneuropathy. A randomized, controlled trial. *Neurology* 2003; **60**: 1284–9.

45 Degner D, Grohmann R, Kropp S, et al. Severe adverse drug reactions of antidepressants: results of the German multicenter drug surveillance program AMSP. *Pharmacopsychiatry* 2004; **37**(Suppl. 1): S39–45.

46 Rowbotham MC, Goli V, Kunz NR, et al. Venlafaxine extended release in the treatment of painful diabetic neuropathy: a double-blind, placebo-controlled study. *Pain* 2004; **110**: 697–706.

47 Sindrup SH, Gram LF, Brøsen K, Eshøj O, Mogensen EF. The selective serotonin reuptake inhibitor paroxetine is effective in the treatment of diabetic neuropathy symptoms. *Pain* 1990a; **42**: 135–44.

48 Backonja M, Beydoun A, Edwards KR, et al. Gabapentin for the symptomatic treatment of painful neuropathy in patients with diabetes mellitus: a randomized controlled trial. *JAMA* 1998; **280**: 1831–6.

49 Lesser H, Sharma U, LaMoreaux L, et al. Pregabalin relieves symptoms of painful diabetic neuropathy. *Neurology* 2004; **63**: 2104–10.

50 Rosenstock J, Tuchmann M, LaMoreaux L, et al. Pregabalin for the treatment of painful diabetic peripheral neuropathy: a double-blind, placebo-controlled trial. *Pain* 2004; **110**: 628–38.

51 Simpson DA. Gabapentin and venlafaxine for the treatment of painful diabetic neuropathy. *J. Clin. Neuromusc. Dis.* 2001; **3**: 53–62.

52 Freynhagen R, Strojek K, Griesing T, et al. Efficacy of pregabalin in neuropathic pain evaluated in a 12-week, randomised, double-blind, multicentre, placebo-controlled trial of flexible- and fixed-dose regimens. *Pain* 2005; **115**: 254–63.

53 Richter RW, Portenoy R, Sharma U, et al. Relief of diabetic peripheral neuropathy with pregabalin: a randomised placebo-controlled trial. *J. Pain* 2005; **6**: 253–60.

54 Morello CM, Leckband SG, Stoner CP, et al. Randomized double-blind study comparing the efficacy of gabapentin with amitriptyline on diabetic peripheral neuropathy pain. *Arch. Intern. Med.* 1999; **159**: 1931–7.

55 Dworkin RH, Corbin AE, Young Jr JP, et al. Pregabalin for the treatment of postherpetic neuralgia: a randomized, placebo-controlled trial. *Neurology* 2003b; **60**: 1274–83.

56 Magenta P, Arghetti S, Di Palma F, et al. Oxcarbazepine is effective and safe in the treatment of neuropathic pain: pooled analysis of seven clinical studies. *Neurol. Sci.* 2005; **26**: 218–26.

57 Dogra S, Beydoun S, Mazzola J, et al. Oxcarbazepine in painful diabetic neuropathy: a randomized, placebo-controlled study. *Eur. J. Pain* 2005; **9**: 543–54.

58 Gomez-Perez FJ, Choza R, Rios JM, et al. Nortriptyline-fluphenazine vs. carbamazepine in the symptomatic treatment of diabetic neuropathy. *Arch. Med. Res.* 1996; **27**: 525–9.

59 Kutluay E, McCague K, D'Souza J, et al. Safety and tolerability of oxcarbazepine in elderly patients with epilepsy. *Epilepsy Behav.* 2003; **4**: 175–80.

60 Eisenberg E, Lurie Y, Braker C, et al. Lamotrigine reduces painful diabetic neuropathy: a randomized, controlled study. *Neurology* 2001; **57**: 505–9.

61 Kochar DK, Jain N, Agarwal RP, et al. Sodium valproate in the management of painful polyneuropathy in type 2 diabetes – a randomized placebo controlled study. *Acta. Neurol. Scand.* 2002; **106**: 248–52.

62 Kochar DK, Rawat N, Agrawal RP, et al. Sodium valproate for painful diabetic neuropathy: a randomised double-blind placebo-controlled study. *QJM* 2004; **97**: 33–8.

63 Otto M, Bach FW, Jensen TS, et al. Valproic acid has no effect on pain in polyneuropathy: a randomized controlled trial. *Neurology* 2004; **62**: 285–8.

64 Raskin P, Donofrio PD, Rosenthal NR, et al. Topiramate vs placebo in painful diabetic polyneuropathy: analgesic and metabolic effects. *Neurology* 2004; **63**: 865–73.

65 Gimbel JS, Richards P, Portenoy RK. Controlled-release oxycodone for pain in diabetic neuropathy. A randomized controlled trial. *Neurology* 2003; **60**: 927–34.

66 Watson CP, Moulin D, Watt-Watson J, et al. Controlled-release oxycodone relieves neuropathic pain: a randomized controlled trial in painful diabetic neuropathy. *Pain* 2003; **105**: 71–8.

67 Harati Y, Gooch C, Swenson M, et al. Double-blind randomized trial of tramadol for the treatment of diabetic neuropathy. *Neurology* 1998; **50**: 1842–6.

68 Sindrup SH, Andersen G, Madsen C, et al. Tramadol relieves pain and allodynia in polyneuropathy: a randomised, double-blind, controlled trial. *Pain* 1999a; **83**: 85–90.

69 Raja SN, Haythornwaite JA, Pappagallo M, et al. Opioids versus antidepressants in postherpetic neuralgia. *Neurology* 2002; **59**: 1015–21.

70 Rowbotham MC, Twilling L, Davies PS, et al. Oral opioid therapy for chronic peripheral and central neuropathic pain. *N. Engl. J. Med.* 2003; **348**: 1223–32.

71 Watson CP, Babul N. Efficacy of oxycodone in neuropathic pain: a randomized trial in postherpetic neuralgia. *Neurology* 1998; **50**: 1837–41.

72 Attal N. Chronic neuropathic pain: mechanisms and treatment. *Clin. J. Pain* 2000; **16**(Suppl. 3): S118–30.

73 Kalso E, Allan L, Dellemijn PL, et al. Recommendations for using opioids in chronic non-cancer pain. *Eur. J. Pain* 2003; **7**: 381–6.

74 Boureau F, Legallicier P, Kabir-Ahmadi M. Tramadol in postherpetic neuralgia: a randomized, double-blind, placebo-controlled trial. *Pain* 2003; **104**: 323–31.

75 Gilron I, Bailey JM, Tu D, et al. Morphine, gabapentin, or their combination for neuropathic pain. *N. Engl. J. Med.* 2005; **352**: 1324–34.

76 Watson CP, Chipman M, Reed K, et al. Amitriptyline versus maprotiline in postherpetic neuralgia: a randomized, double-blind, crossover trial. *Pain* 1992; **48**: 29–36.

77 Rice ASC, Maton S. Post Herpetic Neuralgia Study Group. Gabapentin in postherpetic neuralgia; a randomised, double-blind, controlled study. *Pain* 2001; **94**: 215–24.

78 Rowbotham MC, Harden N, Stacey B, et al. Gabapentin for treatment of postherpetic neuralgia. *JAMA* 1998; **280**: 1837–43.

79 Sabatowski R, Galvez R, Cherry DA, et al. Pregabalin reduces pain and improves sleep and mood disturbances in patients with post-herpetic neuralgia: results of a randomised, placebo-controlled clinical trial. *Pain* 2004; **109**: 26–35.

80 Kochar DK, Garg P, Bumb RA, et al. Divalproex sodium in the management of post-herpetic neuralgia: a randomized double-blind placebo-controlled study. *QJM* 2005; **98**: 29–34.

81 Eisenberg E, Kleiser A, Dortort A, et al. The NMDA (*N*-methyl-D-aspartate) receptor antagonist memantine in the treatment of postherpetic neuralgia: a double-blind, placebo-controlled study. *Eur. J. Pain* 1998; **2**: 321–7.

82 Galer BS, Rowbotham MC, Perander J, et al. Topical lidocaine patch relieves postherpetic neuralgia more effectively than a vehicle topical patch: results of an enriched enrollment study. *Pain* 1999; **80**: 533–8.

83 Wasner G, Kleinert A, Binder A, et al. Postherpetic neuralgia: topical lidocaine is effective in nociceptor-deprived skin. *J. Neurol.* 2005; **252**: 677–86.

84 Watson CP, Tyler KL, Bickers DR, et al. A randomized vehicle-controlled trial of topical capsaicin in the treatment of postherpetic neuralgia. *Clin. Ther.* 1993; **15**: 510–26.

85 Cardenas DD, Warms CA, Turner JA, et al. Efficacy of amitriptyline for relief of pain in spinal cord injury: results of a randomized controlled trial. *Pain* 2002; **96**: 365–73.

86 Leijon G, Boivie J. Central post-stroke pain – a controlled trial of amitriptyline and carbamazepine. *Pain* 1989; **36**: 27–36.

87 Finnerup NB, Sindrup SH, Bach FW, et al. Lamotrigine in spinal cord injury pain: a randomized controlled trial. *Pain* 2002; **96**: 375–83.

88 Drewes AM, Andreasen A, Poulsen LH. Valproate for treatment of chronic central pain after spinal cord injury. A double-blind cross-over study. *Paraplegia* 1994; **32**: 565–9.

89 Svendsen KB, Jensen TS, Bach FW. The cannabinoid dronabinol reduces central pain in multiple sclerosis. A randomised double-blind placebo controlled cross-over trial. *BMJ* 2004; **329**: 253–61.

90 Rog DJ, Nurmikko TJ, Friede T, et al. Randomized, controlled trial of cannabis-based medicine in central pain in multiple sclerosis. *Neurology* 2005; **65**: 812–19.

91 Chiou-Tan FY, Tuel SM, Johnson JC, et al. Effect of mexiletine on spinal cord injury dysesthetic pain. *Am. J. Phys. Med. Rehabil.* 1996; **75**: 84–7.

CHAPTER 8

Vertigo and dizziness: treatment of benign paroxysmal positional vertigo, vestibular neuritis and Menière's disease

Michael Strupp, Thomas Brandt, Christian Daniel Cnyrim

Background

Vertigo and dizziness are not unique disease entities. Sometimes vertigo is attributed to vestibular disorders, while dizziness is not [1]. There is no general agreement about them, and visual stimuli can cause vertigo (e.g. height vertigo or optokinetic vection), just as central vestibular or otolith disorders can cause dizziness. The two terms cover a number of multisensory and sensorimotor syndromes of various aetiologies and pathogeneses. They can be elucidated only within an interdisciplinary approach [2]. After headache, vertigo and dizziness are among the most frequent presenting symptoms, not only in neurology. According to a survey of over 30,000 persons, the prevalence of vertigo as a function of age is around 17%; it rises to 39% in those over 80 years of age [3]. The most frequent forms of peripheral vestibular vertigo and dizziness are benign paroxysmal positioning vertigo (BPPV), vestibular neuritis (VN), and Menière's disease (MD) (Table 8.1).

Table 8.1 Relative frequency of different vertigo/dizziness syndromes diagnosed in a dedicated neurological dizziness unit (*n* = 5353).

Diagnosis	*N*	Frequency (%)
Benign paroxysmal positioning vertigo	992	18.5
Phobic postural vertigo (PPV)	831	15.6
Central vestibular vertigo	669	13.2
Vestibular migraine	553	10.3
Menière's disease	444	8.3
Vestibular neuritis	409	7.6
Bilateral vestibulopathy	193	3.6
Psychogenic vertigo (without PPV)	193	3.6
Vestibular paroxysmia	173	3.2
Perilymph fistula	22	0.4
Unknown aetiology	214	4.0
Others	630	11.8

BPPV is the most common cause of vertigo, not only in the elderly. About one-third of all over the age of 70 years have experienced BPPV at least once. It is characterized by brief attacks of rotatory vertigo and simultaneous positioning rotatory-vertical nystagmus towards the undermost ear, and is elicited by extending the head or positioning the head or body towards the affected ear. BPPV can appear at any time from childhood to senility, but the idiopathic form is typically a disease of old age, peaking in the sixth to seventh decade (women:men = 2:1). It is called benign because it often resolves spontaneously within weeks to months; in some cases, however, it can last for years. The canalolithiasis hypothesis of freely floating 'heavy otoconia' is compatible with all features of BPPV: latency, duration, course of attacks, direction of nystagmus, reversal of nystagmus, fatigability, and, most important, the efficacy of positioning 'liberatory manoeuvres' of the head [4]. Brandt and Daroff [5] were the first to devise an effective exercise programme that required the simple performance of a series of head-positioning movements. Semont et al. [6] recommended that the patient's position should be changed from the inducing position by a tilt of 180° to the opposite side (Figure 8.1). In 1992 Epley proposed another variation that involved turning the patient's trunk and head into a head-hanging position [8]. The efficacy of these manoeuvres can also be explained by the mechanism of canalolithiasis.

VN is the second most common cause of peripheral vestibular vertigo (the first being BPPV). It accounts for 7% of the patients who present at outpatient clinics specializing in the treatment of dizziness [9] and has an incidence of 3.5 per 100,000 population [10]. The key signs and symptoms of VN are the acute onset of sustained rotatory vertigo, horizontal spontaneous nystagmus towards the unaffected ear with a rotational component, postural imbalance with Romberg's sign, that is, falls with the eyes closed towards the affected ear, and nausea. Caloric testing invariably shows ipsilateral hyporesponsiveness or nonresponsiveness. In the past, either

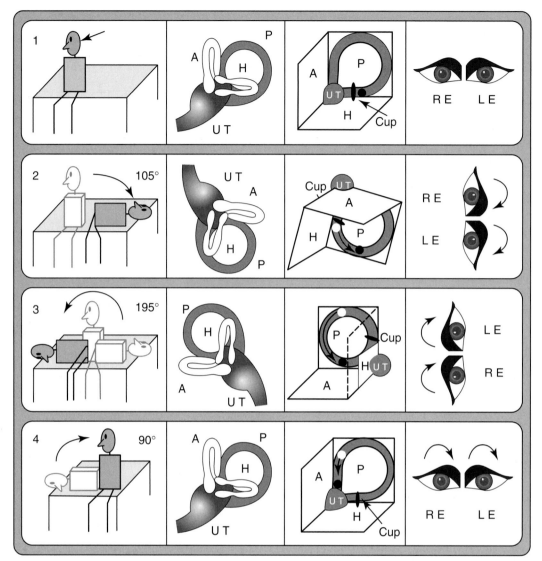

Figure 8.1 Schematic drawing of the Semont liberatory manoeuvre in a patient with typical BPPV of the left ear. Boxes from left to right: position of body and head, position of labyrinth in space, position and movement of the clot in the posterior canal and resulting cupula deflection, and direction of the rotatory nystagmus. The clot is depicted as an open circle within the canal; a black circle represents the final resting position of the clot. (1) In the sitting position, the head is turned horizontally 45° to the unaffected ear. The clot, which is heavier than endolymph, settles at the base of the left posterior semicircular canal. (2) The patient is tilted approximately 105° towards the left (affected) ear. The change in head position, relative to gravity, causes the clot to gravitate to the lowermost part of the canal and the cupula to deflect downward, inducing BPPV with rotatory nystagmus beating towards the undermost ear. The patient maintains this position for 3 min. (3) The patient is then turned approximately 195° with the nose down, causing the clot to move towards the exit of the canal. The endolymphatic flow again deflects the cupula so that the nystagmus beats towards the left ear, now uppermost. The patient remains in this position for 3 min. (4) The patient is slowly moved to the sitting position; this causes the clot to enter the utricular cavity.

A, P, and H: anterior, posterior, and horizontal semicircular canals, respectively; Cup: cupula; UT: utricular cavity; RE: right eye; LE: left eye [7].

inflammation of the vestibular nerve or labyrinthine ischaemia was proposed to cause VN. Currently a viral aetiology is favoured. Herpes simplex virus type 1 (HSV-1) DNA has been detected on autopsy with the use of polymerase chain reaction in about two of three human vestibular ganglia [11–15]. This, as well as the expression of CD8-positive T-lymphocytes, cytokines, and chemokines, indicates that the vestibular ganglia are latently infected with HSV-1 [16]. The evidence, however, remains circumstantial.

The major complaints of vertigo, nausea, imbalance, and a tendency to fall resolve slowly over a few weeks, and within 3–5 weeks the patient is generally free of them when at rest. Recovery is a result of a combination of restoration of peripheral labyrinthine function (frequently incomplete), substitution of the functional loss by the contralateral vestibular system as well as by somatosensory (neck proprioception) and visual afferences, and central compensation of the peripheral vestibular tonus imbalance. In the course of illness only about 40% of patients have complete recovery of peripheral vestibular function after 24 months [17], in 20–30% there is only partial recovery, and the rest have a persisting unilateral defect. Therapeutic measures include symptomatic treatment of vertigo and nausea with antivertiginous drugs and a potentially causal treatment with corticosteroids and antiviral agents.

MD is clinically characterized by recurrent spontaneous attacks of vertigo, fluctuating hearing loss, tinnitus, and aural fullness. The American Academy of Ophthalmology and Otolaryngology, Head and Neck Surgery formulated diagnostic criteria in 1995 for certain, definite, probable, and possible MD. Its incidence varies between 7.5 per 100,000 and 160 per 100,000 persons [18]. While the onset of the disease is unilateral, the other ear can also become affected in time. According to a study on 119 patients with a follow-up of at least 14 years, bilateral involvement was present initially in 13% and developed subsequently in 45% of the patients [19]. Endolymph hydrops is assumed to be the pathological basis of MD, due either to a too high production or a too low absorption of the endolymph. The increased endolymphatic pressure causes periodic rupturing or leakage (by the opening of non-selective, stretch-activated ion channels [20] of the membrane separating the endolymph from the perilymph space). It therefore makes pathophysiological sense to reduce the production and increase the absorption of endolymph. The clinical goals of treating MD are to stop vertigo, reduce or abolish tinnitus, and preserve hearing or even reverse its loss. Most studies focus on the severest symptom of MD: recurrent attacks of vertigo.

A plethora of treatment strategies have been suggested for MD. Destructive procedures involving the lateral semicircular canal and vestibule have been proposed since 1904. The first endolymphatic sac decompression was performed in 1926. This method is still used in some settings despite its evident ineffectiveness. Restricting salt and fluid intake and diuretics were first proposed in 1934. Salt restriction and diuretics are still recommended, although in one double-blind study diuretics did not show any effect [21]. Vestibulotoxic drugs have been in use since 1948; local intratympanic delivery has been performed since 1956 (see Ref. [22]). It is remarkable that despite the high incidence of MD and the large number of studies published on its treatment over the last decades, there are still only very few state-of-the-art prospective, placebo-controlled, double-blind trials. Moreover, there are significant differences in the treatment regimen of MD between Europe and the USA. In the USA low salt diet, diuretics, and intratympanic injection of gentamicin and corticosteroids are preferred. In Europe betahistine is more often used, in the US rarely. In this context it is remarkable that in an article on Menière's disease by Minor et al. [18] from Johns Hopkins the word *betahistine* does not even appear. A national survey among UK otolaryngologists on the treatment of MD revealed that 94% used betahistine, 63% diuretics, 71% salt restriction, 52% sac decompression, and approximately 50% insertion of a grommet [22]. Local gentamicin instillation has become progressively more popular since its introduction in the UK 10 years ago: approximately two-thirds of the otolaryngologists use this method.

Framing answerable clinical questions and general approach to search evidence

A consideration of the most effective treatment for the above three vestibular disorders raises the following questions:

1 Which liberatory manoeuvre is the most effective for patients with BPPV to free the typical posterior canal of the heavy causative clot: Semont's, Epley's, or Brandt/Daroff's?

2 Are there any predictive factors for BPPV recurrences in patients successfully treated by liberatory manoeuvres?

3 Should patients with acute VN be treated with corticosteroids or antiviral agents?

4 What is the evidence that central compensation of the vestibular tonus imbalance in patients with acute VN is facilitated by structured physical exercises?

5 Should patients with MD and frequent attacks be treated with betahistine or intratympanic injections of gentamicin?

To arrive at concrete answers, we searched the literature in the Medline (1966–2005) and PubMed databases.

Critical review of the evidence for each question

1. Liberatory manoeuvres

Which liberatory manoeuvre is the most effective for patients with BPPV to free the typical posterior canal of the causative heavy clot: Semont's, Epley's, or Brandt/Daroff's manoeuvre?

Effectiveness of the manoeuvres

Everyone who uses the liberatory manoeuvres is convinced of their efficacy. It is generally assumed that they are highly effective for the common posterior canal BPPV in 80–99% of patients [5,6,8,23,24], and that they are also very cost-effective procedures [25].

There is, however, no real *class I* evidence (i.e. quality of evidence ratings for therapeutic modalities following Brainin et al. [26]; *class I* evidence is provided by one or more well-designed randomized-controlled clinical trials) on the effectiveness of the different manoeuvres or on a comparison of the three manoeuvres.

In our search for BPPV treatment studies published since 1995 in PubMed and Medline, we found 55 studies that examined the efficacy of various manoeuvres in patients with BPPV of the posterior canal. Only two studies, however, had a prospective, controlled, and single-blinded design.

Simhadri et al. [23] evaluated (in only 40 patients) the efficacy of a modified Epley manoeuvre, proposed by Parnes

Table 8.2 Liberatory manoeuvre for patients with benign paroxysmal positioning vertigo.

Study	Type of study	N (female:male)/ impaired canal	Median age (years)	Follow-up	Type of manoeuvre (N)	Success rate (%)	Duration of treatment Number of manoeuvres Carried out by
Simhadri et al. [23]	Single blinded, randomized controlled, prospective	40 (1:1)/ posterior canal	41	12 months	PRM [27] (20)	90	1 week Every 3rd hour while awake Patients themselves
Lynn et al. [24]	Single blinded, randomized controlled, prospective	33 (24:9)/ posterior canal	68	1 month	Epley (18)	89	One session Mostly four cycles Audiologist
Li [28]	Randomized controlled, prospective	60 n.s./ posterior canal	n.s.	7 days	Epley, partially with mastoid vibration (37)	51	Not specified
Salvinelli et al.[29]	Randomized controlled, prospective	80 (54:26)/ posterior canal	60	6 months	Semont (40)	88	1–3 manoeuvres
Angeli et al. [30]	Randomized controlled, prospective	47 (26:21)/ posterior canal	74	1 month	Modified Epley (28)	64	One session 1–3 manoeuvres
Soto Varela et al. [31]	Randomized controlled, prospective	106 (73:33)/ posterior canal	59	3 months	Brandt Daroff (11) Semont (12) Epley (13)	62 77 93	3/day patients Not specified repeated if necessary
Sherman and Massoud [32]	Randomized controlled, prospective	71 (53:18)/ posterior canal	54	12 months	PRM [27] (18)	83	Not specified
Wolf et al. [33]	Randomized controlled, prospective	41 (23:18)/ posterior canal	46	6 months	Epley (31)	94	Titration manoeuvre performed weekly
Cohen and Kimball [34]	Randomized controlled, prospective	124 (76:48)/ posterior canal	58	6 months	Brandt Daroff (25) CRP (Epley) (24) LM (Semont) (25) Habituation exercise (25)	– – – –	Various parameters analysed
Motamed et al. [35]	Randomized controlled, prospective	84 (70:14)/ posterior canal	49	1–1.5 months	Epley, partially with mastoid vibration (79)	68	Not specified
Asawavichianginda et al. [36]	Randomized controlled, prospective	85 (56:29)/ posterior canal	50	6 months	Epley (42)	92	Not specified Physician
Herdman et al. [37]	Randomized controlled, prospective	60 (44:16)/ posterior canal	58	4 months	Semont (30) Epley (30)	70 57	Not specified
Froehling et al. [38]	Randomized controlled, prospective	50 (32:18)/ posterior canal	64	10 days	Epley (24)	67	Titration

and Price-Jones [27]. They showed that it had a success rate of 95% (versus 15% in the control group) after 1 week. After 6 months the success rate was still 95% (versus 25%) and after 1 year, 90% (versus 15%). Previously Lynn et al. [24] had assessed the effectiveness of the Epley manoeuvre without mastoid vibration and medical treatment in 18 patients with 1-month follow-up and found a success rate of 88.9%. An overview of both trials is presented in Table 8.2. Since both studies defined success as absence of vertigo and nystagmus during the Dix–Hallpike test, the success rates could be averaged. This yielded a value of 90% for a total 38 patients.

Eleven further randomized-controlled prospective studies [28–38] evaluated the efficacy of Epley's (10 trials), Semont's (4 trials), Brandt and Daroff's (2 trials), or habituation manoeuvres (1 trial). They are listed in Table 8.2 but were not included in the meta-analysis presented above because of substantial methodological deficits. Despite their differences in definitions of success, follow-up time, and manoeuvres, we averaged the cited success rates and obtained a value of approximately 70% for 500 evaluated cases of BPPV (range 51–94% success). Even though this result has marginal explanatory power, it nevertheless indicates that positioning manoeuvres in the treatment of BPPV are very efficacious.

Studies that were not of randomized-controlled design are not listed.

A recent critical meta-analysis [39] of the Epley manoeuvre also pointed to the absence of sufficient trials on this topic: 'The 11 studies identified by the search strategy as being trials of the Epley manoeuvre in the treatment of posterior canal BPPV were generally of low methodological quality, particularly in the key areas of allocation concealment and blinding of the assessors to outcome. Nine of the studies were excluded because of concern about a high probability of bias. Only two trials [24,38] were judged to be of sufficient methodological quality to be included in the review' [39]. The meta-analysis of a total of 83 patients in this study revealed that patients who perform the Epley manoeuvre are more likely to have complete resolution of their symptoms (odds ratio 4.92 (95% confidence interval 1.84–13.16)) and more likely to convert from a positive to a negative Dix–Hallpike test (odds ratio 5.67 (95% confidence interval 2.21–14.56)). The authors concluded that further research in this field should consider using a rigorous randomization technique with respect to adequate pre-allocation concealment, the blinding of the outcome assessors, the inclusion of the post-treatment Hallpike manoeuvre as an efficacy criterion, and a long-term follow-up of the patients [39].

In a very careful meta-analysis by White et al. [40] on the Epley manoeuvre a total of nine randomized-controlled trials were identified and included in their analysis; three had a blinded follow-up (141 patients). The nine trials consisted of a total of 505 patients with a mean follow-up time of 16 days. The risk of persistence of BPPV without treatment was 69%, the risk after a single canalith repositioning manoeuvre was 28% ($P < 0.00001$; relative risk reduction 61%). The authors concluded from their analysis that the Epley manoeuvre is a safe and effective treatment of BPPV. A single treatment session resolves BPPV in 72% of the cases.

The following studies dealt with the comparison of different positioning manoeuvres. A recent retrospective study on 840 patients with posterior canal BPPV compared the effectiveness of Epley's with Semont's manoeuvre [41]. The Epley 'repositioning' manoeuvre was performed on 607 (66%) patients; the mean number of treatment sessions was 2.98 (range 1–12), 409 (67%) became symptom free, 164 (27%) were significantly improved, and 34 (6%) had no change of their symptoms; Semont's liberatory manoeuvre was performed on 233 (25%) patients. The mean number of treatment sessions was 4.34 (range 1–19). In this group 144 (62%) of the patients became symptom free, 83 (36%) were significantly improved, and 6 (2%) did not experience any change in their symptoms.

In another study the efficacy of the three manoeuvres was compared in 106 patients 1 week, 1 month, and 3 months after treatment. The success rate after 1 week was 74% with Semont's, 71% with Epley's, and 24% with Brandt–Daroff's manoeuvres and after 3 months 77% with Semont's, 93% with Epley's, and 62% with Brandt–Daroff's manoeuvres [31]. One study on 62 patients retrospectively evaluated whether the success rate of Epley's manoeuvre depends on the aetiology of the BPPV and demonstrated that it was lower in secondary BPPV, for example, due to head injury, MD, or VN [42].

A very recent controlled study compared the efficacy of the Epley, Semont, Brandt and Daroff, and sham manoeuvres and habituation exercises in 124 patients (each group with 24–25 patients, follow-up of 6 months) [34]. It showed that the decrease of vertigo after Epley, Semont, Brandt and Daroff manoeuvres was significantly better than in the sham group (with no difference between the three treatment groups). The effect of habituation exercises was not significantly different neither from the treatment nor the sham group.

Finally, the efficacy of the Epley versus Semont manoeuvre for self-treatment of posterior canal BPPV was evaluated in 70 patients with posterior canal BPPV [43]. The response rate after 1 week was 95% in the Epley group and 58% in the Semont group ($P < 0.01$). Treatment failure, however, was due to incorrect performance of the Semont manoeuvre (see below). This indicates that detailed instruction and monitoring of the correct manoeuvre are necessary in all patients.

All in all, the following conclusions can be drawn: first, so far only a few methodologically high-quality studies on the effectiveness of the different liberatory manoeuvres in BPPV are available; second, the success rate after the first manoeuvre seems to be lower and the recurrence rate higher than previously reported; and third, prospective, randomized, controlled studies in this field are necessary in the future.

Supplementary procedures to the manoeuvres

Li [28] found in a randomized-controlled survey that the success rate improved if the procedure is combined with mastoid vibration; this, however, was not confirmed in a more recent study [44], mainly because the success rate without vibration was already very high in the second study. Semont [6] recommended having the patient maintain the upright position for 48 h following liberation, but we have not found this to be necessary. Our view is supported by two prospective and at least partially controlled studies that showed that post-manoeuvre restrictions are not necessary in posterior canal BPPV to improve effectiveness [45,46].

Side effects of the manoeuvres

A possible complication of liberatory manoeuvres is that the clot leaves the posterior canal but instead of staying in the utricular cavity enters the anterior (via the common crus) or the horizontal canal. Thus, posterior BPPV may convert to horizontal or anterior BPPV. This occurred in 5 of 85 patients who originally had typical posterior BPPV (horizontal canal: 3, anterior canal: 2) after they had undergone liberatory manoeuvres [47]. 'Canalith jam' is another speculative description of hitherto unexplained transient phenomena that rarely occur during physical treatment [48]. Despite successful liberatory manoeuvres, many patients complain of postural vertigo and dizziness when standing and walking after the liberatory manoeuvres. This may last a few or several weeks and can be explained by the partial repositioning of the otoconia towards the otolith organs, namely the utricle (i.e.

most likely an otolithic vertigo). Patients should be informed in advance about this side effect of the manoeuvres, which disappears spontaneously within a few days due to central compensation and can be improved by exercises.

Failure of manoeuvre treatment

There are several reasons for the failure of treatment with the manoeuvres described above. First, the diagnosis may have been wrong, that is, the patient suffered from central positioning or positional vertigo or nystagmus, bilateral BPPV, or BPPV of the horizontal or (very rarely) anterior semicircular canal (see below). Second, the patient may not have performed the manoeuvres correctly, for example, the head rotation in Semont's liberatory manoeuvre is often performed incorrectly when the patient moves the body 180° to the non-affected side or this body movement is performed too slowly so that the clot moves in the 'wrong direction' within the posterior canal. In such cases, the patient should be re-instructed, and if the symptoms persist, he should be admitted to a hospital for a few days until the symptoms resolve.

2. BPPV recurrences

Are there any predictive factors for BPPV recurrences in patients successfully treated by liberatory manoeuvres?

Retrospective [49,50] and prospective [51,52] studies reported a recurrence rate of 26.8–45%. The follow-up time for men was 10.2–51.9 months in the retrospective and 9.4–26 months in the prospective studies. In a recent retrospective long-term follow-up (6–17 years, mean 10 years) of 125 patients the overall recurrence rate of 50% was slightly higher than expected from the previous studies [53]. Eighty per cent of the first relapses occurred in the 1st year following effective physical liberatory manoeuvres for canalolithiasis. This was quite different from conclusions drawn by Nunez et al. [51], who after applying their recurrence data to a Kaplan–Meier estimation reported a 15% recurrence rate per year. Recurrences were more often observed in women (58% versus 39% [49,53], that is, the women:men ratio was 3:2). This correlates well with epidemiological data indicating a higher prevalence for BPPV in women [54,55]. Thus, women appear to be more susceptible to both the first manifestation and to relapses of BPPV. Two more predictive factors were recently disclosed: a history of three or more BPPV attacks prior to the initial liberatory manoeuvre indicate a higher risk of impending multiple recurrences for about two-thirds of the patients. The recurrence rate of patients in the seventh decade of age is about half of those in the sixth decade. Spontaneously vigorous head movements characteristically decrease with increasing age, and this may explain why otoconia are less often loosened from their macula layer in the seventh decade.

3. Cortisteroids for acute VN

Should patients with acute VN be treated with corticosteroids or antiviral agents?

Despite the widely assumed viral cause of VN, the effects of corticosteroids, antiviral agents, or the two in combination were still uncertain. A non-blinded study on 36 patients with VN examined the effects of corticosteroids [56]. Eighteen patients were treated with steroids over 2 years after symptom onset; 18 received no treatment. Caloric irrigation showed that the steroid-treated patients had a better recovery of peripheral vestibular function (13 of 18, 72%) than nonsteroid-treated subjects (10 of 18, 55.6%). Steroids also seemed to improve central vestibular compensation. More recently a prospective, randomized, double-blind, two-by-two factorial trial was performed, in which patients with acute VN were randomly assigned to treatment with placebo, methylprednisolone (100 mg/day, doses tapered by 20 mg every 3rd day), valacyclovir (1 g 3 times daily for 7 days), or methylprednisolone plus valacyclovir. Vestibular function was determined by caloric irrigation, with the use of the vestibular paresis formula (to measure the extent of unilateral caloric paresis), within 3 days after the onset of symptoms and 12 months afterwards. A total of 141 patients underwent randomization. The mean improvement in peripheral vestibular function at 12-month follow-up was 39.6 percentage points in the placebo group, 62.4 percentage points in the methylprednisolone group, 36.0 percentage points in the valacyclovir group, and 59.2 percentage points in the methylprednisolone plus valacyclovir group. Analysis of variance (ANOVA) showed that methylprednisolone had a significant effect, but valacyclovir did not. This study, therefore, showed that methylprednisolone alone significantly improves the recovery of peripheral vestibular function in patients with VN [57]. Symptom outcome after 12 months was not addressed for two reasons. First, animal experiments show that steroids improve central vestibular compensation. Thus, parameters other than vestibular paresis, such as postural imbalance or 'vertigo and dizziness', would not help differentiate between the effects of steroids on the recovery of peripheral vestibular function and on central vestibular compensation. Second, there are no validated scales for measuring vertigo and dizziness. All in all, this inexpensive and well-tolerated therapy can be recommended as the pharmaceutical treatment of choice for VN. An overview of the results of both studies and information about the therapy's side effects is presented in Table 8.3.

4. Physical therapy for vestibular tonus imbalance

What is the evidence that central compensation of the vestibular tonus imbalance in patients with acute VN is facilitated by structured physical exercises?

Animal experiments in the monkey and the cat have shown that spontaneous central vestibular compensation of unilateral peripheral vestibular lesions can be improved by vestibular exercises [59,60]. Several authors empirically (without evidence) advocate the early use of exercises to treat patients for active readjustment of vestibular dysfunctions [61–63]. There

Table 8.3 Treatment of acute vestibular neuritis.

Study	Design of study	Number (female:male)	Follow-up (months)	Treatment group (Number)	Number of patients improved/ number of patients followed	Mean improvement of vestibular excitability (%)*	Significance (comparison to placebo)	Side effects
Kitahara et al. [56]	Prospective, controlled	36 (19:17)	24	No treatment (18)	10/18		–	Not specified
				Methylprednisolone (18)	13/18		P = 0.07	Not specified
Strupp et al. [57]	Double-blind, randomized, controlled	141 (64:77)	12	Placebo (38)	8/30	39.6	–	None
				Methylprednisolone (35)	22/29	62.4	P < 0.001	Gastric ulcer with minor bleeding (one patient) Dyspepsia (three patients) Mood swings (five patients) Hyperglycaemia (two patients)
				Valacyclovir (33)	10/27	36.0	P = 0.43	None
				Methylprednisolone +valacyclovir (35)	22/28	59.2	P < 0.001	None

*Improvement in percentage points according to Jongkees's vestibular paresis formula [58]; significant P-values (alpha = 0.05) underlined.

are, however, only a few clinical studies and only one equivalent prospective randomized-controlled trial on the efficacy of such physiotherapy in humans who originally had a normal vestibular function before onset of an acute peripheral vestibular deficit [64]. To quantify the differential effects of specific vestibular exercises on central compensation in patients with an acute/subacute unilateral vestibular lesion (VN), the authors determined the time course of recovery of (1) ocular torsion (OT) for the vestibulo-ocular system, (2) subjective visual vertical (SVV) for perception, and (3) the sway path (SP) values for postural control in 19 patients with and 20 patients without vestibular exercises. All of these patients had had a persisting peripheral vestibular deficit for at least 30 days (statistical end point). While normalization of OT and SVV was similar in the control and physiotherapy groups, the SP values on day 30 after symptom onset significantly differed: 3.2 ± 1.9 m/min and 16.9 ± 6.1 m/min in the physiotherapy and control groups, respectively (ANOVA, $P < 0.001$). This study proved that specific vestibular exercises improve vestibulospinal compensation in patients with peripheral vestibular lesions. Moreover, these exercise regimens should begin as early as possible.

A recent randomized-controlled study on 54 patients with acute VN who did intensive home exercises demonstrated that *additional* physical therapy (12 times in 10 weeks) did not further improve balance [65].

5. Treatments for MD

Should patients with MD and frequent attacks be treated with betahistine or with intratympanic injections of gentamicin?

Intratympanic injections of gentamicin

Several studies have been published on the application of intratympanic gentamicin to treat MD. Initially, multiple intratympanic injections of gentamicin were given until patients developed vestibular hypofunction. This led to a good control of attacks of vertigo, but it was accompanied by a high rate of sensorineural hearing loss (approximately 50%). Especially after the delayed onset of ototoxic effects had been demonstrated [66], the regimen was changed in two ways: (1) single instillations at fixed interims of several days or weeks or (2) single shot injections and follow-up. After the latter regimen, a prospective, uncontrolled study on 57 patients with a follow-up time of 2–4 years showed that 95% of vertigo attacks could be controlled [67]. Fifty-three per cent of these patients needed only one injection of 12 mg gentamicin, 32% two or three injections.

Of the numerous prospective but not controlled studies published since 1995 and found in our search of PubMed, we considered nine trials to be of sufficient methodological quality (Table 8.4). They all evaluated the success of gentamicin injection in accordance with the criteria proposed by the American

Table 8.4 Intratympanic gentamicin for Menière's disease.

Study	Design of study (AAO criteria from)	Number (female: male)	Mean age years	Follow-up (months)	Rate of complete vertigo control (AAO class A) (%)	Rate of substantial vertigo control (AAO class B) (%)	Recurrence of vertigo (%)	Rate of hearing loss (%)	Mean hearing loss in PTA (dB)	Treatment protocol: Mean number of injections Dosage of gentamicin per injection Interval of injections Remarks
Lange et al. [67]	Prospective (1995)	57 (29:28)	54	≥24	95	5		9	None	1.48 (t) 12 mg Days: 1, 8, 15
Wu and Minor [72]	Prospective (1995)	34 (20:14)	52	≥24	88	9	29	18	None	2.7 (t) 10.7 mg Weekly
Perez et al. [73]	Prospective (1995)	71 (35:36)	54	≥24	69	14	24	16	1.1	3.1 (t) Uncertain (conc.: 26.7 mg/mL) Weekly
Quaranta et al. [74]	Prospective controlled (1995)	15 (6:9)	46	24	86	7	47	7	6	2 (f) 10 mg Weekly
Kaplan et al. [75]	Prospective (1985)	90 (54:46)	48	≥24	84	9		26	None	12 (f) 18.7–21.4 mg 3/day on 4 subsequent days
Minor [76]	Prospective (1995)	34 (21:13)	54	6	74	17	21	32	None	2.8 (t) 8–16 mg Weekly
Silverstein et al. [77]	Prospective (1995)	32 (13:19)	65	1	39			10	None	2.1 (f) 8–13.4 mg Weekly
Kaasinen et al. [78]	Prospective (1985)	93	51	24	71			39	8.8	1.82 (t) 8–13.4 mg Daily *Piece of gelfoam placed at the round window*
Youssef and Poe [79]	Prospective (1995)	37 (17:20)	52	≥24	41	46		43	10.4	3.57 (t) 30 mg Weekly

AAO: Academy of otolaryngology; PTA: pure tone audiogram; (f): fixed number of injections; (t): titration of injections.

Academy of Otolaryngology (AAO) in the version from either 1985 [68] or 1995 [69]. The cited success rates for complete control of vertigo (AAO class A) ranged from 39.3% to 95%, with an average of 73.6% for 463 patients.

A recent meta-analysis by Cohen-Kerem et al. on 15 trials with 627 patients receiving gentamicin injection showed that complete vertigo control was achieved in about 75% of the patients and complete or substantial control in about 93%. The success rate was not affected by the gentamicin treatment regimen (i.e. fixed versus titration) [70]. Hearing level and word recognition were not adversely affected, regardless of treatment regimen. The authors, however, pointed out that the level of evidence reflected in the relevant articles is insufficient, especially because of relatively poor study designs: none of the trials were double blind or had a blinded prospective control. Meanwhile there is good evidence that the beneficial effect of gentamicin is due to its damage to the hair cells. A complete ablation of function, however, does not seem necessary in order to control vertigo [71].

Betahistine

In Europe betahistine is more often used, mainly on the basis of a study by Meyer in 1985 [80] and more recent meta-analyses [81–83]. Betahistine is an H_1 agonist and H_3 antagonist.

It improves the microcirculation by acting on the pre-capillary sphincters of the stria vascularis [84]. There is evidence that it reduces the production and increases the absorption of endolymph. On the basis of our experience with a high dosage of betahistine-dihydrochloride (48 mg 3 times daily), we started an open trial, which is currently in progress. A preliminary interim analysis of the effects of high-dosage betahistine on vertigo attacks showed a significant reduction of attacks after 3 months [85]. These data are the basis for a recently begun prospective, randomized, double-blind dose-finding study comparing placebo with 16 mg betahistine-dihydrochloride 3 times daily and 48 mg, 3 times daily.

Finally, however, it must be pointed out that up to now no state-of-the-art studies have been conducted in this field despite the large number of trials. This was also pointed out by a comprehensive Cochrane Review dedicated exclusively to the efficacy of betahistine on MD [83]. Due to the great variability in the long-term course of MD, clinical trials have to be controlled and double blind; moreover, they require a large number of patients to have any explanatory power.

Conclusion

The initially raised questions can be answered as follows:

1 The treatment of choice for BPPV due to canalolithiasis of a posterior canal is one of the cited positioning manoeuvres. In the majority of studies the Semont and the Epley manoeuvres were preferred, although the efficacy seems to be widely independent of the type of manoeuvre used. Even though the success rates reported in various trials are of the same order of magnitude, only a few studies of sufficient methodological quality have been published.

2 The rate of recurrence of BPPV, albeit in retrospective analyses only, has been explored to a satisfying degree; it ranges in different studies from 26.8% to 50%. About 80% of recurrences occur within the 1st year after successful application of a liberatory manoeuvre.

3 The efficacy of steroids for treatment of VN is evident. The optimal dosage and duration of therapy still have to be determined. Another question to be addressed is whether further improvement can be achieved by administering antiviral agents very early.

4 Physical exercises for central compensation of tonus imbalance in the vestibular system due to VN seem beneficial. When exercises are performed correctly by the patients themselves, no additional physical therapy appears to be necessary.

5 The treatment of MD by intratympanic gentamicin injections has been thoroughly examined. Since complete functional destruction of the inner ear is not necessary to achieve satisfying control of vertigo, a careful titration or single-shot application is preferable to a series of injections. A significant and well-designed study on the treatment of MD with oral betahistine is urgently required.

Acknowledgement

We thank Ms. J. Benson for copy-editing the manuscript.

References

1 Neuhauser H, Lempert T. Vertigo and dizziness related to migraine: a diagnostic challenge. *Cephalalgia* 2004; **24**(2): 83–91.

2 Brandt T, Strupp M. General vestibular testing. *Clin. Neurophysiol.* 2005; **116**(2): 406–26.

3 Davis A, Moorjani P. *The Epidemiology of Hearing and Balance Disorders.* Martin Dunitz, London, 2003.

4 Brandt T, Steddin S. Current view of the mechanism of benign paroxysmal positioning vertigo: cupulolithiasis or canalolithiasis? *J. Vestibul. Res.* 1993; **3**(4): 373–82.

5 Brandt T, Daroff RB. Physical therapy for benign paroxysmal positional vertigo. *Arch. Otolaryngol.* 1980; **106**(8): 484–5.

6 Semont A, Freyss G, Vitte E. Curing the BPPV with a liberatory maneuver. *Adv. Otorhinolaryngol.* 1988; **42**: 290–3.

7 Brandt T, Steddin S, Daroff RB. Therapy for benign paroxysmal positioning vertigo, revisited. *Neurology* 1994; **44**(5): 796–800.

8 Epley JM. The canalith repositioning procedure: for treatment of benign paroxysmal positional vertigo. *Otolaryngol. Head Neck Surg.* 1992; **107**(3): 399–404.

9 Brandt T, Dieterich M, Strupp M. *Vertigo and Dizziness – Common Complaints.* Springer, London, 2005.

10 Sekitani T, Imate Y, Noguchi T, Inokuma T. Vestibular neuronitis: epidemiological survey by questionnaire in Japan. *Acta Otolaryngol. Suppl.* 1993; **503**: 9–12.

11 Schulz P, Arbusow V, Strupp M, Dieterich M, Rauch E, Brandt T. Highly variable distribution of HSV-1-specific DNA in human geniculate, vestibular and spiral ganglia. *Neurosci. Lett.* 1998; **252**(2): 139–42.

12 Arbusow V, Schulz P, Strupp M, Dieterich M, von Reinhardstoettner A, Rauch E, et al. Distribution of herpes simplex virus type 1 in human geniculate and vestibular ganglia: implications for vestibular neuritis. *Ann. Neurol.* 1999; **46**(3): 416–19.

13 Arbusow V, Theil D, Strupp M, Mascolo A, Brandt T. HSV-1 not only in human vestibular ganglia but also in the vestibular labyrinth. *Audiol. Neurootol.* 2001; **6**(5): 259–62.

14 Theil D, Arbusow V, Derfuss T, Strupp M, Pfeiffer M, Mascolo A, et al. Prevalence of HSV-1 LAT in human trigeminal, geniculate, and vestibular ganglia and its implication for cranial nerve syndromes. *Brain Pathol.* 2001; **11**(4): 408–13.

15 Theil D, Derfuss T, Strupp M, Gilden DH, Arbusow V, Brandt T. Cranial nerve palsies: herpes simplex virus type 1 and varizella-zoster virus latency. *Ann. Neurol.* 2002; **51**(2): 273–4.

16 Theil D, Derfuss T, Paripovic I, Herberger S, Meinl E, Schueler O, et al. Latent herpes virus infection in human trigeminal ganglia causes chronic immune response. *Am. J. Pathol.* 2003; **163**(6): 2179–84.

17 Okinaka Y, Sekitani T, Okazaki H, Miura M, Tahara T. Progress of caloric response of vestibular neuronitis. *Acta Otolaryngol. Suppl.* 1993; **503**: 18–22.

18 Minor LB, Schessel DA, Carey JP. Meniere's disease. *Curr. Opin. Neurol.* 2004; **17**(1): 9–16.

19 Green JD Jr, Blum DJ, Harner SG. Longitudinal followup of patients with Meniere's disease. *Otolaryngol. Head Neck Surg.* 1991; **104**(6): 783–8.

20 Yeh TH, Herman P, Tsai MC, Tran Ba Huy P, Van den Abbeele T. A cationic nonselective stretch-activated channel in the Reissner's membrane of the guinea pig cochlea. *Am. J. Physiol.* 1998; **274**(3 Pt 1): C566–76.

21 van Deelen GW, Huizing EH. Use of a diuretic (Dyazide) in the treatment of Meniere's disease. A double-blind cross-over placebo-controlled study. *ORL. J Otorhinolaryngol. Relat. Spec.* 1986; **48**(5): 287–92.

22 Smith WK, Sankar V, Pfleiderer AG. A national survey amongst UK otolaryngologists regarding the treatment of Meniere's disease. *J. Laryngol. Otol.* 2005; **119**(2): 102–5.

23 Simhadri S, Panda N, Raghunathan M. Efficacy of particle repositioning maneuver in BPPV: a prospective study. *Am. J. Otolaryngol.* 2003; **24**(6): 355–60.

24 Lynn S, Pool A, Rose D, Brey R, Suman V. Randomized trial of the canalith repositioning procedure. *Otolaryngol. Head Neck Surg.* 1995; **113**(6): 712–20.

25 Li JC, Li CJ, Epley J, Weinberg L. Cost-effective management of benign positional vertigo using canalith repositioning. *Otolaryngol. Head Neck Surg.* 2000; **122**(3): 334–9.

26 Brainin M, Barnes M, Baron JC, Gilhus NE, Hughes R, Selmaj K, et al. Guidance for the preparation of neurological management guidelines by EFNS scientific task forces – revised recommendations 2004. *Eur. J. Neurol.* 2004; **11**(9): 577–81.

27 Parnes LS, Price-Jones RG. Particle repositioning maneuver for benign paroxysmal positional vertigo. *Ann. Otol. Rhinol. Laryngol.* 1993; **102**(5): 325–31.

28 Li JC. Mastoid oscillation: a critical factor for success in canalith repositioning procedure. *Otolaryngol. Head Neck Surg.* 1995; **112**(6): 670–5.

29 Salvinelli F, Casale M, Trivelli M, D'Ascanio L, Firrisi L, Lamanna F, et al. Benign paroxysmal positional vertigo: a comparative prospective study on the efficacy of Semont's maneuver and no treatment strategy. *Clin. Ther.* 2003; **154**(1): 7–11.

30 Angeli SI, Hawley R, Gomez O. Systematic approach to benign paroxysmal positional vertigo in the elderly. *Otolaryngol. Head Neck Surg.* 2003; **128**(5): 719–25.

31 Soto Varela A, Bartual Magro J, Santos Perez S, Velez Regueiro M, Lechuga Garcia R, Perez-Carro Rios A, et al. Benign paroxysmal vertigo: a comparative prospective study of the efficacy of Brandt and Daroff exercises, Semont and Epley maneuver. *Rev. Laryngol. Otol. Rhinol. (Bord)* 2001; **122**(3): 179–83.

32 Sherman D, Massoud EA. Treatment outcomes of benign paroxysmal positional vertigo. *J. Otolaryngol.* 2001; **30**(5): 295–9.

33 Wolf M, Hertanu T, Novikov I, Kronenberg J. Epley's manoeuvre for benign paroxysmal positional vertigo: a prospective study. *Clin. Otolaryngol. Allied Sci.* 1999; **24**(1): 43–6.

34 Cohen HS, Kimball KT. Effectiveness of treatments for benign paroxysmal positional vertigo of the posterior canal. *Otol. Neurotol.* 2005; **26**(5): 1034–40.

35 Motamed M, Osinubi O, Cook JA. Effect of mastoid oscillation on the outcome of the canalith repositioning procedure. *Laryngoscope* 2004; **114**(7): 1296–8.

36 Asawavichianginda S, Isipradit P, Snidvongs K, Supiyaphun P. Canalith repositioning for benign paroxysmal positional vertigo: a randomized, controlled trial. *Ear Nose Throat J.* 2000; **79**(9): 732–4, 736–7.

37 Herdman SJ, Tusa RJ, Zee DS, Proctor LR, Mattox DE. Single treatment approaches to benign paroxysmal positional vertigo. *Arch. Otolaryngol. Head Neck Surg.* 1993; **119**(4): 450–4.

38 Froehling DA, Bowen JM, Mohr DN, Brey RH, Beatty CW, Wollan PC, et al. The canalith repositioning procedure for the treatment of benign paroxysmal positional vertigo: a randomized controlled trial. *Mayo Clin. Proc.* 2000; **75**(7): 695–700.

39 Hilton M, Pinder D. The Epley (canalith repositioning) manoeuvre for benign paroxysmal positional vertigo. *Cochrane Database Syst. Rev.* 2002; **1**: CD003162.

40 White J, Savvides P, Cherian N, Oas J. Canalith repositioning for benign paroxysmal positional vertigo. *Otol. Neurotol.* 2005; **26**(4): 704–10.

41 Steenerson RL, Cronin GW, Marbach PM. Effectiveness of treatment techniques in 923 cases of benign paroxysmal positional vertigo. *Laryngoscope* 2005; **115**(2): 226–31.

42 Monobe H, Sugasawa K, Murofushi T. The outcome of the canalith repositioning procedure for benign paroxysmal positional vertigo: are there any characteristic features of treatment failure cases? *Acta Otolaryngol. Suppl.* 2001; 545: 38–40.

43 Radtke A, von Brevern M, Tiel-Wilck K, Mainz-Perchalla A, Neuhauser H, Lempert T. Self-treatment of benign paroxysmal positional vertigo: Semont maneuver vs Epley procedure. *Neurology* 2004; **63**(1): 150–2.

44 Hain TC, Helminski JO, Reis IL, Uddin MK. Vibration does not improve results of the canalith repositioning procedure. *Arch. Otolaryngol. Head Neck Surg.* 2000; **126**(5): 617–22.

45 Nuti D, Nati C, Passali D. Treatment of benign paroxysmal positional vertigo: no need for postmaneuver restrictions. *Otolaryngol. Head Neck Surg.* 2000; **122**(3): 440–4.

46 Marciano E, Marcelli V. Postural restrictions in labyrintholithiasis. *Eur. Arch. Otorhinolaryngol.* 2002; **259**(5): 262–5.

47 Herdman SJ, Tusa RJ. Complications of the canalith repositioning procedure. *Arch. Otolaryngol. Head Neck Surg.* 1996; **122**(3): 281–6.

48 Epley JM. Positional vertigo related to semicircular canalithiasis. *Otolaryngol. Head Neck Surg.* 1995; **112**(1): 154–61.

49 Beynon GJ, Baguley DM, da Cruz MJ. Recurrence of symptoms following treatment of posterior semicircular canal benign positional paroxysmal vertigo with a particle repositioning manoeuvre. *J. Otolaryngol.* 2000; **29**(1): 2–6.

50 Sakaida M, Takeuchi K, Ishinaga H, Adachi M, Majima Y. Long-term outcome of benign paroxysmal positional vertigo. *Neurology* 2003; **60**(9): 1532–4.

51 Nunez RA, Cass SP, Furman JM. Short- and long-term outcomes of canalith repositioning for benign paroxysmal positional vertigo. *Otolaryngol. Head Neck Surg.* 2000; **122**(5): 647–52.

52 Macias JD, Ellensohn A, Massingale S, Gerkin R. Vibration with the canalith repositioning maneuver: a prospective randomized study to determine efficacy. *Laryngoscope* 2004; **114**(6): 1011–4.

53 Brandt T, Huppert D, Hecht J, Karch C, Strupp M. Benign paroxysmal positioning vertigo: a long-term follow-up (6–17 years) of 125 patients. *Acta Otolaryngol.* 2006 Feb; **126**(29): 160–163.

54 Katsarkas A, Kirkham TH. Paroxysmal positional vertigo – a study of 255 cases. *J. Otolaryngol.* 1978; **7**(4): 320–30.

55 Baloh RW, Honrubia V, Jacobson K. Benign positional vertigo: clinical and oculographic features in 240 cases. *Neurology* 1987; **37**(3): 371–8.

56 Kitahara T, Kondoh K, Morihana T, Okumura S, Horii A, Takeda N, et al. Steroid effects on vestibular compensation in human. *Neurol. Res.* 2003; **25**(3): 287–91.

57 Strupp M, Zingler VC, Arbusow V, Niklas D, Maag KP, Dieterich M, et al. Methylprednisolone, valacyclovir, or the combination for vestibular neuritis. *N. Engl. J. Med.* 2004; **351**(4): 354–61.

58 Jongkees LB, Maas JP, Philipszoon AJ. Clinical nystagmography. A detailed study of electro-nystagmography in 341 patients with vertigo. *Pract. Otorhinolaryngol. (Basel)* 1962; **24**: 65–93.

59 Igarashi M, Levy JK, Ou T, Reschke MF. Further study of physical exercise and locomotor balance compensation after unilateral labyrinthectomy in squirrel monkeys. *Acta Otolaryngol.* 1981; **92**(1–2): 101–5.

60 Mathog RH, Peppard SB. Exercise and recovery from vestibular injury. *Am. J. Otolaryngol.* 1982; **3**(6): 397–407.

61 Norre ME, Beckers AM. Vestibular habituation training. Specificity of adequate exercise. *Arch. Otolaryngol. Head Neck Surg.* 1988; **114**(8): 883–6.

62 Norre ME, Beckers A. Vestibular habituation training: exercise treatment for vertigo based upon the habituation effect. *Otolaryngol. Head Neck Surg.* 1989; **101**(1): 14–19.

63 Herdman SJ. *Vestibular Rehabilitation.* FA Davis, Philadelphia, 1994.

64 Strupp M, Arbusow V, Maag KP, Gall C, Brandt T. Vestibular exercises improve central vestibulospinal compensation after vestibular neuritis. *Neurology* 1998; **51**(3): 838–44.

65 Kammerlind AS, Ledin TE, Odkvist LM, Skargren EI. Effects of home training and additional physical therapy on recovery after acute unilateral vestibular loss – a randomized study. *Clin. Rehabil.* 2005; **19**(1): 54–62.

66 Magnusson M, Padoan S, Karlberg M, Johansson R. Delayed onset of ototoxic effects of gentamicin in treatment of Meniere's disease. *Acta Otolaryngol. Suppl.* 1991; **481**: 610–12.

67 Lange G, Maurer J, Mann W. Long-term results after interval therapy with intratympanic gentamicin for Meniere's disease. *Laryngoscope* 2004; **114**(1): 102–5.

68 Pearson BW, Brackmann DE. Committee on Hearing and Equilibrium guidelines for reporting treatment results in Meniere's disease. *Otolaryngol. Head Neck Surg.* 1985; **93**(5): 579–81.

69 Committee on Hearing and Equilibrium guidelines for the evaluation of hearing preservation in acoustic neuroma (vestibular schwannoma). American Academy of Otolaryngology-Head and Neck Surgery Foundation, INC. *Otolaryngol. Head Neck Surg.* 1995; **113**(3): 179–80.

70 Cohen-Kerem R, Kisilevsky V, Einarson TR, Kozer E, Koren G, Rutka JA. Intratympanic gentamicin for Meniere's disease: a meta-analysis. *Laryngoscope* 2004; **114**(12): 2085–91.

71 Carey JP, Hirvonen T, Peng GC, Della Santina CC, Cremer PD, Haslwanter T, et al. Changes in the angular vestibulo-ocular reflex after a single dose of intratympanic gentamicin for Meniere's disease. *Ann. NY Acad. Sci.* 2002; **956**: 581–4.

72 Wu IC, Minor LB. Long-term hearing outcome in patients receiving intratympanic gentamicin for Meniere's disease. *Laryngoscope* 2003; **113**(5): 815–20.

73 Perez N, Martin E, Garcia-Tapia R. Intratympanic gentamicin for intractable Meniere's disease. *Laryngoscope* 2003; **113**(3): 456–64.

74 Quaranta A, Scaringi A, Aloidi A, Quaranta N, Salonna I. Intratympanic therapy for Meniere's disease: effect of administration of low concentration of gentamicin. *Acta Otolaryngol.* 2001; **121**(3): 387–92.

75 Kaplan DM, Nedzelski JM, Chen JM, Shipp DB. Intratympanic gentamicin for the treatment of unilateral Meniere's disease. *Laryngoscope* 2000; **110**(8): 1298–305.

76 Minor LB. Intratympanic gentamicin for control of vertigo in Meniere's disease: vestibular signs that specify completion of therapy. *Am. J. Otolaryngol.* 1999; **20**(2): 209–19.

77 Silverstein H, Arruda J, Rosenberg SI, Deems D, Hester TO. Direct round window membrane application of gentamicin in the treatment of Meniere's disease. *Otolaryngol. Head Neck Surg.* 1999; **120**(5): 649–55.

78 Kaasinen S, Pyykko I, Ishizaki H, Aalto H. Intratympanic gentamicin in Meniere's disease. *Acta Otolaryngol.* 1998; **118**(3): 294–8.

79 Youssef TF, Poe DS. Intratympanic gentamicin injection for the treatment of Meniere's disease. *Am. J. Otol.* 1998; **19**(4): 435–42.

80 Meyer ED. [Treatment of Meniere disease with betahistine dimesilate (Aequamen) – double-blind study versus placebo (crossover)]. *Laryngol. Rhinol. Otol. (Stuttg)* 1985; **64**(5): 269–72.

81 Claes J, Van de Heyning PH. Medical treatment of Meniere's disease: a review of literature. *Acta Otolaryngol. Suppl.* 1997; **526**: 37–42.

82 James A, Thorp M. Meniere's disease. *Clin. Evid.* 2004; (11): 664–72.

83 James AL, Burton MJ. Betahistine for Meniere's disease or syndrome. *Cochrane Database Syst. Rev.* 2001; Issue 1. Art. No.: CD001873. DOI: 1002/14641858. CD001873.

84 Dziadziola JK, Laurikainen EL, Rachel JD, Quirk WS. Betahistine increases vestibular blood flow. *Otolaryngol. Head Neck Surg.* 1999; **120**(3): 400–5.

85 Strupp M, Brandt T. Pharmacological advances in the treatment of neuro-otological and eye movement disorders. *Curr. Opin. Neurol.* 2006; **19**(1): 33–40.

CHAPTER 9
Sleep disorders

Michel Billiard

Background

Recent years have been marked by a renewed interest of neurologists in sleep disorders, not only primary sleep disorders such as narcolepsy with or without cataplexy, idiopathic hypersomnia with or without long sleep time, restless legs syndrome, but also sleep disorders associated with neurological conditions such as rapid eye movement (REM) sleep behaviour disorder predominantly in synucleinopathies, obstructive sleep apnoea syndrome in stroke patients or in neurodegenerative conditions, etc.

Framing clinical questions

In this chapter five different issues will be referred to: obstructive sleep apnoea syndrome in stroke patients, due to the high incidence of the phenomenon and the unsettled therapeutic attitude; narcolepsy, given the recent discovery of the role of the loss or dysfunction of hypocretin/orexin neurons, both in animal models and in humans, and the emergence of a renewed treatment, sodium oxybate; idiopathic hypersomnia in consideration of the recent distinction between idiopathic hypersomnia with and without long sleep time; REM sleep behaviour disorder (RBD) due to its frequently outdating appearance of daytime symptoms of Parkinson's disease and other synucleinopathies, and insomnia in Parkinson's disease, because of its numerous aetiological factors and the complexity of treatment.

Critical review of evidence

1. Sleep disordered breathing and stroke

1 *What are the consequences of sleep disordered breathing on the severity and outcome of stroke?*
2 *What is the adequate treatment in a stroke patient diagnosed with obstructive sleep apnoea syndrome?*
3 *What is the outcome of stroke patients with obstructive sleep apnoea syndrome treated with continuous positive airway pressure (CPAP)?*

Stroke is the leading cause of disability among adults and the prevalence of sleep disordered breathing in patients with acute ischaemic stroke is fairly high (30–70%). This is of major importance as it has been evidenced that sleep disordered breathing is strongly associated with increased risk of stroke, independent of other known risk factors.

Scenario

A 66-year-old male shopkeeper was brought into the emergency room after being found on the floor, at the foot of his bed, unable to move his left side. Physical examination revealed a complete left hemiplegia equally involving face, arm and leg, and marked inattention to the left side of the body. Speech was normal and the patient was fully oriented. There appeared to be sensory deficit on the left to pinch, touch and to vibration, although examination was difficult because of neglect of that side. Reflexes were decreased on the left and left plantar response was extensive. General examination was remarkable for slight obesity, 83 kg, 1.72 m, body mass index (BMI) 28.1. Blood pressure was 160/100, pulse 80 and regular. Neck was short and enlarged and spouse's interview disclosed loud snoring, nycturia, marked fatigue on awakening and excessive daytime sleepiness for several years. Early computed tomography (CT) scan revealed a decrease in the size of the right lateral ventricle compatible with early swelling of the right hemisphere. There was no contrast enhancement. Polysomnography demonstrated a high respiratory disturbance index of 44 respiratory events per hour of sleep, mainly obstructive sleep apnoeas, with a mean oxyhemoglobine saturation of 91% and a minimum of 81%.

Evidence

1 Sleep disordered breathing accompanied by arterial oxyhemoglobine desaturation appears to be associated with higher mortality at 1 year and lower Barthel index scores at discharge and at 3 and 12 months after stroke [1].
2 Only a few studies are available on the effects of CPAP in patients with sleep disordered breathing and stroke. In one trial (non-randomized) the effectiveness of nasal CPAP was studied in 105 stroke patients (75 males, 30 females) with a polysomnographically confirmed diagnosis of obstructive sleep apnoea syndrome (respiratory disturbance index >15) [2]. Thirty-one patients (29.5%) rejected CPAP during the titration or shortly after, while 74 (70.5%) tolerated it and continued treatment at home. Subjective well-being was measured with a visual analogue scale in 41 unselected patients, and 24-h

blood pressure in 16 patients before and after 10 days of treatment. Differences were compared between patients who did and did not accept treatment. Among the 41 unselected patients the compliant users ($n = 28$) showed a clear improvement in well-being ($P = 0.021$) in comparison with the 13 patients without acceptance; among the 16 patients, 11 showed a high compliance while 5 did not use CPAP. Only the compliant patients had a reduction in mean nocturnal blood pressure. In a second trial 63 patients consecutively admitted to a stroke rehabilitation unit 2–4 weeks after a stroke, with an apnoea/hypopnoea index ≥15, were randomized to either CPAP treatment ($n = 33$) or a control group ($n = 30$) [3]. Both groups were assessed at baseline and after 7 and 28 nights using the Montgomery-Asberg-Depression-Rating Scale (MADRS), Mini-Mental State Examination (MMSE) scale and Barthel-ADL index. Compared to controls, depressive symptoms (MADRS) improved in patients randomized to CPAP treatment ($P = 0.004$). On the other hand no significant treatment effect was found with regard to delirium, MMSE and Barthel-ADL index. Finally a recent study prospectively analysed the role of long-term CPAP treatment in protecting stroke patients from new vascular events [4]. A total of 51 patients with an apnoea–hypopnoea index (AHI) ≥ 20 were included. Two groups were defined: patients who could tolerate CPAP ($n = 15$) and patients who could not tolerate CPAP after 1 month of initial adaptation ($n = 36$). The incidence of new vascular events, evaluated through a follow-up of 18 months, was 6.7% in the patients who tolerated CPAP and 36% in those who did not tolerate CPAP, indicating that CPAP treatment afforded significant protection against new vascular events after ischaemic stroke. Worth mentioning is an ongoing trial investigating the role of nasal CPAP in the treatment of sleep disordered breathing in patients who have recently suffered a stroke [5].

3 CPAP, the main medical therapy for patients with sleep apnoeas is in theory the most relevant therapy for sleep apnoea in stroke patients. However compliance with CPAP treatment is a problem in stroke patients, specially when delirium and severe cognitive impairment occurs. Also of concern are a low functional status, as measured by the Barthel index, and the presence of aphasia. Generally speaking CPAP treatment in stroke patients requires much support from nurses or family.

In conclusion CPAP treatment brings some improvement in stroke patients affected with sleep-disordered breathing. This improvement concerns well-being, mood and protection against new vascular events. On the other hand delirium, mental state and Barthel-ADL index are not affected by CPAP treatment.

2. Narcolepsy with and without cataplexy

1 *In a subject suspect of narcolepsy with cataplexy, which tests should be performed prior to treatment?*

2 *Which treatment should be implemented? Among patients with narcolepsy with or without cataplexy, how does pharmacological treatments affect the probability for reducing daytime sleepiness and/or cataplexy?*

3 *Which main difficulties can occur with time in relation with the treatment?*

Narcolepsy with cataplexy is primarily characterized by excessive daytime sleepiness and cataplexy. Excessive daytime sleepiness is usually the most disabling symptom and the first one to occur. It is characterized by episodes of naps or lapses into sleep across the daytime. Cataplexy, a unique feature of the condition, is characterized by sudden loss of bilateral muscle tone provoked by strong emotions that are usually positive, such as a fit of laughter, receiving a compliment, humour expressed by the subject, the sight of prey for the hunter, a well-caught ball, and less often negative, that is anger or stress. Sleep paralysis, hypnagogic hallucinations and nocturnal sleep disruption commonly occur in patients with narcolepsy with cataplexy. These three symptoms, however, can occasionally, occur in normal people.

Narcolepsy without cataplexy is a minor phenotype of the same condition. Narcolepsy with cataplexy affects 20–40/100,000 of the European and North-American population, depending on the methodology of the surveys. Studies using both questionnaires and polysomnography find lower prevalence of the condition than those relying on questionnaire only. Both sexes are affected with some preponderance of males. Narcolepsy without cataplexy is less frequent, but no prevalence study is available. The natural history of narcolepsy varies considerably with subjects. In most cases excessive daytime sleepiness and irresistible sleep episodes persist throughout the lifetime, although they tend to improve with advancing age. Cataplexy may vanish with age and even spontaneously disappear in some patients. Nocturnal sleep does not improve with age.

Clinical scenario

A 32-year-old secretary complained of excessive daytime sleepiness and irresistible episodes of sleep occurring daily or almost daily for the last year. The interview quickly showed that she had cataplexy at a rate of approximately one attack per week and hypnagogic hallucinations. The diagnosis of narcolepsy with cataplexy was confirmed by an all-night polysomnography followed by a multiple sleep latency test (MSLT) showing three sleep onset REM periods (SOREMPs). This woman is on the verge of being fired due to falling asleep at work.

Evidence

1 Narcolepsy can be diagnosed on purely clinical grounds. However additional tests are useful to confirm the diagnosis. Most commonly, nocturnal polysomnography followed by a MSLT is recommended, and, in a few selected cases, measurement of cerebrospinal fluid (CSF) levels of hypocretin-1. In all-night polysomnography, a SOREMP is observed in 25–50%

Table 9.1 Treatment of excessive daytime sleepiness.

Reference	Methods	Participants	Interventions	Outcome measures	Outcome
Billiard et al. (1994)	12-week, placebo-controlled trial. Crossover design	50 narcolepsy with cataplexy subjects	Modafinil, 300 mg (2 divided doses) 100 mg in a.m. and 200 mg at noon or vice versa	Maintenance of Wakefulness Test (MWT) Global Symptoms Index (GSI)	Modafinil improves daytime sleepiness
Broughton et al. (1997)	6-week, randomized placebo-controlled trial. Crossover design	75 narcoleptic subjects	Modafinil 200 or 400 mg in divided doses (morning and noon), versus placebo	MWT Epworth Sleepiness Scale (ESS)	Modafinil effective in keeping narcolepy patients awake
US Modafinil in Narcolepsy Study Group (1998)	9-week, randomized placebo-controlled trial	283 narcoleptic subjects	Modafinil 200 or 400 mg, versus placebo, followed by an open-label treatment period	ESS MSLT MWT GSI	Modafinil 200 mg and 400 mg significantly reduced all measures of sleepiness
US Modafinil in Narcolepsy Study Group (2000)	9-week, randomized placebo-controlled trial	271 narcoleptic subjects	Modafinil 200 or 400 mg versus placebo	MSLT MWT ESS	Effective for treatment of daytime sleepiness in narcolepsy for 9 weeks
US Xyrem Multicenter Study Group (2002)	4-week, randomized placebo-controlled trial	136 narcolepsy with cataplexy subjects	Sodium oxybate, 3, 6, or 9 g, versus placebo	Daily diaries (n° of inadvertent naps/sleep attacks) ESS Clinical Global Impression of Change (CGI-c)	Frequency of inadvertent naps/sleep attacks and nightime awakenings, reduced at all doses, becoming significant at the 9 g dose ESS reduced at all doses, becoming significant at the 9 g dose CGI-c demonstrated a dose-related improvement, significant at the 9 g dose
US Xyrem Multicenter Study Group (2003)	12-month, open-label trial	118 narcolepsy with cataplexy subjects previously enrolled in a 4-week double-blind sodium oxybate trial	Sodium oxybate 6 g nightly, taken in equally divided doses at bedtime and 2.5–4 h later. The study protocol permitted the dose to be increased or decreased in 1.5 g increments at 2 week intervals, based on efficacy response or adverse experiences, but staying within the range of 3–9 g nightly	Daily diaries (n° of inadvertent naps/sleep attacks) ESS CGI-c	Overall improvement in excessive daytime sleepiness, which were significant at 4 weeks and maximal after 8 weeks

Table 9.2 Treatment of cataplexy.

Reference	Methods	Participants	Interventions	Outcome measures	Outcome
The US Xyrem Multicenter Study Group (2002)	4-week, randomized placebo-controlled trial	136 narcolepsy with cataplexy subjects	Sodium oxybate, 3, 6, or 9 g, versus placebo	Daily diaries (n° of cataplectic attacks) CGI-c	Weekly cataplectic attacks were decreased by sodium oxybate at the 6 g dose and significantly at the 9 g dose CGI-c demonstrated a dose-related improvement, significant at the 9 g dose
US Xyrem Multicenter Study Group (2003)	Method: 12-month, open-label trial	118 narcolepsy subjects previously enrolled in a 4-week double-blind sodium oxybate trial	Sodium oxybate 6 g nightly, taken in equally divided doses at bedtime and 2.5–4 h later. The study protocol permitted the dose to be increased or decreased in 1.5 g increments at 2-week intervals based on efficacy response or adverse experiences, but staying within the range of 3–9 g nightly	Daily diaries (n° of cataplexy attacks) CGI-c	Significant decrease in frequency of cataplexy attacks
US Xyrem Multicenter Study Group (2004)	Double-blind treatment withdrawal paradigm in patients who had received continuous treatment with sodium oxybate for 7–44 months (mean 21 months)	55 narcolepsy with cataplexy subjects	Subjects enrolled in a 2-week single-blind sodium oxybate treatment phase to establish a baseline for the weekly occurrence of cataplexy, followed by a 2-week double-blind phase in which patients were randomized to receive unchanged drug therapy versus placebo	Daily diaries (n° of cataplexy attacks)	The abrupt cessation of sodium oxybate therapy in the placebo patients resulted in a significant increase in the number of cataplexy attacks compared to patients who remained on sodium oxybate
Xyrem International Study Group (2005)	8-week, double-blind, placebo-controlled	22 narcolepsy with cataplexy subjects	Subjects randomized to receive 4.5, 6 or 9 g sodium oxybate nightly for 8 weeks versus placebo	Daily diaries (n° of cataplexy attacks)	Compared to placebo, nightly doses of 4.5, 6 and 9 g sodium oxybate resulted in statistically significant median decreases in weekly cataplexy attacks of 57.0%, 65.0% and 84.7%, respectively. The decrease in cataplexy at the 4.5 g dose represented a novel finding

of cases of narcolepsy with cataplexy and is a highly specific finding. In addition a disruption of the normal sleep pattern with repeated awakenings is a frequent feature. The MSLT demonstrates a mean sleep latency of less than 8 min and two or more SOREMPs. However a few typical cases of narcolepsy may have only one SOREMP or even none, specially in elderly subjects. Measuring CSF levels of hypocretin-1 is highly specific and sensitive for the diagnosis of narcolepsy with cataplexy. Values below 110 pg/mL are found in approximately 90% of cases of narcolepsy with cataplexy. However due to the limited number of laboratories providing this service, the test should be used in a few selected indications only: need to objectively document a diagnosis when the MSLT cannot be used; already treated patients if the diagnosis is in doubt; in young children and in cases with associated psychiatric or neurological disorders. This test is of much less value in narcolepsy without cataplexy as only 10% of patients show low values [6].

2 The two more recently introduced treatments of excessive daytime sleepiness, modafinil and sodium oxybate, are the most commonly used agents in newly diagnosed narcoleptic patients (Table 9.1, [7–12]). Modafinil is given at a daily dose of 400 mg (range 100–400 mg), with one dose in the morning and one dose early in the afternoon. One of the major advantages of modafinil is its relative lack of adverse effects. It can be administered concurrently with anticataplectic medications without problems. Sodium oxybate (not yet registered for excessive daytime sleepiness in Europe) is taken orally upon getting into bed and again 2.5–4 h later. The current recommended starting dose is 4.5 g/day divided into two equal dose of 2.25 g. The dose may be increased to a maximum of 9 g/day by increments of 1.5 g. Two weeks are recommended between dosage increments. In addition to either modafinil or sodium oxybate, behavioural measures are always advisable, the main recommandation being to take naps during the day, on a patient-by-patient basis. Previous treatments included methylphenidate, 10–60 mg/day, and in case of non-response, dextroamphetamine or methamphetamine under close control.

Treatment of cataplexy relies on sodium oxybate with the same mode of administration already recommended for excessive daytime sleepiness (Table 9.2, [11–14]). Second line treatments include tricyclic antidepressants, mainly clomipramine selective serotonine reuptake inhibitors (SSRIs), such as fluoxetine or fluvoxamine, a norepinephrine uptake inhibitor, viloxazine, a norepinephrine and serotonine uptake inhibitor, venlafaxine. However the use of these drugs is based on no or few randomized, placebo-controlled clinical trials, and none of them is registered forcataplexy except clomipramine in few European countries.

Benzodiazepines or non-benzodiazepine hypnotics may be effective in consolidating sleep. Unfortunately objective evidence is lacking over intermediate or long-term follow-up. According to US Xyrem studies [11–12], a significant decrease

of nighttime awakenings is obtained with sodium oxybate 3–9 g, given in two doses, one at bedtime and another one during the night.

3 As already pointed out adverse effects are limited with modafinil. Headache is the most common complaint followed by nausea, rhinitis and nervousness. As for sodium oxybate most commonly reported adverse effects include vomiting, incontinence, sleepwalking and confusion, in a limited number of cases. However some patients do not respond to stimulants or to anticataplectic drugs or both; some patients show an insufficient response and in some patients an originally good response progressively fades out with time. This is the reason why novel therapies are in a phase of research, either hypocretin-based therapies (peptide agonists, non-peptide agonists and cell transplantation or gene therapy) or immune-based therapies (steroid therapies, intravenous-immunoglobulins or plasmapheresis [15].

3. Idiopathic hypersomnia with and without long sleep time

1 *In a subject complaining of excessive daytime sleepiness, prolonged night sleep and difficulty in awakening, which diagnosis should be evoked and which tests should be performed?*
2 *Which treatment should be established?*
3 *What is the outcome of the treatment of idiopathic hypersomnia with long sleep time?*

There are two types of idiopathic hypersomnia, idiopathic hypersomnia with long sleep time and idiopathic hypersomnia without long sleep time. Idiopathic hypersomnia with long sleep time is remarkable for three symptoms: a complaint of constant or recurrent daily excessive sleepiness and unwanted nap(s), longer and less irresistible than in narcolepsy and non-refreshing regardless of their duration; night sleep is sound, uninterrupted and prolonged; morning awakening is laborious and sometimes referred to as sleep drunkenness; associated symptoms suggesting an autonomic nervous system dysfunction, such as cold hands and feet, light headedness on standing up, fainting episodes and headache, are not uncommon. Idiopathic hypersomnia without long sleep time stands as isolated excessive daytime sleepiness. Daytime sleep episodes may be more irresistible and more refreshing than in idiopathic hypersomnia with long sleep time, establishing a bridge with narcolepsy without cataplexy. Abnormally long sleep or sleep drunkenness are not features of the condition.

Due to long standing nosological uncertainty and the relative rarity of the condition, prevalence studies have not been conducted so far. However a ratio of one to two patients with idiopathic hypersomnia, either with or without long sleep time, for every 10 with narcolepsy, is suggested from clinical series.

Clinical scenario
A 24-year-old department manager working on morning shift (6:00–14:00) was referred for great difficulty waking up in the

morning. He first got remarks from his superiors and is now on the verge of being fired. This is all the more upsetting to him as he had good marks in his job when he was working on the afternoon shift and had no problem being in time at his work. The subject developed excessive daytime sleepiness and difficulty waking up in the morning during late adolescence. He reports having to be awakened by his parents with major difficulty. Today he lives alone. He does not wake up to the ringing of the alarm clock or to the wake up call. He has to use a repeating alarm clock and when he eventually wakes up he is almost confused, very slow and unable to react adequately to any event. During daytime he complains of being more or less drowsy, and when he takes an afternoon nap he may sleep for up to 3–4 h experiencing the same difficulty to wake up.

Evidence

1 The scenario refers to a typical case of idiopathic hypersomnia with long sleep time. However laboratory tests are essential to confirm the diagnosis and rule out other hypersomnia conditions. Polysomnographic monitoring of nocturnal sleep demonstrates normal sleep except for its prolonged duration. Non-REM (NREM) sleep and REM sleep are in normal proportions. The MSLT demonstrates a mean sleep latency less than 8 min, with some exceptions however, and less than two SOREMPs. However the MSLT seems questionable. Indeed, awakening the patient in the morning in view of the first session of the test precludes documenting the abnormally prolonged night sleep, and the MSLT sessions preclude recording of prolonged unrefreshing daytime sleep episode(s) of major diagnostic value. Thus other procedures are of potential interest: a 1-week actigraphy or a 24-h continuous polysomnography on an ad-lib sleep/wake protocol. Differential diagnosis includes upper airway resistance syndrome, hence the need for monitoring oesophageal pressure during sleep in the case of multiple arousals documented on polysomnography; narcolepsy without cataplexy characterized by the presence of two or more SOREMPs on the MSLT; hypersomnia associated with psychiatric disorder, in which the complaint of excessive daytime sleepiness is rather similar to that of idiopathic hypersomnia with long sleep time, with the exception of frequent poor sleep at night and normal sleep latency on the MSLT; post-traumatic hypersomnia in which past-history is remarkable for recent severe head traumatism; hypersomnia following a viral infection such as pneumonia, infectious mononucleosis or Guillain–Barré syndrome, where hypersomnia develops within months after the infection; chronic fatigue syndrome characterized by persistent or relapsing fatigue not resolving with sleep or rest and polysomnography with frequent evidence of alpha intrusion into sleep electroencephalogram (EEG).

2 Historically the only medications, that have often brought partial or intermittent relief, have been the stimulants, particularly methylphenidate and amphetamine. Randomized, placebo-controlled trials are lacking in idiopathic hypersomnia

with long sleep time and idiopathic hypersomnia without long sleep time. The only available study is an open-label study of modafinil in 18 patients with idiopathic hypersomnia taken globally, dating back to 1988 [16]. In this study the clinical diagnosis was confirmed by a 24-h polysomnography. Drowsiness and sleep episodes were evaluated through sleep diary data. During the second month of treatment drowsiness and sleep episodes were significantly reduced. However duration of night sleep and difficulty in awakening were not considered. Apart from this study there are some clinical reports of morning sleep drunkenness being reduced by administering a small dose of stimulant in the evening or immediately after morning awakening. In addition a recent study reported decreased sleep drunkenness, shortened nocturnal sleep duration and relieved daytime sleepiness in five out of ten subjects with idiopathic hypersomnia with long sleep time treated with melatonin (2 mg of slow release melatonin administered at bedtime) [17].

Behavioural treatment possibilities are limited. Naps are of no help as they are both lengthy and non-refreshing. 'Saturating' the subjects with sleep on weekends has been recommended, but does not seem to have a sustained effect.

3 The prognosis for spontaneous improvement of idiopathic hypersomnia is poor. The condition almost always has a stationary course and persists into old age. Clinical experience indicates that modafinil has a sustained effect in some subjects while its effects vanish with time in others.

4. RBD in Parkinson's disease

1 *In a subject with RBD what are the main actions to engage before starting a treatment?*

2 *What are the available treatments of RBD?*

3 *What is the outcome of RBD with the various treatments available?*

RBD is characterized by abnormal behaviours emerging during REM sleep that cause injury or sleep disruption. RBD is associated with electromyographic (EMG) abnormalities during REM sleep. The EMG demonstrates an excess of muscle tone or phasic EMG twitching activity during REM sleep. There are two forms of RBD, an idiopathic form and a form associated with neurological disorders, mainly synucleinopathies, narcolepsy and other neurological conditions. The most remarkable aspect of the association between synucleinopathies and RBD is that the latter can precede the development of the former by years. Idiopathic RBD is becoming progressively scarce (and may cease to exist) as more patients with RBD are being thoroughly evaluated and meticulously followed for prolonged periods. RBD is a male predominant disorder that usually emerges after the age of 50 years. The prevalence is not known. In a study aimed at evaluating the frequency of RBD in a large group of unselected patients with Parkinson's disease, one-third of patients with Parkinson's disease met the diagnostic criteria of RBD based on polysomnographic recordings. Only one half of these cases could have been detected by history.

Clinical scenario

A 66-year-old architect was referred for a 7-year history of progressively severe and injurious dream-enacting behaviour. He would frequently kick the wall, punch his pillow and sometimes bit his wife in bed or grab her by the hair while dreaming that he was confronted or attacked by unfamiliar people or animals. One night while dreaming that his daughter was attacked by a man he violently punched his wife. This patient was diagnosed recently with Parkinson's disease. Overnight polysomnography demonstrated classic RBD findings with intermittent loss of REM atonia and increased phasic twitching during REM sleep of the submental, anterior tibialis, and extensor digitorum muscles.

Evidence

1 Thorough evaluation for an underlying neurological disorder, particularly synucleinopathy (Parkinson's disease, multiple system atrophy and dementia with Lewy bodies) that may develop years later, narcolepsy or another neurological-condition. Also, given medications being recognized as an increasingly precipitating factor, to screen for venlafaxine, SSRI, mirtazapine and other antidepressant agents.

2 The most frequently prescribed treatment of RBD is clonazepam. Treatment is usually immediately active at a dose of 0.5–1.0 mg at bedtime [18]. Despite the dramatic control of clinical symptoms, clonazepam has little effect on the characteristic polysomnographic REM sleep abnormalities. Clonazepam is generally effective and safe. All instances of drug discontinuation result in prompt relapse. An alternative treatment is desirable for those with RBD refractory to clonazepam, for those who experience disturbing adverse effects, mainly excessive daytime sleepiness or ataxia, for those who develop tolerance and for those in whom clonazepam aggravates obstructive sleep apnoea syndrome. In these subjects melatonin is of definite value. According to Boeve et al. RBD was either controlled or significantly improved in 10 out of 14 patients, at doses of 3–12 mg [19]. The mean duration of follow-up was 14 months (range 9–25 months), with eight patients experiencing continued benefit with melatonin beyond 12 months of therapy. However five patients reported adverse effects, morning headaches in two, morning sleepiness in two and delirium/hallucinations in one. These symptoms resolved with decreased dosage. Another possibility is pramipexole, a dopaminergic D2–D3 receptor agonist, which was shown to be active in five out of eight patients with apparent idiopathic RBD [20].

3 Long-term outcome of RBD with available medications are the following. The main risk of clonazepam is the development of tolerance although little evidence of it was reported in the clinical outcome of 70 consecutive cases with RBD [18]. As for melatonin the actual risk of protracted consumption remains unknown. Preliminary observations suggest that long-term melatonin administration is associated with decreased semen quality, but the antigonadal effects of exogenous melatonin on the reproductive hormones are not conclusively established.

5. Insomnia in Parkinson's disease

1 *In Parkinson's disease patients what should be done first for those complaining of insomnia?*
2 *In this particular patient which therapeutic programme can be proposed?*
3 *What is the outcome of insomnia?*

Parkinson's disease is primarily a disease of the elderly. The prevalence increases with age from 0.9% among persons 65–69 years old to 5% among persons 80–84 years old. Sleep problems are common. In one series of insomniac patients with Parkinson's disease, 67% had difficulty initiating sleep and 88% had difficulty maintaining sleep. Insomnia in Parkinson's disease patients may depend on several factors, including Parkinson's disease related motor symptoms occurring at night, use of drugs altering sleep, psychiatric symptoms and specially depression, dementia and other sleep disorders.

Scenario

A 65-year-old retired bus driver, affected with Parkinson's disease for 7 years, was referred for insomnia. The subject complained of frequent awakenings throughout the night, specially in the second half of it, of decreased total sleep time and of daytime fatigue. Moreover, the interview of the subject revealed awakenings associated with paraesthesias of the legs forcing him to get up and walk around. On examination the subject was very slow in his movements and often sat motionless with an expressionless face. His right hand shook. There was cogwheel rigidity of his right wrist and a shuffling gait. Wearing off had developed within the last 6 months. There was no obvious cognitive impairment but some degree of depression. The treatment was carbidopa/levodopa (Sinemet) 250 mg × 4, ropinirole 3 mg × 4 and zolpidem one tablet at night.

Evidence

1 Given the plurality of possible contributing factors, it is of utmost importance to assess the respective part of each of the factors involved in the insomnia of a Parkinson's disease patient. Parkinson's disease related nocturnal motor symptoms most often reflect the presence of motor fluctuations («on off» phenomena, «wearing off») during the day and are often due to nocturnal underdosage of dopamine drugs. In addition nocturia and urinary incontinence may participate in the disturbance of sleep. Accordingly, a careful description from both the patient and his (her) spouse is essential to determine the behaviour of the patient during the night. Drug regimen and the time of day when drugs are taken must be considered, given their ability to alter sleep patterns in patients with Parkinson's disease. Another issue is a frequent underlying depression and/or cognitive impairment which are associated with sleep fragmentation and sleep-wake cycle disruption. Finally Parkinson's disease patients may suffer from other sleep disorders such as restless legs syndrome, obstructive sleep apnoea syndrome or RBD. Polysomnography may be indicated in some cases.

2 The severity of nocturnal disturbances in Parkinson's disease patients contrasts with the paucity of clinical trials specifically designed for the treatment of these Parkinson's disease related sleep disturbances. In the above referred scenario Parkinson's disease related motor symptoms were obviously important, particularly in the second half of the night. Consequently, adding a small dose of dopaminergic medication at bedtime such as 100 mg of L-dopa combined with 25 mg of carbidopa (Sinemet 25/100), with a second similar dose at 2 or 3 a.m. if the patient awakens is a possible option. Alternatively a bedtime dose of a controlled release formulation containing 200 mg of L-dopa and 50 mg of carbidopa can be proposed [21–22]. Moreover, adding a catechol-O-methyltransferase (COMT) inhibitor may be useful to provide a long-acting antiparkinsonism benefit. Due to the variability of response to dopaminergic medications, trials of several different agents in varying doses are usually warranted if sleep is not improved. Of note is that dopaminergic medications may induce sleep problems such as vivid dreams or nightmares. In addition, this patient was probably affected with restless legs syndrome responsible for awakenings with paraesthesias of the legs. However, the patient was already under dopamine agonists which have been proved to be effective in treating restless legs syndrome and the dose required to treat restless legs syndrome tends to be lower than that used to treat motor symptoms of Parkinson's disease [23]. Finally treatment of the associated depression may lead to an improvement of nocturnal disturbances. One possibility is tricyclic antidepressants. SSRIs can also be an option but they have an activating effect and tend to increase disruption of normal sleep architecture [24].

3 The global evaluation of nocturnal disturbances and the chosen therapeutic intervention should improve the nocturnal disturbances experienced by this patient. However it must be kept in mind that management of nocturnal disturbances may sometimes be at the expense of some other symptoms of Parkinson's disease, to the point that it may be advisable in some cases not to treat nocturnal disturbances.

Conclusion

Much effort has been put in further identifying sleep disorders and sleep disorders associated with neurological conditions, and in designing relevant laboratory tests. On the other hand most of the available therapeutic interventions refer to common sense-based practice and there is still an urgent need for randomized-controlled trials in many areas of sleep disorders, to assess the validity of the current interventions.

References

1 Good DC, Henkle JQ, Gelber D, et al. Sleep-disordered breathing and poor functional outcome after stroke. *Stroke* 1996; **27**: 252–9.

2 Wessendorf TE, Wang YM, Thilmann AF, et al. Treatment of obstructive sleep apnoea with nasal continuous positive airway pressure in stroke. *Eur. Respir. J.* 2001; **18**: 623–9.

3 Sandberg O, Franklin KA, Bucht G, et al. Nasal continuous positive airway pressure in stroke patients with sleep apnoea: a randomized treatment study. *Eur. Respir. J.* 2001; **18**: 630–4.

4 Martinez-Garcia MA, Galiano-Blancart R, Roman-Sanchez P, et al. Continuous positive airway pressure treatment in sleep apnea prevents new vascular events after ischemic stroke. *Chest* 2005; **128**: 2123–9.

5 Douglas NJ. Investigating the role of nasal continuous positive airway pressure (nCPAP) in the treatment of sleep disordered breathing (SDB) in patients who have recently suffered a stroke. *National Research Register Document* 2001, Issue 1.

6 Mignot E, Lammers GJ, Ripley B, et al. The role of cerebrospinal fluid hypocretin measurement in the diagnosis of narcolepsy and other hypersomnias. *Arch. Neurol.* 2002; **59**: 1553–62.

7 Billiard M, Besset A, Montplaisir J, et al. Modafinil: a double blind multicenter study. *Sleep* 1994; **17**(Suppl.): S107–12.

8 Broughton R, Fleming JAE, Georges CFP, et al. Randomized, double blind, placebo-controlled crossover trial of modafinil in the treatment of excessive daytime sleepiness in narcolepsy. *Neurology* 1997; **49**: 444–51.

9 US Modafinil in Narcolepsy Multicenter Study Group. Randomized trial of modafinil for the treatment of pathological somnolence in narcolepsy. *Ann. Neurol.* 1998; **434**: 88–97.

10 US Modafinil in Narcolepsy Multicenter Study Group. Randomized trial of modafinil as a treatment for the excessive daytime somnolence of narcolepsy. *Neurology* 2000; **54**: 1166–75.

11 US Xyrem Multicenter Study Group. A randomized, double-blind, placebo-controlled multicenter trial comparing the effects of three doses of orally administered sodium oxybate with placebo for the treatment of narcolepsy. *Sleep* 2002; **25**: 42–9.

12 US Xyrem Multicenter Study Group. A 12-month, open-label multi-center extension trial of orally administered sodium oxybate for the treatment of narcolepsy. *Sleep* 2003; **26**: 31–5.

13 US Xyrem Multicenter Study Group. Sodium oxybate demonstrates long-term efficacy for the treatment of cataplexy in patients with narcolepsy. *Sleep Med.* 2004; **5**: 119–23.

14 Xyrem International Study Group. Further evidence supporting the use of sodium oxybate for the treatment of cataplexy: a double-blind placebo-controlled study in 228 patients. *Sleep Med.* 2005; **6**: 415–21.

15 Mignot E, Nishino S. Perspectives for new treatments. In: Bassetti C, Billiard M & Mignot E, eds., *Narcolepsy and Hypersomnias*, Marcel Dekker, in press.

16 Bastuji H, Jouvet M. Successful treatment of idiopathic hypersomnia and narcolepsy with modafinil. *Prog. Neuropsychopharmacol. Biol. Psychiat.* 1988; **12**: 695–700.

17 Montplaisir J, Fantini L. Idiopathic hypersomnia. A diagnostic dilemma. *Sleep Med. Rev.* 2001; **5**: 361–2.

18 Schenck CH, Mahowald MW. Polysomnographic, neurologic, psychiatric, and clinical outcome report on 70 consecutive cases with REM sleep behavior disorder (RBD): sustained clonazepam efficacy in 89.5% of 57 treated patients. *Cleve. Clin. J. Med.* 1990; **57**(Suppl.): S9–S23.

19 Boeve BF, Silber MH, Ferman TJ. Melatonin for treatment of REM sleep behaviour disorder in neurologic disorders: results in 14 patients. *Sleep Med.* 2003; **4**: 281–4.

20 Fantini ML, Gagnon JF, Filipini MD, et al. The effects of pramipexole in REM sleep behavior disorder. *Neurology* 2003; **61**: 1418–20.

21 Jansen EN, Meerwaldt JD. Madopar HBS in nocturnal symptoms of Parkinson's disease. *Adv. Neurol.* 1990; **53**: 527–31.

22 Pahwa R, Busenbark K, Huber SJ, et al. Clinical experience with controlled-release carbidopa/levodopa in Parkinson's disease. *Neurology* 1993; **43**: 677–81.

23 Garcia-Borreguero D, Odin P, Serrano C. Restless legs syndrome and PD: a review of the evidence for a possible association. *Neurology* 2003; **61**(Suppl. 3): S49–55.

24 Movement Disorders Task Force. Management of Parkinson's disease: an evidence based review. *Mov. Disord.* 2002; **17**(Suppl. 4): S1–165.

10

CHAPTER 10

Cognitive rehabilitation of non-progressive neuropsychological disorders

Stefano F. Cappa, Thomas Benke, Stephanie Clarke, Bruno Rossi, Brigitte Stemmer, Caroline M. van Heugten

Background

Disorders of language, spatial perception, attention, memory, calculation and praxis are a frequent consequence of acquired brain damage (in particular, stroke and traumatic brain injury (TBI)) and a major determinant of long-term disability. The possibility to effectively rehabilitate aphasia and other cognitive disorders can thus be expected to have a considerable impact on the burden of neurological disease. Many different treatment approaches have been suggested. While the early treatments were developed on a purely empirical basis, in recent years there has been an effort to propose rehabilitation procedures based on the limited available knowledge of the neuroscience of recovery and on models of learning. Evidence about the effectiveness of cognitive rehabilitation is limited, with only a small number of randomized controlled trials (RCTs) which are generally of low quality. There is a need for adequately designed studies in this area, which should take into account specific problems such as patient heterogeneity, and the difficulties in the standardization of treatment techniques.

Framing clinical questions and general approach to search evidence

The review deals with the rehabilitation of non-progressive neuropsychological disorders due to stroke and traumatic brain damage (TBI):
- Aphasia
- Unilateral neglect (ULN)
- Attention disorders
- Memory problems
- Apraxia
- Acalculia.

Other relevant areas, such as the non-pharmacological treatment of dementia and of psychiatric disorders, and the rehabilitation of developmental cognitive disorders, are not considered here. The present chapter is largely based on the recent update and revision of the Guidelines on Cognitive Rehabilitation produced by the Task Force on Cognitive Rehabilitation under the auspices of the European Federation of Neurological Societies [1].

Critical review of the evidence for each question

1. Rehabilitation of aphasia

Among patients with aphasia due to stroke or TBI how does language therapy (professional) compared to no-therapy (or non-specific treatment provided by non-professionals) improve language and communication? Is more intensive treatment compared to less intensive treatment better in improving language function?

The rehabilitation of speech and language disorders following brain damage is the area of intervention for acquired cognitive deficits with the longest tradition, dating back to the 19th century [2]. It has been shown that 38% of patients who present with an acute stroke demonstrate an aphasic syndrome [3]. The most important prognostic factors for recovery are severity, lesion size and time post-onset. Severity of aphasia in stroke patients is associated with poor functional outcome and an increased (doubled) mortality rate at follow-up [4,5]. Age does not appear to play a role independent of other factors, such as co-morbidity [6]. Less is known about aphasia associated to closed head injury and other lesions, such as tumours and tumour resections that involve the language areas of the brain. Language disorders appear to be milder in tumour patients, in comparison with strokes of similar location and extent, and complete recovery is more likely in traumatic than in vascular aphasia [7]. Some degree of spontaneous recovery can be observed in most patients with aphasia due to non-progressive brain diseases.

A variety of approaches have been applied to the rehabilitation of aphasia [8]. Stimulation-facilitation is based on the assumption that language abilities, rather than lost, become inaccessible after brain damage. The treatment approach is centred on language comprehension, in particular in the auditory modality, and aphasia is considered as a unitary disorder, with individual patients differing in term of the severity of impairment, rather than on the specific features of linguistic breakdown. Behavioural modification emphasizes the behavioural approach to the learning process, and is an application to aphasia treatment of programmed instruction based on operant conditioning. The techniques include shaping and fading, and other principles of behaviour modification, which are incorporated in many other treatment approaches. Neo-associationism includes several treatment programs, which focus on a detailed psycholinguistic and neurological description of the classic aphasic syndromes [9], and comprise very heterogeneous approaches, such as Melodic Intonation Therapy and Treatment of Aphasic Perseveration. The neurolinguistic-cognitive approach originates from the early attempts to apply linguistic theory to aphasia in the sixties and seventies, and flourished with the development of cognitive neuropsychology. The emphasis is on detailed assessment of language in single cases, and analysis of the pattern of linguistic dysfunction on the basis of a model of normal processing, resulting in a 'functional' diagnosis. The assumption is that a precise identification of the locus of functional damage provides the grounds for a rational intervention [10]. Finally, pragmatic approaches aim at improving the patient's ability to communicate, regardless of the linguistic or non-linguistic strategies. In the most widely known programme, Promoting Aphasics' Communicative Effectiveness (PACE) [11], therapist and patient are engaged in situations in which they exchange 'real' information. Pragmatic principles are now incorporated in many eclectic treatment programmes, with a particular indication for severe aphasia.

The need to establish the effectiveness of aphasia rehabilitation has stimulated a number of investigations that are based on a variety of methodologies. There is one systematic review of studies limited to post-stroke aphasia that addresses the effectiveness of language rehabilitation and covers articles about speech and language rehabilitation up to January 1999 [12]. The conclusion of the review is that 'speech and language therapy treatment for people with aphasia after a stroke has not been shown either to be clearly effective or clearly ineffective within an RCT. Decisions about the management of patients must therefore be based on other forms of evidence. Further research is required to find out if speech and language therapy for aphasic patients is effective. If researchers choose to do a trial, this must be large enough to have adequate statistical power, and be clearly reported.' This conclusion is based on 12 studies all of which were considered of poor quality.

Including lower classes of evidence has led other authors to different conclusions [13,14]. The findings of three large studies all indicate significant benefits of treatment [15,16,17]. Single case studies have also shown large treatment effects

in aphasic patients [18]. Some of the RCT comparing therapy with unstructured stimulation were based on a very limited number of treatment sessions. A recent meta-analysis [19] found a significant treatment effect if treatment was frequent and intensive over a short period of time (8.8 h of therapy per week for 11.2 weeks), compared to less frequent and intensive treatment over a long period of time (approximately 2 h per week for 22.9 weeks). Total length of therapy was significantly inversely correlated with mean change in Porch Index of Communicative Abilities (PICA) scores. The number of hours of therapy provided in a week was significantly correlated to greater improvement on the PICA and the Token Test. These results indicate that an intense therapy programme provided over a short period of time can improve outcomes of speech and language therapy for stroke patients with aphasia.

2. Rehabilitation of ULN

Among patients with unilateral spatial neglect due to stroke how does the visual or visuo-spatial training improve attentional skill or general disability?

ULN is a frequent manifestation of damage to the right hemisphere. In the Copenhagen study, ULN was present in 23% of stroke patients in the acute stage [20]. The presence of ULN beyond the acute stage has been associated with poor outcome in terms of independence [21] and considerable effort has therefore been devoted to its rehabilitation. Several recent reviews are available [22,23,24], including the Cochrane Systematic Review [25]. The latter analysed 15 studies and found evidence that ULN rehabilitation resulted in significant and persisting improvements in performance on impairment level assessments. There was, however, insufficient evidence to confirm or exclude an effect of cognitive rehabilitation at the level of disability or return to home following discharge from hospital. Several different approaches are currently used for neglect rehabilitation. Visual scanning training was shown to improve significantly neglect in one class I study [26]. Spatiomotor or visuospatiomotor cueing improved neglect significantly in another class I study [27]. There is less evidence for the effectiveness of combined training of visual scanning, reading, copying and figure description, visual cueing with kinetic stimuli, video feedback and visuomotor feedback, training of sustained attention, increasing of alertness or cueing of spatial attention.

Several studies investigated effects that aimed at influencing multisensory representations. Generally, these studies demonstrated transient effects, lasting little longer than the end of the appropriate stimulation. The methods include vestibular stimulation by cold-water infusion into the left outer ear canal [28], galvanic vestibular stimulation, transcutaneous electrical stimulation of the left neck muscles, neck muscle vibration and changes in trunk orientation. The use of prism goggles deviating by 10 degrees to the right, introduced relatively recently, was shown to improve significantly, in a transient fashion, neglect symptoms [29,30]. Computer training was note effective in one class I study [31]. A more recent class II study showed statistically significant improvement in wheel chair mobility [32].

In conclusion, there is evidence for the effectiveness of visual scanning training and of visuo-spatio-motor training in ULN. Lower levels of evidence are available for the combined training of visual scanning, reading, copying and figure description, trunk orientation, neck vibration and forced use of left eye. Other treatments need to be tested in further studies such as the use of prism goggles, video feedback, training of sustained attention and alertness, chaloric or galvanic vestibular stimulations as well as transcutaneous electrical stimulation of neck muscles. Visual cueing with kinetic stimuli and the use of computers in neglect rehabilitation remain controversial.

3. Rehabilitation of attention disorders

Among patient with attention disorders due to acute or sub-acute TBI or stroke, how does attentional training improve concentration and alertness or reduce general disability?

Attention deficits follow many types of brain damage, including stroke and TBI [33]. The Cochrane Review [34] identified two studies [35] showing that attention training improved sustained attention in stroke. A very important distinction is between studies conducted in the acute and post-acute stage. In the acute stage, one class I study [36] compared the effectiveness of focused treatment consisting of sequential, hierarchical interventions directed at specific attention mechanisms versus unstructured intervention consisting of non-sequential, non-hierarchical activities requiring memory or reasoning skills. Both groups improved to a similar degree and the observed improvements are probably due to spontaneous recovery. One class II study [37] used a multiple baseline design across subjects and evaluated a programme for the remediation of processing speed deficits in patients with severe TBI. Although the authors reported no benefit or generalization of effects of attention training there was improvement in some patients when practice on attention training tasks was combined with therapist feedback and praise. In another class II study [38], subjects with lateralized stroke showed beneficial effects of attention training on five of 14 outcome measures, especially on measures of perceptual speed and selective attention in left hemisphere lesions. Three class I studies assessed the attention treatment effectiveness during the post-acute period of rehabilitation [39,40,42]. In one study [39] patients with attention dysfunction showed marked improvement immediately after training on two measures of attention; however, when premorbid intelligence score and time since injury were added as covariates, the treatment effect was no longer significant. At 6-month follow-up, the treatment group showed continued improvement and superior performance compared to the control group

on tests involving auditory-verbal working memory. The authors suggested that the improvement, continuing over the follow-up period, was consistent with a strategy-training model, as it becomes increasingly automated and integrated into a wider range of behaviours. Another post-acute class I study [40] dealt with community dwelling patients with moderate to severe brain injury. The experimental attention training group improved significantly more than the alternative (memory) treatment group on four attention measures administered throughout the treatment period, although the effects did not generalize to the second set of neuropsychological measures. Two other studies using a crossover design [41,42] reported superiority of 'attention process training' compared to therapeutic support. In addition, the 'time pressure management' programme demonstrated greater improvement compared to a generic 'concentration' programme. Several attempts were made to establish the differential role for effectiveness of training of specific components of attention. A Class II study [43] on TBI investigated four different sub-processes of attention: cognitive flexibility, speed of processing, interference and working memory. The findings support the view that there are different sub-processes of attention that can be trained specifically and this may have implications for neuropsychological assessment and rehabilitation and may have implications for neuropsychological assessment and rehabilitation. Improvements in speed of processing appear to be less robust than improvements on non-speeded tasks [37]. Moreover, several studies suggest greater benefits of attention training on more complex tasks requiring selective or divided attention than on basic tasks of reaction time or vigilance [38,39].

In conclusion, there is class I evidence for attention training in the post-acute phase after TBI. On the other hand, there is insufficient evidence to distinguish the effects of specific attention training from spontaneous recovery or more general cognitive interventions during the acute period of recovery and inpatient rehabilitation for patients with moderate-to-severe TBI and stroke.

4. Rehabilitation of memory

Among patients with memory problems due to TBI or stroke how does memory rehabilitation (internal and external memory aids) improve memory function or general disability?

In the US, the prevalence of TBI is 5.3 million and there is an incidence of over 1.7 million cases per year. However, information on the prevalence of memory impairment after TBI is scarce. One study reported that nearly a fourth (25%) of those having sustained TBI suffer from memory problems [44]. The prevalence of stroke in the US is 4.5 million and there is an incidence of 600,000 cases per year. On an international basis, the prevalence of stroke is over 35 million with an incidence of over 6 million cases annually. Although memory problems are commonly reported after TBI they are often neglected in stroke patients although a comprehensive assessment frequently shows memory problems also after stroke. Reliable statistics for stroke patients, however, is virtually non-existent, and even less is known about the efficacy of intervention of memory problems in these patients. Overall, clinical observation shows that some degree of spontaneous recovery or improvement of memory usually occurs but not much is known about the interaction between spontaneous recovery and intervention. The need to establish the effectiveness of memory rehabilitation has stimulated a wide range of studies. Unfortunately, however, only few of these studies meet the critical standards for evaluating scientifically proven measures of prevention and treatment of neurological diseases and disability. Generally, approaches to memory rehabilitation either target to restore or optimize damaged or residual functions, or they are directed towards compensating for lost or deficient functions (for a summary see Ref. [45]). Evidence-based studies have most frequently investigated techniques in memory rehabilitation that include the use of internal and external memory aids, assistive electronic technologies and pharmacological agents. In what follows a summary of the findings of memory rehabilitation techniques reported in controlled studies is provided. The summary is based on two recommendations [1,13] and two systematic reviews [14–46]. It should be noted that the criteria according to which authors have included studies in their reviews and the recommendations based on the reviews differ.

The use of internal memory aids

For patients with mild memory impairment compensatory memory training has been recommended [1,13,14]. It seems, however, unlikely that this pertains to all patient groups and types of memory impairment. For example, there is only one controlled study investigating the effectiveness of training compensatory memory strategies in a few (six) stroke patients, and this study did not report positive effects [47]. Although for TBI patients there are more evidence-based reports on the use of memory strategies, the findings are controversial possibly due to the difference in the training techniques used and the heterogeneity of the groups investigated. For example, one randomized-controlled study reported positive effects of visual imagery training on memory functioning in TBI patients [48]. The interpretability of this study is, however, severely hampered by the small sample size (12 patients in each experimental group with 3 dropouts) and the little or no control over external variables such as patient distribution over seven different rehabilitation centres and patients being either in- or outpatients. Another technique that has shown some beneficial effects is the errorless learning technique. In this technique people are prevented from making errors and this is compared to errorful learning where people are allowed to make mistakes (e.g. trial-and-error learning) (for a summary see Ref. [49]). It seems, however, that the benefit of errorless learning depends on the type of task used, the way in which

memory is tested and on the severity of the memory impairment. Finally, the spacing-of-repetitions procedure has also shown some efficacy in improving learning in TBI patients [50,51]. This technique is based on the spacing effect, which has been shown to improve learning and memory when repeated trials are distributed over time (spaced repetitions).

The use of external memory aids

Controlled studies generally support the efficacy of external non-electronic memory aids such as calendars, lists, notebooks and diaries (for a summary see Ref. [1]). The effectiveness of these memory aids seems to be boosted by combining them with internal memory strategy training. However, there is some indication that not all aids or strategies are similarly beneficial [52].

The use of assistive electronic technologies

Computers, paging systems, voice organizers and virtual environments have all been used to enhance memory performance. A few well controlled studies have demonstrated the efficacy of paging systems and voice organizers to enhance learning and improve activities of daily living (ADL) particularly in patients with moderate to severe memory impairments (for a summary see Ref. [1,13,14]). Despite the generally reported success of using memory assisted computer training and virtual environments, it is currently not clear whether they are superior to conventional methods as a comparison with conventional methods is still missing.

5. Rehabilitation of apraxia

Among patients with apraxia due to acquired brain damage, how does behavioural training programmes or teaching compensatory strategies improve praxis or reduce general disability?

Although apraxia occurs frequently after acquired brain damage [53], the literature on recovery and treatment is minimal. Several reasons for this lack of evidence can be identified [54]. First, patients with apraxia often seem to be unaware of their deficit and rarely complain. Second, many researchers believe that recovery from apraxia is spontaneous and treatment is not necessary. Finally, some authors believe that apraxia only occurs when performance is requested of patients in testing situations, and that correct behaviour is displayed in natural settings. There is agreement that apraxia hinders ADL independence [55,56,57].

There are two recent RCTs on the rehabilitation of apraxia. One study [58] found that a behavioural training programme with gesture-production exercises led to a significant improvement of limb apraxia with better performance and a reduction of errors in both ideational and ideomotor apraxia tests. Another study [59] assessed the effectiveness of strategy training in left hemisphere stroke patients with apraxia. After 8 weeks of treatment, patients who received strategy training improved significantly more than patients in the usual treatment group on standardized ADL observations and the Barthel ADL index. However, at follow-up 5 months later no beneficial effects of strategy training were found. A some what less well-controlled study investigated a therapy programme for teaching patients strategies to compensate for the presence of apraxia [60]. Large improvements in ADL functioning were reported in all measures and small improvements on the apraxia test and motor functioning test.

In sum, there is evidence that behavioural training programmes improve limb apraxia and the teaching of compensatory strategies enables apraxic patients to function more independently. The evidence supports the view that treatment of apraxia should be part of the overall neuro-rehabilitation programme after brain damage.

6. Rehabilitation of acalculia

Among patients with acalculia due to acquired brain damage, how does a re-teaching approach, or exploiting of residual resources improve calculation abilities?

Though often unnoticed, many neurological disorders are associated with impairments of number processing and calculation (INPC). Depending on the underlying disease and on lesion location, the frequency of calculation disorders in patients with neurological disorders has been estimated to range between 10% and 90% [61]. Furthermore, no group studies exist which have compared different treatment strategies in larger patient samples. Studies are mostly 'quasi-experimental' using a single-case or small-group approach guided by the principles of cognitive neuropsychology [62–65] and single-subject research [66,67]. Two main types of rationales have been applied to improve INPC. The 'reconstitution' or 'reteaching' approach consists of extensive lost or damaged abilities by way of extensive practice. The indirect approach promotes the use of 'back-up' strategies based on the patient's residual resources. In this case, the treatment would not merely point to restore the functionality of the impaired component but rather to exploit the preserved abilities to compensate for the deficit. Both types of remediation employ step-by-step training consisting in presentation of problems of increasing difficulty, facilitation cues and other types of assistance which are eventually faded with progressive recovery; in all cases direct feedback is provided to the patient on his/her accuracy and errors. Outcome measures typically entail a comparison of the individual's pre- and post-treatment performance in transcoding tasks, simple and complex calculation. The amount of functional disability on daily life is rarely assessed or estimated in this corpus of studies. Rehabilitation of INPC may be grouped into several areas of intervention [68]. Rehabilitation of transcoding ability (the ability to translate numerical stimuli between different formats) has been successfully performed in several studies (see, e.g. [69,70]), mostly by re-teaching the patient the required set of rules. Impairments of arithmetical facts (simple multiplication, addition, subtraction or division solved directly from memory) were the target of several rehabilitation studies (see, e.g. [68,71,72]). In all studies, extensive practice with the defective domain of knowledge (i.e. multiplication tables determined significant improvement). A positive outcome was reached also by a rehabilitation programme based on the strategic use of the patient's residual knowledge of arithmetic [73]. This specific case suggests that the integration of declarative, procedural and conceptual knowledge critically mediates the re-acquisition process. Deficient arithmetical problem solving (the ability to provide a solution for complex, multi-step arithmetical text problems) has also been treated in one study [74]. The study was rated as partly successful by the authors, as patients benefited from the cueing procedure engaged and generated a higher number of correct solution steps, but did not show a prominent effect on the actual execution process. Overall, the available evidence suggests that rehabilitation procedures used to treat selected variants of INPC were successful at the single-subject or small group level. Notably, significant improvements were observed even in severely impaired and chronic patients. Several caveats need to be mentioned in this context. At present, little is known about the prognosis and spontaneous recovery of INPC, thus, the effects of different interventions in the early stages of numerical disorders may be difficult to evaluate. Moreover, different underlying neurological disorders (e.g. stroke, dementia and trauma) have only partly been compared as to their specific effects on INPC. Furthermore, it has not been studied in detail how impairments of attention or executive functions influence the rehabilitation process of INPC.

Conclusion

The evidence findings (systematic reviews, randomized-clinical trials) are summarized in Table 10.1. These results clearly indicate that many methodological issues remain to be solved. The prevalence and relevance of cognitive disorders in terms of functional outcome after stroke and TBI dictates the need to establish recommendations for good practice of cognitive rehabilitation. This need was formally recognized by a subcommittee of the Brain Injury-Interdisciplinary Special Interest Group of the American Congress of Rehabilitation Medicine. The initial recommendations of the Committee were published in 1992 as the Guidelines for Cognitive Rehabilitation [75] and were based on expert opinions that did not consider evidence-based empirical support of the effectiveness of cognitive rehabilitation. In 2000, an evidence-based review of the scientific literature for cognitive rehabilitation was published by the same group [13], and an update from 1998 to 2002 has appeared recently [14]. The update process will result in regular publications (K.D. Cicerone, personal communication). There are other systematic reviews that address only TBI patients. The NIH Consensus Development Panel [76]

Table 10.1 Systematic reviews (SR) and randomized controlled trials (RCTs) on cognitive rehabilitation.

Type of study (reference)	Impairment patients	Number of participants (number of trials)	Intervention	Outcome	Main findings	Comment
SR [12]	Aphasia stroke	950 (12)	Treatment (professional) versus no treatment (non-professional)	Aphasia tests disability	Absence of evidence	
SR [19]	Aphasia stroke	864 (10)	Intensive treatment versus less intensive treatment	Aphasia tests	Intensive treatment better	
SR [25]	Neglect stroke	400 (15)	Visual scanning and visuo-spatial motor training versus standard rehabilitation	Neglect tests disability	Improvement of neglect No evidence of impact on disability	
SR [34]	Attention stroke	56 (2)	Attention task versus standard rehabilitation	Concentration and alertness disability	Improvement No evidence of impact on disability	
RCT [39]	Attention post acute TBI	31 (1)	Attentional training versus no specific treatment	Attention tests	'Minor' effects	
RCT [40]	Attention post acute TBI	29 (1)	Attention training versus memory training	Attention tests	Improvement	Multiple baseline design; no evidence of generalization
RCT cross over [42]	Attention acute TBI	22 (1)	Time pressure management versus generic concentration training	Attention and memory tests	Improvement	
SR [14]	Memory	132 (6)	Internal memory aids	Memory tests	Improvement only in 'mild' patients	
SR [49]	Memory	147 (11)	Errorless learning	Memory tests	Large effect size for errorless learning treatment; no significant effect of vanishing cues	Quantitative systematic review
SR [46]	Memory stroke	12 (1)	Internal and external aids	Memory tests disability	Absence of evidence	
RCT [58]	Apraxia	13 (1)	Apraxia training	Apraxia tests	Improvement	
RCT [59]	Apraxia stroke	113 (1)	Apraxia training versus standard rehabilitation	Disability	Short-term (no long-term) improvement	
SR [77]	TBI	? (32)	Cognitive rehabilitation	Disability	Absence of evidence	

reviewed studies published from January 1988 through August 1998 (including 11 RCTs), and concluded that data on the effectiveness of cognitive rehabilitation programmes were limited by the heterogeneity of subjects, interventions and outcomes studied. Another review published by the Evidence-based Practice Center at Oregon Health Sciences University [77] concluded that the durability and clinical relevance of the reported rehabilitation effects was not established.

Although the situation has changed since the first recommendations for cognitive rehabilitation were published, we strongly agree with the view that the current status of studies on the effectiveness of cognitive rehabilitation is unsatisfactory. As pointed out previously, many RCTs in neurological rehabilitation are of poor methodological quality: the sample size is often insufficient, a control condition is frequently missing, and/or there is a failure to assess the outcome at the disability level. There is definitely a need for large-scale RCTs evaluating well-defined methodologies of intervention in common clinical conditions (e.g. the assessment of the efficacy of an intervention for ULN after right hemispheric stroke on long-term motor disability). The question of the efficacy of cognitive rehabilitation 'in general' is clearly ill-posed for a number of reasons. First, we are dealing with heterogeneous clinical manifestations of different diseases. For example, it is questionable whether the same standardized aphasia treatment would be similarly effective for a patient with a fluent neologistic jargon due to closed head injury and for a patient with agrammatic nonfluent production associated with a fronto-parietal infarction. Asking whether aphasia therapy is 'generally' effective is like organizing a RCT to assess the effectiveness of a given treatment of skin rashes. At the same time the attempt to assess the effectiveness of a treatment only in patients with a complete genome screening, in which a specific mutation associated with the precise type of skin rash has been identified, would not be realistic. Research in neuropsychology has focused on the assessment of specific, theoretically driven treatments on well-defined areas of impairment, usually by means of single-case methodology (e.g. the effect of a linguistically driven intervention compared with simple stimulation of the ability to retrieve lexical items belonging to a defined class). It must be underlined that the randomization procedure per se does not guarantee the adequacy of the study unless the sample is large enough to control for the effect of known or unknown confounding variables [78]. When targeting a large sample size of patients, a realistic level of description should be chosen. It is conceivable that despite a careful clinical specification of the target group there is still a residual heterogeneity. In such a case clinical labels such as agrammatism or anomia may represent an acceptable compromise. The second problem concerns the standardization of the treatment. In the case of a behavioural intervention, it is clear that a number of factors, such as dosage, frequency of intervention, etc. are more difficult to standardize than in the case of a

pharmacological treatment. Moreover, given the length and complexity of the interaction between treatment provider and client, personality factors and, in general, interpersonal dynamics can be expected to interfere. Again, a large sample size rather than an attempt to control beyond a reasonable degree may solve this problem. Computer-based approaches seem to simplify this problem; however, the evidence about their usefulness in the absence of constant human (therapist) intervention is not encouraging. Finally, we are facing the problem of feasibility of a true placebo double-blind controlled intervention. It is often difficult if not impossible to conceal the intervention condition from the therapist and the patient. Furthermore, ethically it is usually not justified to withhold treatment from a patient group (the 'placebo' condition). However, such a situation is easily solved by crossover designs.

In sum, high standards for performing well-controlled studies, as they are obligatory in pharmacological and surgical intervention, also need to be developed for and applied to intervention studies in neurological rehabilitation. In particular, it is necessary to show that rehabilitation is effective not only in modifying the impairment but also in having sustained effects at the disability level.

Acknowledgements

We would like to thank Prof. Klaus Willmes von Hinckeldey for discussions and useful suggestions, and Prof. Livia Candelise for her revision of the manuscript and help with the evidence table.

References

1 Cappa SF, Benke T, Clarke S, Rossi B, Stemmer B, van Heugten CM. Task Force on Cognitive Rehabilitation. EFNS guidelines on cognitive rehabilitation: report of an EFNS task force. *Eur. J. Neurol.* 2005; **12**: 665–80.

2 Howard D, Hatfield FM. *Aphasia therapy: historical and contemporary issues.* Hove and London, Lawrence Erlbaum Associates, 1987.

3 Pedersen PM, Jorgensen HS, Nakayama H, Raaschou HO, Olsen TS. Aphasia in acute stroke: incidence, determinants, and recovery. *Ann. Neurol.* 1995; **38**: 659–66.

4 Paolucci S, Antonucci G, Gialloreti LE, Traballesi M, Lubich S, Pratesi L, et al. Predicting stroke inpatient rehabilitation outcome: the prominent role of neuropsychological disorders. *Eur. Neurol.* 1996; **36**: 385–90.

5 Laska AC, Hellblom A, Murray V, Kahan T, Von Arbin M. Aphasia in acute strike and relation to outcome. *J. Internal Med.* 2004; **249**: 413–22.

6 Cappa SF. Spontaneous recovery from aphasia. In: Stemmer B & Whitaker H, eds., *Handbook of Neurolinguistics*. Academic Press, San Diego 1998.

7 Kertesz A, McCabe P. Recovery patterns and prognosis in aphasia. *Brain* 1977; **100** Part 1: 1–18.

8 Basso A. *Aphasia and its therapy.* Oxford University Press, Oxford, 2003.

9 Helm-Eastabrooks N, Albert MA. *Manual of Aphasia Therapy.* Pro-Ed Publishers, Austin TX, 1991.

10 Hillis AEE. *The Handbook of Adult Language Disorders.* Psychology Press, New York, 2002.

11 Davis GA, Wilcox MJ. Incorporating parameters of normal conversation in aphasia. In: *Language intervention strategies in adult aphasia.* William and Wilkins, Baltimore, 1981: pp. 169–94.

12 Greener J, Enderby P, Whurr R. Speech and language therapy for aphasia following stroke. *Cochrane Database Sys. Rev.* 1999; 4: CD000425. DOI: 10.1002/14651858.CD000425.

13 Cicerone KD, Dahlberg C, Kalmar K, Langenbahn DM, Malec JF, Berquist TF, Felicetti T, Giacino J, Harley JP, Harrington DE, Herzog J, Kneipp S, Laatsch L, Morse PA. Evidence-based cognitive rehabilitation: recommendations for clinical practice. *Arch. Phys. Med. Rehabil.* 2000; **81**: 1596–615.

14 Cicerone KD, Dahlberg C, Malec JF, Langenbahn DM, Felicetti T, 13. Kneipp S, Ellmo W, Kalmar K, Giacino JT, Harley JP, Laatsch L, Morse PA, Catanese J. Evidence-based cognitive rehabilitation: updated review of the literature from 1998 through 2002. *Arch. Phys. Med. Rehabil.* 2005; **86**: 1681–92.

15 Basso A, Capitani E, Vignolo LA. Influence of rehabilitation on language skills in aphasic patients. A controlled study. *Arch. Neurol.* 1979; **36**: 190–6.

16 Shewan CM, Kertesz, A. Effects of speech language treatment on recovery from aphasia. *Brain Lang.* 1985; **23**: 272–99.

17 Poeck, K, Huber, W, Willmes K. Outcome of intensive language treatment in aphasia. *J. Speech Hear. Dis.* 1989; **54**: 471–9.

18 Robey RR, Schultz MC, Crawford AB, Sinner CA. Single-subject clinical-outcome research: designs, data, effect sizes, and analyses. *Aphasiology* 1999; **13**: 445–73.

19 Bhogal SK, Teasell R, Speechley M. Intensity of aphasia therapy, impact on recovery. *Stroke* 2003; **34**: 987–93.

20 Pedersen PM, Jorgensen HS, Nakayama H, Raaschou HO, Olsen TS. Hemineglect in acute stroke–incidence and prognostic implications. The Copenhagen Stroke Study. *Am. J. Phys. Med. Rehabil.* 1997; **76**: 122–7.

21 Denes G, Semenza C, Stoppa E, Lis A. Unilateral spatial neglect and recovery from hemiplegia: A follow-up study. *Brain* 1982; **105**: 543–52.

22 Pierce SR, Buxbaum LJ. Treatments of unilateral neglect: a review. *Arch. Phys. Med. Rehabil.* 2002; **83**: 256–68.

23 Kerkhoff G. Modulation and rehabilitation of spatial neglect by sensory stimulation. *Prog Brain Res.* 2003; **142**: 257–71.

24 Paton A, Malhortra P, Husain M. Hemispatial neglect. *J. Neurol. Neurosurg. Psychiatr.* 2004; **75**: 13–21.

25 Bowen A, Lincoln NB, Dewey M. Cognitive rehabilitation for spatial neglect following stroke. *Cochrane Database Syst. Rev.* 2002; 2: CD003586. DOI: 10.1002/14651858.CD003586.

26 Weinberg J, Diller L, Gordon WA, Gerstman lJ, Liebermann A, Lakin P, Hodges G, Ezrachi O. Visual scanning training effect on reading-related tasks in acquired right brain damage. *Arch. Phys. Med. Rehabil.* 1977; **58**: 479–86.

27 Kalra L, Perez I, Gupta S, Wittink M. The influence of visual neglect on stroke rehabilitation. *Stroke* 1997; **28**: 1386–91.

28 Rode G, Perenin MT. Temporary remission of representational hemineglect through vestibular stimulation. *NeuroReport* 1994; **5**: 869–72.

29 Rossetti Y, Rode G, Pisella L, Farné A, Li L, Boisson D, Perenin M-T Prism adaptation to rightward optical deviation rehabilitates left hemispatial neglect. *Nature* 1998; **395**: 166–9.

30 Frassinetti F, Angeli V, Meneghello F, Avanzi S, Ladavas E. Long-lasting amelioration of visuospatial neglect by prism adaptation. *Brain* 2002; **125**: 608–23.

31 Robertson IH, Gray J, Pentland B, Waite LJ. Microcomputer-based rehabilitation for unilateral left visual neglect: a randomized controlled trial. *Arch. Phys. Med. Rehabil.* 1990; **71**: 663–8.

32 Webster JS, McFarland PT, Rapport LJ, Morrill B, Roades LA, Abadee PS. Computer assisted training for improving wheelchair mobility in unilateral neglect patients. *Arch. Phys. Med. Rehabil.* 2001; **82**: 769–75.

33 Van Zomeren AH, Van DenBurg W. Residual complaints of patients two years after severe head injury. *J. Neurol. Nurosurg. Psychiatr.* 1985; **48**: 21–8.

34 Lincoln NB, Majid MJ, Weyman N. Cognitive rehabilitation for attention deficits following stroke (Cochrane Review). *Cochrane Database Syst. Rev.* 2000; 3: CD002842. DOI: 10.1002/14651858. CD002842.

35 Schoettke H. Rehabilitation von Aufmerksamkeitsstörungen nach einem Schlagenfall. Effektivität eines verhaltensmedizinisch-neuropsychologischen Aufmerksamkeitstrainings. *Verhaltenstherapie* 1997; **7**: 21–23.

36 Novack TA, Caldwell SG, Duke LW, Bergquist TF. Focused versus unstructured intervention for attention deficits after traumatic brain injury. *J. Head Trauma Rehabil.* 1996; **11**: 52–60.

37 Ponsford JL, Kinsella G. Evaluation of a remedial programme far attentional deficits following closed-head injury. *J. Clin. Exp. Neuropsychol.* 1988; **10**: 693–708.

38 Sturm W, Willmes K. Efficacy of a reaction training on various attentional and cognitive functions in stroke patients. *Neuropsychol. Rehabil.* 1991; **1**: 259–80.

39 Gray JM, Robertson I, Pentland B, Anderson S. Microcomputer-based attentional retraining after brain damage: a randomised group controlled trial. *Neuropsychol. Rehabil.* 1992; **2**: 97–115.

40 Niemann H, Ruff RM, Baser CA. Computer assisted attention retraining in head injured individuals: a controlled efficacy study of an out-patient program. *J. Consult. Clin. Psychol.* 1990; **58**: 811–7.

41 Sohlberg MM, McLaughlin KA, Pavese A, Heidrich A, Posner MI. Evaluation of attention process training and brain injury education in persons with acquired brain injury. *J. Clin. Exp. Neuropsychol.* 2000; **22**: 656–76.

42 Fasotti L, Kovacs F, Eling PA, Brouwer WH. Time pressure management as a compensatory strategy training after closed head injury. *Neuropsychol. Rehabil.* 2000; **10**: 47–65.

43 Rios M, Perianez JA, Munoz-Cespedes JM. Attentional control and slowness of information processing after severe traumatic brain injury. *Brain Injury* 2004; **18**: 257–72.

44 Walker R, Logan TK, Leukefeld C, Stevenson E. Kentucky traumatic brain injury prevalence study. *CDAR Technical Report* No. 2004-01. University of Kentucky, Center on Drug and alcohol Research, Lexington, Kentucky.

45 Glisky EL, Glisky ML. Learning and memory impairments. In: PJ Eslinger ed., *Neuropsychological Interventions: Clinical Research and Practice*. Guilford Press, New York, NY, 2002; pp. 137–62.

46 Majid MJ, Lincoln NB, Weyman N. Cognitive rehabilitation for memory deficits following stroke. *Cochrane Database Syst. Rev.* 2001; 2: CD003586. DOI: 10.1002/14651858.CD003586 2001.

47 Doornhein K, de Haan EHF. Cognitive training for memory deficits in stroke patients. *Neuropsychol. Rehabil.* 1998; **8**: 393–400.

48 Kaschel R, Della Sala S, Cantagallo A, Fahlbock A, Laaksonen R, Kazen M. Imagery mnemonics for the rehabilitation of memory: a randomised group controlled trial. *Neuropsychol. Rehabil.* 2002; **12**: 127–53.

49 Kessels RPC, de Haan EHF. Implicit learning in memory rehabilitation: a meta-analysis on errorless learning and vanishing cues methods. *J. Clin. Exp. Neuropsychol.* 2003; **25**: 805–14.

50 Hillary FG, Schultheis MT, Challis BH, Millis SR, Carnevale GJ. Spacing of repetitions improves learning and memory after moderate and severe TBI. *J. Clin. Exp. Neuropsychol.* 2003; **25**: 49–58.

51 Schacter DL, Rich SA, Stampp MS. Remediation of memory disorders: experimental evaluation of the spaced retrieval techniques. *J. Clin. Exp. Neuropsychol.* 1985; **7**: 79–96.

52 Evans JJ, Wilson BA, Needham P, Brentnall S. Who makes good use of memory aids? Results of a survey of people with acquired brain injury. *J. Int. Neuropsychol. Soc.* 2003; **9**: 925–35.

53 Pedersen PM, Jorgensen HS, Kammersgaard LP, Nakayama H, Raaschou HO, Olsen TS. Manual and oral apraxia in acute stroke, frequency and influence on functional outcome: The Copenhagen Stroke Study. *Am. J. Phys. Med. Rehabil.* 2001; **80**: 685–92.

54 Maher ML, Ochipa C. Management and treatment of limb apraxia. In: Rothi LG & Heilman K, eds., A*praxia: The Neuropsychology of Action*. Psychology Press, Hove, UK, 1997.

55 Goldenberg G, Daumuller M, Hagman S. Assessment and therapy of complex activities of daily living in apraxia. *Neuropsychol. Rehabil.* 2001; **11**: 147–69.

56 Hanna-Paddy B, Heilman KM, Foundas AL. Ecological implications od ideomotor apraxia: evidence from physical activities of daily living. *Neurology* 2003; **60**: 487–90.

57 Walker CM, Sunderland A, Sharma J, Walker MF. The impact of cognitive impairments on upper body dressing difficulties after stroke: a video analysis of patterns of recovery. *J. Neurol. Neurosurg. Psychiatr.* 2004; **75**: 43–8.

58 Smania N, Girardi F, Domenciali C, Lora E, Aglioti S. The rehabilitation of limb apraxia: a study in left brain damaged patients. *Arch. Phys. Med. Rehabil.* 2000; **81**: 379–88.

59 Donkervoort M, Dekker J, Stehmann-Saris J, Deelman BG. Efficacy of strategy training in left-hemisphere stroke patients with apraxia: a randomized clinical trial. *Neuropsychol. Rehabil.* 2002; **11**: 549–66.

60 Van Heugten CM, Dekker J, Deelman BG, van Dijuk AJ, Stehmann-Saris JC, Kinebanian A. Outcome of strategy training in stroke patients: a phase-II study. *Clin. Rehabil.* 1998; **2**: 294–303.

61 Jackson M, Warrington EK. Arithmetic skills in patients with unilateral cerebral lesions. *Cortex* 1986; **22**: 611–20.

62 Shallice T. Case-study approach in neuropsychological research. *J. Clin. Neuropsychol.* 1979; **1**: 3–211.

63 Caramazza A. Cognitive neuropsychology and rehabilitation: an unfulfilled promise? In: Seron X & Deloche G, eds., *Cognitive Approach in Neuropsychological Rehabilitation*. Lawrence Erlbaum Associates Ltd, Hillsdale, N.J., 1989.

64 Riddoch MJ, Humphreys GW. eds. *Cognitive Neuropsychology and Cognitive Rehabilitation*. Lawrence Erlbaum Associates, Hove, 1994.

65 Seron X. Effectiveness and specificity in neuropsychological therapies: a cognitive point of view. *Aphasiology* 1997; **11**: 105–23.

66 Kratochwill TR, Levin LR, eds. *Single-Case Research Design and Analysis*. Lawrence Erlbaum Associates, Hove, 1992.

67 Randall RR, Schultz MC, Crawford AB, Sinner CA. Single-subject clinical outcome research: designs, data, effect sizes, and analyses. *Aphasiology* 1999; **13**: 445–73.

68 Girelli L, Delazer M. Subtraction bugs in an alcalculic patient. *Cortex* 1996; **32**: 547–55.

69 Deloche G, Ferrand I, Naud E, Baeta E, Vendrell J, Claros-Salinas D. Differential effects of covert and overt training of the syntactic component of verbal processing and generalisations to other tasks: a single-case study. *Neuropsychol. Rehabil.* 1992; **2**: 257–81.

70 Sullivan KS, Macaruso P, Sokol SM. Remediation of Arabic numeral processing in a case of development dyscalculia. *Neuropsychol. Rehabil.* 1996; **6**: 27–53.

71 Domahs F, Bartha L, Delazer M. Rehabilitation of arithmetical abilities: different intervention strategies for multiplication. *Brain Lang.* 2003; **87**: 165–6.

72 Domahs F Lochy A, Eibl G, Delazer M. Adding colour to multiplication: rehabilitation of arithmetical fact retrieval in a case of traumtaic brain injury. *Neuropsychol. Rehabil.* 2004; **14**: 303–28.

73 Girelli L, Bartha L, Delazer M. Strategic learning in the rehabilitation of semantic knowledge. *Neuropsychol. Rehabil.* 2002; **12**: 41–61.

74 Delazer M, Bodner T, Benke T. Rehabilitation of arithmetical text problem solving. *Neuropsychol. Rehabil.* 1998; **8**: 401–12.

75 Harley JP, Allen C, Braciszeski TL, Cicerone KD, Dahlberg C, Evans S. Guidelines for cognitive rehabilitation. *NeuroRehabil itation* 1992; **2**: 62–7.

76 NIH Consensus Development Panel on Rehabilitation of Persons with Traumatic Brain Injury. Rehabilitation of persons with traumatic brain injury. *J. Am. Med. Assoc.* 1999; **282**: 974–83.

77 Carney N, Chesnut RM, Maynard H, Mann NC, Hefland M. Effect of cognitive rehabilitation on outcomes for persons with traumatic brain injury: a systematic review. *J. Head Trauma Rehabil.* 1999; **14**: 277–307.

78 Hsu LM. Random sampling, randomization, and equivalence of contrasted groups in psychotherapy outcome research. In: Kazdin AE, ed., *Methodological Issues and Strategies in Clinical Research*. American Psychological Association, Washington DC, 1992, pp. 91–106.

CHAPTER 11

Management and pharmaceutical treatment of central and spinal spasticity

David T. Shakespeare

Background

Spasticity has been defined as 'a motor disorder characterized by a velocity-dependent increase in tonic stretch reflexes that results from abnormal intraspinal processing of primary afferent input' [1]. However, the velocity- and length-dependent increase in stretch reflexes elicitable at rest as resistance to passive movement is only one of the features of the upper motor neurone (UMN) syndrome. Other features (such as weakness, lack of selective voluntary movement and various types of involuntary spasms) are often of more symptomatic and functional relevance to the patient, and may not be well correlated with the diagnostic sign described above [2]. Structural alterations within affected musculo-skeletal structures (often referred to as contracture) also contribute to resistance to active and passive movement [3]. Other neurological problems (e.g. myoclonus, dystonia, 'shooting-type' neuropathic pain) can also mimic UMN phenomena and may require different treatment.

Different patterns of UMN phenomena (e.g. the typical hemiplegic posture, paraplegia in flexion, paraplegia in extension) are likely to reflect impairment of different combinations of pyramidal and parapyramidal motor pathways at different central nervous system (CNS) levels [2]. However changes in UMN patterns caused by nociceptive input (e.g. from constipation, bladder problems, pressure sores) and physical measures suggest that the level of sensory input also plays a key role. Successful spasticity treatment requires integration of the physical, psychological and medical aspects of management [4].

Spasticity affects around 60–70% of people with multiple sclerosis (MS) or spinal cord injury (SCI) and 40% with stroke (cerebrovascular accident, CVA), and can often worsen with time. This chapter summarizes the available evidence for physical and medical management of spasticity for adults with acquired brain injury, SCI and MS. A summary of evidence for the management of spasticity in children with cerebral palsy has been recently published [5].

Framing clinical questions

UMN phenomena are thought to develop because of deficiencies in the descending control of voluntary motor function from higher centres [2]. However, suppression of these phenomena (e.g. by physical therapeutic measures or drugs acting on different neurotransmitter systems) may not lead to recovery of good quality voluntary movement. It is therefore important to identify the relevant and feasible goals for each patient, for example:
- To improve active voluntary movement.
- To improve passive range of movement (PROM, to allow easier passive functions such as positioning or being dressed).
- To reduce spasticity-related pain and spasms.

A variety of different outcome measures have been used in spasticity treatment trials in an attempt to cover some or all of these possible treatment goals. The original and modified Ashworth scales (AS [6] and MAS [7]) are the most commonly used impairment-level outcome measures, but these are really only ordinal-level measures of PROM (which could be due to spasticity or contracture) [8] and they do not assess spasms, pain or active function. Other outcome measures (e.g. Penn spasm scale [9], global assessments of spasticity) have limited validation, particularly as UMN phenomena can vary so much at different times of the day [10]. Standard activity-level outcome measures (e.g. Barthel score, walking time) may lack sensitivity for the types of changes likely to be seen due to reduction in spasticity. These methodological difficulties limit the amount of quantitative comparison that can be carried out between trials with differing methodologies, so in the tables below I have merely indicated whether the trials gave a statistically significant result under each of the goal headings with whatever outcome measures were used.

Critical review of evidence

1. Physiotherapy

Do physiotherapeutic interventions lead to functional or symptomatic improvements in adults with spasticity?

Physical approaches to the management of spasticity include teaching self-management techniques, mobilization and stretching exercises, standing and transfer techniques, locomotor training, constraint-induced movement therapy and the use of splinting, orthoses and functional electrical stimulation. Table 11.1 summarizes randomized-controlled studies and meta-analyses of physical interventions for UMN problems, which can be read in conjunction with the studies of medical interventions summarized in the following sections. However as this table shows, research into physical interventions often views them as generic rehabilitation interventions rather than just spasticity treatments, so impairment-level outcome measures for spasticity or spasms are often not included. These studies show that PROM can be improved or maintained by casting and functional electrical stimulation, but passive stretches alone may be ineffective (particularly if carried out for only short periods). Physiotherapeutic treatment, exercise therapy and functional electrical stimulation can lead to improvements in active voluntary movement.

2. Oral anti-spasticity drugs

Do oral anti-spasticity drugs lead to functional or symptomatic improvements in adults with spasticity?

Baclofen, tizanidine, benzodiazepines, gabapentin, clonidine, cannabinoids and tolperisone all act on various central neurotransmitters, whereas dantrolene predominantly has a peripheral action on calcium flux within muscle fibres [19]. All can cause drowsiness and weakness to varying degrees, and other specific side effects include hepatotoxicity (tizanidine, dantrolene), exacerbation of urinary symptoms (baclofen), urine discolouration (dantrolene) and weight gain (gabapentin). The placebo-controlled randomized-controlled trial (RCT) evidence for efficacy of these agents is summarized in Table 11.2. This indicates that evidence for improvement in active voluntary movement with oral anti-spasticity treatment is very limited. Most drugs (except cannabinoids) have at least one RCT showing evidence of improvement in PROM. There is evidence for some drugs leading to improvements in spasticity-related pain (baclofen, cannabinoids, gabapentin) and spasms (baclofen, dantrolene, tizanidine, cannabinoids, gabapentin), although many trials did not assess these two outcomes separately. Methodological quality has improved since the 1970s studies, where unvalidated outcome measures were often used, no measures were taken to standardize Ashworth score grading between assessors, and control for physical factors (e.g. posture and positioning, physical activity, physiotherapy regimes) that can have a significant impact on spasticity during the trial was limited.

3. Intrathecal drugs

Does intrathecal (IT) drug infusion lead to functional or symptomatic improvements in adults with spasticity?

Baclofen can also be infused via a subcutaneous pump directly into the subarachnoid space for those with severe spasticity that is unresponsive to less complex treatments. Although mainly suitable for wheelchair-bound patients with severe lower limb (LL) spasticity, some mobile patients can gain significant benefit and higher catheter placement can lead to useful effects on upper limb (UL) spasticity [44]. Risks include infection, haemorrhage and pump failure. The likely effect of IT baclofen therapy can be evaluated before pump placement by a bolus test dose through a standard lumbar puncture or infusion through a temporary lumbar catheter.

The evidence for benefit from IT baclofen therapy consists of placebo-controlled RCTs of (mostly) bolus test doses, together with longer-term case series of infusion treatment via implanted pump for patients with both spinal and cerebral spasticity (Table 11.3). This confirms improvement in PROM, spasticity-related pain and spasms in appropriately selected patients, together with improvements in active voluntary movement in some.

Phenol can also be injected via standard lumbar puncture to cause a chemical neurolysis, with profound (potentially permanent) suppression of LL spasticity. As this treatment is not selective for motor nerves, it is unsuitable for those who retain control of bowel and bladder emptying, and sexual function. No RCTs have been carried out of this palliative procedure but published case series indicate significant improvement in PROM (Ashworth score and seating), spasms and spasticity-related pain [49,50].

4. Butulinum toxin

Does local injection of botulinum toxin (BTX) lead to functional or symptomatic improvements in adults with spasticity?

Intramuscular BTX injections can be used to selectively weaken overactive, spastic muscles by preventing the release of acetylcholine from presynaptic nerve endings [51]. The effect takes approximately 2 weeks to develop and lasts for 2–6 months, but the maximum dose that can be administered at any one time is limited. Preparations of two serotypes are currently available (in UK: Type A Botox® and Dysport®, Type B Neurobloc®), but the doses of the different formulations (even of the same serotype) are not equivalent. A good therapeutic outcome depends on careful selection of target muscles and a realistic appraisal of the possible rehabilitation goals (often requiring a detailed, multi-disciplinary assessment) [52]. Electromyography (EMG) or ultrasound localization can improve injection accuracy.

The placebo-controlled RCT evidence for the use of BTX in adult spasticity is summarized in Table 11.4. All studies to date have used BTX Type A, except Ref. [53] which used Type B. These studies showed good evidence that BTX Type A can lead to improvements in PROM (and functions such as passive dressing), together with some evidence for improvements in spasticity-related pain and spasms, and active

Table 11.1 Physical interventions for spasticity and other upper motor neurone phenomena.

Reference	Study type (reference)	Patients (n)	Intervention	Intensity	Improvement in active voluntary movement	Improvement in PROM	Reduction in spasticity-related pain	Reduction in spasms
[11]	RCT Single blind	SCI (14)	Passive stretching of one ankle versus other ankle not stretched	30 min daily	No	No		
[12]	RCT crossover Single blind	TBI (9)	Ankle casts and stretching versus no casts	7 days each arm		Yes Torque-controlled PROM		
[13]	RCT crossover	TBI (15)	Serial elbow and/or wrist casts versus traditional therapy	1 month	No	Yes Goniometry		
[14]	RCT crossover Single blind	Stroke (44, 21 with spasticity)	Bobath versus orthopaedic physiotherapy approach	20 sessions over 4 weeks	Bobath was superior at motor assessment and stroke impact scales			
[15]	SR of 6 RCTs	MS (164)	Exercise therapy versus normal activity		Strong evidence for mobility-related activities Moderate evidence for arm/hand use			
[16]	SR of 11 RCTs	Stroke (458)	Treadmill training with body weight support versus usual activity		No Walking speed Walking dependence			
[17]	RCT Single blind	Stroke (28)	Functional electrical stimulation (UL) versus usual activity	30 min daily for 3 weeks	Yes Upper extremity functioning test Drawing Test Motor activity log	Yes Higher functioning group only Ashworth score		
[18]	RCT	Stroke (32)	Functional electrical stimulation (LL) versus usual activity	12 sessions of physiotherapy to train use of FES	Yes Walking speed Physiological cost index	Yes Wartenberg pendulum test		

UL: upper limbs; LL: lower limbs; SCI: Spinal cord injury; MS: Multiple sclerosis; PROM: Passive range of movement; SR: systematic review; TBI: traumatic brain injury.

Table 11.2 Oral drug treatments for spasticity.

Reference	Study type	Patients (n)	Intervention	Improvement in active voluntary movement	Improvement in PROM	Reduction in spasticity-related pain	Reduction in spasms
[20]	RCT	Stroke (20)	Baclofen (30 mg) versus placebo		Yes Ashworth		
[21]	RCT crossover	MS (23)	Baclofen (up to 80 mg) versus placebo		Yes Unvalidated score	Yes	Yes
[22]	Four-way crossover study with no washout period between treatment arms	MS (38)	Baclofen (20 mg) and/or stretching exercises		Yes Ashworth score and angle of flexion		
[23]	RCT	MS (166)	Baclofen (60–80 mg) versus placebo		Yes Unvalidated score		Yes
[24]	RCT crossover	Stroke (38)	Dantrolene (50–200 mg) versus placebo	No	No		
[25]	RCT	Stroke (18)	Dantrolene (average dose 165.4 mg/day)		Yes Novel spasticity grading scale		
[26]	RCT	Spinal cord disease (25)	Dantrolene (up to 400 mg) versus placebo	Yes Walking speed only	Yes Unvalidated tone score		Yes
[27]	RCT	Various with spastic paraparesis (13)	Tizanidine (up to 10 mg/day) versus placebo		No		
[28]	RCT crossover	Stroke (9) and TBI (8)	Tizanidine (up to 36 mg) versus placebo		Yes Ashworth score		Yes For LL only
[29]	RCT	SCI (124)	Tizanidine (4–36 mg) versus placebo		Yes Ashworth score		Yes
[30]	RCT	MS (257)	Tizanidine (2–36 mg) versus placebo	No	No	No	No
[31]	RCT	MS (187)	Tizanidine (up to 36 mg) versus placebo	No	Yes Composite Ashworth score	No	No
[32]	RCT	MS (66)	Tizanidine (up to 36 mg) versus placebo	No	Yes in some muscle groups Unvalidated tone score	No	No

Ref	Study design	Patients (n)	Comparison				
[33]	RCT crossover	MS (16)	Cannabinoids versus placebo	No. Worsening in timed walk and 9-hole peg test in THC treated group	No		
[34]	RCT crossover with no washout period	MS (24) and SCI (4)	Cannabinoids versus placebo	No	No	Yes VAS	Yes VAS
[35]	RCT	MS (611)	Cannabinoids versus placebo	Yes. Timed walk in THC group	No	Yes	Yes
[36]	RCT crossover with unequal treatment periods	MS (50)	Cannabinoids versus placebo	Yes. Mobility in those who received >90% prescribed dose	No		Yes in those who received >90% prescribed dose
[37]	RCT	MS (160)	Cannabinoids versus placebo	No	No		No
[38]	RCT crossover	Stroke (19)	Diazepam (6–15 mg) versus placebo	No. Grip strength worse	No		
[39]	RCT crossover	Stroke (12)	Diazepam versus placebo	No	Yes. Knee passive movement		
[40]	RCT	Stroke (120)	Tolperisone (300–900 mg) versus placebo	? Yes for walking distance (graph but not statistics shown)	Yes. Modified Ashworth score		
[41]	RCT crossover	SCI (6 paraplegic, 3 paraparetic)	Clonidine (0.1–0.5 mg) versus placebo	Yes – in only 1 paraparetic patient	Yes in 5 of 9. Ashworth score		
[42]	RCT crossover with 2-day treatment periods	SCI (25)	Gabapentin (2400 mg) versus placebo	Yes	Yes. Ashworth score		Yes
[43]	RCT crossover	MS (22)	Gabapentin (900 mg) versus placebo	Yes	Yes. Ashworth score	Yes	Yes

LL: lower limbs; TBI: traumatic brain injury; SCI: Spinal cord injury; MS: Multiple sclerosis; PROM: Passive range of movement; VAS: Visual analogue scale.

Table 11.3 Intrathecal baclofen treatment for spasticity.

Reference	Study type	Patients (n)	Intervention	Improvement in active voluntary movement	Improvement in PROM	Reduction in spasticity-related pain	Reduction in spasms
[45]	RCT	Hemiplegia due to TBI or CVA (6)	Test dose of IT baclofen versus saline		Yes Ashworth score		Yes Penn scale
[46]	RCT	Stroke (21)	Test dose of IT baclofen versus saline		Yes Ashworth score		Yes Penn scale
[47]	RCT	Spinal spasticity (93)	Test dose of IT baclofen versus saline		Yes (88 responded, but outcome measure results not reported)		
[48]	RCT	Spinal spasticity (22)	Infusion of IT baclofen versus saline for 13 weeks	Mobility subscale of sickness Impact profile	Yes (effect size 1.40) Modified Ashworth score	Yes (effect size 0.94) 10-point scale	Slight (effect size 0.20) Penn scale

TBI: traumatic brain injury; CVA: cerebrovascular accident; IT: intrathecal.

Table 11.4 Intramuscular botulinum toxin injections for spasticity.

Reference	Study type	Patients (*n*)	Intervention	Improvement in active voluntary movement	Improvement in PROM and function	Reduction in spasticity-related pain	Reduction in spasms
[55]	RCT	CVA (39)	BTX versus placebo for arm and forearm spasticity	No	Yes Ashworth in 300 units group only	No	
[56]	RCT	CVA or TBI (21)	BTX versus placebo for arm and forearm spasticity	No	Yes Ashworth Finger curl distance PROM at wrist but not fingers		
[57]	RCT	CVA (82)	BTX versus placebo for arm spasticity	No	Yes – for all doses Modified Ashworth		
[58]	RCT	CVA (40)	BTX versus placebo for arm and forearm spasticity	No	Yes Ashworth Disability and carer burden scales	No	
[59]	RCT	CVA (59)	BTX versus placebo for arm spasticity	No	Yes Modified Ashworth Elbow PROM	No	
[60]	RCT	CVA (126)	BTX versus placebo for forearm spasticity	No	Yes Ashworth Disability assessment scale	Yes	
[53]	RCT	CVA (15)	BTX Type B versus placebo for arm and forearm spasticity	No	No Ashworth	No	
[61]	RCT	CVA (91)	BTX versus placebo for arm and forearm spasticity	No	Yes Ashworth	No	
[62]	RCT	CVA (50)	BTX versus placebo for arm and forearm spasticity with some residual active movement	Yes Action research arm test (500 unit group only)	Yes MAS	Yes VAS	
[63]	RCT	MS (74)	BTX versus placebo for hip adductor spasticity		Yes Distance between knees for highest dose (1500 units Dysport) only		

(*Continued* p. 96)

Table 11.4 (Continued.)

Reference	Study type	Patients (n)	Intervention	Improvement in active voluntary movement	Improvement in PROM and function	Reduction in spasticity-related pain	Reduction in spasms
[64]	RCT	Chair or bed bound MS (9)	BTX versus placebo for hip adductor spasticity	No	Yes Adduction angle Nursing care		No
[65]	RCT crossover	(23) 19 CVA 4 TBI	BTX versus placebo for foot spasticity	Yes for active dorsiflexion Reduced use of walking aids in 6 patients	Yes Ashworth		
[66]	RCT	CVA (234)	BTX versus placebo for calf spasticity	Yes – use of walking aids only No – 2 min walking distance or stepping rate	Yes MAS	Yes	
[67]	RCT	CVA (45)	BTX versus placebo for foot spasticity	Yes Gait speed	Yes Ashworth	Yes	
[54]	RCT	Early after TBI (35)	Casting alone versus casting plus BTX versus stretches to prevent loss of ankle dorsiflexion range		Yes – for casting and/or BTX Ankle PROM		
[68]	RCT crossover	Various (12)	BTX versus placebo for UL (8) or LL (4) spasticity		Yes Ashworth		Yes
[69]	RCT	Various (52)	BTX versus placebo for UL (32) or LL (20) spasticity	Yes for LL group Rivermead mobility index only	Yes Ashworth Range of movement		Yes

TBI: traumatic brain injury; BTX: Botulinumtoxin; UL: upper limbs; LL: lower limbs; MS: Multiple sclerosis; CVA: cerebrovascular accident; MAS: Modified Ashworth Scale; PROM: passive range of movement.

55 Simpson DM, Alexander DN, O'Brien CF, et al. Botulinum toxin type A in the treatment of upper extremity spasticity: a randomized, double-blind, placebo-controlled trial. *Neurology* 1996; **46**: 1306–10.

56 Smith SJ, Ellis E, White S, Moore AP. A double-blind placebo-controlled study of botulinum toxin in upper limb spasticity after stroke or head injury. *Clin. Rehabil.* 2000; **14**: 5–13.

57 Bakheit AM, Thilmann AF, Ward AB, et al. A randomized, double-blind, placebo-controlled, dose-ranging study to compare the efficacy and safety of three doses of botulinum toxin type A (Dysport) with placebo in upper limb spasticity after stroke. *Stroke* 2000; **31**: 2402–6.

58 Bhakta BB, Cozens JA, Chamberlain MA, Bamford JM. Impact of botulinum toxin type A on disability and carer burden due to arm spasticity after stroke: a randomised double blind placebo controlled trial. *J. Neurol. Neurosurg. Psychiatr.* 2000; **69**: 217–21.

59 Bakheit AM, Pittock S, Moore AP, et al. A randomized, double-blind, placebo-controlled study of the efficacy and safety of botulinum toxin type A in upper limb spasticity in patients with stroke. *Eur. J. Neurol.* 2001; **8**: 559–65.

60 Brashear A, Gordon M, Elovic E, et al. Intramuscular injection of botulinum toxin for the treatment of wrist and finger spasticity after a stroke. *N. Engl. J. Med.* 2002; **347**: 395–400.

61 Childers MK, Brashear A, Jozefczyk P, et al. Dose-dependent response to intramuscular botulinum toxin type A for upper-limb spasticity in patients after a stroke. *Arch. Phys. Med. Rehabil.* 2004; **85**: 1063–9.

62 Suputtitada A, Suwanwela NC. The lowest effective dose of botulinum A toxin in adult patients with upper limb spasticity. *Disabil. Rehabil.* 2005; **27**: 176–84.

63 Hyman N, Barnes M, Bhakta B, et al. Botulinum toxin (Dysport) treatment of hip adductor spasticity in multiple sclerosis: a prospective, randomised, double blind, placebo controlled, dose ranging study. *J. Neurol. Neurosurg. Psychiatr.* 2000; **68**: 707–12.

64 Snow BJ, Tsui JK, Bhatt MH, Varelas M, Hashimoto SA, Calne DB. Treatment of spasticity with botulinum toxin: a double-blind study. *Ann. Neurol.* 1990; **28**: 512–5.

65 Burbaud P, Wiart L, Dubos JL, et al. A randomised, double blind, placebo controlled trial of botulinum toxin in the treatment of spastic foot in hemiparetic patients. *J. Neurol. Neurosurg. Psychiatr.* 1996; **61**: 265–9.

66 Pittock SJ, Moore AP, Hardiman O, et al. A double-blind randomised placebo-controlled evaluation of three doses of botulinum toxin type A (Dysport) in the treatment of spastic equinovarus deformity after stroke. *Cerebrovasc. Dis.* 2003; **15**: 289–300.

67 Mancini F, Sandrini G, Moglia A, Nappi G, Pacchetti C. A randomised, double-blind, dose-ranging study to evaluate efficacy and safety of three doses of botulinum toxin type A (Botox) for the treatment of spastic foot. *Neurol. Sci.* 2005; **26**: 26–31.

68 Grazko MA, Polo KB, Jabbari B. Botulinum toxin A for spasticity, muscle spasms, and rigidity. *Neurology* 1995; **45**: 712–7.

69 Richardson D, Sheean G, Werring D, et al. Evaluating the role of botulinum toxin in the management of focal hypertonia in adults. *J. Neurol. Neurosurg. Psychiatr.* 2000; **69**: 499–506.

12

CHAPTER 12
Background to neurorehabilitation

Kathryn McPherson, Paula Kersten, Lynne Turner-Stokes

Background

Neurological illness and injury are major causes of disability. With an ageing population and more people surviving what would have until relatively recently been fatal neurological insults, utilizing best evidence for rehabilitation is increasingly important. Rehabilitation emphasizes adaptive and restorative strategies across the many aspects of human life and performance. Whilst management and prevention of pathology and impairment remain crucial, promoting functional improvement, assisting people to participate in a meaningful life and helping them and their families attain or maintain the best quality of life (QoL) are rehabilitation's real goals.

Data on incidence and prevalence of different neurological disability vary greatly according to the way data are collected. The USA Centre for Disease Control[1] suggests 1 in every 10 people has major activity limitation due to a chronic condition with two recent household surveys (in the UK and New Zealand [1,2]) suggesting that around one in every five adults and one in every ten children have some sort of disability, with the most common disability being difficulties resulting from neurological origin. The Neurological Alliance recently estimated that around 6% of people have a neurological condition where they need daily help with activities [3]. Disability arising from neurological conditions is therefore no small issue.

Despite some very clear gaps in knowledge, research in rehabilitation has advanced significantly over recent years. New technologies are being applied (including advanced neuroimaging, robotics and virtual reality) and the critique that rehabilitation interventions have lacked a firm theoretical basis [4] is increasingly being challenged. For instance, recent advances in motor learning theory are being applied to develop novel physiotherapeutic interventions [5,6], self-regulation theory being utilized to challenge perhaps the most ubiquitous intervention in neurorehabilitation – goal setting [7–10] and neurobiology findings influencing a wide range of developments across conditions and strategies given the emerging potential that neural 'reorganization' shows in contributing to recovery, restoration and adaptation [11].

Along with technological and theoretical advance, many aspects of rehabilitation now having increasing evidence that they work: specialized stroke units are effective [12,13]; specialist neurological rehabilitation teams can improve outcome after traumatic brain injury [14]; interventions from specialist rehabilitation teams are beneficial for people with multiple sclerosis [15,16] as well as younger people with physical and complex disabilities [17]. There is also a growing body of evidence for the cost-effectiveness of neurorehabilitation [13,18,19].

Despite these advances, evaluating the impact of rehabilitation remains complex [20]. It is not a synonym for any one type of intervention (such as surgery/medication) nor is it the domain of any one health professional group (such as medicine, physiotherapy or occupational therapy). Further, rehabilitation strategies aim to achieve outcomes that are wide ranging and difficult to operationalize and the interventions themselves can be difficult to describe. Subtle differences in the way interventions are delivered may very well influence the impact of those interventions (i.e. the process of care/management [21]).

One of the frustrations for clinicians, patients and their families is that as a result of this complexity, trial data (and therefore meta-analyses) concerning rehabilitation has frequently yielded equivocal findings. Whilst improved rehabilitation trials are a clear priority, it is arguable that in addition, practical tools are required to help determine best practice and best decision making in the absence of 'gold standard' results from randomized trials [20,22]. Further, for some questions that need to be confronted, (such as what type of therapeutic interventions are most acceptable to specific populations, what barriers and facilitators exist in relation to promoting active engagement in rehabilitation) methodologies including qualitative work have a clear role. With these cautions in mind, advances over the very recent past about 'what works', mean there is reason to feel optimistic about the knowledge base of neurorehabilitation.

Outcomes in neurorehabilitation[2]

In order to evaluate evidence about the effectiveness of interventions, it is crucial to be specific about the outcomes

---

[1] http://www.cdc.gov/nccdphp/overview.htm

[2] The World Health Organisation models utilized in rehabilitation to specify outcome are outlined in full elsewhere http://www3.who.int/icf/ and so are only be touched on briefly to provide context for considering the topic.

aimed for and to ensure measures used are both appropriately targeted and psychometrically robust. Whilst these questions are an issue across healthcare, they are of particular concern in rehabilitation where mortality and morbidity are clearly insufficient descriptors. Two key frameworks have advanced our ability to think about and measure outcomes of relevance in rehabilitation.

The first of these frameworks is the International Classification of Impairments, Disabilities and Handicaps (ICIDH), and more latterly the International Classification of Health and Functioning (ICF) [23,24]. These frameworks aimed to facilitate explicit consideration of the consequences of chronic or disabling conditions to guide treatment and provide a comprehensive focus for evaluation. Whilst the models do consider *pathology* and/or *impairment*, they expand their focus to include and specify *body functions, activity limitations* and social roles that individuals held – handicap (in the ICIDH) and *participation* (in the ICF). Whilst these frameworks are not without criticism [25], they have been extraordinarily influential in the development of outcome measures in rehabilitation and in helping us understand what really matters to patients [26].

For rehabilitation interventions to be considered effective, change at the level of impairment (say increased range of motion in the lower limbs) is arguably of limited benefit if that is all that is achieved. Whilst it may have every relevance in that it alleviates secondary impairments (such as pain, skin breakdown and so on), the aim of rehabilitation is to help people maintain or improve the ability to perform related activities (being able to move about) and/or participate (being able to engage in the roles where that mobility is necessary – say manoeuvre within a work location or attend family celebrations). This factor is of importance when considering rehabilitation 'evidence' as functional and social outcomes are considered just as, and sometimes even more important than, curing pathology or reducing impairment.

The second area of focus in outcome measurement relevant to rehabilitation has been in the field of QoL. Early developments here considered that what might truly define a 'good outcome' was that the quality of a person's life may be just as, or in some cases more, important than its quantity [27]. Whilst QoL is not explicitly listed in the ICF, its core constructs (such as body function, activity and participation within the context of environmental facilitators and barriers) comprise aspects of some definitions of QoL.

However, debate about what QoL really means prevails and measures purporting to address QoL frequently lack a clear definition of the concept and may in reality be symptom checklists, measures of activity, and/or health status measures. Difficulties in defining the concept persist, perhaps in part due to the quite different basis for interest among the various stakeholders in health. Patients, family and indeed healthcare providers are frequently driven to understand effectiveness of interventions from individual or humanistic aspects of QoL (i.e. what matters most to the patient themselves) whilst those driven more by economic perspectives on outcome are clearly looking to establish effectiveness largely in relation to 'cost' to society. These two very different perspectives result in quite different types of QoL measure [28]. Despite these persisting issues, what was famously called the missing measurement in healthcare [29] has become an essential component of rehabilitation evaluations [30,31].

Determining the effectiveness of rehabilitation therefore depends on considering outcomes related to the specific activity or function being targeted, the roles in life that are being facilitated, and/or the aspects of QoL that are being enhanced.

Framing clinical questions in neurorehabilitation

Neurological injury or illness can affect the ability to perform or participate in any activity or life role. Given the aim of this book and the other diagnostically specific chapters, we focus on three questions facing clinicians and patients across a range of neurological conditions:

1 When should rehabilitation be initiated and how intense does it need to be?
2 Who will benefit from rehabilitation – can we accurately predict response?
3 What are the components of an effective specialist rehabilitation service?

General approach to searching evidence

The above complexity concerning the breadth of populations, the diversity of interventions, and the potential range of outcomes means searching for evidence about effectiveness in rehabilitation is somewhat difficult when compared to that for a relatively discreet interventions with a specific outcome (such as use of a novel medication aiming for reduction in seizure or mortality rates). Nevertheless the same principles apply whereby a precise definition of each term is required. Therefore a key step in rehabilitation research is to identify all possible acronyms and alternate words for each term. The search presented here also utilized reference list searching within specific papers and citation index of key papers.

Critical review of the evidence for each question

1. Timing and intensity of rehabilitation
When should rehabilitation be initiated and how intense does it need to be?

There has long been debate about how much rehabilitation is needed to produce the best outcomes. This section considers whether patients (as an exemplar considering those with acute stroke and moderate severe TBI) benefit from early

Table 12.1 Intensity and rehabilitation.

Types of study (reference)	Intervention intensity	Patients	Outcome	Number of participants/ trials	Main findings	Comments
Kwakkel et al. [37]	Physiotherapy and occupational therapy. On average twice as much therapy time for intervention versus control.	Stroke	ADL, Instrumental ADL (e.g. activities such as shopping) walking and dexterity.	2686/20	Experimental participants received on average twice as much therapy with a weighted average of 16 h total additional therapy time per patient. SES χ^2 = 28.61 significant (0.15 SD units CI 0.06 to 0.23, Z = 3.24, $P < 0.001$) for ADL in favour of those receiving enhanced therapy when therapy initiated in the first 6 months after stroke (but not for those initiated after 6 months – only three studies).	20 trials, mixed quality rating from 2 to 10 (out of 14) on self-developed quality rating tool. Limited pooling of data possible due to the variability of outcomes evaluated. Effect size negatively associated with study quality ($r = -0.438$, $P < 0.05$).
Van Peppen et al. [38]	Physiotherapy. Difference between intervention and control ranging from 132 to 6816 min.	Stroke	Function, impairment	?/151	SES ranged from 0.13 (95% CI 0.03–0.23) for effects of high intensity of exercise training in functional outcomes to 0.92 (95% CI 0.54–1.29) for impairment (improving symmetry when moving from sitting to standing).	Very informative review with other findings of interest regarding specific therapeutic interventions. Methodological quality of all RCTs a median of 5 points on the 10-point PEDro scale (range 2–8 points).
Bhogal et al. [39]	Speech and language therapy. Intensity – variable therapy time difference between intervention and control.	Stroke	Aphasia – Porch Index of Communicative Abilities (PICA) and the Token test (T test) (verbal comprehension of commands of increasing complexity).	833/8	The four trials demonstrating improved outcome had intensive practice per week (mean = 8.8 h compared with 2 h/week) over a shorter period of time (mean 11.2 weeks compared 22.9 weeks). T test = 8.79, $P > 0.001$ (PICA) and 2.561, $P < 0.05$ (T test).	Although 10 trials were considered, quality evaluation removed two trials. Clear description of each trial. Utilized PEDro scale.
Turner-Stokes et al. [19]	Multidisciplinary rehabilitation across a broad range of interventions. Intensity – variable time difference between intervention and control.	Brain injury (TBI, stroke, mixed)	Wide range of outcomes including symptoms, function, carer strain, QoL, mood, and social integration.	?/15	Synthesis limited to descriptive due to heterogeneity of studies. Intensity recorded in four of the 15 studies included. Three of the four studies found faster functional gain in the enhanced group and reduced length of stay in rehabilitation.	This systematic review covers many issues relating to TBI rehabilitation. Mixed quality of trial data a restriction in determining difference. Utilized Van Tulder quality screening scores. No trials explored 'adverse effects'.

ADL: activities of daily living; SES: summary effect size; TBI: traumatic brain injury.

commencement of therapy and/or greater intensity (hours of therapeutic intervention) in terms of decreased impairment and/or improved function, participation or QoL?

Langhorne and colleagues [32] published one of the early studies investigating this issue and suggested that although further research was needed, early and intense rehabilitation was important – not just for improved function but as it decreased the rate of death/deterioration. Teasell et al. [33] recently offered an in depth descriptive review of the topic highlighting that getting this 'window of opportunity' right is crucial in stroke rehabilitation. One might reasonably assume this to be so across other conditions with discrete events causing damage to the brain such as in acquired brain injury from trauma or illness. Whilst animal studies have indicated intense rehabilitation initiated within hours following stroke actually increases the size of the lesion, therapy initiated shortly thereafter (within days) appears to result in enhanced recovery of function when compared with delayed rehabilitation [34]. It does appear that the acute phase post-stroke is when the brain is most primed for recovery and that this effect diminishes over time.

A series of studies (focused on both primary trial data and secondary analyses in a systematic review) by Gert Kwakkel et al. [35–38] have done much to advance knowledge in physical rehabilitation. In addition, there have been a number of recent reviews including that by Bhogal et al. [39] in the field of aphasia, Turner-Stokes et al. [19] in traumatic brain injury and Cicerone et al. [40] in cognitive rehabilitation. The most persuasive evidence so far is in relation to stroke, at least in part due to the focused investment in research that has taken place. A selection of recent reviews focused on intensity and timing of rehabilitation is provided in Table 12.1.

Most evidence about timing and intensity of rehabilitation would support early, targeted and more intense interventions than that routinely delivered. However, there are of course caveats to this: firstly, Page et al. [41] highlight that lasting cortical changes have been demonstrated in task specific therapies that are relatively non-intense; secondly, some intense therapies such as constraint induced therapy are up to 6 h a day which is difficult to absorb into clinical practice and lastly; in more chronic phases of disability, rehabilitation therapy may well be of benefit in stroke [42,43], traumatic brain injury [44] and conditions such as multiple sclerosis [45]. So despite some evidence, definitive guidance about intensity and timing of rehabilitation is yet to be determined.

2. Who will benefit from rehabilitation?

Who will benefit from rehabilitation – can we accurately predict response?

With limited resources and increasing demand, important choices are constantly being made concerning service provision. Given the above arguments for providing more targeted, intense rehabilitation at the appropriate windows of need

and opportunity, the question as to who should have priority in accessing services in the face of limited availability is daunting. This section considers in particular which patients (with acute stroke, moderate severe TBI and those in vegetative state) benefit from rehabilitation interventions in terms of decreased impairment and/or improved function, participation or QoL?

Whilst across the board increases in funding clearly have an important part to play in facilitating access to services, being able to accurately predict who will gain most is also important. This is not just because of resource limitation, but also so as to promote access to the rehabilitation services/interventions that are most appropriate for individual patients. But how 'evidence based' are decisions about referral and discharge from neurorehabilitation? Table 12.2 presents findings of some recent reviews in the field.

Accurate prediction of who will benefit from rehabilitation remains problematic. Variables such as premorbid function, degree of neurological damage and deficit, age, mood and behavioural disturbance, functional performance at discharge, and presence of social support emerge in many of the models predicting improved long-term outcome. Whilst useful for informing patients and their families about possible prognosis, how useful are these models for targeting priority for specific patients? Well the current answer has to be – not as useful as we need them to be. Most variables are either aspects of being human (age) or features of the neurological condition itself (level of deficit) and the variance accounted for by even quite complex multifactorial models is only around 60%.

It may be that this is as good as our predictive models can be given the variability of human kind and heterogeneous presentation of neurological illness or injury. On the other hand, perhaps some of the big issues impacting on outcome in neurorehabilitation are yet to be well understood. For instance, whilst 'motivation' to participate in rehabilitation has been identified as key to achieving good outcomes [46–49], the concept is poorly understood and problematic for clinicians and patients [50]. In particular, motivation in neurological rehabilitation is a far more complex concept than many interventions, and much of rehabilitation practice, would seem to reflect [9,51]. If, as would appear likely given the nature of executive functioning deficit, motivation is a skill set rather than a personality trait, intervention at this level may well be a core component of the gains that need to be made in rehabilitation, not only in enhancing motivation itself but in achieving the core rehabilitation outcomes suggested earlier [7,8,10,52]. Finally, plateau has become a frequent rationale for discharge from rehabilitation, particularly where services are contracted according to continued functional gain. However, recent work would suggest that even in areas where the phrase has become common such as in stroke rehabilitation, it is of questionable meaning and value [53,54].

Evidence to guide decisions about who should receive which rehabilitation strategies is advancing. However, accurate

Table 12.2 Predicting who will benefit more from rehabilitation (observational non-controlled studies).

Type of study (reference)	Population	Outcome	Number of participants/trials	Main findings	Comments
Observational. Whyte et al. [89]	Vegetative state and minimally conscious state after TBI	Disability rating scale (DRS) at 16 weeks post injury and time until commands first followed	Seven acute inpatient rehabilitation centres across USA and Europe (124 patients)	Initial disability (DRS), time between injury and enrolment in the study, rate of DRS change during the first 2 weeks of the study were predictive of both outcomes ($P < 0.001$ – multivariate modelling). The second model excluded rate of change but included hypothesized psychoactive medication exposure. Both initial DRS and later admission stayed in the model with exposure to Amantadine associated with positive outcome ($P < 0.001$) Dantroline worse ($P = 0.011$).	Observational research design. Authors note inconsistent findings of the nature of pathology on outcome and call for prospective trials.
Observational. Schepers et al. [90]	1 year post-stroke	Social activity measured by the Frenchay activities index (FAI). Disability and impairment – Motricity Index and Barthel Index, The Trunk Control Test (TCT) and Utrecht Communication Observation (UTO).	Four rehabilitation centres – (250 patients)	The highest correlation coefficient was found for the Multivariate analysis showed that gender sex (female) B = 2.82 $P = 0.010$ and age B = –0.16, $P = 0.001$; followed Motricity Index (B = 0.1, $P = 0.001$); UCO (B = 0.92, $P = 0.058$) and Barthel score (B = 0.41, $P = 0.031$). The ROC curve had an AUC of 0.85 (95% confidence interval, 0.80–0.90). Claim to have developed a score chart that is easy to use in clinical practice for the identification of patients at risk for social inactivity 1 year post-stroke. The chart includes sex, age, marital status, Motricity Index.	The authors note that 'social activity' is difficult to define. Utilized the FAI as it is commonly used in stroke. This measure has been criticized elsewhere. Numerous variables that might impact on outcome not measured.
Cicerone et al. [40]. More detail in Chapter 10.	Stroke and TBI	Cognitive rehabilitation – mainly measures of cognitive impairment	87 studies. 291 TBI patients and 247 with stroke	Substantial evidence that people with language deficit after stroke benefit from cognitive-linguistic therapies and recent evidence supporting training for those with apraxia after left hemisphere stroke. Also for training those with mild memory impairment and strategy training for those with post-acute attention deficit. 17 of the studies considered class 1 with 16 of these studies supporting cognitive rehabilitation.	Useful review and descriptive synthesis of cognitive rehabilitation. Reiterates the difficulty of synthesising 'evidence' in rehabilitation due to lack of standardization of interventions, measures and methods. Also identifies need to consider broader range of outcomes including activities and participation.

prediction of prognosis and for targeting strategies is likely to require greater knowledge of variables such as motivation and decreased reliance on outdated notions of 'plateau'. Until then, we may be able to 'rule in' who might benefit from rehabilitation, but 'ruling out' is at best imprecise.

3. Specialist rehabilitation service

What are the key components of an effective specialist rehabilitation service?

Given the emergent evidence that specialist rehabilitation is effective [12–19], a key goal of research has been to determine just exactly what components of those services are crucial for achieving better outcomes. It is perhaps unsurprising that there has therefore been a growth in focus on this 'black box' of neurorehabilitation [55–64]. This section considers in particular whether patients (with acute stroke) benefit from any one aspect of the rehabilitation 'black box' in terms of decreased impairment and/or improved function, participation or QoL?

Recent steps to more fully identify, define and operationalize these components in stroke [63–66] have been undertaken in the Post-Stroke Rehabilitation Outcomes Project (PSROP)[3] with findings recently published in a special issue of the Archives of Physical Medicine and Rehabilitation [67–75]. The key goal of PSROP is to determine the impact that each stroke rehabilitation 'activity or intervention' of itself and collectively has on patient outcomes on discharge [65]. This is of course no small endeavour given the complexity of rehabilitation *p*opulations, *i*nterventions, *c*ontrol groups and *o*utcome measures (i.e. each level of the PICO format [76,77]). However, the framework proposed and the methodological developments undertaken show very real potential for leading to a better understanding of separate *and* interdependent components/attributes of successful rehabilitation. DeJong highlights a number of cautions in interpreting the findings of PSROP [65], in particular the limited follow-up into the community and the observational/clinical practice improvement (CPI) rather than experimental nature of the work (meaning association but not causation is examined). However, the second criticism (concerning a CPI methodology) must sit alongside the fact that the randomized clinical trial format has fallen short in answering some of the important questions in neurorehabilitation [22,66].

A very real strength of PSROP is that it has proposed and validated a taxonomy concerning what goes on in rehabilitation after stroke. Whilst individual professions have proposed checklists of input (e.g. physiotherapists [78]), there has been little consensus about the nature of contributions between and across the different disciplines. The clear specification of both interventions and activities (the purpose for which interventions are delivered) is an advance in the specification of rehabilitation. As a result, there seems very real potential to determine the patterns of delivery of rehabilitation services across different settings and countries, and to find out the proportional effects of the various components of what is by definition, an interdisciplinary and holistic process. In their commentaries about PSROP, Ottenbacher [79] and Jette [80] reiterate that caution is needed in interpreting and acting on findings prior to replication and hopefully in studies where bias and confounding are more controlled. However, they too acknowledge the black box of rehabilitation has been at least partially illuminated by PRSOP with such findings as:

- Fewer days from stroke symptom onset to rehabilitation admission being associated with better functional outcomes at discharge and shorter length of stay [74].
- Despite recognition that the environment influences task performance, little time was spent in community mobility activities by physiotherapists before discharge [73].
- More occupational therapy time spent on higher-level activities such as community integration, functional mobility, home management, and leisure activities and greater use of high level and complex speech and language therapy activities linked with better functional outcome at discharge. However, in both instances, these tend to be the least common activities focused on during inpatient rehabilitation [69,75].
- The nature, duration and intensity of rehabilitation interventions and actions varied across sites [68,69,72–75,81]. In particular, poorer outcome were found in the site where greater time was spent on administrative versus treatment/therapeutic activities [81].

As noted by DeJong [65], there are aspects of rehabilitation that were not fully evaluated in the PRSOP study. Such processes include team coherence and organizational milieu and whilst other research would suggest they too are part of the 'black box' of effective rehabilitation [21,82,83]. There is undoubtedly more work to be done in this area if the crucial components of specialist rehabilitation are to be determined and prioritized.

Conclusion

Implications for health service organization and policy

The need for neurorehabilitation provision is escalating and evidence that more targeted and timely rehabilitation is the most appropriate provision is also accumulating. However, for health policy, a number of pieces in the jigsaw puzzle are still missing. When is the timeliest provision for people with conditions such as multiple sclerosis and Parkinson's disease? What is the best approach to utilizing goals in rehabilitation?

---

[3]The study involved seven centres and 1291 patients where stroke rehabilitation practice was documented in a standardized format, and its relationship to inpatient outcomes investigated.

A European study investigating similar issues is currently running – The Collaborative Evaluation of Rehabilitation in Stroke Across Europe (CERISE).

Is the provision of one rehabilitation strategy compared to another (or no treatment) cost effective? We have few answers to these questions and until we do, evidence based policy in rehabilitation will probably remain a rare beast. The knowledge base gained from stroke research is a real warning that inadequate rehabilitation results in preventable death, deterioration and harm [84]. These are not inconsequential findings. For society to manage prioritization in provision of services, it is clear that investment in research is crucial. Whilst calls for this are frequent [85] and increasingly societies appears cognizant of this need, without an increase in good rehabilitation research answering the important questions, decisions will be made on the absence of evidence and that is unlikely to be in patient's best interests.

Implications for research

There is certainly no shortage of research that needs to be done in rehabilitation. Despite the advances that have been noted, we need to facilitate research that:
- Has better specification of experimental and alternate interventions.
- Utilizes, and where required develops, more robust measures of outcome appropriate to those interventions and to what matters most to patients (in particular 'participation' or role fulfilment).
- Adopts more rigorous approaches to research methodology including appropriate power in studies so that definitive results are determined when they actually do exist along with appropriate blinding and randomization in RCTs.
- Is not deterred from developing and utilizing appropriate methodologies to answer important questions, not all of which will be answered by trial data.

It is also important to note in considering and devising rehabilitation research, that lifelong neurological conditions pose a number of challenges for traditional research methods including [22]:

(a) The effects of a long-term condition unfold over many years – a time scale beyond the scope of most clinical trials.

(b) Interventions are complex and played out over a long period, changing progressively in the light of the individual's response to what has gone before. They are frequently multidisciplinary in nature, and any one intervention will often overlap and interact with others.

(c) The effect of any clinical intervention must be assessed not only in the context of other clinical care, but also against a complex background of social and environmental factors, which are not adequately described by existing quantitative techniques. To control properly for these 'unseen confounders' potentially requires a much larger sample than the total affected population. This may be particularly so for the less common conditions.

(d) By definition, in the context of a long-term condition, 'cure' or reversal of pathology is rarely a goal for treatment. Instead, the intended outcomes focus on reducing the impact of the disease – for example on QoL or societal participation. Whilst a variety of standardized 'measures' have been developed to evaluate these issues, many appear to provide a less than satisfactory reflection of real life experiences in chronic conditions [28,86].

(e) Response shift is likely to occur throughout the trajectory of a long-term condition and may confound evaluative efforts [87].

These issues are not small but they are ones we need to confront and respond to. Without doing so, it is likely that patients and their families will get less than they should from rehabilitation despite the efforts of those doing their best to deliver evidence-based, high-quality interventions/services.

In conclusion recent advances in neurorehabilitation are exciting and the evidence base to inform decision making in practice is growing. Less than 10 years ago, rehabilitation was arguably a 'Cinderella' of medicine and of research [88]. This is no longer the case with it increasingly recognized as an important area of management in neurology, and as making a difference. There is much to learn from the gains made in stroke rehabilitation where much hard work, focused attention and collaboration between leading clinicians and researchers across a range of medical and non-medical disciplines has seen clear answers emerging in response to a number of important questions. Such gains are vital for those patients with other neurological conditions where disability is frequent, but definitive answers less so.

References

1 Department of Health (UK). *Health Survey for England*. The Stationery Office, London, 2004.

2 New Zealand Ministry of Health. *Living with Disability in New Zealand*. New Zealand Ministry of Health, Wellington, 2004.

3 The Neurological Alliance. *Neuro Numbers – a Brief Review of the Numbers of People in the UK with a Neurological Condition*. The Neurological Alliance, London, 2003.

4 Siegert RJ, McPherson KM, Dean S. Theory development and a science of rehabilitation. *Disabil. Rehabil.* 2005; **27**(24): 1493–1501.

5 Cauraugh JH, Summers JJ. Neural plasticity and bilateral movements: a rehabilitation approach for chronic stroke. *Prog. Neurobiol.* 2005; **75**(5): 309–20.

6 Cauraugh JH, Kim SB. Stroke motor recovery: active neuromuscular stimulation and repetitive practice schedules. *J. Neurol. Neurosurg. Psychiatr.* 2003; **74**(11): 1562–6.

7 Ylvisaker M, Jacobs HE, Feeney T. Positive supports for people who experience behavioral and cognitive disability after brain injury: a review. *J. Head Trauma Rehabil.* 2003; **18**(1): 7–32.

8 Ylvisaker M, Feeney T. Executive functions, self-regulation, and learned optimism in paediatric rehabilitation: a review and implications for intervention. *Pediatr. Rehabil.* 2002; **5**(2): 51–70.

9 Siegert RJ, McPherson KM, Taylor WJ. Toward a cognitive-affective model of goal-setting in rehabilitation: is self-regulation theory a key step? *Disabil. Rehabil.* 2004; **26**(20): 1175–83.

10 Levine B, Robertson IH, Clare L, Carter G, Hong J, Wilson BA, et al. Rehabilitation of executive functioning: an experimental–clinical validation of goal management training. *J. Int. Neuropsychol. Soc.* 2000; **6**(3): 299–312.

11 Dobkin BH. Neurobiology of rehabilitation. *Ann. New York Acad. Sci.* 2004; **1038**: 148–70.

12 Langhorne P, Dey P, Woodman M, Kalra L, Wood-Dauphinee S, Patel N, et al. Is stroke unit care portable? A systematic review of the clinical trials. *Age Ageing* 2005; **34**(4): 324–30.

13 Kalra L, Evans A, Perez I, Knapp M, Swift C, Donaldson N. A randomised controlled comparison of alternative strategies in stroke care. *Health Technol. Assess.* 2005; **9**(18): 1–94.

14 Shiel A, Burn JP, Henry D, Clark J, Wilson BA, Burnett ME, et al. The effects of increased rehabilitation therapy after brain injury: results of a prospective controlled trial. *Clin. Rehabil.* 2001; **15**(5): 501–14.

15 Patti F, Ciancio MR, Cacopardo M, Reggio E, Fiorilla T, Palermo F, et al. Effects of a short outpatient rehabilitation treatment on disability of multiple sclerosis patients – a randomised controlled trial. *J. Neurol.* 2003; **250**(7): 861–6.

16 Patti F, Ciancio MR, Reggio E, Lopes R, Palermo F, Cacopardo M, et al. The impact of outpatient rehabilitation on quality of life in multiple sclerosis. *J. Neurol.* 2002; **249**(8): 1027–33.

17 Bent N, Tennant A, Swift T, Posnett J, Scuffham P, Chamberlain MA. Team approach versus ad hoc health services for young people with physical disabilities: a retrospective cohort study. *Lancet* 2002; **360**(9342): 1280–6.

18 Turner-Stokes L. The evidence for the cost-effectiveness of rehabilitation following acquired brain injury. *Clin. Med.* 2004; **4**(1): 10–2.

19 Turner-Stokes L, Disler PB, Nair A, Wade DT. Multi-disciplinary rehabilitation for acquired brain injury in adults of working age. *Cochrane Database Syst. Rev.* 2005; 3: CD004170.

20 Turner-Stokes L. The national service framework for long term conditions: a novel approach for a 'new style' NSF. *J. Neurol. Neurosurg. Psychiatr.* 2005; **76**(7): 901–2.

21 McNaughton H, McPherson K, Taylor W, Weatherall M. Relationship between process and outcome in stroke care. *Stroke* 2003; **34**(3): 713–7.

22 Turner-Stokes L, Harding R, Sergeant J, Lupton C, McPherson KM. Generating the evidence base for the National Service Framework (NSF) for long term conditions: a new research typology. *Clin. Med.* 2006; **6**(1): 91–7.

23 World Health Organisation. *International Classification of Impairments, Disabilities and Handicaps.* WHO, Geneva, 1980.

24 World Health Organisation. *International Classification of Functioning Disability and Health* (Final Draft). WHO, Geneva, 2001.

25 McPherson KM, Levac W, Kersten P. Using the International Classification of Functioning, Disability and Health (ICF) as a basis for understanding outcomes in illness and injury. *Hosp. Med.* 2005; **66**(4): 210–4.

26 McPherson KM, Brander P, Taylor WJ, McNaughton HK. Consequences of stroke, arthritis and chronic pain – are there important similarities? *Disabil. Rehabil.* 2004; **26**(16): 988–999.

27 Armstrong D, Ogden J, Lilford R, Wessley S. *Quality of Life As an Innovative Health Technology.* Swindon, UK, 2005.

28 McPherson K, Myers J, Taylor WJ, McNaughton HK, Weatherall M. Self-valuation and societal valuations of health state differ with disease severity in chronic and disabling conditions. *Med. Care* 2004; **42**(11): 1143–51.

29 Fallowfield L. *The Quality of Life. The Missing Measurement in Health Care.* Souvenir Press, London, 1990.

30 Haacke C, Althaus A, Spottke A, et al. Long-term outcome after stroke: evaluating health-related quality of life using utility measurements. *Stroke* 2006; **37**(1): 193–8.

31 Johnston MV, Miklos CS. Activity-related quality of life in rehabilitation and traumatic brain injury. *Arch. Phys. Med. Rehabil.* 2002; **83**(12 Suppl. 2): S26–38.

32 Langhorne P, Wagenaar R, Partridge C. Physiotherapy after stroke: more is better? *Physiother. Res. Int.* 1996; **1**(2): 75–88.

33 Teasell R, Bitensky J, Salter K, Bayona NA. The role of timing and intensity of rehabilitation therapies. *Topics Stroke Rehabil.* 2005; **12**(3): 46–57.

34 Biernaskie J, Chernenko G, Corbett D. Efficacy of rehabilitative experience declines with time after focal ischemic brain injury. *J. Neurosci.* 2004; **24**(5): 1245–54.

35 Kwakkel G, Wagenaar RC, Koelman TW, Lankhorst GJ, Koetsier JC. Effects of intensity of rehabilitation after stroke. A research synthesis. *Stroke* 1997; **28**(8): 1550–6.

36 Kwakkel G, Kollen BJ, Wagenaar RC. Long term effects of intensity of upper and lower limb training after stroke: a randomised trial [see comment]. *J. Neurol. Neurosur. Psychiatr.* 2002; **72**(4): 473–9.

37 Kwakkel G, van Peppen R, Wagenaar RC, Wood Dauphinee S, Richards C, Ashburn A, et al. Effects of augmented exercise therapy time after stroke: a meta-analysis. *Stroke* 2004; **35**(11): 2529–39.

38 Van Peppen RP, Kwakkel G, Wood-Dauphinee S, Hendriks HJ, Van der Wees PJ, Dekker J. The impact of physical therapy on functional outcomes after stroke: what's the evidence? *Clin. Rehabil.* 2004; **18**(8): 833–62.

39 Bhogal SK, Teasell R, Speechley M. Intensity of aphasia therapy, impact on recovery [see comment]. *Stroke* 2003; **34**(4): 987–93.

40 Cicerone KD, Dahlberg C, Malec JF, Langenbahn DM, Felicetti T, Kneipp S, et al. Evidence-based cognitive rehabilitation: updated review of the literature from 1998 through 2002. *Arch. Phys. Med. Rehabil.* 2005; **86**(8): 1681–92.

41 Page SJ. Intensity versus task-specificity after stroke: how important is intensity? *Am. J. Phys. Med. Rehabil.* 2003; **82**(9): 730–2.

42 Kwakkel G, Kollen B, Lindeman E. Understanding the pattern of functional recovery after stroke: facts and theories. *Restorat. Neurol. Neurosci.* 2004; **22**(3–5): 281–99.

43 Teasell RW, Kalra L. What's new in stroke rehabilitation: back to basics. *Stroke* 2005; **36**(2): 215–7.

44. Ylvisaker M, Adelson PD, Braga LW, Burnett SM, Glang A, Feeney T, et al. Rehabilitation and ongoing support after pediatric TBI: twenty years of progress. *J. Head Trauma Rehabil.* 2005; **20**(1): 95–109.

45. Kesselring J, Beer S. Symptomatic therapy and neurorehabilitation in multiple sclerosis. *Lancet Neurol.* 2005; **4**(10): 643–52.

46. Lenze EJ, Munin MC, Quear T, Dew MA, Rogers JC, Begley AE, et al. Significance of poor patient participation in physical and occupational therapy for functional outcome and length of stay. *Arch. Phys. Med. Rehabil.* 2004; **85**(10): 1599–601.

47. Grahn BE, Borgquist LA, Ekdahl CS. Rehabilitation benefits highly motivated patients: a six-year prospective cost-effectiveness study. *Int. J. Technol. Assess. Health Care* 2004; **20**(2): 214–21.

48. Maclean N, Pound P, Wolfe C, Rudd A. Qualitative analysis of stroke patients' motivation for rehabilitation. *BMJ* 2000; **321**(7268): 1051–4.

49. Maclean N, Pound P, Wolfe C, Rudd A. The concept of patient motivation: a qualitative analysis of stroke professionals' attitudes. *Stroke* 2002; **33**(2): 444–8.

50. Maclean N, Pound P. A critical review of the concept of patient motivation in the literature on physical rehabilitation. *Soc. Sci. Med.* 2000; **50**(4): 495–506.

51. Siegert RJ, Taylor WJ. Theoretical aspects of goal-setting and motivation in rehabilitation. *Disabil. Rehabil.* 2004; **26**(1): 1–8.

52. Levin HS, Hanten G. Executive functions after traumatic brain injury in children. *Pediatr. Neurol.* 2005; **33**(2): 79–93.

53. Page SJ, Gater DR, Bach YRP. Reconsidering the motor recovery plateau in stroke rehabilitation. *Arch. Phys. Med. Rehabil.* 2004; **85**(8): 1377–81.

54. Demain S, Wiles R, Roberts L, McPherson K. Recovery plateau following stroke: fact or fiction? *Disabil. Rehabil.* 2005 (In Press).

55. Bode RK, Heinemann AW, Semik P, Mallinson T. Patterns of therapy activities across length of stay and impairment levels: peering inside the 'black box' of inpatient stroke rehabilitation. *Arch. Phys. Med. Rehabil.* 2004; **85**(12): 1901–8.

56. Messina N, Nemes S, Wish E, Wraight B. Opening the black box. The impact of inpatient treatment services on client outcomes. *J. Subst. Abuse Treat.* 2001; **20**(2): 177–83.

57. Pientka L. Health services research in geriatrics and geriatric rehabilitation from the national and international viewpoint. *Z. Gerontol. Geriatr.* 2001; **34**(Suppl. 1): 57–62.

58. Pincus HA, Zarin DA, West JC. Peering into the 'black box'. Measuring outcomes of managed care. *Arch. Gen. Psychiatr.* 1996; **53**(10): 870–7.

59. Pomeroy VM, Niven DS, Barrow S, Faragher EB, Tallis RC. Unpacking the black box of nursing and therapy practice for post-stroke shoulder pain: a precursor to evaluation. *Clin. Rehabil.* 2001; **15**(1): 67–83.

60. Thompson AJ. The effectiveness of neurological rehabilitation in multiple sclerosis. *J. Rehabil. Res. Dev.* 2000; **37**(4): 455–61.

61. Wade DT. Research into the black box of rehabilitation: the risks of a Type III error. *Clin. Rehabil.* 2001; **15**(1): 1–4.

62. Ballinger C, Ashburn A, Low J, Roderick P. Unpacking the black box of therapy – a pilot study to describe occupational therapy and physiotherapy interventions for people with stroke. *Clin. Rehabil.* 1999; **13**(4): 301–9.

63. DeJong G, Horn SD, Gassaway JA, Slavin MD, Dijkers MP. Toward a taxonomy of rehabilitation interventions: Using an inductive approach to examine the 'black box' of rehabilitation. *Arch. Phys. Med. Rehabil.* 2004; **85**(4): 678–86.

64. Conroy BE, Hatfield B, Nichols D. Opening the black box of stroke rehabilitation with clinical practice improvement methodology. *Top Stroke Rehabil.* 2005; **12**(2): 36–48.

65. DeJong G, Horn SD, Conroy B, Nichols D, Healton EB. Opening the black box of post-stroke rehabilitation: stroke rehabilitation patients, processes, and outcomes. *Arch. Phys. Med. Rehabil.* 2005; **86**(12 Suppl. 2): S1–S7.

66. Horn SD, DeJong G, Ryser DK, Veazie PJ, Teraoka J. Another look at observational studies in rehabilitation research: going beyond the holy grail of the randomized controlled trial. *Arch. Phys. Med. Rehabil.* 2005; **86**(12 Suppl. 2): S8–15.

67. Horn SD, DeJong G, Smout RJ, Gassaway J, James R, Conroy B. Stroke rehabilitation patients, practice, and outcomes: Is earlier and more aggressive therapy better? *Arch. Phys. Med. Rehabil.* 2005; **86**(12 Suppl. 2): S101–14.

68. James R, Gines D, Menlove A, Horn SD, Gassaway J, Smout RJ. Nutrition support (tube feeding) as a rehabilitation intervention. *Arch. Phys. Med. Rehabil.* 2005; **86**(12 Suppl. 2): S82–92.

69. Hatfield B, Millet D, Coles J, Gassaway J, Conroy B, Smout RJ. Characterizing speech and language pathology outcomes in stroke rehabilitation. *Arch. Phys. Med. Rehabil.* 2005; **86**(12 Suppl. 2): S61–72.

70. Gassaway J, Horn SD, DeJong G, Smout RJ, Clark C, James R. Applying the clinical practice improvement approach to stroke rehabilitation: methods used and baseline results. *Arch. Phys. Med. Rehabil.* 2005; **86**(12 Suppl. 2): S16–33.

71. DeJong G, Horn SD, Smout RJ, Ryser DK. The early impact of the inpatient rehabilitation facility prospective payment system on stroke rehabilitation case mix, practice patterns, and outcomes. *Arch. Phys. Med. Rehabil.* 2005; **86**(12 Suppl. 2): S93–100.

72. Conroy B, Zorowitz R, Horn SD, Ryser DK, Teraoka J, Smout RJ. An exploration of central nervous system medication use and outcomes in stroke rehabilitation. *Arch. Phys. Med. Rehabil.* 2005; **86**(12 Suppl. 2): S73–81.

73. Latham NK, Jette DU, Slavin M, Richards LG, Procino A, Smout RJ, et al. Physical therapy during stroke rehabilitation for people with different walking abilities. *Arch. Phys. Med. Rehabil.* 2005; **86**(12 Suppl. 2): S41–50.

74. Maulden SA, Gassaway J, Horn SD, Smout RJ, DeJong G. Timing of initiation of rehabilitation after stroke. *Arch. Phys. Med. Rehabil.* 2005; **86**(12 Suppl. 2): S34–40.

75. Richards LG, Latham NK, Jette DU, Rosenberg L, Smout RJ, DeJong G. Characterizing occupational therapy practice in stroke rehabilitation. *Arch. Phys. Med. Rehabil.* 2005; **86**(12 Suppl. 2): S51–60.

76. Sackett DL, Strauss SE, Richardson WS, Rosenberg W, Haynes RB. *Evidence-Based Medicine: How to Practice and Teach EBM*, 2nd edn. Churchill Livingstone, 2000.

77. Demner-Fushman D, Linn J. *Knowledge Extraction for Clinical Question Answering: Preliminary Results*. American Association for Artificial Intelligence; 2004.

78. Tyson SF, Selley A. The development of the Stroke Physiotherapy Intervention Recording Tool (SPIRIT). *Disabil. Rehabil.* 2004; **26**(20): 1184–8.

79. Ottenbacher KJ. The post-stroke rehabilitation outcomes project. *Arch. Phys. Med. Rehabil.* 2005; **86**(12 Suppl. 2): S121–S123.

80. Jette AM. The post-stroke rehabilitation outcomes project. *Arch. Phys. Med. Rehabil.* 2005; **86**(12 Suppl. 2): S124–S125.

81. McNaughton H, DeJong G, Smout RJ, Melvin JL, Brandstater M. A comparison of stroke rehabilitation practice and outcomes between New Zealand and United States facilities. *Arch. Phys. Med. Rehabil.* 2005; **86**(12 Suppl. 2): S115–20.

82. McPherson K, Headrick L, Moss F. Working and learning together: good quality care depends on it, but how can we achieve it? *Qual. Health Care* 2001; **10**(Suppl. 2): ii46–53.

83. Strasser DC, Falconer JA, Herrin JS, Bowen SE, Stevens AB, Uomoto J. Team functioning and patient outcomes in stroke rehabilitation. *Arch. Phys. Med. Rehabil.* 2005; **86**(3): 403–9.

84. Langhorne, P., Williams, B., Gilchrist, W. and Howie, K. Do stroke units save lives? *Lancet* 1993; **342**: 395–7.

85. Weinrich M, Stuart M, Hoyer T. Rules for rehabilitation: an agenda for research. *Neurorehabil. Neural. Repair.* 2005; **19**(2): 72–83.

86. Carr AJ, Higginson IJ. Measuring quality of life: Are quality of life measures patient centred? *BMJ* 2001; **322**(7298): 1357–60.

87. Ahmed S, Mayo NE, Wood-Dauphinee S, Hanley JA, Cohen SR. Response shift influenced estimates of change in health-related quality of life poststroke. *J. Clin. Epidemiol.* 2004; **57**(6): 561–70.

88. Tesio L, Gamba C, Capelli A, Franchignoni FP. Rehabilitation: the Cinderella of neurological research? A bibliometric study. *Ital. J. Neurol. Sci.* 1995; **16**(7): 473–7.

89. Whyte J, Katz D, Long D, DiPasquale MC, Polansky M, Kalmar K, et al. Predictors of outcome in prolonged posttraumatic disorders of consciousness and assessment of medication effects: a multicenter study. *Arch. Phys. Med. Rehabil.* 2005; **86**(3): 453–62.

90. Schepers VP, Visser-Meily AM, Ketelaar M, Lindeman E. Prediction of social activity 1 year poststroke. *Arch. Phys. Med. Rehabil.* 2005; **86**(7): 1472–6.

PART 3
Neurological diseases

13 CHAPTER 13

Acute stroke management and prevention of recurrences

Gord Gubitz

Background

Stroke refers to the clinical syndrome of sudden onset of focal or global disturbance of central nervous system function, with no apparent cause other than a vascular one [1]. Ischaemic stroke is responsible for about 80% of all strokes, intracerebral haemorrhage for 15%, and subarachnoid haemorrhage for 5%. A *transient ischaemic attack (or TIA)*, has the same symptom complex as a stroke, but with a resolution of these symptoms within 24 h [2]. Most TIAs resolve within 1 h. It is increasingly understood that TIAs and minor strokes represent a continuum of disease; some now suggest that the time-based definition of TIA yield to a tissue-based definition, as approximately one third of people with clinically diagnosed TIAs will actually have structural changes visible on neuroimaging, such as diffusion-weighted MRI scanning (DWI) [3,4]. Other terms used in the past to describe stroke and TIA, such as *cerebrovascular accident (CVA)* and *reversible ischaemic neurological deficit (RIND)*, lack specificity, and have generally fallen out of common use.

Mechanism and pathophysiology

Strokes and TIAs occur when the blood supply to the brain is disrupted, usually for one of the following reasons:

- Occlusion of the lumen of an artery by a blood clot that develops as a local thrombus, often in relation to atherosclerotic plaque rupture and endothelial injury, with activation of the local coagulation cascade.
- Distal occlusion of the lumen of an artery by a blood clot that has embolized from the heart (atrial fibrillation), aortic arch or arterial system.
- Local or embolic blood clots related to hypercoagulable states (hereditary or, secondary to systemic disease or malignancy).
- Occlusion of the arterial lumen following the dissection of an arterial wall.
- Narrowing of smaller arteries due to arteriosclerosis.
- Rupture of a blood vessel wall (artery or vein), leading to haemorrhage.
- Hypotension secondary to cardiac arrest or decreased circulating blood volume.

During stroke or TIA, normal cellular function is lost in the affected area of the brain, leading to the presenting symptoms.

If normal blood flow is not restored quickly, a *infarct core* of dead cells will form; these cells do not recover. In many cases of stroke, there also exists an area of tissue around the infarct core (*the ischaemic penumbra*), which is metabolically threatened, but theoretically viable [5]. If blood flow can be restored quickly, this penumbral tissue may be salvagable, hopefully resulting in a better clinical outcome for the patient.

Epidemiology

Each year, about 15 million people around the world experience a stroke; of these, 5 million die and 5 million are left permanently disabled [6]. In developed countries stroke is a leading cause of death and dementia, and is the number one cause of adult disability [6]. In general, stroke is a disease of the elderly, and so these trends will increase over the next several decades as the result of an aging population combined with the disturbing persistence of many well understood 'modifiable' risk factors, including hypertension, dyslipidemia, smoking, diabetes, obesity, physical inactivity, excessive alcohol intake and diets high in saturated fats and low in fruits and vegetables.

Clinical scenario

A 67-year-old woman is brought to your local emergency room by ambulance. Her family, who accompany her, tell you that exactly 1 h and 15 min ago, she experienced a sudden onset of complete paralysis of her left arm and leg, with an associated facial droop, while having her evening meal. There was no associated loss of consciousness, and the patient is not aware that anything in particular is the matter, apart from a slight headache. Her physical examination confirms a dense left sided hemiparesis, with associated neglect phenomena, including a left visual field cut. You have been able to ascertain that she has hypertension, dyslipidemia, and normally smokes one package of cigarettes per day. She is not taking aspirin; her only medication is a diuretic. An emergency computed tomography (CT) head scan does not demonstrate any obvious abnormality. An electrocardiograph (ECG) shows her to be in atrial fibrillation.

Framing clinical questions and general approach to search evidence

In general, four goals for the management of the patient with acute stroke can be defined:
(1) minimize brain damage and restore perfusion, (2) restore functional independence, (3) prevent complications, and (4) reduce the risk of stroke recurrence.

This chapter will address the following main clinical questions:

1 Among patients with hyper-acute ischaemic stroke, how do intravenous (IV) thrombolysis, intra-arterial (IA) thrombolysis, and mechanical clot retrieval within the first few hours affect the probability of long-term outcomes such as death or dependency and of short-term adverse events such as death and symptomatic intracranial haemorrhage (ICH)?

2 Among patients with acute ischaemic stroke, how does the pharmacological treatment, the management of complications, and the organization of care affect the probability of long-term outcomes such as death or dependence, and of short-term adverse events?

3 Among patients with acute ischaemic stroke with brain oedema, what treatment options affect the probability of long-term outcomes such as death or dependence, and of short-term adverse events?

4 Among patients with acute haemorrhagic stroke, are there surgical treatments or drug therapies that influence the probability of long-term outcomes such as death or dependence, and of short-term adverse events?

5 What can be done to prevent further strokes in stroke survivors?

The search strategy conducted to provide the best available evidence to answer these questions included a review of the Cochrane Library (using standard search terms) for completed systematic reviews and randomized controlled trials, as well as a search of the Internet Stroke Center's Stroke Trials Directory (http://www.strokecenter.org/trials/) for completed clinical trials not yet included in relevant systematic reviews, as well as ongoing clinical trials.

Critical review of the evidence for each question

The main results of acute stroke treatment and management are summarized on Table 13.1 that gives the relative risk (RR) and the absolute risk reduction for each intervention.

1. Thrombolysis and clot retrieval

Among patients with hyper-acute ischaemic stroke, how do IV thrombolysis, IA thrombolysis, and mechanical clot retrieval within the first few hours affect the probability of long-term outcomes such as death or dependency and of short-term adverse events such as death and symptomatic ICH?

IV thrombolysis

A Cochrane Systematic Review has demonstrated that thrombolytic therapy with recombinant tissue plasminogen activator (rt-PA) administered IV within 3 h of stroke onset for highly selected patients who meet strict eligibility criteria has been shown to save lives and reduce disability despite an early risk of intracerebral haemorrhage [8]. The systematic review included 18 randomized controlled trials, with 5727 patients; 16 trials were double-blind. About 50% of the data (patients and trials) come from trials testing IV tissue plasminogen activator, with few data from patients aged over 80 years. Overall, thrombolytic therapy, administered up to 6 h after ischaemic stroke, significantly reduced the proportion of patients who were dead or dependent (modified Rankin 3–6) at the end of follow-up at 3–6 months (odds ratio (OR) 0.84, 95% confidence interval (CI) 0.75–0.95). This was in spite of a significant increase in: the odds of death within the first 10 days (OR 1.81, 95% CI 1.46–2.24), the main cause of which was fatal ICH (OR 4.34, 95% CI 3.14–5.99). Symptomatic ICH was increased following thrombolysis (OR 3.37, 95% CI 2.68–4.22). Thrombolytic therapy also increased the odds of death at the end of follow-up at 3–6 months (OR 1.33, 95% CI 1.15–1.53). For patients treated within 3 h of stroke, thrombolytic therapy appeared more effective in reducing death or dependency (OR 0.66, 95% CI 0.53–0.83) with no statistically significant adverse effect on death (OR 1.13, 95% CI 0.86–1.48). There was heterogeneity between the trials that could have been due to many trial features including: thrombolytic drug used, variation in the use of aspirin and heparin, severity of the stroke (both between trials and between treatment groups within trials), and time to treatment. It was the opinion of the authors of the systematic review that the data are promising and may justify the use of thrombolytic therapy with IV recombinant tissue plasminogen activator in experienced centres in highly selected patients where a licence exists. A subsequent individual patient data meta-analysis has suggested that the time window for IV rt-PA may extend beyond 3 h [18].

At the present time, two large scale randomized controlled trials are ongoing, and hope to identify whether the time window for thrombolysis may be extended beyond the 3-h time interval. These two trials include the European cooperative acute stroke study-3 (ECASS-3): (http://www.strokeconference.org/sc_includes/pdfs/CTP34.pdf), and the IST-3: (http://www.dcn.ed.ac.uk/ist3/).

IA thrombolysis

No systematic review was identified; the practice is presently of limited clinical application, except in highly specialized centres, where research continues. One ongoing research trial (the Interventional Management of Stroke Study (IMS-3) is attempting to provide data concerning the risks and benefits of combined intravenous and intra-arterial (IV/IA) rt-PA in

Table 13.1 Treatment and management of acute stroke.

Type of study (reference)	Intervention	Outcome	No of patients (no of trials)	Control group risk (range)	Relative risk (95% CI)	Absolute risk reduction	Comment
SR [7]	Stroke unit versus conventional care	Death or dependency	3935 (23)	59% (39–100)	0.91 (0.86–0.96)	5% (2–8)	Organized stroke care better
SR [8]	Thrombolysis IV versus control	Death or dependency	4807 (14)	56% (41–80)	0.93 (0.88–0.98)	4% (1–7)	Thrombolysis better Heterogeneity
	Thrombolysis IV versus control	Symptomatic haemorrhage	5675 (19)	2.5% (0–6.5)	3.54 (2.74–4.58)	+7% (5–8)	Thrombolysis worse
	Thrombolysis IV within 3 h versus control	Death or dependency	1311 (10)	60% (46–70)	0.83 (0.75–0.92)	10% (5–15)	Thrombolysis better
	rt-PA IV within 3 h versus Placebo	Symptomatic haemorrhage	306 (4)	3.3% (0–5)	3.27 (1.36–7.89)	+9% (3–15)	rt-PA worse
See text	IA thrombolysis	Currently being evaluated in research studies					
See text	Mechanical clot retrieval	Approved for use in some jurisdictions based on a phase II non-randomized study, involving (only) 141 patients (9).					
SR [9]	Aspirin (160–300 mg daily) versus control	Death or dependency	41,207 (5)	47% (31–68)	0.97 (0.95–0.99)	1% (0–2)	Aspirin better
		Symptomatic haemorrhage	41,399 (9)	0.1% (0–0.8)	1.23 (1.00–1.50)	+2/1000	Aspirin worse
SR [10]	Anticoagulants versus control	Death or dependency	21,966 (6)	59% (26–65)	1.00 (0.97–1.02)	0 (ns)	Anticoagulant worse
		Symptomatic haemorrhage		0.5% (0–0.8)	2.63 (1.95–3.55)	+1% (1–1)	
SR [11]	Mannitol versus control	Just one small trials of 77 patients. Mortality outcome is not reported.					
SR [12]	Glycerol versus control	Death	945 (10)	53% (0–47)	0.83 (0.67–1.04)	4% (ns)	Glycerol better
SR [13]	Corticosteroid versus control	Death	453 (7)	32% (0–79)	1.04 (0.83–1.29)	+1% (ns)	Corticosteroids worse
SR [14]	Surgery craniotomy versus medical	No RCT trials					
SR [15]	Surgery for intracerebral haemorrhage versus medical	Death at 6 months	254 (3)	52% (40–84)	1.17 (0.87–1.57)	+9% (ns)	Surgery worse Heterogeneity
RCT [16]	Surgery for intracerebral haemorrhage versus medical	Favourable outcome	1033 (1)	24%	OR 0.89 (0.66–1.19)		Surgery better
RCT [17]	Factor VII within 3 h versus placebo	Volume ICH increase	399 (1)				31% Placebo 14% Factor VII
		Death (3 months)	399 (1)				29% Placebo 18% Factor VII

SR: systematic review; RCT: randomized controlled trial; ns: not statistically significant; ICH: intracranial haemorrhage.

patients with ischaemic stroke http://www.strokecenter.org/trials/.

Mechanical clot retrieval

Mechanical embolectomy has also been studied in the acute stroke population, but no systematic review or randomized controlled trials have been published. The Mechanical embolus removal in cerebral ischaemia (MERCI) trial [19], a phase II non-randomized study, involved 141 patients treated within 8 h of symptom onset; patients were not eligible for rt-PA. The primary outcomes were recanalization and safety. In the study, recanalization of treatable vessels with the study device was achieved in 48% ($P < 0.0001$) patients treated. Investigators used adjuvant therapy in 51 instances after deployment of the device. Clinically significant procedural complications occurred in 10 of 141 (7%) patients; symptomatic ICH was observed in 11 of 141 (7.8%) patients. Three percent of the devices used during the trial fractured, possibly causing the death of 2 patients.

2. Organization of care
Among patients with acute ischaemic stroke, how does the organization of care affect the probability of long-term outcomes such as death or dependence and of short-term adverse events?

Reliable evidence from systematic reviews of randomized trials strongly supports a policy of caring for *all* patients with acute stroke on a geographically defined stroke unit with a coordinated multidisciplinary team [7]. Organized stroke unit care is provided by multidisciplinary teams that either manage stroke patients in a dedicated ward (stroke ward), with a mobile team (stroke team) or within a generic disability service (a mixed rehabilitation ward). Twenty-three trials were included in the systematic review. Compared with alternative services, stroke unit care showed reductions in the odds of death recorded at final (median 1 year) follow-up (OR 0.86, 95% CI 0.71–0.94, $P = 0.005$), the odds of death or institutionalized care (0.80, 0.71–0.90, $P = 0.0002$) and death or dependency (0.78, 0.68–0.89, $P = 0.0003$). Subgroup analyses indicated that the observed benefits remained when the analysis was restricted to truly randomized trials with blinded outcome assessment. Outcomes were independent of patient age, sex, and stroke severity but appeared to be better in stroke units based in a discrete ward. There was no indication that organized stroke unit care resulted in increased hospital stay. The authors concluded that patients who receive organized inpatient care in a stroke unit are more likely to be alive, independent, and living at home 1 year after the stroke. The benefits were most apparent in units based in a discrete ward. No systematic increase was observed in the length of inpatient stay. On a population basis, such an approach will result in less death and dependency than thrombolytic therapy because far more patients are eligible for stroke unit care.

3. Treatment of acute ischaemic stroke
Among patients with acute ischaemic stroke, how does the pharmacological treatment affect the probability of long-term outcomes such as death or dependence, and of short-term adverse events?

Antiplatelet agents (predominantly aspirin)
The use of antiplatelet agents in the acute stroke period has been evaluated in one Cochrane Systematic Review [9]. Nine trials involving 41,399 patients were included. Two trials testing aspirin 160–300 mg once daily started within 48 h of onset contributed 98% of the data. The maximum follow-up was 6 months. With treatment, there was a significant decrease in death or dependency at the end of follow-up (OR = 0.94, 95% CI 0.91–0.98). In absolute terms, 13 more patients were alive and independent at the end of follow-up for every 1000 patients treated. Furthermore, treatment increased the odds of making a complete recovery from the stroke (OR = 1.06, 95% CI 1.01–1.11). In absolute terms, 10 more patients made a complete recovery for every 1000 patients treated. Antiplatelet therapy was associated with a small but definite excess of 2 symptomatic ICH for every 1000 patients treated, but this was more than offset by a reduction of 7 recurrent ischaemic strokes and about 1 pulmonary embolus for every 1000 patients treated. The authors concluded that antiplatelet therapy with aspirin 160–300 mg daily, given orally (or per rectum in patients who cannot swallow), and started within 48 h of onset of presumed ischaemic stroke reduces the risk of early recurrent ischaemic stroke without a major risk of early haemorrhagic complications and improves long-term outcome. Further information regarding the appropriate dose of aspirin has been provided by a non-Cochrane meta-analysis, which had suggested that a policy of administering aspirin (75–150 mg/day) within the first few days after stroke will reduce the RR of stroke (and other adverse vascular events) by about 20% [20].

Anticoagulants
The use of anticoagulants in acute stroke has been evaluated in one Cochrane Systematic Review [10]. Twenty-two trials involving 23,547 patients were included in the review. The quality of the trials varied considerably. The anticoagulants tested were standard unfractionated heparin (UFH), low-molecular-weight heparins, heparinoids, oral anticoagulants, and thrombin inhibitors. Based on nine trials (22,570 patients) there was no evidence that anticoagulant therapy reduced the odds of death from all causes (OR = 1.05, 95% CI 0.98–1.12) at the end of follow-up. Similarly, based on six trials (21,966 patients), there was no evidence that anticoagulants reduced the odds of being dead or dependent at the end of follow-up (OR = 0.99, 95% CI 0.93–1.04). Although anticoagulant therapy was associated with about 9 fewer recurrent ischaemic strokes per 1000 patients treated (OR = 0.76, 95% CI 0.65–0.88), it was also associated with a similar sized 9 per 1000 increase in symptomatic ICH (OR = 2.52, 95% CI 1.92–3.30). Similarly, anticoagulants avoided about 4 pulmonary emboli per 1000 (OR = 0.60, 95% CI 0.44–0.81), but this benefit was offset by an extra 9 major extracranial haemorrhages per 1000 (OR = 2.99, 95% CI 2.24–3.99). Sensitivity analyses did not identify a particular type of anticoagulant regimen or patient characteristic associated with net benefit, including those with: cardioembolic stroke, 'stroke in progression', vertebrobasilar territory stroke, or following thrombolysis for acute ischaemic stroke to prevent re-thrombosis of the treated cerebral artery. The authors concluded that immediate anticoagulant therapy in patients

with acute ischaemic stroke is not associated with net short- or long-term benefit. The data from this review do not support the routine use of any type of anticoagulant in acute ischaemic stroke. It was also suggested that people treated with anticoagulants had less chance of developing deep vein thrombosis (DVT) and pulmonary embolism (PE) following their stroke, but these sorts of blood clots are not very common, and may be prevented in other ways.

Anticoagulants versus antiplatelet agents

One Cochrane Systematic Review sought to assess the effectiveness of anticoagulants compared with antiplatelet agents in acute ischaemic stroke, and to assess whether the addition of anticoagulants to antiplatelet agents offers any net advantage over antiplatelet agents alone [21]. A total of 16,558 patients from four trials contributed to the analyses. The methodological quality was high in all four trials. The anticoagulants tested were UFH and low-molecular-weight heparin. Aspirin was used as control in all trials. Overall, there was no evidence that anticoagulants were superior to aspirin in reducing 'death or dependency' at long-term follow-up (OR 1.07, 95% CI 0.98–1.15). Compared with aspirin, anticoagulants were associated with a small but significant increase in the number of deaths at the end of follow-up (OR 1.10, 95% CI 1.01–1.29), equivalent to 20 more deaths (95% CI 0–30) per 1000 patients treated; a significant increased risk of symptomatic ICH (OR 2.35, 95% CI 1.49–3.46); and a non-significant increased risk of 'any recurrent stroke' during treatment (OR 1.20, 95% CI 0.99–1.46). These neutral or adverse effects outweighed a small, but significant effect on symptomatic DVT (OR 1.20, 95% CI 0.07–0.58), equivalent to 10 fewer (95% CI 0–30) DVTs by 14 days per 1000 patients treated with anticoagulants instead of aspirin. Subgroup analysis could not identify any type, dose, or route of administration of anticoagulants associated with net benefit, or any benefit in patients with atrial fibrillation. Overall, the combination of UFH and aspirin did not appear to be associated with a net advantage over aspirin alone. A subgroup analysis showed that, compared with aspirin, the combination of low-dose UFH and aspirin was associated with a marginally significant reduced risk of 'any recurrent stroke' (OR 0.75, 95% CI 0.56–1.03) and a marginally significant reduced risk of death at 14 days (OR 0.84, 95% CI 0.69–1.01), and with no clear adverse effect on death at end of follow-up (OR 0.98, 95% CI 0.85–1.12). The authors concluded that anticoagulants offered no net advantages over antiplatelet agents in acute ischaemic stroke. The combination of low-dose UFH and aspirin appeared in a subgroup analysis to be associated with net benefits compared with aspirin alone, and this merits further research.

HMG CoA reductase inhibitors (statins)

No systematic review was identified. The role that statins might play within the first hours of acute stroke is being addressed in the ongoing Fast Assessment of Stroke and Transient ischemic attack to prevent Early Recurrences (FASTER) trial, a multi-centre, randomized, double-blind, controlled trial involving patients over the age of 40 with reported or ongoing symptoms lasting at least 5 min and having included either weakness and/or language disturbance at time of TIA/minor stroke. All patients will be treated with aspirin. Patients will be randomized to clopidogrel (300 mg loading dose + 75 mg/day) or placebo and to simvastatin (40 mg/day) or placebo within 24 h of onset of TIA or minor stroke. The primary outcomes are stroke at 90 days and stroke severity. Further information is available on the FASTER website: http://www.faster.ca/.

Neuroprotective agents

A number of different agents acting at various points in the ischaemic cascade to potentially protect vulnerable neurons or salvage the ischaemic penumbra have been developed. Cochrane Systematic Reviews have evaluated excitatory amino acid antagonists [22], gangliosides [23], calcium channel antagonists [24], lubeluzole [25], methylxanthine derivatives [26], and tirilazad [27]. Unfortunately, none of these agents has been proven to be effective in the treatment of acute ischaemic stroke, and some of them may actually cause harm. A number of clinical trials involving agents with different suspected neuroprotective mechanisms are ongoing (http://www.strokecenter.org/trials/).

Haemodilution

Once Cochrane Review has evaluated the role of haemodilution in acute ischaemic stroke [28]. Haemodilution is thought to improve the flow of blood to the affected areas of the brain and thus reduce infarct size. Eighteen trials were included in the review. A combination of venesection and plasma volume expander was used in eight trials. Ten trials used plasma volume expander alone. The plasma volume expander was dextran 40 in 12 trials, hydroxyethyl starch (HES) in 5 trials and albumin in 1 trial. Two trials tested haemodilution in combination with another therapy. Evaluation was blinded in 11 trials. Five trials probably included some patients with intracerebral haemorrhage. Overall, haemodilution *did not significantly reduce* deaths within the first 4 weeks (OR 1.09, 95% CI 0.86–1.38). Similarly, haemodilution *did not influence deaths* within 3–6 months (OR 1.01, 95% CI 0.84–1.22), *or death and dependency or institutionalization* (OR 0.98, 95% CI 0.84–1.15). The results were similar in confounded and unconfounded trials, and in trials of isovolaemic and hypervolaemic haemodilution. No statistically significant benefits were documented for any particular type of haemodiluting agents, but the statistical power to detect effects of HES and albumin was weak. Six trials reported venous thromboembolic events. There was a tendency towards reduction in deep venous thrombosis and/or PE at 3–6 months follow-up (OR 0.59, 95% CI 0.33–1.06). There was no increased risk of serious cardiac events among haemodiluted patients. One ongoing randomized, double-blind, placebo controlled clinical trial (ALIAS) http://www.strokecenter.org/trials/ with a planned recruitment size of 1800 patients is attempting to determine if human serum albumin at 2 g/kg given over 2 h, to ischaemic stroke patients, within 5 h of stroke onset results in improved outcome at 3 months.

Hyperbaric oxygen

It has been postulated that hyperbaric oxygen therapy (HBOT) may reduce the volume of brain that will die by greatly increasing the oxygen available, and it may further improve outcome by reducing brain swelling. One systematic review was identified [29]. Three randomized controlled trials (106 participants) satisfied the inclusion criteria. The methodological quality of the trials varied but was generally high. Data could be pooled for a limited number of clinically important outcomes. There were no significant differences in mortality rate at 6 months in those receiving HBOT compared to the control group (RR 0.61, 95% CI 0.17–2.2, $P = 0.45$). Two of 15 scale measures of disability and functional indicated an improvement following HBOT, both at 1-year follow up: the mean Trouillas Disability Scale was lower with HBOT (mean difference (MD) 2.2 points reduction with HBOT, 95% CI 0.15–4.3, $P = 0.04$) and the mean Orgogozo Scale was higher (MD 27.9 points, 95% CI 4.0–51.8, $P = 0.02$). These improvements were not reflected in other trials or functional scales. The authors concluded that there was insufficient evidence to show that HBOT improves clinical outcomes when applied during the acute presentation of ischaemic stroke. While evidence from the three randomized controlled trials is insufficient to provide clear guidelines for practice, clinical benefit does not seem likely. Further research is required to better define the role of HBOT in acute stroke.

Cooling

Hyperthermia has been associated with poor outcome after stroke. One Cochrane Systematic Review has evaluated the role of cooling in patients with acute stroke [30]. The objective of the systematic review was to assess the effects of cooling when applied to patients with acute ischaemic stroke or primary intracerebral haemorrhage (PICH). No completed randomized trials or controlled trials were identified. The Nordic Cooling Stroke Study (NOCSS), a multi-centre randomized controlled trial with an anticipated recruitment of 1000 patients, is presently evaluating the safety and possibleneuroprotective efficacy of induced mild hypothermia in non-anaesthetized patients who present within 6 h of a moderate-to-severe acute hemispheric stroke (http://www.strokeconference.org/sc_includes/pdfs/CTP8.pdf).

4. Management of complications

Among patients with acute ischaemic stroke, how does the management of complications affect the probability of long-term outcomes such as death or dependence, and of short-term adverse events?

People with acute stroke are at higher risk of complications, such as deep venous thrombosis, PE, infection, pneumonia, and skin breakdown. In general, all of these are preventable with excellent nursing care [31]. In addition, there is at least some evidence supporting the maintenance adequate oxygenation, treating fevers with antipyretics, and maintaining a normal blood glucose level [31].

Prevention of deep venous thrombosis

One area that has been studied in more detail is involves the prevention of deep venous thrombosis and PE. One Cochrane Review evaluated the effectiveness and safety of physical methods of preventing the onset of DVT and fatal or non-fatal PE in patients with recent stroke [32]. Symptomatic DVT and resulting PE are uncommon but important complications of stroke. There is good evidence that anticoagulants can reduce the risk of DVT and PE after stroke, but this benefit is offset by a small but definite risk of serious haemorrhages. Physical methods to prevent DVT and PE (such as compression stockings applied to the legs) are not associated with any bleeding risk and are effective in some categories of medical and surgical patients. Two small trials which included 123 patients were identified. In one trial of 97 patients, compression stockings were associated with a non-significant trend towards a reduction in DVT detected by Doppler ultrasound. In one trial of 26 patients, an intermittent pneumatic compression device was not associated with a significant reduction in DVT detected by 125-I-fibrinogen scanning. Overall, physical methods were not associated with a significant reduction in DVT during the treatment period in survivors (OR 0.54, 95% CI 0.18–1.57) or death (OR 1.54, 95% CI 0.5–4.77). The authors concluded that there was insufficient evidence from randomized trials to support the routine use of physical methods for preventing DVT in acute stroke.

CLOTS (Clots in Legs or TEDS after Stroke), is an ongoing two-part, multi-centre, randomized, partially blinded, controlled trial with a planned enrolment of 2000 patients in each trial is evaluating the role of graduated compression stockings in patients presenting within 7 days of stroke, who are not independently mobile (i.e. who are unable to get up and walk across the room), and who can be randomized within 3 days of hospital admission. In trial one, patients for whom the responsible clinician is unsure about the value of graduated compression stockings are eligible for this study. In trial two, patients requiring graduated compression stockings for whom the responsible clinician is unsure of the optimum stocking length, are eligible for this study. The primary outcome is incidence at 30 days of DVT's in the popliteal or more proximal veins, detected on either Doppler ultrasound or venography. Further information is available at the CLOTS trial website: http://www.clotstrial.com/.

Blood pressure

Acute blood pressure (BP) alteration has been evaluated in one Cochrane Systematic Review [33], which sought to assess the effect of lowering or elevating BP in people with acute stroke, and the effect of different vasoactive drugs on BP in acute stroke. Data were obtained for 32 trials (5368 patients).

Calcium channel blockers (CCBs) and prostacyclin. Significant imbalances in baseline BP were present across trials of IV CCBs and prostacyclin. Major imbalances in baseline BP between treatment and control groups have made the interpretation of these results difficult. IV CCBs and oral CCBs. Significantly lowered late BP as compared to controls. Systolic/diastolic BP: IV CCBs −8.2/−6.7 mmHg (95% CI −12.6 to −3.8)/(95% CI −9.2 to −4.3); oral CCBs −3.2/−2.1 mmHg (95% CI −5.0 to −1.3)/(95% CI −3.0 to −1.0). CCBs also significantly reduced heart rate by −2.8 beats/min (95% CI −3.9 to −1.7).

Beta blockers significantly lowered late diastolic BP but not significantly late systolic BP; −5.0/−4.5 mmHg (95% CI −10.2–0.4)/(95% CI −7.8 to −1.15). Beta blockers also significantly reduced heart rate by −9.3 beats/min (95% CI −12.0 to −6.6).

Angiotensin-converting enzyme (ACE) inhibitors and prostacyclin non-significantly reduced late BP as compared to the controls by −5.4/−3.0 mmHg (95% CI −16.5–5.8)/(95% CI −11.1–5.0) and −7.4/−3.9 mmHg (95% CI −15.6–0.2)/(95% CI −8.1–0.4), respectively. Prostacyclin significantly increased late heart rate by +5.6 beats/min (95% CI 0.8–10.4).

Magnesium, naftidrofuryl and piracetam had no significant effect on BP.

None of the drug classes significantly altered outcome apart from beta blockers and streptokinase which increased early case fatality (OR 1.77, 95% CI 1.05–3.00) and 2.27 (95% CI 1.4–3.67). The authors concluded that there was not enough evidence to reliably evaluate the effect of altering BP on outcome after acute stroke. CCBs, beta blockers, and probably ACE inhibitors, prostacyclin and nitric oxide, each lowered BP during the acute phase of stroke. In contrast, magnesium, naftidrofuryl, and piracetam had little or no effect on BP. A number of randomized controlled clinical trials are ongoing in this area, including:

COSSACS (Continue or Stop post-Stroke Antihypertensives Collaborative Study: http://www.le.ac.uk/cv/research/COSSACS/COSSACShome.html);

CHHIPPS (Controlling Hypertension and Hypotension Immediately Post-Stroke Trial: http://www.le.ac.uk/cv/research/CHHIPS/HomePage.html);

HASTE (Hypertension in Acute Stroke TrEatment: http://www.strokecenter.org/trials/);

ENOS (Efficacy of Nitric Oxide in Stroke: http://www.enos.ac.uk/).

Blood glucose control

Hyperglycaemia is associated with poor outcome after stroke, suggesting that may be beneficial. One Cochrane Systematic Review [34] is available in abstract form, and proposes to determine whether maintaining serum glucose

within a specific normal range (4–7 mmol/L) in the first 24 h of acute ischaemic stroke influences outcome, but no definitive clinical trial data are available. An ongoing multi-centre randomized controlled trial (the United Kingdom Glucose Insulin in Stroke Trial (GIST-UK http://www.strokeconference.org/sc_includes/pdfs/CTP35.pdf) plans to enroll 2400 patients presenting within 24 h of CT-proven acute stroke, and a baseline plasma glucose of either >6.0 mmol/L or <17 mmol/L. The treatment group will receive a single 24-h continuous infusion of 10% glucose, 20 mMol KCl, and variable-dose actrapid insulin adjusted to maintain capillary whole blood glucose at 4–7 mmol/L. The control group will be infused with normal saline at 100 mL/h for 24 h.

5. Brain oedema

Among patients with acute ischaemic stroke and significant brain oedema, what treatment options affect the probability of long-term outcomes such as death or dependence, and of short-term adverse events?

Several treatment strategies have been identified that attempt to deal specifically with brain oedema in the early stages of ischaemic stroke, but support for their routine use has not been confirmed by the evidence.

Mannitol

One Cochrane Systematic Review evaluated the use of mannitol in acute ischaemic stroke [11]. It has been theorized that since mannitol is an osmotic agent and a free radical scavenger, it might decrease oedema and tissue damage in stroke. Unfortunately, only one trial fulfilled the inclusion criteria. The number of included patients was small (36 treated and 41 controls) and the follow up was short. Neither beneficial nor harmful effects of mannitol could be proved. Case fatality, the proportion of dependent patients at the end of the follow up and side effects were not reported and were not available from the investigators. The planned outcome analyses and sensitivity analyses could not be performed due to lack of appropriate trials. The authors concluded that there is currently not enough evidence to decide whether the routine use of mannitol in acute stroke would result in any beneficial or harmful effect.

Glycerol

One Cochrane Systematic Review evaluated the role of IV glycerol treatment in acute stroke [12]. A 10% solution of glycerol is a hyperosmolar agent that is thought to reduce brain oedema. The review sought to determine whether IV glycerol treatment in acute stroke, either ischaemic or haemorrhagic, influences death rates and functional outcome in the short or long term, and whether the treatment is safe. Eleven completed, randomized trials comparing IV glycerol and control were considered. Analysis of death during the scheduled treatment period for acute ischaemic and/or haemorrhagic stroke was possible in 10 trials where 482 glycerol treated patients were compared with 463 control patients. Glycerol was associated with a *non-significant* reduction in the odds of death within the scheduled treatment period (OR 0.78, 95% CI 0.58–1.06). Among patients with definite or probable ischaemic stroke, glycerol was associated with a significant reduction in the odds of death during the scheduled treatment period (OR 0.65, 95% CI 0.44–0.97). However, at the end of the scheduled follow up period, there was no significant difference in the odds of death (OR 0.98, 95% CI 0.73–1.31). Functional outcome was reported in only two studies but there were non-significantly more patients who had a good outcome at the end of scheduled follow up (OR 0.73, 95% CI 0.37–1.42). Haemolysis seems to be the only relevant adverse effect of glycerol treatment. The authors concluded that there was the suggestion of a favourable effect of glycerol treatment on short-term survival in patients with probable or definite ischaemic stroke, but the CI were wide and the magnitude of the treatment effect may be only minimal. The lack of evidence of benefit in long-term survival does not support the routine or selective use of glycerol treatment in patients with acute stroke.

Corticosteroids

Corticosteroids have been used to reduce brain swelling to help limit damage and speed recovery. Although studies of their use in acute stroke have been disappointing many physicians continue to treat stroke with corticosteroids. One Cochrane Systematic Review [13] included seven trials involving 453 people. No difference was shown in the odds of death within 1 year (OR 1.08, 95% CI 0.68–1.72). Treatment did not appear to improve functional outcome in survivors. Six trials reported neurological impairment but pooling the data was impossible because no common scale or time interval was used. The results were inconsistent between individual trials. The only adverse effects reported were small numbers of gastrointestinal bleeds, infections, and deterioration of hyperglycaemia across both groups. There is not enough evidence to evaluate corticosteroid treatment for people with acute presumed ischaemic stroke.

Craniectomy

The high mortality that follows large cerebral infarctions is in part due to brain oedema, with mass effect leading to herniation. Craniectomy is sometimes performed on patients with massive infarcts whose level of consciousness is declining in an attempt to improve survival and hopefully longer-term outcome. One Cochrane Systematic Review [14] evaluated the role of decompressive surgery with medical therapy alone on the outcomes death and 'death or dependency' in patients with an acute ischaemic stroke complicated by clinical and radiologically confirmed cerebral oedema. Over 9000 citations were retrieved and inspected for relevance in this systematic review. No randomized controlled trials were identified to include in a meta-analysis. Five observational studies reporting comparative data were found along with a number of small series and single case reports. The authors concluded that there was no evidence from randomized controlled trials to support the use of decompressive surgery for the treatment of cerebral oedema in acute ischaemic stroke. At the present time, there are several ongoing randomized controlled trials ongoing in this area, including the DECIMAL (DEcompressive Craniectomy In MALignant Middle Cerebral Artery Infarcts) trial, which plans to evaluate 60 consecutive patients presenting with patients who present within 24 h of a malignant MCA infarct (http://www.strokecenter.org/trials/); the DESTINY (Decompressive Surgery for the Treatment of Malignant Infarction of the Middle Cerebral Artery) trial, which plans to randomize 68 patients with onset of symptoms between 12 and 36 h to hemicraniectomy versus best medical management (http://www.strokecenter.org/trials/); the HAMLET (*Hemicraniectomy After MCA infarction with Life-threatening Edema Trial*), a multi-centre, open, randomized clinical trial of 112 patients with space-occupying infarct in the territory of the middle cerebral artery in either hemisphere leading to a decrease in consciousness randomized to surgery or best medical management (http://www.strokecenter.org/trials/); and the HeMMi (*Hemicraniectomy For Malignant Middle Cerebral Artery Infarcts*) trial, an pen randomized clinical trial of patients diagnosed clinically and radiographically with ischaemic stroke in the middle cerebral artery territory, who will be randomized to surgery or best medical management (http://www.strokecenter.org/trials/).

In clinical practice, patients with large cerebellar infarcts with volume effects such as compression of the fourth ventricle may benefit from surgical intervention, but there are no randomized clinical trials to support this.

6. Treatments for acute haemorrhagic stroke

Among patients with acute haemorrhagic stroke, are there surgical treatments and hyper-drug therapies that influence the probability of long-term outcomes such as death or dependence, and of short-term adverse events?

Surgery

One Cochrane Systematic Review was identified that assessed the effects of surgery plus routine medical management, compared with routine medical management alone, in patients with primary supratentorial intracerebral haematoma [15]. Four trials were included. No trial had blinded outcome assessment. Craniotomy and endoscopic evacuation were analysed separately. Craniotomy showed a non-significant trend towards increased odds of death and dependency among survivors (OR 1.99, 99% CI 0.92–4.31). The result was inconclusive in the two trials with patients confirmed as having primary supratentorial intracerebral haematoma by CT. Endoscopic evacuation was not shown to significantly decrease the odds of death and dependency among survivors in one trial involving 100 patients (OR 0.45, 99% CI 0.15–1.33). The authors concluded that there is not enough evidence to evaluate the effect of craniotomy or stereotactic surgery, or endoscopic evacuation in patients with supratentorial intracerebral haematoma.

Since this Cochrane Systematic Review was updated, an additional randomized controlled trial comparing surgical intervention versus a non-surgical approach for treating supratentorial haemorrhages has been published [16]. In this trial, 1033 patients from 83 centres in 27 countries were randomized to early surgery (503) or initial conservative treatment (530). At 6 months, 51 patients were lost to follow-up, and 17 were alive with unknown status. Of 468 patients randomized to early surgery, 122 (26%) had a favourable outcome compared with 118 (24%) of 496 randomized to initial conservative treatment (OR 0 89, 95% CI 0 66–1 19, P = 0.414). The authors concluded that patients with spontaneous supratentorial intracerebral haemorrhage in neurosurgical units show no overall benefit from early surgery when compared with initial conservative treatment.

Although no clinical trial evidence has been provided, it is common practice to consider patients with infratentorial haemorrhages for surgical decompression if mass-effect is a consideration.

Drugs for acute haemorrhagic stroke

One Cochrane Systematic Review aimed to determine whether corticosteroid therapy reduces the proportion of patients who die or have a poor outcome at 1–6 months after the onset of ICH and to determine the frequency of adverse effects of corticosteroid therapy in patients with ICH within 6 months of the onset of the event [35]. Eight trials that fulfilled the eligibility criteria were identified, with a total of 206 patients in five PICH trials. The studies differed substantially with regard to the study populations and drugs, and methodological quality. The number of patients allocated to dexamethasone treatment in patients with PICH, was too small to make any definitive conclusions (CI were wide for any of the outcome estimates). The authors concluded that there was no evidence of a beneficial or adverse effect of corticosteroids in patients with PICH. CI are wide and include clinically significant effects in both directions.

A recent phase II study of 399 patients evaluating different doses of recombinant activated factor VII (VIIa), a pro-coagulant drug, demonstrated a significant reduction in the size of post-treatment haematoma volume when compared to placebo [17]. One phase III randomized, double-blind, placebo controlled trial has recently completed enrollment. The study aims to determine if the use of recombinant factor VIIa in patients with acute intracerebral bleeding will help more patients recover without severe permanent disability by reducing further intracerebral bleeding. Patients with spontaneous ICH within 3 h after first symptom will be included. The primary outcome is clinical outcome after 3 months, with secondary outcomes including haematoma volume and mortality. Further information is available from the FAST website, http://www.clinicaltrials.gov/ct/show/NCT00127283?order=1.

7. Secondary prevention

What can be done to prevent further strokes in stroke survivors?

The major evidence findings are summarized in Table 13.2 that reports the available RR and absolute risk reduction.

Risk factor modification

Hypertension: It is generally accepted that hypertension is the most important modifiable risk factor for stroke, and must be treated to acceptable standards. One systematic review [36] assessed the effectiveness of lowering BP in preventing recurrent vascular events in patients with previous stroke (ischaemic or haemorrhagic) or TIA. Seven randomized controlled trials, with eight comparison groups, were included. The results of the meta-analysis indicated that lowering BP or treating hypertension with a variety of antihypertensive agents reduced a number of outcome events, including: stroke (OR 0.76, 95% CI 0.63–0.92), non-fatal stroke (OR 0.79, 95% CI 0.65–0.95), myocardial infarction (MI) (OR 0.79, 95% CI 0.63–0.98), and total vascular events (OR 0.79, 95% CI 0.66–0.95). Importantly, heterogeneity was present for several outcomes and was partly related to the class of antihypertensive drugs used. The meta-analysis indicated that ACE inhibitors and diuretics separately, *and especially together*, reduced vascular events, while beta-receptor antagonists had no discernable effect. The reduction in stroke was related to the difference in systolic BP between treatment and control groups (P = 0.002). The authors of the systematic review indicated that the trial evidence supported the use of antihypertensive agents in lowering BP for the prevention of vascular events in patients with previous stroke or TIA. In addition, vascular prevention was associated positively with the magnitude by which BP is reduced. Many countries now have national hypertension guidelines with specific targets for stroke prevention.

Serum lipids: One systematic review was identified, which investigated the effect of altering serum lipids in the prevention of cardiovascular disease and stroke recurrence in subjects with a history of stroke [45]. Five studies involving 1700 patients were included in the review. Fixed effects analysis showed no evidence of a difference in stroke recurrence between the treatment and placebo groups for those with a previous history of stroke or TIA (OR 0.96, 95% CI 0.71–1.30). In addition there was also no evidence, based on two studies, that intervention reduced the odds of all cause mortality (OR 0.87, 95% CI 0.55–1.39) nor, from one study, that there was any effect on subsequent vascular events (OR 1.27, 95% CI 0.84–1.89). Data from these trials do not provide strong evidence for benefit, or harm, from interventions

Table 13.2 Secondary prevention after an acute stroke.

Type of study (reference)	Patients	Intervention	Outcome (follow-up time)	No of participants (No. of trials)	Control group risk (Range)	Relative risk (95% CI)	Absolute risk reduction (95% CI)	Comment
SR [36]	Stroke and TIA hypertension	Diuretics ACE inhibitors Beta blockers versus control	Vascular events (2–5 years)	15,428 (6)	16%	0.79* (0.66–0.95)	3%	Lowering BP better Heterogeneity Due to types of drugs
SR (37)	Stroke and TIA	Drugs for lowering lipid levels versus placebo	Stroke (1–5 years)	1448 (4)	15% (13–38)	0.97 (0.76–1.23)	1% (ns)	
RCT [37]	Stroke or TIA also with normal cholesterol	Simvastatin 40 mg versus placebo	Vascular events (5 years)	3280 (1)	25%	0.80 (0.71–0.92)	5%	Statin better Subgroup of large RCT
SR [38]	Stroke or TIA atrial fibrillation	Oral anticoagulants INR 2.4–1.8 versus control	Vascular events (2 years)	485 (2)	33% (31–44)	0.64 (0.48–0.87)	12% (4–19)	Anticoagulant better
			Major extracranial bleeding (2 years)	439 (1)	1%	6.18 (1.41–27.07)	+5% (2–8)	Anticoagulant worse
SR [39]	Stroke or TIA non-cardioembolic	Oral anticoagulants (INR 3–4.5) versus Aspirin 30 mg	Vascular events (1 year)	1316 (1)	5%	2.30 (1.58–3.35)	+7% (4–10)	Anticoagulant worse
SR [40]	Stroke or TIA	Aspirin versus control	Vascular events (3 years)	18,270 (21)	21%	0.78* (0.73–0.85)	3%	Aspirin better
SR [41]	Stroke and TIA	Ticlopidine or clopidogrel versus Aspirin	Vascular events 2 years	9840 (3)	18% (9–26)	0.92 (0.85–1.00)	1% (0–3)	Ticlopidine or clopidogrel better
RCT [42]	Stroke and TIA plus one risk factor	Clopidogrel 75 mg plus aspirin 75 mg versus Clopidogrel 75 mg	Vascular events (1.5 year)	7599 (1)	13%	0.94 (0.83–1.07)	0.7% (ns)	Clopidogrel plus aspirin better
			Major bleeding (1.5 year)		1.3%	0.34 (0.21–0.57)	+1.3% (0.6–1.9)	Clopidogrel plus aspirin worse
SR [43]	Symptomatic carotid stenosis 70–99% (NASCET)	Endarterectomy versus control	Disabling stroke and death (2–6 years)	1247 (2)	14% (11–16)	0.52 (0.37–0.73)	7% (3–10)	Endarterectomy better
			Disabling stroke and death (30 days)		0.6% (0–1)	3.52 (1.11–11.13)	+2% (1–3)	Endarterectomy worse
SR [44]	Carotid stenosis	Endovascular versus endarterectomy	Death and stroke (1 year)	723 (2)	9% (4–13)	1.38 (0.88–1.95)	+3% (ns)	Increased risk heterogeneity
			Death and stroke (30 days)	1157 (5)	7% (0–10)	1.23 (0.83–1.81)	+2% (ns)	Increased risk heterogeneity
See text	See text	Other risk factors	Although systematic reviews are lacking, what evidence is available would strongly support regular monitoring of blood glucose levels in diabetics, that smoking cessation strategies employed wherever possible, and that patients adopt a healthy diet and active lifestyle.					

SR: systematic review; RCT: randomized controlled trial; ns: not statistically significant. *OR instead of RR.

to alter serum lipid levels in patients with a history solely of cerebrovascular disease. Their use, therefore, cannot yet be recommended routinely in this patient group, but ischaemic stroke patients with a history of MI should receive statin therapy along the lines of the previous recommendations for those patients with a history of myocardial ischaemia. This systematic review had not been updated to include the results of the Heart Protection Study [37]. This trial enrolled 20,536 patients, 40–80 years, at elevated risk of coronary heart disease death because of past history of MI or other coronary heart disease, occlusive disease of non-coronary arteries, diabetes mellitus or treated hypertension, or had baseline blood total cholesterol of 3.5 mmol/L or greater. The trial demonstrated benefit in patients with prior stroke and TIA, even if their low density lipoprotein (LDL) cholesterol level was not significantly elevated. Simvastatin significantly reduced the first event rate of stroke versus placebo (444 versus 585, $P < 0.0001$). There was no significant difference in strokes attributed to haemorrhage (51 versus 53, $P = 0.8$). Simvastatin also reduced the number of patients having transient cerebral ischaemic attacks alone (2.0% versus 2.4%, $P = 0.02$) or requiring carotid endarterectomy or angioplasty (0.4% versus 0.8%, $P = 0.0003$). Stroke reduction was not significant in the 1st year, but was highly significant by the end of the 2nd year ($P = 0.0004$) and continued through the 5-year follow-up.

Other risk factors: Although systematic reviews are lacking, what evidence is available would strongly support regular monitoring of blood glucose levels in diabetics, that smoking cessation strategies employed wherever possible, and that patients adopt a healthy diet and active lifestyle.

Antithrombotic agents

Anticoagulants for patients with atrial fibrillation: It is known that people with non-rheumatic atrial fibrillation (NRAF) who have had a TIA or a minor ischaemic stroke are at high risk of recurrent stroke. One Cochrane Systematic Review sought to assess the effect of anticoagulants for secondary prevention, after a stroke or TIA, in patients with NRAF [38]. Two trials involving 485 people were included. Follow-up time was 1.7 years in one trial and 2.3 years in the other. Anticoagulants reduced the odds of recurrent stroke by two-thirds (OR 0.36, 95% CI 0.22–0.58). The odds of all vascular events was shown to be almost halved by treatment (OR 0.55, 95% CI 0.37–0.82). The odds of major extracranial haemorrhage was increased (OR 4.32, 95% CI 1.55–12.10). No intracranial bleeds were reported among people given anticoagulants. The authors concluded that anticoagulants are beneficial, without serious adverse effects, for people with NRAF and recent cerebral ischaemia.

Anticoagulants versus antiplatelet agents for patients with atrial fibrillation: One Cochrane Systematic Review compared the effect of anticoagulants with antiplatelet agents, for secondary prevention, in people with NRAF and previous cerebral

ischaemia [46]. Two trials were identified. The European Atrial Fibrillation Trial (EAFT) involving 455 patients, who received either anticoagulants (International Normalized Ratio (INR) 2.5–4.0), or aspirin (300 mg/day). Patients joined the trial within 3 months of TIA or minor stroke. The mean follow up was 2.3 years. In the Studio Italiano Fibrillazione Atriale (SIFA) trial, 916 patients with NRAF and a TIA or minor stroke within the previous 15 days were randomized to open label anticoagulants (INR 2.0–3.5) or indobufen (a reversible platelet cyclooxygenase inhibitor, 100 or 200 mg bid). The follow-up period was 1 year. The combined results show that anticoagulants were significantly more effective than antiplatelet therapy both for all vascular events (Peto odds ratio (Peto OR) 0.67, 95% CI 0.50–0.91) and for recurrent stroke (Peto OR 0.49, 95% CI 0.33–0.72). Major extracranial bleeding complications occurred more often in patients on anticoagulants (Peto OR 5.16, 95% CI 2.08–12.83), but the absolute difference was small (2.8% per year versus 0.9% per year in EAFT and 0.9% per year versus 0% in SIFA). Warfarin did not cause a significant increase of intracranial bleeds. The authors concluded that the evidence from two trials suggests that anticoagulant therapy is superior to antiplatelet therapy for the prevention of stroke in people with NRAF and recent non-disabling stroke or TIA. The risk of extracranial bleeding was higher with anticoagulant therapy than with antiplatelet therapy.

Anticoagulants for patients with non-cardiac stroke: One Cochrane Systematic Review sought to determine the effect of prolonged anticoagulant therapy (compared with placebo or open control) following presumed non-cardioembolic ischaemic stroke or TIA [47]. Eleven trials involving 2487 patients were included. The quality of the nine trials which predated routine computerized tomography scanning and the use of the INR to monitor anticoagulation was poor. There was no evidence of an effect of anticoagulant therapy on either the odds of death or dependency (two trials, OR 0.83, 95% CI 0.52–1.34) or of 'non-fatal stroke, MI, or vascular death' (four trials, OR 0.96, 95% CI 0.68–1.37). Death from any cause (OR 0.95, 95% CI 0.73–1.24) and death from vascular causes (OR 0.86, 95% CI 0.66–1.13) were not significantly different between treatment and control. The inclusion of two recent completed trials did not alter these conclusions. There was no evidence of an effect of anticoagulant therapy on the risk of recurrent ischaemic stroke (OR 0.85, 95% CI 0.66–1.09). However, anticoagulants increased fatal ICH (OR 2.54, 95% CI 1.19–5.45), and major extracranial haemorrhage (OR 3.43, 95% CI 1.94–6.08). This is equivalent to anticoagulant therapy causing about 11 additional fatal ICH and 25 additional major extracranial haemorrhages per year for every 1000 patients given anticoagulant therapy. The authors concluded that, compared with control, there was no evidence of benefit from long-term anticoagulant therapy in people with presumed non-cardioembolic ischaemic stroke or TIA, but there was a significant bleeding risk.

Anticoagulants versus aspirin for patients with non-cardiac stroke: One Cochrane Systematic Review [39] evaluated five trials, with a total of 4076 patients. The available data do not allow a robust conclusion on whether anticoagulants (in any intensity) are more efficacious in the prevention of vascular events than antiplatelet therapy (medium intensity anticoagulation RR 0.96, 95% CI 0.38–2.42, high intensity anticoagulation RR 1.02, 95% CI 0.49–2.13). There is no evidence that treatment with low or medium intensity anticoagulation gives a higher bleeding risk than treatment with antiplatelet agents. The RR for major bleeding complications for low intensity anticoagulation was 1.27 (95% CI 0.79–2.03) and for medium intensity anticoagulation 1.19 (95% CI 0.59–2.41). However, it was clear that high intensity oral anticoagulants with INR 3.0–4.5 were not safe, because they yielded a higher risk of major bleeding complications (RR 9.0, 95% CI 3.9–21).

Antiplatelet agents other than aspirin: The most widely studied and prescribed antiplatelet agent for the prevention of stroke and other serious vascular events among high vascular risk patients is aspirin [40]. One Cochrane Systematic Review sought to determine the effectiveness and safety of thienopyridine derivatives (ticlopidine and clopidogrel) versus aspirin for the prevention of serious vascular events (stroke, MI or vascular death) in patients at high risk of such events, and specifically in patients with a previous TIA or ischaemic stroke [41]. Four trials involving a total of 22,656 high vascular risk patients were included. The trials were of high quality and comparable. Aspirin was compared with ticlopidine in three trials (3471 patients) and with clopidogrel in one trial (19,185 patients). Allocation to a thienopyridine was associated with a modest, yet statistically significant, reduction in the odds of a serious vascular event (12.0% versus 13.0%, OR 0.91, 95% CI 0.84–0.98, 2P = 0.01), corresponding to the avoidance of 11 (95% CI 2–19) serious vascular events per 1000 patients treated for about 2 years. There was also a reduction in stroke (5.7% versus 6.4%, OR 0.88, 95% CI 0.79–0.98, 7 (95% CI 1–13) strokes avoided per 1000 patients treated for 2 years). Compared with aspirin, thienopyridines produced a significant reduction in the odds of gastrointestinal haemorrhage and other upper gastrointestinal upset, but a significant increase in the odds of skin rash and of diarrhoea. However, the increased odds of skin rash and diarrhoea were greater for ticlopidine than for clopidogrel. Allocation to ticlopidine, but not clopidogrel, was associated with a significant increase in the odds of neutropenia (2.3% versus 0.8%, OR 2.7, 95% CI 1.5–4.8). In the subset of patients with TIA/ischaemic stroke, the results were similar to those for all patients combined. However, since these patients are at particularly high risk of stroke, allocation to a thienopyridine was associated with a larger absolute reduction in stroke (10.4% versus 12.0%, OR 0.86, 95% CI 0.75–0.97, 16 (95% CI 3–28) strokes avoided per 1000 patients treated for 2 years). The authors concluded that the thienopyridine derivatives are modestly but significantly more effective than aspirin in preventing serious vascular events in patients at high risk (and specifically in TIA/ischaemic stroke patients), but there is uncertainty about the size of the additional benefit. The thienopyridines are also associated with less gastrointestinal haemorrhage and other upper gastrointestinal upset than aspirin, but an excess of skin rash and diarrhoea. The risk of skin rash and diarrhoea is greater with ticlopidine than with clopidogrel. Ticlopidine, but not clopidogrel, is associated with an excess of neutropenia and of thrombotic thrombocytopenic purpura.

Combinations of antiplatelet agents (in the non-acute phase): No Cochrane Systematic Review is available. The combination of ASA and clopidogrel for secondary stroke prevention has been studied in two randomized controlled trials. The MATCH trial determined that adding aspirin to clopidogrel in high-risk patients with recent ischaemic stroke or TIA was associated with an increased risk of bleeding and a non-significant reduction in major ischaemic vascular events [42]. The combination of ASA and clopidogrel for the secondary prevention of stroke was further studied in the CHARISMA study, which investigated clopidogrel and aspirin versus aspirin alone in lower and higher risk patients [48]. In this trial, there was a suggestion of benefit with clopidogrel treatment in patients with symptomatic atherothrombosis and a suggestion of harm in patients with multiple risk factors but no vascular symptoms. Overall, clopidogrel plus aspirin was not significantly more effective than aspirin alone in reducing the rate of MI, stroke, or death from cardiovascular causes. The combination of these antiplatelet agents is also being evaluated in the FASTER trial (http://www.faster.ca/trials).

Endarterectomy for symptomatic carotid stenosis
One Cochrane Review sought to summarize the evidence from randomized trials on the balance of risks and benefits of carotid endarterectomy in adults with symptomatic carotid stenosis [43]. Data on death or disabling stroke were available from two trials, which included 5950 patients: the North American Symptomatic Carotid Endarterectomy Trial (NASCET), and the European Carotid Surgery Trial (ECST). The two trials used different methods to measure stenosis, but a simple formula can be used to convert between the two methods. For patients with severe stenosis (ECST >80% = NASCET >70%), surgery reduced the RR of disabling stroke or death by 48% (95% CI 27–73%). The number of patients needed to be operated on (number needed to treat (NNT)) to prevent one disabling stroke or death over 2–6 years follow-up was 15 (95% CI 10–31). For patients with less severe stenosis (ECST 70–79% = NASCET 50–69%), surgery reduced the RR of disabling stroke or death by 27% (95% CI 15–44%). The number of patients needed to be operated on to prevent one disabling stroke or death was 21 (95% CI 11–125). Patients with lesser degrees of stenosis were harmed by surgery. Surgery increased the risk of disabling stroke or death by 20% (95% CI 0–44%). The number of

patients needed to be operated on to cause one disabling stroke or death was 45 (95% CI 22–infinity). The authors concluded that carotid endarterectomy reduced the risk of disabling stroke or death for patients with stenosis exceeding ECST-measured 70% or NASCET-measured 50%. This result is generalizable only to surgically-fit patients operated on by surgeons with low complication rates (less than 6%).

Subsequent to this review, an analysis of pooled data from the randomized trials of endarterectomy for symptomatic carotid stenosis has demonstrated that the benefits of surgery are greatest in men, for patients aged 75 years or older, and for patients operated on soonest after their symptoms took place [49]. The benefit of surgery is lost after 4 weeks for patients with 50–69% stenosis, and after 12 weeks for patients with stenosis >70%. Delaying carotid endarterectomy therefore exposes these patients to an unnecessary risk of recurrent stroke.

Endovascular treatment for carotid stenosis

Two randomized trials comparing endovascular treatment with carotid endarterectomy for patients with carotid stenosis (symptomatic and asymptomatic) were evaluated on one Cochrane Systematic Review [44]. In addition there were two trials which fulfilled the inclusion criteria and which were stopped early, and a third trial which has completed only the 30-day follow up. The odds of death or disabling stroke at 30 days were similar in the endovascular and surgical group (OR 1.22, CI 0.61–2.41). At 1 year following procedure, there was no significant difference between the two groups in preventing any stroke or death (OR 1.36, CI 0.87–2.13). Endovascular treatment significantly reduced the risk of cranial neuropathy (OR 0.12, CI 0.06–0.25). There was substantial heterogeneity between the trials renders the overall estimates of effect somewhat unreliable. There is also uncertainty about the potential for restenosis to develop and cause recurrent stroke after endovascular treatment. Additional trials are ongoing (http://www.strokecentre.org.trials/).

References

1 Warlow CP, Dennis MS, van Gijn J, et al. What caused this transient or persisting ischaemic event? In: *Stroke: A Practical Guide to Management*. Blackwell Science, Oxford, 2001: pp. 223–300.

2 Special report from the National Institute of Neurological Disorders and Stroke. Classification of cerebrovascular diseases III. *Stroke* 1990; **21**: 637–76.

3 Albers G, Caplan L, Easton D, et al. Transient ischemic attack: proposal for a new definition. *N. Engl. J. Med.* 2002; **347**: 1713–16.

4 Warach S, Kidwell C. The redefinition of TIA: the uses and limitations of DWI in acute ischemic cerebrovascular syndromes. *Neurology* 2004; **62**: 359–60.

5 Lassen NA. Pathophysiology of brain ischemia as it relates to the therapy of acute ischemic stroke [Review]. *Clin. Neuropharmacol.* 1990; **13**(Suppl. 3): S1–8.

6 World Health Organization. *The Atlas of Heart Disease and Stroke.* Accessed via the internet at: http://www.who.int/cardiovascular_diseases/resources/atlas/en

7 Stroke Unit Trialists' Collaboration. Organised inpatient (stroke unit) care for stroke. *Cochrane Database Syst. Rev.* 2001; 3: CD000197. DOI: 10.1002/14651858.CD000197.

8 Wardlaw JM, del Zoppo G, Yamaguchi T, Berge E. Thrombolysis for acute ischaemic stroke. *Cochrane Database Syst. Rev.* 2003, 3: CD000213. DOI: 10.1002/14651858.CD000213.

9 Sandercock P, Gubitz G, Foley P, Counsell C. Antiplatelet therapy for acute ischaemic stroke. *Cochrane Database Syst. Rev.* 2003; 2: CD000029. DOI: 10.1002/14651858.CD000029.

10 Gubitz G, Sandercock P, Counsell C. Anticoagulants for acute ischaemic stroke. *Cochrane Database Syst. Rev.* 2004; 2: CD000024. pub2. DOI: 10.1002/14651858.CD000024.pub2.

11 Bereczki D, Liu M, Fernandes do Prado G, Fekete I. Mannitol for acute stroke. *Cochrane Database Syst. Rev.* 2001; 1: CD001153. DOI: 10.1002/14651858.CD001153.

12 Righetti E, Celani MG, Cantisani T, Sterzi R, Boysen G, Ricci S. Glycerol for acute stroke. *Cochrane Database Syst. Rev.* 2004; 2: CD000096. DOI: 10.1002/14651858.CD000096.pub2.

13 Qizilbash N, Lewington SL, Lopez-Arrieta JM. Corticosteroids for acute ischaemic stroke. *Cochrane Database Syst. Rev.* 2002; 3: CD000064. DOI: 10.1002/14651858.CD000064.

14 Morley NCD, Berge E, Cruz-Flores S, Whittle IR. Surgical decompression for cerebral oedema in acute ischaemic stroke. *Cochrane Database Syst. Rev.* 2002; 3: CD003435. DOI: 10.1002/14651858.CD003435.

15 Prasad K, Shrivastava A. Surgery for primary supratentorial intracerebral haemorrhage. *Cochrane Database Syst. Rev.* 1999; 2: CD000200. DOI: 10.1002/14651858.CD000200.

16 Mendelow A, Gregson B, Fernandes H, et al. Early surgery versus initial conservative treatment in patients with spontaneous supratentorial intracerebral haematomas in the International surgical Trial in Intracerebral Haemorrhage (STICH): a randomised trial. *Lancet* 2005; **365**(9452): 387–97.

17 Mayer, S, Brun N, Begtrup M, et al. Recombinant activated factor VII for acute intracerebral hemorrhage. *N. Engl. J. Med.* 2005; **352**: 777–85.

18 Hacke W, Donnan G, Fieschi C, et al. Association of outcome with early stroke treatment: pooled analysis of ATLANTIS, ECASS, and NINDS rt-PA stroke trials. ATLANTIS Trials Investigators; ECASS Trials Investigators; NINDS rt-PA Study Group Investigators. *Lancet* 2004; **363**: 768–74.

19 Wade S. Smith, Gene Sung, Sidney Starkman, Jeffrey L. Saver, Chelsea S. Kidwell, Pierre Gobin Y., Helmi L. Lutsep, Gary M. Nesbit, Thomas Grobelny, Marilyn M. Rymer, Isaac E. Silverman, Randall T. Higashida, Ronald F. Budzik, Michael P. Marks for the MERCI Trial Investigators. *Stroke* 2005; **36**: 1432–8.

20 Antithrombotic Trialists' Collaboration. Collaborative meta-analysis of randomised trials of antiplatelet therapy for the prevention of death, myocardial infarction, and stroke in high risk patients. *BMJ* 2002; **324**: 71–86.

21 Berge E, Sandercock P. Anticoagulants versus antiplatelet agents for acute ischaemic stroke. *Cochrane Database Syst. Rev.* 2002; 4: CD003242. DOI: 10.1002/14651858.CD003242.

22 Muir KW, Lees KR. Excitatory amino acid antagonists for acute stroke. *Cochrane Database Syst. Rev.* 2003; 3: CD001244. DOI: 10.1002/14651858.CD001244.

23 Candelise L, Ciccone A. Gangliosides for acute ischaemic stroke. *Cochrane Database Syst. Rev.* 2001; 4: CD000094. DOI: 10.1002/14651858.CD000094.

24 Horn J, Limburg M. Calcium antagonists for acute ischemic stroke. *Cochrane Database Syst. Rev.* 2000; 1: CD001928. DOI: 10.1002/14651858.CD001928.

25 Gandolfo C, Sandercock P, Conti M. Lubeluzole for acute ischaemic stroke. *Cochrane Database Syst. Rev.* 2002; 1: CD001924. DOI: 10.1002/14651858.CD001924.

26 Bath PMW, Bath-Hextall FJ. Pentoxifylline, propentofylline and pentifylline for acute ischaemic stroke. *Cochrane Database Syst. Rev.* 2004; 3: CD000162. DOI: 10.1002/14651858.CD000162.pub2.

27 The Tirilazad International Steering Committee. Tirilazad for acute ischaemic stroke. *Cochrane Database Syst. Rev.* 2001; 4: CD002087. DOI: 10.1002/14651858.CD002087.

28 Asplund K. Haemodilution for acute ischaemic stroke. *Cochrane Database Syst. Rev.* 2002; 4: CD000103. DOI: 10.1002/14651858. CD000103.

29 Bennett MH, Wasiak J, Schnabel A, Kranke P, French C. Hyperbaric oxygen therapy for acute ischaemic stroke. *Cochrane Database Syst. Rev.* 2005; 3: CD004954. DOI: 10.1002/14651858. CD004954.pub2.

30 Correia M, Silva M, Veloso M. Cooling therapy for acute stroke. *Cochrane Database Syst. Rev.* 1999; 4: CD001247. DOI: 10.1002/ 14651858.CD001247.

31 Langhorne P, Pollock A in conjunction with the Stroke Unit Trialists Collaboration. What are the components of effective stroke unit care? *Age Ageing* 2002; **31**: 365–71.

32 Mazzone C, Chiodo Grandi F, Sandercock P, Miccio M, Salvi R. Physical methods for preventing deep vein thrombosis in stroke. *Cochrane Database Syst. Rev.* 2004; 4: CD001922. DOI: 10.1002/ 14651858.CD001922.pub2.

33 The Blood pressure in Acute Stroke Collaboration (BASC). Vasoactive drugs for acute stroke. *Cochrane Database Syst. Rev.* 2000; 4: CD002839. DOI: 10.1002/14651858.CD002839.

34 Stead LG, Gilmore RM, Anand N, Weaver AL. Interventions for controlling hyperglycaemia in acute ischaemic stroke (Protocol). *Cochrane Database Syst. Rev.* 2005; 3: CD005346. DOI: 10.1002/ 14651858.CD005346.

35 Feigin VL, Anderson N, Rinkel GJE, Algra A, van Gijn J, Bennett DA. Corticosteroids for aneurysmal subarachnoid haemorrhage and primary intracerebral haemorrhage. *Cochrane Database Syst. Rev.* 2005; 3: CD004583. DOI: 10.1002/14651858. CD004583.pub2.

36 Rashid P, Leonardi-Bee J, Bath P. Blood pressure reduction and secondary prevention of stroke and other vascular events. A systematic review. *Stroke* 2003; **34**: 2741–9.

37 Heart Protection Study Collaborative Group. Effects of cholesterol-lowering with simvastatin on stroke and other major vascular events in 20,536 people with cerebrovascular disease or other high-risk conditions. *Lancet* 2004; **363**: 757–67.

38 Saxena R, Koudstaal PJ. Anticoagulants for preventing stroke in patients with nonrheumatic atrial fibrillation and a history of stroke or transient ischaemic attack. *Cochrane Database Syst. Rev.* 2004; 2: CD000185. DOI: 10.1002/14651858.CD000185.pub2.

39 Algra A, De Schryver ELLM, van Gijn J, Kappelle LJ, Koudstaal PJ. Oral anticoagulants versus antiplatelet therapy for preventing further vascular events after transient ischaemic attack or minor stroke of presumed arterial origin. *Cochrane Database Syst. Rev.* 2001; 4: CD001342. DOI: 10.1002/14651858.CD001342.

40 Antithrombotic Trialists' Collaboration. Collaborative meta-analysis of randomised trials of antiplatelet therapy for prevention of death, myocardial infarction, and stroke in high risk patients. *BMJ* 2002; **324**: 71–86.

41 Hankey GJ, Sudlow CLM, Dunbabin DW. Thienopyridine derivatives (ticlopidine, clopidogrel) versus aspirin for preventing stroke and other serious vascular events in high vascular risk patients. *Cochrane Database Syst. Rev.* 2000; 1: CD001246. DOI: 10.1002/14651858.CD001246.

42 Diener H, Bogousslavsky J, Brass L for the MATCH Investigators. Aspirin and clopidogrel compared with clopidogrel alone after recent ischaemic stroke or transient ischaemic attack in high-risk patients (MATCH): randomised, double-blind, placebo-controlled trial. *Lancet* 2004; **364**: 331–7.

43 Cina CS, Clase CM, Haynes RB. Carotid endarterectomy for symptomatic carotid stenosis. *Cochrane Database Syst. Rev.* 1999; 3: CD001081. DOI: 10.1002/14651858.CD001081.

44 Coward LJ, Featherstone RL, Brown MM. Percutaneous transluminal angioplasty and stenting for carotid artery stenosis. *Cochrane Database Syst. Rev.* 2004; 2: CD000515.pub2. DOI: 10.1002/14651858.CD000515.pub2.

45 Manktelow B, Gillies C, Potter JF. Interventions in the management of serum lipids for preventing stroke recurrence. *Cochrane Database Syst. Rev.* 2002; 3: CD002091. DOI: 10.1002/14651858. CD002091.

46 Saxena R, Koudstaal PJ. Anticoagulants versus antiplatelet therapy for preventing stroke in patients with nonrheumatic atrial fibrillation and a history of stroke or transient ischemic attack. *Cochrane Database Syst. Rev.* 2004; 4: CD000187. DOI: 10.1002/ 14651858.CD000187.pub2.

47 Sandercock P, Mielke O, Liu M, Counsell C. Anticoagulants for preventing recurrence following presumed non-cardioembolic ischaemic stroke or transient ischaemic attack. *Cochrane Database Syst. Rev.* 2003; 1: CD000248. DOI: 10.1002/14651858.CD000248.

48 Bhatt D, Fox K, Hacke W, et al., for the Charisma Investigators. Clopidogrel and aspirin versus aspirin alone for the prevention of atherothrombotic events. *N Engl. J. Med.* 2006; **354**(16): 1706–17.

49 Rothwell, P, Eliasziw M, Gutnikov S, et al., for the Carotid Endarterectomy Trialists Collaboration. Endarterectomy for symptomatic carotid stenosis in relation to clinical subgroups and timing of surgery. *Lancet* 2004; **363**: 915–24.

14

CHAPTER 14

Aneurysmal subarachnoid haemorrhage

Jan van Gijn, Gabriel J.E. Rinkel

Background

Aneurysms of the cerebral vessels are not congenital but almost invariably develop during the course of life, usually after the second decade [1]. In a systematic review of studies reporting the prevalence of all intracranial aneurysms in patients studied for reasons other than subarachnoid haemorrhage (SAH), the best estimate of the frequency for an average adult without specific risk factors was 2.3% (95% confidence interval (CI) 1.7–3.1%); this proportion tended to increase with age [1]. Rupture of these aneurysms occurs in only a small fraction of these subjects: the incidence is 6–10 per 100,000 per year in most western countries, but in Finland and Japan the incidence is twice as high [2]. In terms of attributable risk, the modifiable risk factors alcohol, smoking and hypertension account for half of first SAH episodes, genetic factors for only 11% [3]. Only in patients with multiple aneurysms genetic factors predominate, given the finding that these patients are younger at the time of rupture than patients with a SAH and a single aneurysm [4].

Framing clinical questions

The essence of managing patients with aneurysmal SAH is deceptively simple: make the diagnosis, locate the aneurysm and occlude it. Yet, in the latest population-based studies, up to the mid-1990s, the case fatality rate was still as high as 50% [5], including the 10–15% who die before receiving medical attention [6]. Of the 50% who survive the episode after operative aneurysm clipping, again half report an incomplete recovery [7]. The poor outcome can for a large part be attributed to the many complications that beset the course of the disease: rebleeding, delayed cerebral ischaemia, hydrocephalus and a variety of systemic disorders [8]. Thus, occlusion of the ruptured aneurysm by the interventional radiologist or the neurosurgeon is an important but by far not the only part in the management of patients with SAH.

First of all, the patient should be transferred as quickly as possible to a centre where a multidisciplinary team including neurosurgeons and interventional radiologists is continuously available and where the volume of such patients is large enough to maintain and improve standards of care [9]. Continuous observation in a high dependency unit is the basis of management in these patients, before but also after interventions to occlude the aneurysm. The neurologist is well suited to fulfil a central role, in day-to-day mutual consultation with the other team members.

The need for referral applies also and perhaps especially to patients who are infelicitously designated as 'poor grade cases'. These may be the very patients that need urgent intervention because of, for example, early rebleeding, progressive brain shift from a haematoma, acute hydrocephalus or hypovolaemia.

Despite the considerable proportion of patients who die before reaching medical attention and the many complications that can occur, the prognosis for patients with SAH has gradually improved over the last decades [5].

Critical review of the evidence for each question

1. Patients in poor clinical condition

How to manage patients in poor clinical condition on admission.

The following sections provide a guideline for the management of patients in poor clinical condition on admission.

Intracerebral haematoma

Intraparenchymal haematomas occur in approximately 30% of patients with ruptured aneurysms [10]. Not surprisingly, the average outcome is worse than in patients with purely subarachnoid blood [11]. When the most likely cause of a deterioration in the level of consciousness is a large temporal haematoma, usually from a ruptured aneurysm of the middle cerebral artery, immediate occlusion of the aneurysm should be considered. The intervention traditionally consists in evacuation of the haematoma (with simultaneous clipping of the aneurysm if it can be identified, usually only by magnetic resonance (MR) angiography or computed tomography (CT) angiography); this course of action is backed up by a small randomized study, in which 11 of 15 patients in the operated group survived, against three of 15 in the conservatively treated group (relative risk (RR) 0.27; 95% CI 0.09–0.74) [12]. Nowadays of course coiling of the aneurysm followed by clot occlusion is often a good alternative strategy [13]. Another approach is an extensive hemicraniectomy that allows external expansion of the brain [14].

Acute subdural haematoma

An acute subdural haematoma complicates rupture of an intracerebral aneurysm in approximately 2% of cases [15,16]. Subdural haematomas secondary to a ruptured aneurysm may be life threatening, in which cases immediate evacuation seems called for, despite the lack of controlled studies [17,18].

Acute hydrocephalus and intraventricular haemorrhage

Gradual obtundation within 24 h of haemorrhage, sometimes accompanied by slow pupillary responses to light and downward deviation of the eyes, is fairly characteristic for acute hydrocephalus [19,20]. If the diagnosis is confirmed by CT this can be a reason for lumbar puncture or early ventricular drainage [21,22], although some patients improve spontaneously in the first 24 h. This is an area badly in need of controlled studies.

Acute hydrocephalus with large amounts of intraventricular blood is often associated with a poor clinical condition from the outset. In patients with ruptured aneurysms, that is an arterial source of bleeding, intraventricular haemorrhage with a volume of 20 mL or more is invariably lethal [23]. An indirect comparison of observational studies suggests that insertion of an external ventricular catheter is not very helpful in these patients, but that a strategy where such drainage is combined with fibrinolysis through the drain results in a good outcome in half the patients [24]. This needs to be confirmed in studies with concurrent, randomized controls [25]. Surgical evacuation of a 'packed' intraventricular haemorrhage, especially from the fourth ventricle, is pointless according to some [26], while others disagree [27].

2. General care

How to distinguish facts from fiction.

The following sections will briefly describe how to distinguish facts from fiction.

Blood pressure

Aggressive treatment of high blood pressure entails a definite risk of ischaemia in brain areas with loss of autoregulation. The rationalistic approach is therefore to advise against treating hypertension following aneurysmal rupture. There is no evidence from clinical trials to support this, but observational studies tend to support the avoidance of antihypertensive drugs. In a comparison of patients in whom hypertension had been newly treated with normotensive controls, the rate of rebleeding was lower but the rate of cerebral infarction was higher than in untreated patients, despite the blood pressures being, on average, still higher than in the controls [28]. This suggests that hypertension after SAH is a compensatory phenomenon, at least to some extent, and one that

should not be interfered with. In keeping with this, a further observational study from the same centre (Rotterdam) suggested that the combined strategy of avoiding antihypertensive medication and increasing fluid intake may decrease the risk of cerebral infarction [29]. Therefore it seems best only to use antihypertensive therapy in patients with extreme elevations of blood pressure (mean arterial pressure of 130 mmHg or over) as well as in those with evidence of rapidly progressive end organ deterioration.

Fluids and electrolytes

Fluid management in SAH is important to prevent a reduction in plasma volume, which may contribute to the development of cerebral ischaemia. Nevertheless, the arguments for a liberal (some might say aggressive) regimen of fluid administration are indirect. Fluid restriction in patients with hyponatraemia, applied in the past because it was erroneously attributed to water retention, via inappropriate secretion of antidiuretic hormone, is associated with an increased risk of cerebral ischaemia [30].

Two randomized studies of prophylactic hypervolaemia have been published. One included only 30 patients [31]. Treatment allocation was not blinded (personal information obtained from the authors), and outcome was not assessed beyond the time of operation (day 7–10); at that time, the rate of delayed ischaemia had been reduced by two thirds (67%; 95% CI 1–89%). The second trial included 32 patients after operation and allocated 16 of them to hypervolaemic hypertensive haemodilution fluid therapy, according to a pseudo-randomized design; not surprisingly, given the small numbers, after 1 year there was no difference in outcome with the 16 patients who had been kept normovolaemic [32]. Despite the incomplete evidence, it seems reasonable to prevent hypovolaemia. Therefore a reliable intravenous route should be maintained for sufficient administration of fluids (and drugs).

Analgesics and general nursing care

Headache can sometimes be managed with mild analgesics such as paracetamol (acetaminophen); salicylates should be avoided until the aneurysm has been clipped because of their inhibitory effect on haemostasis. However, usually the pain is so severe that codeine needs to be added, which will not mask neurological signs. Sometimes, pain can be alleviated with anxiolytic drugs such as midazolam (5 mg via an infusion pump). Often a synthetic opiate such as tramadol may be needed to obtain relief. As a last resort, severe headache can be treated with piritramide. The blood pressure should be checked frequently until the pain has subsided. Constipation is a common disadvantage of all opiates. Coughing and straining must be rigorously prevented because of the attendant overshoots in arterial blood pressure. Stool softeners should therefore be prescribed routinely.

As long as the aneurysm has not been occluded the patient is traditionally restricted to complete bed rest, flat and in a surrounding that is as quiet as possible, on the assumption that any form of excitement increases the risk of rebleeding. Some centres prefer to maintain complete bed rest even after aneurysm occlusion until after the period that secondary ischaemia can occur, on the assumption that because of the impaired autoregulation drops in blood pressure induced by raising from bed may induce cerebral ischaemia. However, the entire notion of bed rest for patients with SAH is an evidence free zone.

Continuous assessment of the level of consciousness is essential. This should preferably be recorded by means of the Glasgow Coma Scale, since any change in the level of consciousness may signify a treatable complication.

The body temperature should be frequently measured, up to 4 times per day, depending on the interval after SAH and the level of consciousness. After the first few hours mild fever (up to 38.5°C) often occurs, probably resulting from the inflammatory reaction in the subarachnoid space [33]; in that case the pulse rate is characteristically normal [34]. Infection should be suspected if the temperature exceeds 38.5°C, if the pulse rate is elevated as well, or if the patient has vomited. An elevated white cell count is not helpful in distinguishing infection from non-infective causes of pyrexia [35].

Deep venous thrombosis

Deep venous thrombosis (DVT) is not as common after SAH as in patients with ischaemic stroke, presumably because the patients are restless, mostly younger and, most important, have no paralysed leg; in a large and prospective series DVT was clinically diagnosed in only 4% [36]. In general, DVT can be prevented by subcutaneous low-dose heparin or heparinoids, but the obvious qualm is that anticoagulation will not be confined to the venous system. In a randomized trial comparing the low molecular weight heparin enoxaparin given after aneurysm occlusion with placebo, intracranial bleeding complications occurred more often in the treatment group, while there were no differences in overall outcome or the chance of delayed cerebral ischaemia [37]. In the absence of proof of effectiveness many physicians do not prophylactically institute treatment with heparin or its low molecular heparinoids.

Graduated compression stockings are of confirmed benefit in preventing DVT in patients undergoing general surgical, neurosurgical or orthopaedic procedures, according to a Cochrane Review [38]. They are also the preferred form of thrombosis prevention in patients with SAH before aneurysm occlusion – though admittedly this piece of advice lacks support from a controlled trial in this specific situation.

3. Preventing rebleeding?

How to prevent rebleeding.

The main results are included in Table 14.1.

Table 14.1 Treatment for preventing rebleeding in aneurysmal SAH.

Type of study (reference)	Intervention	Outcome (follow-up time)	Number of patients (number of trials)	Control group risk (range)	Relative risk (95% CI)	Absolute risk reduction (95% CI)	Comment
SR [41]	Coiling versus clipping	Death or dependency (1 year)	2243 (3)	31% (24–50)	0.76 (0.67–0.84)	7% (4–11)	Coiling better. The evidence comes mainly from one large trial
		Rebleeding (1 year)	2272 (3)	1.2% (0–3)	2.00 (1.08–3.70)	+1% (0–2)	Coiling worse Heterogeneity
SR [56]	Early versus intermediate surgery	Death or dependency (3 months)	141 (1)	21%	0.3 (0.16–0.36)	13% (1–25)	Early surgery better Just one small trial
	Early versus late surgery	Death or dependency (3 months)	141 (1)	20%	0.47 (0.17–1.04)	12% (ns)	Early surgery better
SR [62]	Antifibrinolytic versus control	Death or severe disability (3 months)	1041 (3)	45% (40–47)	1.02 (0.93–1.21)	+3% (ns)	Antifibrinolytic worse
		Rebleeding	1399 (9)	27% (15–34)	0.62 (0.50–0.76)	10% (6–14)	Antifibrinolytic better
		Cerebral ischaemia	1166 (5)	23% (4–36)	1.27 (1.05–1.53)	+6% (1–11)	Antifibrinolytic worse Heterogeneity
RCT [63]	Antifibrinolytic versus control	Death or disability (6 months)	505 (1)	29%		4%	Not appreciable improvement

SR: systematic review; RCT: randomized controlled trial; CI: confidence intervals; ns: not statistically significant.

Endovascular occlusion

Over the last decade, endovascular occlusion of aneurysms has largely replaced surgical occlusion as the preferred intervention of choice for the prevention of rebleeding. The technique consists of packing the aneurysm with platinum coils, with a system for controlled detachment [39]. Numerous observational studies have reflected this development [40]. A Cochrane Review of randomized trials (one large trial and two small trials, of which one was still unpublished) included a total of 2272 patients [41]. Most of the patients were in good clinical condition and had an aneurysm on the anterior circulation. After 1 year of follow-up, the RR of poor outcome for coiling versus clipping was 0.76 (95% CI 0.67–0.88). The absolute risk reduction of poor outcome was 7% (95% CI 4–11%). For patients with anterior circulation aneurysm the RR of poor outcome was 0.78 (95% CI 0.68–0.90) and the absolute risk decrease was 7% (95% CI 3–10%). For those with a posterior circulation aneurysm the RR was 0.41 (95% CI 0.19–0.92) and the absolute decrease in risk 27% (95% CI 6–48%).

Several qualifications are needed to avoid the impression that these numbers fully define the relative merits of endovascular and surgical occlusion of aneurysms. Firstly, aneurysms in some locations are more suitable for occlusion by one or the other technique. Basilar artery aneurysms and many other types of posterior circulation aneurysms are relatively easy to access by the endovascular route [42], whereas surgical treatment is often complicated. Conversely, aneurysms at the trifurcation of the middle cerebral artery are relatively easy to occlude via a surgical approach, whereas it is often difficult to coil them without interfering with major arterial branches. Secondly, patients over 70 years were underrepresented in the largest study, the international subarachnoid aneurysm trial (ISAT) trial [43], reflecting a preference for coiling – or perhaps for no treatment – in many aged patients with SAH. It is not an unrealistic guess that the relative advantages of coiling over surgical treatment are even greater in patients over 70 than in younger patients, given that the risk of complications for treatment of unruptured aneurysms is in older patients much higher for surgery than for coiling [44].

A third and last concern is the durability of the occlusion with coils, given that the early rebleeding rate after surgical occlusion is rather low. Reanalysis of the ISAT trial after 1 year showed that the rate of rebleeding from the target aneurysms between the procedure and the end of the first year was somewhat higher after coiling than after clipping (2.6% versus 1.2%; risk ratio 2.0, 95% CI 1.08–3.70), but that the initial 7.4% absolute gain in the avoidance of death or dependence was maintained after 1 year, while the early survival advantage was maintained for up to 7 years [45]. Data on long-term durability are thus far scarce. The risk of late rebleeding after coiling should be weighed up against the background risk of late rebleeding or bleeding from new aneurysms in patients treated surgically. This risk is around 3% in the first 10 years after surgical treatment of ruptured aneurysms [46,47].

The lack of data on long-term durability also causes uncertainty about the length of time during which patients need to be followed up with imaging beyond the period of 6 months that is fairly standard. A related question is the most suitable method of imaging. Conventional angiography is the current standard but carries a small but definite risk of complications and is time consuming. MR angiography is feasible and gives good imaging quality [48], but its test characteristics and effectiveness have not yet been studied in large series of patients.

A last area of uncertainty is the need to perform a second procedure for aneurysm necks that have recanalized by impaction of the coils, through recoiling [49] or surgical occlusion [50].

Surgical occlusion

Craniotomy for occlusion of the aneurysm has now become second choice, at least for most patients and aneurysms. Surgical clipping has never been tested in a randomized controlled study; in the only trials in which operation was compared with conservative management, the interventions consisted in carotid ligation [51,52]. A statistical modelling exercise that weighed the benefit that rebleeding is prevented against the complications of the operation at current standards estimated an absolute reduction in the risk of poor outcome of almost 10% and a RR reduction of 0.81 [53].

Nowadays, neurosurgeons preferably clip aneurysms early, that is within 3 days of the initial bleed – if possible within 24 h [54]. The only randomized trial of the timing of operation, performed in Finland, allocated 216 patients to one of three groups: operation within 3 days, after 7 days, or in the intermediate period [55]. The outcome tended to be better after early than intermediate or late surgery, but as the difference was not statistically significant a disadvantage of early surgery could not be excluded [55,56]. The same result – no difference in outcome after early or late operation – emerged from observational studies [57–59].

It should not be assumed that surgical treatment is always definitive. To begin with, in the surgical arm of the ISAT trial rebleeding occurred in 1% of operated patients within the first year [45]. In the long term, the rebleed rate after initially successful clipping is around 3% after 10 years [46,47]. Despite all this, a modelling study estimated that repeated screening and preventive treatment of newly detected aneurysms could not be recommended, because the prevented episodes of rebleeding are outweighed by the complications of diagnostic and therapeutic procedures [60].

Pharmacological treatment

Because rebleeding is attributed to dissolution of the clot at the tear in the aneurysm wall, prevention by drug treatment is a logical aim.

Antifibrinolytic agents: The clot dissolution probably results from fibrinolytic activity in the cerebrospinal fluid (CSF) after SAH. Antifibrinolytic agents reduce fibrinolytic activity and cross the blood–brain barrier rapidly after SAH and might so reduce the risk of rebleeding [61]. Ten randomized trials with antifibrinolytic agents in SAH have so far been performed. The most recent Cochrane Review included nine of these, involving 1399 patients. Death from all causes was not significantly influenced by treatment across all nine trials (odds ratio 0.99, 95% CI 0.79–1.24). Poor outcome (death, vegetative state or severe disability) was recorded in 1041 patients in three trials, antifibrinolytic treatment did not show any evidence of benefit (risk ratio 1.02, 95% CI 0.93–1.21). On the other hand, the analysis of specific event rates did show striking differences. Antifibrinolytic treatment reduced the risk of rebleeding reported at the end of follow-up, with some heterogeneity between the trials (risk ratio 0.62, 95% CI 0.50–0.76). Conversely, treatment increased the risk of cerebral ischaemia in five trials (risk ratio 1.27, 95% CI 1.05–1.53) with considerable heterogeneity between the most recent study, in which specific treatments to prevent cerebral ischaemia were used [62], and the four older studies. The 10th trial was subsequently performed in Sweden and included 505 patients; again the overall outcome did not appreciably improve in patients treated with TEA, despite an impressive reduction in the rate of rebleeding [63].

Recombinant factor VIIa: Theoretically, an activated coagulation factor might also prevent rebleeding. An open label, dose escalation safety study of recombinant factor VIIa showed no evidence of ischaemic complications in the first nine patients but was suspended when the tenth patient developed middle cerebral artery branch occlusion contralateral to the aneurysm [64].

4. Preventing cerebral ischaemia
How to prevent delayed cerebral ischaemia.

The main results are summarized in Table 14.2.

Calcium antagonists
Arterial narrowing ('vasospasm') is one of the factors involved in the complex pathogenesis of delayed cerebral ischaemia. Calcium antagonists have been used because they inhibit the contractile properties of smooth muscle cells, particularly those in cerebral arteries, and also because they may, to some extent, protect neurones against the deleterious effect of calcium influx after ischaemic damage.

A Cochrane Review of calcium antagonists in SAH included 12 trials, totalling 2844 patients with SAH (1396 in the treatment group and 1448 in the control group) [65]. The drugs analysed were: nimodipine (eight trials, 1574 patients), nicardipine (two trials, 954 patients), AT877 (one trial, 276 patients) and magnesium (one trial, 40 patients). Overall, calcium antagonists reduced the risk of poor outcome: RR 0.82 (95% CI 0.72–0.93); the absolute risk reduction was 5.1%, the corresponding number of patients needed to treat

Table 14.2 Treatment for preventing ischaemia.

Type of study (reference)	Intervention	Outcome (follow-up time)	Number of patients (number of trials)	Control group risk (range)	Relative risk (95% CI)	Absolute risk reduction (95% CI)	Comment
SR [65]	Calcium antagonists versus control	Death or dependency (3/6 months)	2507 (8)	30% (13–69)	0.82 (0.72–0.93)	5% (2–9)	Calcium antagonists better Mainly nimodipine 60 mg orally every 4 h Heterogeneity
		Secondary ischaemia	2187 (11)	40% (17–65)	0.67 (0.60–0.76)	13% (9–17)	Calcium antagonists better
RCT [73]	Magnesium versus placebo	Death or dependency (3 months)	283 (1)	35%	0.77 (0.54–1.09)	8% (ns)	Magnesium better
SR [89]	Volume expansion versus control	Death or severe disability	114 (2)	17% (11–19)	1.00 (0.45–2.22)	0% (ns)	
		Secondary ischaemia	114 (2)	21% (19–22)	1.08 (0.54–2.16)	+2% (ns)	Volume expansion worse
SR [95]	Intracisternal fibrinolysis versus control	Death or disability	652 (9)	24%		9.5% (4.2–14.8)	Only one RCT
		Secondary ischaemia	652 (9)	30%		14.4% (6.5–22.5)	

SR: systematic review; RCT: randomized controlled trial; CI: confidence intervals; ns: not statistically significant.

to prevent a single poor outcome event was [20]. For oral nimodipine alone the RR was 0.70 (0.58–0.84). The RR of death on treatment with calcium antagonists was 0.90 (95% CI 0.76–1.07), that of clinical signs of secondary ischaemia 0.67 (95% CI 0.60–0.76), and that of CT or MR confirmed infarction 0.80 (95% CI 0.71–0.89).

In brief, the risk reduction for 'poor outcome' is statistically robust, but depends mainly on trials with oral nimodipine, and especially on a single large trial, in which patients received 60 mg orally every 4 h, for 3 weeks [66]. The intermediate factors through which nimodipine exerts its beneficial effect after aneurysmal SAH remain uncertain. Interestingly, several studies with nimodipine found there was no difference between treated patients and controls with regard to the frequency of arterial narrowing on a repeat angiogram [66–68].

If the patient is unable to swallow, the tablets should be crushed and washed down a nasogastric tube with normal saline. Intravenous administration is advocated by the producer but there is no evidence from trials that intravenous administration of nimodipine is beneficial [65]. Moreover, intravenous administration of nicardipine does not improve outcome [65]. The lack of effectiveness of intravenous nicardipine is probably explained by the increased risk of hypotension, which also occurs after intravenous administration of nimodipine [69]. Hypotension may even be a problem even if nimodipine is given orally. If no blood loss has occurred or any other cause for hypotension is found, the dose of nimodipine can be at first halved (to 60 mg tds) and subsequently discontinued if the blood pressure does not come back to initial levels.

Magnesium sulphate

Hypomagnesaemia occurs in more than 50% of patients with SAH and is associated with the occurrence of delayed cerebral ischaemia and poor outcome [70]. Its administration reduced infarct volume after experimental SAH in rats [71]. Its putative modes of action consist in inhibition of the release of excitatory amino acids and blockade of the N-methyl-D-aspartate-glutamate receptor. Magnesium is also a non-competitive antagonist of voltage-dependent calcium channels and it has a dilatatory effect on cerebral arteries.

Two controlled trials have studied the efficacy of magnesium sulphate in preventing delayed cerebral ischaemia and poor outcome. The smallest one, including 40 patients and necessarily inconclusive [72], was provisionally included in the most recent Cochrane Review of calcium antagonists. A larger trial included 283 patients but was still intended as a preliminary ('phase II') study, with delayed cerebral ischaemia and not overall outcome as primary measure of efficacy [73]. Magnesium treatment consisting of a continuous intravenous dose of 64 mmol/L per day reduced the risk of delayed cerebral ischaemia (defined as the occurrence of a new hypodense lesion on CT, compatible with clinical features of delayed cerebral ischaemia, analysed according to the 'on-treatment principle') by 34% (hazard ratio 0.66, 95%

CI 0.38–1.14). After 3 months, the risk reduction for poor outcome (analysed according to the 'intention-to-treat' principle) was 23% (risk ratio 0.77, 95% CI 0.54–1.09). At that time, 18 patients in the treatment group and 6 in the placebo group had an excellent outcome (risk ratio 3.4, 95% CI 1.3–8.9). A phase III trial is now ongoing.

Aspirin and other antithrombotic agents

Several studies have found that blood platelets are activated from day three after SAH. This was mostly inferred from increased levels of thromboxane B2, the stable metabolite of thromboxane A2, which promotes platelet aggregation and vasoconstriction [74,75].

Two small trials with aspirin have been performed in patients with SAH, and three with antiplatelet agents other than aspirin. In a systematic overview of these five trials, the rate of delayed cerebral ischaemia (reported in only three of the five studies) was decreased (RR 0.65, 95% CI 0.47–0.89), but poor outcome was not significantly different between patients treated with antiplatelet agents and controls [76]. A still unpublished trial aiming to include 200 patients did not confirm a beneficial effect of aspirin (van den Bergh, for the MASH study group). The trial was prematurely stopped after the second interim analysis, because by then the chances of a positive effect were negligible. Aspirin did indeed not reduce the risk of delayed cerebral ischaemia (HR 1.83, 95% CI 0.85–3.9). The RR reduction for poor outcome was 21% (RR 0.79, 95% CI 0.38–1.6). It is unknown whether other platelet aggregation inhibitors are more beneficial.

A low-molecular-weight heparinoid, enoxaparin (40 mg subcutaneously once a day after aneurysm occlusion), was tested in a trial of 170 patients [37]; the treatment did not improve outcome and was associated with haemorrhages in 4 of 85 patients in the experimental group.

Statins

HMG-CoA reductase inhibitors or statins are primarily used because these drugs lower LDL-cholesterol levels, but they also have anti-inflammatory, immunomodulatory, antithrombotic and vascular effects. It has often been claimed that these 'pleiotropic effects' contribute to cardiovascular risk reduction beyond that expected from LDL-cholesterol reduction alone, but this is not confirmed by a meta-regression analysis of clinical trials [77].

In patients with SAH, two controlled trials have been performed so far. One included only 39 patients and found that 80 mg simvastatin given within 48 h after the ictus reduced 'vasospasm' (undefined) [78], the other enrolled 80 patients and found that 40 mg pravastatin given within 72 h reduced angiographic vasospasm and impairment of autoregulatory responses as well as vasospasm-related ischaemic complications [79]. On the other hand, an observational study found that previous use of statins increased the risk of angiographic vasospasm though not that of associated ischaemic complications [80]. In conclusion, the evidence for a beneficial effect of statins after SAH is still rather meagre.

Free radical scavengers

Tirilazad mesylate, a 21-aminosteroid free radical scavenger, has so far failed to show consistent improvement of outcome in four randomized controlled trials, with a total of more than 3500 patients [81–84]. The only beneficial effect on overall outcome was seen in a single subgroup of a single trial, that is, those treated with 6 mg/kg/day (two other groups received 0.2 mg/kg/day or 2 mg/kg/day) [81]. Delayed cerebral ischaemia was reduced in only one of the four trials, although there was no effect on overall outcome [83]. A formal overview of the complete clinical evidence is not yet available, but the case for the drug seems weak, for any dose and either sex.

A single trial with another hydroxyl radical scavenger, N'-propylenedinicotinamide (nicaraven) in 162 patients, showed a decreased rate of delayed cerebral ischaemia but not of poor outcome at 3 months after SAH [85]. Curiously enough, the reverse was found a trial of 286 patients with ebselen, a seleno-organic compound with antioxidant activity through a glutathione peroxidase-like action: improved outcome at 3 months after SAH, but without any reduction in the frequency of delayed ischaemia [86].

Other drugs

Nizofenone, an anionic channel blocker believed to inhibit glutamate release, was studied in a randomized trial of 100 patients, of whom only 90 were included in the analysis [87]; the occurrence of angiographic vasospasm was not influenced by the drug, poor outcome only in a complicated subgroup analysis.

The endothelin A/B receptor antagonist TAK-044 was tested in a multicentre phase II trial (influence on the occurrence of delayed ischaemic deficits) in 420 patients; there was a non-significant risk reduction of 0.8 (95% CI 0.61–1.06) [88].

Increasing plasma volume

The usefulness of circulatory volume expansion to prevent delayed ischaemia after SAH was assessed in a recent Cochrane Review [89]. Three trials were identified. One truly randomized trial and one quasi-randomized trial with comparable baseline characteristics for both groups were included in the analyses. Preventive volume expansion therapy did not improve outcome (RR 1.0, 95% CI 0.5–2.2), nor the occurrence of secondary ischaemia (RR 1.1, 95% CI 0.5–2.2), but tended to increase the rate of complications (RR 1.8, 95% CI 0.9–3.7). In another quasi-randomized trial, outcome assessment was done only at the day of operation (7–10 days after SAH). In the period before operation, treatment resulted in a reduction of secondary ischaemia (RR 0.33, 95% CI

0.11–0.99) and case fatality (RR 0.20, 95% CI 0.07–1.2). In conclusion, the effects of preventive volume expansion therapy have been studied properly in only two trials of patients with aneurysmal SAH, with very small numbers, and there is no sound evidence for the use of volume expansion therapy in patients with aneurysmal SAH.

Because of its mineralocorticoid activity (reabsorption of sodium in the distal tubules of the kidney) fludrocortisone might, in theory, prevent a negative sodium balance, hypovolaemia and ischaemic complications [90]. A randomized study in which 91 patients with SAH were entered soon after admission showed that fludrocortisone acetate indeed significantly reduced natriuresis in the first 6 days after the haemorrhage. Reductions in the occurrence of plasma volume depletion and of ischaemic complications were not statistically significant [91]. These results were confirmed by a smaller trial in 30 patients [92]. Finally, also hydrocortisone was shown in a small trial (28 patients) with an explanatory design to prevent hyponatraemia and a drop in central venous pressure [93]. The evidence from these studies is insufficiently conclusive to warrant routine administration of fludrocortisone to all patients with SAH.

Cisternal drainage and intracisternal fibrinolysis

On the assumption that vasospasm increases the risk of delayed cerebral ischaemia and that extravasated blood induces vasospasm, removal of the subarachnoid blood by drainage or fibrinolysis has been studied in several trials. In a comparison of two cohorts the patients treated with lumbar drainage of CSF had less often cerebral infarction and more often returned home than patients with no lumbar drainage [94]. A more aggressive method in removing subarachnoid blood is intracisternal fibrinolysis. A meta-analysis on this treatment strategy included 9 trials of which only one was randomized [95]. Pooled results demonstrated beneficial effects of treatment, with absolute risk reductions of 14.4% (95% CI 6.5–22.5%, $P < 0.001$) for delayed cerebral ischaemia, and 9.5% (95% CI 4.2–14.8%, $P < 0.01$) for poor clinical outcome. There was no difference between the type of thrombolytic agent used (tissue plasminogen activator versus urokinase) or the method of administration (intraoperative versus postoperative). However, the results of the analysis are limited by the predominance of non-randomized studies. A open, randomized, controlled trial not yet included in the meta-analysis studied the effect of fibrinolysis in 110 patients treated with endovascular coiling [96]. Urokinase was administered into the cisterna magna through a microcatheter inserted via a lumbar puncture. The primary outcome measure was clinical vasospasm, defined as clinical deterioration combined with evidence of vasospasm on angiography. Treatment resulted in a statistical significant reduction of this primary outcome measurement. Case fatality was not reduced, but patients in the treated group had more often a good clinical outcome. Larger studies with overall outcome as primary measurement of outcome are needed before this treatment can be implemented in clinical practice.

5. Management of rebleeding
How to manage rebleeding.

The following sections will briefly describe the procedures required.

To resuscitate or not?
The question whether patients with rebleeding should be resuscitated and artificially ventilated if respiratory arrest occurs is not academic: in a series of 39 patients with a CT-confirmed rebleeding, 14 had initial respiratory abnormalities that called for assisted ventilation. Spontaneous respiration returned within 1 h in eight of these 14 patients, and in three more between 1 and 24 h [97]. Many patients with initial apnoea who were successfully resuscitated later died from subsequent complications, but the crucial point is that survival without brain damage is possible even after respiratory arrest. After resuscitation, it will usually become clear within a matter of hours whether the patient will indeed survive the episode or whether dysfunction of the brain stem will persist. There are no grounds to fear that the intervention will only result in prolongation of a vegetative state. In patients who progress to a state of brain death, the resuscitation procedure at least allows organ donation to be considered, with some benefits to others.

Emergency occlusion of the aneurysm
A large haematoma that causes brain shift without gross intraventricular haemorrhage is an infrequent finding after rebleeding, occurring in around 10% [98]. In these rare cases, emergency evacuation of the haematoma after occlusion of the aneurysm can be indicated, depending on the patient's clinical condition, as in patients who are admitted in a poor condition caused by an intracerebral haematoma associating with the aneurysma rupture (see above). A more common reason for urgent intervention after rebleeding is the concern that amongst the survivors, 50–75% suffer a further rebleed [97,99]. This implies that emergency clipping or coiling of the aneurysm should be seriously considered in patients who regain consciousness after rebleeding. Of course, the risk of the operation is increased after rebleeding but the risks of a wait-and-see policy at that stage seem even more intimidating.

6. Management of cerebral ischaemia
How to manage patients with cerebral ischaemia.

The following sections provide a guideline for the management of patients with cerebral ischaemia.

Induced hypertension and volume expansion
Since the 1960s, induced hypertension has been used to combat ischaemic deficits in patients with SAH. Induced hypertension has often been combined with volume expansion, but only in uncontrolled case series, of which only one had an acceptable definition of outcome events [100]. Another case series argued that hypertensive and hypervolaemic therapy was unlikely to be successful in patients with a Glasgow Coma Score of 11 or less as well as with hydrocephalus [101]. Controlled trials are sadly missing. If raising the blood pressure and increasing plasma volume can indeed reverse ischaemic deficits – which remains to be proven beyond doubt – the most plausible explanation for these phenomena is a defect of cerebral autoregulation that makes the perfusion of the brain passively dependent on the systemic blood pressure. The benefit of adding haemodilution to hypertensive and hypervolaemic treatment (the so-called 'triple-H' regimen) is not only uncertain but also frankly controversial [102].

The risks of deliberately increasing the arterial pressure and plasma volume include rebleeding of an untreated aneurysm, increased cerebral oedema, or haemorrhagic transformation in areas of infarction [103], myocardial infarction and congestive heart failure. At any rate, the circulatory system should be closely monitored, though arterial lines and pulmonary artery catheters carry their own risks: infection, pneumothorax, haemothorax, ventricular arrhythmia and pulmonary infarction [104–106].

Transluminal angioplasty
Only a few centres have reported on the endovascular approach in the treatment of 'symptomatic vasospasm' after SAH. These reports document sustained improvement in more than half the cases, but the series were uncontrolled and evidently there must be publication bias [107]. Some of these studies reported results only for arteries, and not for patients. Vessel rupture is precipitated by this procedure in about 1%, even after the aneurysm has been occluded, and other complications such as hyperperfusion injury in 4% [107]. In an uncontrolled series not included in the review cited above, of patients treated with transluminal angioplasty, papaverine injection or both, overall clinical outcome was poor despite successful arterial dilatation. Half the patients died or remained disabled, and half of the survivors had permanent deficits from cerebral infarction [108]. In view of the risks, the high costs and the lack of controlled trials, transluminal angioplasty should still be regarded as a strictly experimental procedure [109].

The same caution applies to uncontrolled reports of improvement of ischaemic deficits after intra-arterial infusion of drugs through super-selective catheterisation. Papaverine has gained undeserved popularity [110], the more so because not all impressions are positive [111,112]; intra-arterial milrinone, verapamil or nicardipine dilate vessels but whether these agents improve outcome is equally uncertain [113–115].

Pharmacological intervention

Calcitonin gene-related peptide (CGRP) is a potent vasodilator in the carotid vascular bed, but a randomized, multicentre, single-blind clinical trial in 62 patients with ischaemic complications after SAH failed to bear out any benefit in terms of overall outcome: the RR of a poor outcome in CGRP-treated patients was 0.88 (95% CI 0.60–1.28) [116].

7. Management of acute hydrocephalus

How to manage acute hydrocephalus.

A policy of *wait-and-see for 24 h* is eminently justified in patients with dilated ventricles who are alert, because only about one-third of them will become symptomatic in the next few days [117]. Postponing interventions for 1 day can also be rewarding if the level of consciousness is decreased. The reason is that spontaneous improvement within this period has been documented in half the patients (7 of 13) with acute hydrocephalus who were only drowsy, and also in almost half the patients (19 of 43) who had a Glasgow Coma Score of 12/14 or worse but no massive intraventricular haemorrhage [117]. On the other hand, it is not always easy to make a definitive decision on the need for surgical measures even after 1 day has elapsed, because patients may temporarily improve to some extent but then reach a plateau phase or again deteriorate; such fluctuations are encountered in about one-third of patients with symptomatic hydrocephalus [117]. Any further deterioration in the level of consciousness warrants active intervention.

Lumbar puncture was suggested as a therapeutic measure a long-time ago [118], but formal studies are scarce. In a prospective but uncontrolled study, 17 patients were treated in this way because they had acute hydrocephalus with neither a haematoma nor gross intraventricular haemorrhage [21]. Between 1 and 7 spinal taps per patient were performed in the first 10 days, the number depending on the rate of improvement; each time a maximum of 20 mL of CSF was removed, the aim being a closing pressure of 15 cmH$_2$O. Of the 17 patients, 12 showed initial improvement: six fully recovered, two showed incomplete improvement but fully recovered after insertion of an internal shunt and four patients died of other complications several days after the lumbar punctures had been started. Of the five remaining patients in whom lumbar puncture had no effect, two recovered after an internal shunt and three died of other complications.

Whether the risk of rebleeding is increased by lumbar punctures or drainage is uncertain [119]. Until controlled trials are available, and we think these are still needed and ethically justifiable, the tentative conclusion is that lumbar puncture seems a safe and reasonably effective way of treating those forms of acute hydrocephalus that are not obviously caused by intraventricular obstruction.

External drainage of the cerebral ventricles by a catheter inserted through a burr hole is, in many centres, the most common method of treating acute hydrocephalus. Internal drainage, to the right atrium or the peritoneal cavity, is rarely considered in the first few days because the blood in the CSF will almost inevitably block the shunt system. After insertion of an external catheter, the improvement is usually rapid and sometimes dramatic [19,117]. Unfortunately other problems tend to intervene soon, particularly rebleeding and ventriculitis.

Rebleeding after insertion of an external drain occurs significantly more often than in patients with acute hydrocephalus who are not shunted or in patients without hydrocephalus, according to most but not all prospective studies [120]. None of these studies had a randomized design for assessing the effect of shunt insertion, and it is possible that the development of acute hydrocephalus is associated with a more severely disrupted aneurysm which is more prone to rebleeding as part of its natural history.

Ventriculitis is a frequent complication after external drainage, especially if drainage is continued for more than 3 days [117]. Regular exchange of the intraventricular catheter, in a controlled study, did not decrease the rate of infection [121]. Some advocate extra rigid antiseptic techniques [122], prophylactic antibiotics or a long subcutaneous tunnel [123], but these measures have not been subjected to a controlled study. External lumbar drainage probably carries a lower risk of infection than ventricular drainage [124], but obviously cannot be used in patients with large intracerebral haematomas of extensive intraventricular haemorrhage.

To shorten the period in which ventricular catheterisation is necessary, test occlusion is often applied. Gradual weaning by sequential height elevations of the external ventricular drainage (EVD) system over 4 days preceding drain closure conferred no advantage, according to a randomized study of 81 patients [125].

8. Management of complications

How to manage systemic complications.

Neurologists and neurosurgeons are regularly confronted by non-neurological complications in patients with aneurysmal SAH. Life-threatening complications occurred in 40% of 451 consecutive patients enrolled in a drug trial [126], and in another study a similar proportion of medical complications contributed to fatal outcomes [127]. Hyponatraemia is the most common of these but several other systemic disorders may cause secondary deterioration. Clinical detection of these metabolic derangements requires a high index of suspicion.

Hyponatraemia

Hyponatraemia, with or without intravascular volume change, is the most common electrolyte disturbance following aneurysmal rupture. The frequency depends on the cut off point that is chosen; if defined as a sodium level of 134 mmol or less on at least two consecutive days, it occurs in about one-third of patients [91]. It develops most commonly between the 2nd and 10th day [128].

Clinical manifestations of hyponatraemia usually do not occur until the plasma sodium is less than 125 mmol/L, but irritability, restlessness and confusion can result from a rapid decline of sodium, particularly if the downward trend continues over a few days. Sodium levels below 100 mmol/L almost always give rise to seizures and, rarely, ventricular tachycardia or fibrillation [129]. But in patients with SAH the most dreaded complication of hyponatraemia is the precipitation of delayed ischaemia, through associated hypovolaemia and poor outcome in general [130].

In general, the causes of hyponatraemia vary according to the patient's volume status. In most, but not all cases, the total body sodium has remained constant but the water content of the extracellular volume is at fault; therefore hyponatraemia can be best classified according to the extracellular volume status. After the syndrome of inappropriate secretion of antidiuretic hormone (SIADH) had been initially described in the 1950s [131], hyponatraemia in SAH has often been incorrectly attributed to this condition, in which dilutional hyponatraemia ensues. In contrast, hyponatraemia after SAH results from excessive natriuresis, or cerebral salt wasting [128,132]. Predisposing factors for the development of hyponatraemia are hydrocephalus, particularly enlargement of the third ventricle [133], and ruptured aneurysms of the anterior communicating artery [134]. Mechanical pressure on the hypothalamus can perhaps disturb sodium and water homeostasis.

Correction of hyponatraemia in SAH is actually a problem of correcting volume depletion. Acute symptomatic hyponatraemia is rare and requires urgent treatment with hypertonic saline (1.8% or even 3%). On the other hand, over-rapid infusion of sodium may precipitate myelinolysis in the pons and in the white matter of the hemispheres [135]. If possible, correction should not be faster than 8 mmol/L/day [136,137]. A mild degree of hyponatraemia (125–134 mmol/L) is usually well tolerated, self-limiting and need not be treated in itself. Hyponatraemia in patients with evidence of a negative fluid balance or excessive natriuresis is corrected with saline (0.9%; sodium concentration 150 mmol/L).

Disorders of heart rhythm

Aneurysmal rupture is commonly associated with cardiac arrhythmias and electrocardiographic (ECG) abnormalities. This is one of the reasons why patients with SAH are sometimes initially misdiagnosed as acute myocardial infarction and admitted to coronary care units. Left ventricular dysfunction may occur [138], even cardiogenic shock, usually in combination with pulmonary oedema.

Generally, severe ventricular arrhythmias are of short duration. Beta-blockade has been proposed as preventive treatment aimed at lowering the sympathetic tone. In patients with SAH, routine administration of beta-blockers is not warranted until there is evidence of improved overall outcome; the net benefits may be disappointing because beta-blockers also lower blood pressure.

Neurogenic pulmonary oedema

Pulmonary oedema occurs to some degree in approximately one-third of patients with SAH [139,140], but the fulminant variety is much more rare (2% in the largest series to date) [141]. The onset is usually rapid, within hours. What triggers pulmonary oedema is unclear.

The typical clinical picture consists of unexpected dyspnoea, cyanosis and production of pink and frothy sputum. Many patients are pale, sweat excessively and are hypertensive. A chest X-ray usually demonstrates impressive pulmonary oedema which may disappear in a matter of hours following positive end-expiratory pressure ventilation. A problem is that liberal administration of fluids is beneficial for brain perfusion but may delay recovery of pulmonary oedema and hence impair brain oxygenation, and that positive end-expiratory pressure ventilation increases intracranial pressure.

In case of associated left ventricular failure, clinically manifested by sudden hypotension following initially elevated blood pressures, transient lactic acidosis and mild elevation of the creatine kinase MB fraction [142,143], inotropic agents are indicated (dobutamine, 5–15 μg/kg/min) [144].

Conclusion

We think we have distinguished in this chapter, explicitly or at least implicitly, between (a) solid evidence, from several well-performed clinical trials; (b) less reliable evidence, from single trials, case series or observational studies; and (c) pathophysiological reasoning, with all its fallacies. In everyday practice a multitude of management decisions must still be taken without good evidence. There are several reasons for this: there is no trial at all; trial results may be equivocal; patients may be different from those enrolled in trials; new procedures require practice, or a trial may not be feasible. 'Logical reasoning' may be maligned and reviled in the present era but paradoxically it is still indispensable – not only to fill the gaps in empirical knowledge but also to interpret existing evidence and to plan new trials. In fact, the generation of new knowledge is a continuous, cyclical process in which newly gained insights in pathophysiology give rise to new therapeutic experiments, the results of which generate fresh hypotheses, and so on. Compassion, curiosity and doubt are the essential forces that keep the cycle moving [145].

References

1 Rinkel GJE, Djibuti M, Algra A, van Gijn J. Prevalence and risk of rupture of intracranial aneurysms – a systematic review. *Stroke* 1998; **29**: 251–6.

2 Linn FHH, Rinkel GJE, Algra A, van Gijn J. Incidence of sub-arachnoid hemorrhage – role of region, year, and rate of computed tomography: a meta-analysis. *Stroke* 1996; **27**: 625–9.

3 Ruigrok YM, Buskens E, Rinkel GJE. Attributable risk of common and rare determinants of subarachnoid hemorrhage. *Stroke* 2001; **32**: 1173–5.

4 Pleizier CM, Ruigrok YM, Rinkel GJE. Relation between age and number of aneurysms in patients with subarachnoid haemorrhage. *Cerebrovasc. Dis.* 2002; **14**: 51–3.

5 Hop JW, Rinkel GJE, Algra A, van Gijn J. Case-fatality rates and functional outcome after subarachnoid hemorrhage – a systematic review. *Stroke* 1997; **28**: 660–4.

6 Huang J, Van Gelder JM. The probability of sudden death from rupture of intracranial aneurysms: a meta-analysis. *Neurosurgery* 2002; **51**: 1101–5.

7. Hackett ML, Anderson CS, for the ACROSS Group. Health outcomes 1 year after subarachnoid hemorrhage – an international population-based study. *Neurology* 2000; **55**: 658–62.

8 Roos YBWEM, de Haan RJ, Beenen LFM, Groen RJM, Albrecht KW, Vermeulen M. Complications and outcome in patients with aneurysmal subarachnoid haemorrhage: a prospective hospital based cohort study in the Netherlands. *J. Neurol. Neurosurg. Psychiatr.* 2000; **68**: 337–41.

9 Bardach NS, Zhao SJ, Gress DR, Lawton MT, Johnston SC. Association between subarachnoid hemorrhage outcomes and number of cases treated at California hospitals. *Stroke* 2002; **33**: 1851–6.

10 van Gijn J, van Dongen KJ. The time course of aneurysmal haemorrhage on computed tomograms. *Neuroradiology* 1982; **23**: 153–6.

11 Hauerberg J, Eskesen V, Rosenorn J. The prognostic significance of intracerebral haematoma as shown on CT scanning after aneurysmal subarachnoid haemorrhage. *Br. J. Neurosurg.* 1994; **8**: 333–9.

12 Heiskanen O, Poranen A, Kuurne T, Valtonen S, Kaste M. Acute surgery for intracerebral haematomas caused by rupture of an intracranial arterial aneurysm. A prospective randomized study. *Acta Neurochir. (Wien)* 1988; **90**: 81–3.

13 Niemann DB, Wills AD, Maartens NF, Kerr RS, Byrne JV, Molyneux AJ. Treatment of intracerebral hematomas caused by aneurysm rupture: coil placement followed by clot evacuation. *J. Neurosurg.* 2003; **99**: 843–7.

14 Smith ER, Carter BS, Ogilvy CS. Proposed use of prophylactic decompressive craniectomy in poor-grade aneurysmal subarachnoid hemorrhage patients presenting with associated large sylvian hematomas. *Neurosurgery* 2002; **51**: 117–24.

15 Gelabert-Gonzalez M, Iglesias-Pais M, Fernandez-Villa J. Acute subdural haematoma due to ruptured intracranial aneurysms. *Neurosurg. Rev.* 2004; **27**: 259–62.

16 Inamasu J, Saito R, Nakamura Y, et al. Acute subdural hematoma caused by ruptured cerebral aneurysms: diagnostic and therapeutic pitfalls. *Resuscitation* 2002; **52**: 71–6.

17 O'Sullivan MG, Whyman M, Steers JW, Whittle IR, Miller JD. Acute subdural haematoma secondary to ruptured intracranial aneurysm: diagnosis and management. *Br. J. Neurosurg.* 1994; **8**: 439–45.

18 Sasaki T, Sato M, Oinuma M, et al. Management of poor-grade patients with aneurysmal subarachnoid hemorrhage in the acute stage: importance of close monitoring for neurological grade changes. *Surg. Neurol.* 2004; **62**: 531–5.

19 van Gijn J, Hijdra A, Wijdicks EFM, Vermeulen M, van Crevel H. Acute hydrocephalus after aneurysmal subarachnoid hemorrhage. *J. Neurosurg.* 1985; **63**: 355–62.

20 Rinkel GJE, Wijdicks EFM, Ramos LMP, van Gijn J. Progression of acute hydrocephalus in subarachnoid haemorrhage: a case report documented by serial CT scanning. *J. Neurol. Neurosurg. Psychiatr.* 1990; **53**: 354–5.

21 Hasan D, Lindsay KW, Vermeulen M. Treatment of acute hydrocephalus after subarachnoid hemorrhage with serial lumbar puncture. *Stroke* 1991; **22**: 190–4.

22 Suzuki M, Otawara Y, Doi M, Ogasawara K, Ogawa A. Neurological grades of patients with poor-grade subarachnoid hemorrhage improve after short-term pretreatment. *Neurosurgery* 2000; **47**: 1098–104.

23 Roos YBWEM, Hasan D, Vermeulen M. Outcome in patients with large intraventricular haemorrhages: a volumetric study. *J. Neurol. Neurosurg. Psychiatr.* 1995; **58**: 622–4.

24 Nieuwkamp DJ, de Gans K, Rinkel GJE, Algra A. Treatment and outcome of severe intraventricular extension in patients with subarachnoid or intracerebral hemorrhage: a systematic review of the literature. *J. Neurol.* 2000; **247**: 117–21.

25 Naff NJ, Carhuapoma JR, Williams MA, et al. Treatment of intraventricular hemorrhage with urokinase – effects on 30-day survival. *Stroke* 2000; **31**: 841–7.

26 Shimoda M, Oda S, Shibata M, Tominaga J, Kittaka M, Tsugane R. Results of early surgical evacuation of packed intraventricular hemorrhage from aneurysm rupture in patients with poor-grade subarachnoid hemorrhage. *J. Neurosurg.* 1999; **91**: 408–14.

27 Lagares A, Putman CM, Ogilvy CS. Posterior fossa decompression and clot evacuation for fourth ventricle hemorrhage after aneurysmal rupture: case report. *Neurosurgery* 2001; **49**: 208–11.

28 Wijdicks EFM, Vermeulen M, Murray GD, Hijdra A, van Gijn J. The effects of treating hypertension following aneurysmal subarachnoid hemorrhage. *Clin. Neurol. Neurosurg.* 1990; **92**: 111–17.

29 Hasan D, Vermeulen M, Wijdicks EFM, Hijdra A, van Gijn J. Effect of fluid intake and antihypertensive treatment on cerebral ischemia after subarachnoid hemorrhage. *Stroke* 1989; **20**: 1511–15.

30 Wijdicks EFM, Vermeulen M, Hijdra A, van Gijn J. Hyponatremia and cerebral infarction in patients with ruptured intracranial aneurysms: is fluid restriction harmful? *Ann. Neurol.* 1985; **17**: 137–40.

31 Rosenwasser RH, Delgado TE, Buchheit WA, Freed MH. Control of hypertension and prophylaxis against vasospasm in cases of subarachnoid hemorrhage: a preliminary report. *Neurosurgery* 1983; **12**: 658–61.

32 Egge A, Waterloo K, Sjoholm H, Solberg T, Ingebrigtsen T, Romner B. Prophylactic hyperdynamic postoperative fluid therapy after aneurysmal subarachnoid hemorrhage: a clinical,

prospective, randomized, controlled study. *Neurosurgery* 2001; **49**: 593–605.

33 Takagi K, Tsuchiya Y, Okinaga K, Hirata M, Nakagomi T, Tamura A. Natural hypothermia immediately after transient global cerebral ischemia induced by spontaneous subarachnoid hemorrhage. *J. Neurosurg.* 2003; **98**: 50–6.

34 Rousseaux P, Scherpereel R, Bernard MH, Graftieaux JP, Guyot JF. Fever and cerebral vasospasm in intracranial aneurysms. *Surg. Neurol.* 1980; **14**: 459–65.

35 Oliveira-Filho J, Ezzeddine MA, Segal AZ, et al. Fever in subarachnoid hemorrhage: relationship to vasospasm and outcome. *Neurology* 2001; **56**: 1299–304.

36 Vermeulen M, Lindsay KW, Murray GD, et al. Antifibrinolytic treatment in subarachnoid hemorrhage. *N. Engl. J. Med.* 1984; **311**: 432–7.

37 Siironen J, Juvela S, Varis J, et al. No effect of enoxaparin on outcome of aneurysmal subarachnoid hemorrhage: a randomized, double-blind, placebo-controlled clinical trial. *J. Neurosurg.* 2003; **99**: 953–9.

38 Amaragiri SV, Lees TA. Elastic compression stockings for prevention of deep vein thrombosis. *Cochrane Database Sys. Rev.* 2000: CD001484.

39 Guglielmi G, Vinuela F, Duckwiler G, et al. Endovascular treatment of posterior circulation aneurysms by electrothrombosis using electrically detachable coils. *J. Neurosurg.* 1992; **77**: 515–24.

40 Brilstra EH, Rinkel GJE, van der Graaf Y, van Rooij WJJ, Algra A. Treatment of intracranial aneurysms by embolization with coils – a systematic review. *Stroke* 1999; **30**: 470–6.

41 van der Schaaf I, Algra A, Wermer M, et al. Endovascular coiling versus neurosurgical clipping for patients with aneurysmal subarachnoid haemorrhage. *Cochrane Database Sys. Rev.* 2005; **4**: CD003085.

42 Lozier AP, Connolly Jr ES, Lavine SD, Solomon RA. Guglielmi detachable coil embolization of posterior circulation aneurysms – a systematic review of the literature. *Stroke* 2002; **33**: 2509–18.

43 Molyneux A, Kerr R, Stratton I, et al. International Subarachnoid Aneurysm Trial (ISAT) of neurosurgical clipping versus endovascular coiling in 2143 patients with ruptured intracranial aneurysms: a randomised trial. *Lancet* 2002; **360**: 1267–74.

44 Wiebers DO, Whisnant JP, Huston III J, et al. Unruptured intracranial aneurysms: natural history, clinical outcome, and risks of surgical and endovascular treatment. *Lancet* 2003; **362**: 103–10.

45 Molyneux AJ, Kerr RS, Yu LM, et al. International subarachnoid aneurysm trial (ISAT) of neurosurgical clipping versus endovascular coiling in 2143 patients with ruptured intracranial aneurysms: a randomised comparison of effects on survival, dependency, seizures, rebleeding, subgroups, and aneurysm occlusion. *Lancet* 2005; **366**: 809–17.

46 Tsutsumi K, Ueki K, Usui M, Kwak S, Kirino T. Risk of recurrent subarachnoid hemorrhage after complete obliteration of cerebral aneurysms. *Stroke* 1998; **29**: 2511–13.

47 Wermer MJ, Greebe P, Algra A, Rinkel GJ. Incidence of recurrent subarachnoid hemorrhage after clipping for ruptured intracranial aneurysms. *Stroke* 2005; **36**: 2394–9.

48 Majoie CB, Sprengers ME, Van Rooij WJ, et al. MR angiography at 3T versus digital subtraction angiography in the follow-up of intracranial aneurysms treated with detachable coils. *AJNR Am. J. Neuroradiol.* 2005; **26**: 1349–56.

49 Slob MJ, Sluzewski M, Van Rooij WJ, Roks G, Rinkel GJE. Additional coiling of previously coiled cerebral aneurysms: clinical and angiographic results. *AJNR Am. J. Neuroradiol.* 2004; **25**: 1373–6.

50 Zhang YJ, Barrow DL, Cawley CM, Dion JE. Neurosurgical management of intracranial aneurysms previously treated with endovascular therapy. *Neurosurgery* 2003; **52**: 283–93.

51 McKissock W, Richardson A, Walsh L. 'Posterior-communicating aneurysms'. A controlled trial of conservative and surgical treatment of ruptured aneurysms of the internal carotid artery at or near the point of origin of the posterior communicating artery. *Lancet* 1960; **i**: 1203–6.

52 McKissock W, Richardson A, Walsh L. Anterior communicating aneurysms. A trial of conservative and surgical treatment. *Lancet* 1965; **i**: 873–6.

53 Brilstra EH, Algra A, Rinkel GJE, Tulleken CAF, van Gijn J. Effectiveness of neurosurgical clip application in patients with aneurysmal subarachnoid hemorrhage. *J. Neurosurg.* 2002; **97**: 1036–41.

54 Laidlaw JD, Siu KH. Ultra-early surgery for aneurysmal subarachnoid hemorrhage: outcomes for a consecutive series of 391 patients not selected by grade or age. *J. Neurosurg.* 2002; **97**: 250–8.

55 Öhman J, Heiskanen O. Timing of operation for ruptured supratentorial aneurysms: a prospective randomized study. *J. Neurosurg.* 1989; **70**: 55–60.

56 Whitfield PC, Kirkpatrick PJ. Timing of surgery for aneurysmal subarachnoid haemorrhage. *Cochrane Database Syst. Rev.* 2001; CD001697.

57 de Gans K, Nieuwkamp DJ, Rinkel GJE, Algra A. Timing of aneurysm surgery in subarachnoid hemorrhage: a systematic review of the literature. *Neurosurgery* 2002; **50**: 336–40.

58 Ross N, Hutchinson PJ, Seeley H, Kirkpatrick PJ. Timing of surgery for supratentorial aneurysmal subarachnoid haemorrhage: report of a prospective study. *J. Neurol. Neurosurg. Psychiatr.* 2002; **72**: 480–4.

59 Nieuwkamp DJ, de GK, Algra A, et al. Timing of aneurysm surgery in subarachnoid haemorrhage – an observational study in The Netherlands. *Acta Neurochir. (Wien)* 2005; **147**: 815–21.

60 Wermer MJ, Buskens E, van der Schaaf I, Bossuyt PM, Rinkel GJE. Yield of screening for new aneurysms after treatment for subarachnoid hemorrhage. *Neurology* 2004; **62**: 369–75.

61 Fodstad H, Pilbrant A, Schannong M, Stromberg S. Determination of tranexamic acid (AMCA) and fibrin/fibrinogen degradation products in cerebrospinal fluid after aneurysmal subarachnoid haemorrhage. *Acta Neurochir. (Wien)* 1981; **58**: 1–13.

62 Roos YBWEM, for the STAR Study Group. Antifibrinolytic treatment in subarachnoid hemorrhage – a randomized placebo-controlled trial. *Neurology* 2000; **54**: 77–82.

63 Hillman J, Fridriksson S, Nilsson O, Yu Z, Saveland H, Jakobsson KE. Immediate administration of tranexamic acid

and reduced incidence of early rebleeding after aneurysmal subarachnoid hemorrhage: a prospective randomized study. *J. Neurosurg.* 2002; **97**: 771–8.

64 Pickard JD, Kirkpatrick PJ, Melsen T, et al. Potential role of NovoSeven(R) in the prevention of rebleeding following aneurysmal subarachnoid haemorrhage. *Blood Coagul. Fibrinol.* 2000; **11**: S117–20.

65 Rinkel GJE, Feigin VL, Algra A, Van den Bergh WM, Vermeulen M, van GJ. Calcium antagonists for aneurysmal subarachnoid haemorrhage. *Cochrane Database Syst. Rev.* 2005; CD000277.

66 Pickard JD, Murray GD, Illingworth R, et al. Effect of oral nimodipine on cerebral infarction and outcome after subarachnoid haemorrhage: British aneurysm nimodipine trial. *BMJ* 1989; **298**: 636–42.

67 Philippon J, Grob R, Dagreou F, Guggiari M, Rivierez M, Viars P. Prevention of vasospasm in subarachnoid haemorrhage. A controlled study with nimodipine. *Acta Neurochir. (Wien)* 1986; **82**: 110–4.

68 Petruk KC, West M, Mohr G, et al. Nimodipine treatment in poor-grade aneurysm patients. Results of a multicenter double-blind placebo-controlled trial. *J. Neurosurg.* 1988; **68**: 505–17.

69 Ahmed N, Nasman P, Wahlgren NG. Effect of intravenous nimodipine on blood pressure and outcome after acute stroke. *Stroke* 2000; **31**: 1250–5.

70 Van den Bergh WM, Algra A, Van der Sprenkel JWB, Tulleken CAF, Rinkel GJE. Hypomagnesemia after aneurysmal subarachnoid hemorrhage. *Neurosurgery* 2003; **52**: 276–81.

71 Van den Bergh WM, Zuur JK, Kamerling NA, et al. Role of magnesium in the reduction of ischemic depolarization and lesion volume after experimental subarachnoid hemorrhage. *J. Neurosurg.* 2002; **97**: 416–22.

72 Veyna RS, Seyfried D, Burke DG, et al. Magnesium sulfate therapy after aneurysmal subarachnoid hemorrhage. *J. Neurosurg.* 2002; **96**: 510–4.

73 Van den Bergh WM, on behalf of the MASH study group. Magnesium sulfate in aneurysmal subarachnoid hemorrhage. A randomized controlled trial. *Stroke* 2005; **36**: 1011–15.

74 Juvela S, Kaste M, Hillbom M. Platelet thromboxane release after subarachnoid hemorrhage and surgery. *Stroke* 1990; **21**: 566–71.

75 Ohkuma H, Suzuki S, Kimura M, Sobata E. Role of platelet function in symptomatic cerebral vasospasm following aneurysmal subarachnoid hemorrhage. *Stroke* 1991; **22**: 854–9.

76 Dorhout Mees SM, Rinkel GJE, Hop JW, Algra A, van Gijn J. Antiplatelet therapy in aneurysmal subarachnoid hemorrhage: a systematic review. *Stroke* 2003; **34**: 2285–9.

77 Robinson JG, Smith B, Maheshwari N, Schrott H. Pleiotropic effects of statins: benefit beyond cholesterol reduction? A meta-regression analysis. *J. Am. Coll. Cardiol.* 2005; **46**: 1855–62.

78 Lynch JR, Wang H, McGirt MJ, et al. Simvastatin reduces vasospasm after aneurysmal subarachnoid hemorrhage: results of a pilot randomized clinical trial. *Stroke* 2005; **36**: 2024–6.

79 Tseng MY, Czosnyka M, Richards H, Pickard JD, Kirkpatrick PJ. Effects of acute treatment with pravastatin on cerebral vasospasm, autoregulation, and delayed ischemic deficits after

aneurysmal subarachnoid hemorrhage: a phase II randomized placebo-controlled trial. *Stroke* 2005; **36**: 1627–32.

80 Singhal AB, Topcuoglu MA, Dorer DJ, Ogilvy CS, Carter BS, Koroshetz WJ. SSRI and statin use increases the risk for vasospasm after subarachnoid hemorrhage. *Neurology* 2005; **64**: 1008–13.

81 Kassell NF, Haley Jr EC, Apperson-Hansen C, et al. Randomized, double-blind, vehicle-controlled trial of tirilazad mesylate in patients with aneurysmal subarachnoid hemorrhage: a cooperative study in Europe, Australia, and New Zealand. *J. Neurosurg.* 1996; **84**: 221–8.

82 Haley Jr EC, Kassell NF, Apperson-Hansen C, Maile MH, Alves WM. A randomized, double-blind, vehicle-controlled trial of tirilazad mesylate in patients with aneurysmal subarachnoid hemorrhage: a cooperative study in North America. *J. Neurosurg.* 1997; **86**: 467–74.

83 Lanzino G, Kassell NF, Dorsch NWC, et al. Double-blind, randomized, vehicle-controlled study of high-dose tirilazad mesylate in women with aneurysmal subarachnoid hemorrhage. Part I. A cooperative study in Europe, Australia, New Zealand, and South Africa. *J. Neurosurg.* 1999; **90**: 1011–17.

84 Lanzino G, Kassell NF. Double-blind, randomized, vehicle-controlled study of high-dose tirilazad mesylate in women with aneurysmal subarachnoid hemorrhage. Part II. A cooperative study in North America. *J. Neurosurg.* 1999; **90**: 1018–24.

85 Asano T, Takakura K, Sano K, et al. Effects of a hydroxyl radical scavenger on delayed ischemic neurological deficits following aneurysmal subarachnoid hemorrhage: results of a multicenter, placebo-controlled double-blind trial. *J. Neurosurg.* 1996; **84**: 792–803.

86 Saito I, Asano T, Sano K, et al. Neuroprotective effect of an antioxidant, ebselen, in patients with delayed neurological deficits after aneurysmal subarachnoid hemorrhage. *Neurosurgery* 1998; **42**: 269–77.

87 Saito I, Asano T, Ochiai C, Takakura K, Tamura A, Sano K. A double-blind clinical evaluation of the effect of Nizofenone (Y-9179) on delayed ischemic neurological deficits following aneurysmal rupture. *Neurol. Res.* 1983; **5**: 29–47.

88 Shaw MDM, Vermeulen M, Murray GD, Pickard JD, Bell BA, Teasdale GM. Efficacy and safety of the endothelin A/B receptor antagonist TAK-044 in treating subarachnoid hemorrhage: a report by the Steering Committee on behalf of the UK/Netherlands/Eire TAK-044 Subarachnoid Haemorrhage Study Group. *J. Neurosurg.* 2000; **93**: 992–7.

89 Rinkel GJE, Feigin VL, Algra A, van Gijn J. Circulatory volume expansion therapy for aneurysmal subarachnoid haemorrhage. *Cochrane Database Syst. Rev.* 2004; CD000483.

90 Wijdicks EFM, Vermeulen M, van Brummelen P, van Gijn J. The effect of fludrocortisone acetate on plasma volume and natriuresis in patients with aneurysmal subarachnoid hemorrhage. *Clin. Neurol. Neurosurg.* 1988; **90**: 209–14.

91 Hasan D, Lindsay KW, Wijdicks EFM, et al. Effect of fludrocortisone acetate in patients with subarachnoid hemorrhage. *Stroke* 1989; **20**: 1156–61.

92 Mori T, Katayama Y, Kawamata T, Hirayama T. Improved efficiency of hypervolemic therapy with inhibition of natriuresis by fludrocortisone in patients with aneurysmal subarachnoid hemorrhage. *J. Neurosurg.* 1999; **91**: 947–52.

93 Moro N, Katayama Y, Kojima J, Mori T, Kawamata T. Prophylactic management of excessive natriuresis with hydrocortisone for efficient hypervolemic therapy after subarachnoid hemorrhage. *Stroke* 2003; **34**: 2807–11.

94 Klimo Jr P, Kestle JR, MacDonald JD, Schmidt RH. Marked reduction of cerebral vasospasm with lumbar drainage of cerebrospinal fluid after subarachnoid hemorrhage. *J. Neurosurg.* 2004; **100**: 215–24.

95 Amin-Hanjani S, Ogilvy CS, Barker FG. Does intracisternal thrombolysis prevent vasospasm after aneurysmal subarachnoid hemorrhage? A meta-analysis. *Neurosurgery* 2004; **54**: 326–34.

96 Hamada J, Kai Y, Morioka M, et al. Effect on cerebral vasospasm of coil embolization followed by microcatheter intrathecal urokinase infusion into the cisterna magna: a prospective randomized study. *Stroke* 2003; **34**: 2549–54.

97 Hijdra A, Vermeulen M, van Gijn J, van Crevel H. Rerupture of intracranial aneurysms: a clinicoanatomic study. *J. Neurosurg.* 1987; **67**: 29–33.

98 Hijdra A, Braakman R, van Gijn J, Vermeulen M, van Crevel H. Aneurysmal subarachnoid hemorrhage. Complications and outcome in a hospital population. *Stroke* 1987; **18**: 1061–7.

99 Inagawa T, Kamiya K, Ogasawara H, Yano T. Rebleeding of ruptured intracranial aneurysms in the acute stage. *Surg. Neurol.* 1987; **28**: 93–9.

100 Kassell NF, Peerless SJ, Durward QJ, Beck DW, Drake CG, Adams Jr HP. Treatment of ischemic deficits from vasospasm with intravascular volume expansion and induced arterial hypertension. *Neurosurgery* 1982; **11**: 337–43.

101 Qureshi AI, Suarez JI, Bhardwaj A, Yahia AM, Tamargo RJ, Ulatowski JA. Early predictors of outcome in patients receiving hypervolemic and hypertensive therapy for symptomatic vasospasm after subarachnoid hemorrhage. *Crit. Care. Med.* 2000; **28**: 824–9.

102 Sen J, Belli A, Albon H, Morgan L, Petzold A, Kitchen N. Triple-H therapy in the management of aneurysmal subarachnoid haemorrhage. *Lancet Neurol.* 2003; **2**: 614–21.

103 Amin-Hanjani S, Schwartz RB, Sathi S, Stieg PE. Hypertensive encephalopathy as a complication of hyperdynamic therapy for vasospasm: report of two cases. *Neurosurgery* 1999; **44**: 1113–16.

104 Rosenwasser RH, Jallo JI, Getch CC, Liebman KE. Complications of Swan-Ganz catheterization for hemodynamic monitoring in patients with subarachnoid hemorrhage. *Neurosurgery* 1995; **37**: 872–5.

105 Harvey S, Harrison DA, Singer M, et al. Assessment of the clinical effectiveness of pulmonary artery catheters in management of patients in intensive care (PAC-Man): a randomised controlled trial. *Lancet* 2005; **366**: 472–7.

106 Shah MR, Hasselblad V, Stevenson LW, et al. Impact of the pulmonary artery catheter in critically ill patients: meta-analysis of randomized clinical trials. *JAMA* 2005; **294**: 1664–70.

107 Hoh BL, Ogilvy CS. Endovascular treatment of cerebral vasospasm: transluminal balloon angioplasty, intra-arterial papaverine, and intra-arterial nicardipine. *Neurosurg. Clin. N. Am.* 2005; **16**: 501–16.

108 Rabinstein AA, Friedman JA, Nichols DA, et al. Predictors of outcome after endovascular treatment of cerebral vasospasm. *AJNR Am. J. Neuroradiol.* 2004; **25**: 1778–82.

109 Polin RS, Coenen VA, Hansen CA, et al. Efficacy of transluminal angioplasty for the management of symptomatic cerebral vasospasm following aneurysmal subarachnoid hemorrhage. *J. Neurosurg.* 2000; **92**: 284–90.

110 Fandino J, Kaku Y, Schuknecht B, Valavanis A, Yonekawa Y. Improvement of cerebral oxygenation patterns and metabolic validation of super-selective intraarterial infusion of papaverine for the treatment of cerebral vasospasm. *J. Neurosurg.* 1998; **89**: 93–100.

111 Polin RS, Hansen CA, German P, Chadduck JB, Kassell NF. Intra-arterially administered papaverine for the treatment of symptomatic cerebral vasospasm. *Neurosurgery* 1998; **42**: 1256–64.

112 Smith WS, Dowd CF, Johnston SC, et al. Neurotoxicity of intra-arterial papaverine preserved with chlorobutanol used for the treatment of cerebral vasospasm after aneurysmal subarachnoid hemorrhage. *Stroke* 2004; **35**: 2518–22.

113 Arakawa Y, Kikuta K, Hojo M, Goto Y, Ishii A, Yamagata S. Milrinone for the treatment of cerebral vasospasm after subarachnoid hemorrhage: report of seven cases. *Neurosurgery* 2001; **48**: 723–8.

114 Feng L, Fitzsimmons BF, Young WL, et al. Intraarterially administered verapamil as adjunct therapy for cerebral vasospasm: safety and 2-year experience. *Am. J. Neuroradiol.* 2002; **23**: 1284–90.

115 Badjatia N, Topcuoglu MA, Pryor JC, et al. Preliminary experience with intra-arterial nicardipine as a treatment for cerebral vasospasm. *Am. J. Neuroradiol.* 2004; **25**: 819–26.

116 European CGRP in Subarachnoid Haemorrhage Study Group. Effect of calcitonin-gene-related peptide in patients with delayed postoperative cerebral ischaemia after aneurysmal subarachnoid haemorrhage. *Lancet* 1992; **339**: 831–4.

117 Hasan D, Vermeulen M, Wijdicks EFM, Hijdra A, van Gijn J. Management problems in acute hydrocephalus after subarachnoid hemorrhage. *Stroke* 1989; **20**: 747–53.

118 Kolluri VR, Sengupta RP. Symptomatic hydrocephalus following aneurysmal subarachnoid hemorrhage. *Surg. Neurol.* 1984; **21**: 402–4.

119 Ruijs AC, Dirven CM, Algra A, Beijer I, Vandertop WP, Rinkel G. The risk of rebleeding after external lumbar drainage in patients with untreated ruptured cerebral aneurysms. *Acta Neurochir. (Wien)* 2005; **147**: 1157–62.

120 Fountas KN, Kapsalaki EZ, Machinis T, Karampelas I, Smisson HF, Robinson JS. Review of the literature regarding the relationship of rebleeding and external ventricular drainage in patients with subarachnoid hemorrhage of aneurysmal origin. *Neurosurg. Rev.* 2005; **29**: 14–18.

121 Wong GKC, Poon WS, Wai S, Yu LM, Lyon D, Lam JMK. Failure of regular external ventricular drain exchange to reduce cerebrospinal fluid infection: result of a randomised controlled trial. *J. Neurol. Neurosurg. Psychiatr.* 2002; **73**: 759–61.

122 Choksey MS, Malik IA. Zero tolerance to shunt infections: can it be achieved? *J. Neurol. Neurosurg. Psychiatr.* 2004; **75**: 87–91.

123 Khanna RK, Rosenblum ML, Rock JP, Malik GM. Prolonged external ventricular drainage with percutaneous long-tunnel ventriculostomies. *J. Neurosurg.* 1995; **83**: 791–4.

124 Coplin WM, Avellino AM, Kim DK, Winn HR, Grady MS. Bacterial meningitis associated with lumbar drains: a retrospective cohort study. *J. Neurol. Neurosurg. Psychiatr.* 1999; **67**: 468–73.

125 Klopfenstein JD, Kim LJ, Feiz-Erfan I, et al. Comparison of rapid and gradual weaning from external ventricular drainage in patients with aneurysmal subarachnoid hemorrhage: a prospective randomized trial. *J. Neurosurg .*2004; **100**: 225–9.

126 Solenski NJ, Haley Jr EC, Kassell NF, et al. Medical complications of aneurysmal subarachnoid hemorrhage: a report of the multicenter, cooperative aneurysm study. *Crit. Care. Med.* 1995; **23**: 1007–17.

127 Gruber A, Reinprecht A, Görzer H, et al. Pulmonary function and radiographic abnormalities related to neurological outcome after aneurysmal subarachnoid hemorrhage. *J. Neurosurg.* 1998; **88**: 28–37.

128 Wijdicks EFM, Vermeulen M, ten Haaf JA, Hijdra A, Bakker WH, van Gijn J. Volume depletion and natriuresis in patients with a ruptured intracranial aneurysm. *Ann. Neurol.* 1985; **18**: 211–6.

129 Arieff AI. Hyponatremia, convulsions, respiratory arrest, and permanent brain damage after elective surgery in healthy women. *N. Engl. J. Med.* 1986; **314**: 1529–35.

130 Qureshi AI, Suri MFK, Sung GY, et al. Prognostic significance of hypernatremia and hyponatremia among patients with aneurysmal subarachnoid hemorrhage. *Neurosurgery* 2002; **50**: 749–55.

131 Bartter FC, Schwarz WB. The syndrome of inappropriate secretion of antdiuretic hormone. *Am. J. Med.* 1967; **42**: 790–806.

132 Harrigan MR. Cerebral salt wasting syndrome: a review. *Neurosurgery* 1996; **38**: 152–60.

133 Wijdicks EFM, van Dongen KJ, van Gijn J, Hijdra A, Vermeulen M. Enlargement of the third ventricle and hyponatraemia in aneurysmal subarachnoid haemorrhage. *J. Neurol. Neurosurg. Psychiatr.* 1988; **51**: 516–20.

134 Sayama T, Inamura T, Matsushima T, Inoha S, Inoue T, Fukui M. High incidence of hyponatremia in patients with ruptured anterior communicating artery aneurysms. *Neurol. Res.* 2000; **22**: 151–5.

135 Martin RJ. Central pontine and extrapontine myelinolysis: the osmotic demyelination syndromes. *J. Neurol. Neurosurg. Psychiatr.* 2004; **75**(Suppl. 3): iii22–8.

136 Adrogué HJ, Madias NE. Hyponatremia. *N. Engl. J. Med.* 2000; **342**: 1581–9.

137 Adrogué HJ. Consequences of inadequate management of hyponatremia. *Am. J. Nephrol.* 2005; **25**: 240–9.

138 Schuiling WJ, Dennesen PJ, Rinkel GJE. Extracerebral organ dysfunction in the acute stage after aneurysmal subarachnoid hemorrhage. *Neurocrit. Care.* 2005; **3**: 1–10.

139 Vespa PM, Bleck TP. Neurogenic pulmonary edema and other mechanisms of impaired oxygenation after aneurysmal subarachnoid hemorrhage. *Neurocrit. Care.* 2004; **1**: 157–70.

140 McLaughlin N, Bojanowski MW, Girard F, Denault A. Pulmonary edema and cardiac dysfunction following subarachnoid hemorrhage. *Can. J. Neurol. Sci.* 2005; **32**: 178–85.

141 Friedman JA, Pichelmann MA, Piepgras DG, et al. Pulmonary complications of aneurysmal subarachnoid hemorrhage. *Neurosurgery* 2003; **52**: 1025–31.

142 Mayer SA, Fink ME, Homma S, et al. Cardiac injury associated with neurogenic pulmonary edema following subarachnoid hemorrhage. *Neurology* 1994; **44**: 815–20.

143 Parr MJ, Finfer SR, Morgan MK. Reversible cardiogenic shock complicating subarachnoid haemorrhage. *BMJ* 1996; **313**: 681–3.

144 Deehan SC, Grant IS. Haemodynamic changes in neurogenic pulmonary oedema: effect of dobutamine. *Intens. Care. Med.* 1996; **22**: 672–6.

145 Van Gijn J. From randomised trials to rational practice. *Cerebrovasc. Dis.* 2005; **19**: 69–76.

15

CHAPTER 15

Acute traumatic brain injury

Miguel F. Arango, Walter Videtta, Corina Puppo

Background and clinical questions

Acute traumatic brain injury (TBI) is an important public health problem. According from the US National Centre for Injury Prevention and Control, only in the US 1,500,000 people are affected by acute head injury each year. From this 500,000 die, 230,000 require long-term hospitalization and between 80,000 and 90,000 develop some kind of long-term neurological disability [1].

Even under the best circumstances the mortality for acute severe head injury is around 36%, for severe disability in 15%, for moderate disability 20% and for complete recovery 25%, although these patients can remain with significant emotional and significant alterations preventing the normal reintegration in to the society [2].

Evidence about best clinical management, monitoring and follow-up is limited and contradictory. Recently several issues among the management of acute subdural haematoma (ASDH), computed tomography scan (CTS) scan follow-up, intracranial pressure (ICP) and antiepileptic management had been a matter of discussion.

We searched in the following databases: Cochrane Injuries Group Specialised Register, Cochrane Central Register of Controlled Trials, MEDLINE and LILACS.

Critical review of the evidence for each question

1. Non-operative treatment for traumatic ASDH

How does conservative treatment in an intensive care unit (ICU) with respect to immediate surgery affect the short- and long-term outcome?

ASDH, defined as a haematoma within 14 days after trauma, is a common finding after acute TBI. It is diagnosed using head CTS based on revealing extra cranial, hyperdense, and dynamic collections between the dura and the brain parenchyma. Normally all types of ASDH are managed surgically, either by craniotomy or burr holes, but in the past few years there had been an increasing trend towards conservative, medical therapy, despite lack of data supporting such therapeutic strategy.

Several authors [3,4] have reported some clinical and radiological characteristics in patients with traumatic ASDH,

which allow for non-operative management. Irrespective of ASDH, surgical treatment may also be required for other evolving traumatic brain lesions. Due to the frequent association of ASDH with other types of parenchyma injury, non-surgical management decisions should also take into consideration the recommendations for the other lesion types. The subset of ASDH patients that would benefit from medical management still requires definition.

To determine whether or not traumatic ASDH can be managed conservatively, we searched for randomized-controlled trials (RCTs) comparing surgical versus non-surgical management of post-traumatic ASDH in adult patients. We did not find RCTs but only two prospective and five retrospective studies (Table 15.1).

In a prospective study [4] Servadei analyzed 65 patients with large traumatic ASDH. Of a total of 65 patients with Glasgow Coma Scale (GCS) ≤ 8, 15 patients were initially managed conservatively based on a clinical protocol using CTS and ICP parameters. Two CTSs were performed within the first 6 h of injury. Of the 15 cases initially treated conservatively, 7 showed improved GCS compared to admission, 4 remained in stable clinical condition, and 4 showed a decrease in the neurological status not related to the SDH itself. Requirements for non-surgical management were as follows: clinical improvement or stability from the scene of the accident, haematoma thickness <10 mm, midline shift (MLS) <5 mm and ICP <20 mmHg or 20–30 mmHg, if the cerebral perfusion pressure was >75 mmHg. Two patients failed non-operative management and as a result underwent a craniotomy after the sequential CTS was performed. When comparing the different parameters between the surgical group and the patients initially managed conservatively, haematoma thickness and shift of the midline structures were predictive of the need for surgery. Outcomes for the conservatively treated group were as follows: mortality 20% (15 patients), severe disability 13.3% (2 patients) and good recovery 66.7% (10 patients). The authors concluded that GCS scoring at the scene of the accident and in the emergency room combined with early and subsequent CT scanning is crucial when making the decision for non-operative management for selected cases with ASDH with a thickness ≤ 10 mm and with a shift of the midline structures ≤ 5 mm.

Table 15.1 Conservative treatment versus surgical evacuation of acute subdural haematoma in patients with acute severe TBI.

Reference	Type of study	Patients	Intervention	Outcome	Results
Servadei [4]	Non-randomized, non-controlled, prospective	65 patients severe acute TBI, GCS ≤8	–15 patients conservative treatment CTS: haematoma <10 mm and MLS <5 mm ICP: <20 mmHg or between 20 and 30 mmHg if CPP >75 mmHg –50 patients surgical evacuation of haematoma	GOS at 6 months post trauma	Conservative treatment: – mortality 20%, – severe disability 13%, – good recovery 67% Surgery: – mortality 48% – severe disability 22% – good recovery 28%
Servadei [5]	Non-randomized, observational study, prospective	206 patients with TBI and GCS >3 and ASDH ≥5 mm	Conservative treatment: Serial CT scan. First within 3 h of admission, second within 12 h of admission. Subsequent according to the clinical condition	GOS at 6 months post trauma	– mortality 46%, – vegetative state 2%, – severe disability 6%, – favourable outcome 46% First CTS findings associated with poor neurological outcome

GCS: Glasgow Coma Scale; CTS: computed tomographic scan; ICP: intracranial pressure; CPP: cerebral perfusion pressure; ICU: intensive care unit; ASDH: acute subdural haematoma; TBI: traumatic brain injury; MLS: midline shift; GOS: Glasgow Outcome scale.

In an prospective observational study also published by Servadei et al. [5], reported 206 patients (all age groups) with TBI with GCS ≥3 presenting with ASDH ≥5 mm thickness. The study investigates the effects on prognosis of patients with ASDH and other findings on admission which could predict worsening of brain lesions and prognosis. There was no treatment protocol; the authors conclude that haematoma thickness, MLS, status of basal cisterns and presence of sub-arachnoid haemorrhage (SAH) on the initial CTS were related to poor neurological outcome.

In summary there is insufficient information regarding the operative and non-operative management in patients with traumatic ASDH. The prognosis of traumatic ASDH seems to be clinically related: age, pupillary status, ICP; and initial CTS variables: MLS, haematoma thickness, patency of the basal cisterns, and SAH. Sometimes surgical treatment is required for other evolving traumatic brain lesions different from the ASDH. Some subgroups of patients with traumatic ASDH would benefit from initial conservative management.

In conclusion patients with GCS ≤8, and traumatic ASDH, with haematoma thickness <10 mm, MLS <5 mm, and patent basal cisterns admitted in to hospitals, with CT scanner, 24 h neurosurgery and an ICU with ICP monitoring, could be considered as candidates to be treated non-surgically.

Prospective trials including adult patients with mild, moderate, and severe closed TBI with MLS <5 mm, different status of the basal cisterns, SAH, and a clot thickness <10 mm must address whether or not patients with traumatic ASDH can be managed conservatively.

2. Serial CTSs in acute patients

Among patients with acute TBI without clinical deterioration or ICP elevation, how does the practice of serial CTSs affect the indication for surgery treatment, the short-term mortality and the probability of acute complications?

CTS is the current standard imaging method for diagnosing intracranial pathology following acute traumatic head injury. It is well known that intracranial lesions after TBI are not static and develop over time. As a result of the improvements in the trauma system, emergency transport practices and reduced times between trauma and initial CTS, the chances of finding an intracranial lesion very early in its course and evolution are high. The use of sequential CTS to evaluate progression of injury is considered common practice [6] even though the evidence of its impact in outcome is unknown. The utility of repeated head CT performed solely for routine follow-up has not yet been defined [7].

Given the conflicting results regarding the indication for a second scheduled head CT in patients with severe closed brain injury, it is disappointing that we did not find any RCTs evaluating the utility of routine repeated CTS in these patients. Only eight prospective non-RCTs, were identified (Table 15.2).

Lobato et al. [8] reported a prospective study of 56 patients. The author's intention was to determine the incidence of pathological ICP changes during the acute post-traumatic period in patients with severe acute TBI presenting with diffuse injury (DI) I–II (TCDB classification) on the admission CTS. The aim was to define the most appropriate strategy of sequential CTS and ICP monitoring for detecting new intracranial

Table 15.2 Effect on outcome and management of serial brain CTS policy.

Reference	Type of study	Patients	Intervention	Outcome	Results
Lobato [8]	Non-randomized, prospective	56 patients acute severe TBI, diffuse CTS damage, ICP monitoring	Serial CTS admission, 24, 48, and 72 h	Surgery, clinical deterioration and death	CTS add information respect to ICP monitoring alone
Brown [6]	Non-randomized, prospective	100 patients moderate–severe acute TBI, CTS abnormality at admission	68 repeated CTS (no protocol). 32 patients only one CTS on admission.	Surgery	None patient with repeated CTS had surgery
Oertel [9]	Non-randomized, prospective	142 patients acute TBI any severity, mean GCS = 8	Early repeated CTS in patients with 'progressive shift and brain swelling'	Progression of intracranial haemorrhagic injury (PHI)	50% had PHI and 25% required surgery
Servadei [5]	Non-randomized, prospective	206 patients TBI and GCS between >3 and ASDH ⩾5 mm	Serial CTS. First within 3 h, second within 12 h Subsequent according to the clinical condition	CTS worsening	CTS evolution: DI I I 4%, DI II–IV 13–20%
Lubillo [10]	Non-randomized, prospective	82 patients intracranial haematoma and surgery	CTS within 2–12 h after surgery	Mortality and long-term outcome	CTS findings associated with final outcome
Cope [11]	Non-randomized, prospective	47 patients acute TBI traumatic head injuries	CTS at admission, 1 month, and 3 months later	Surgery	CTS allows early diagnosis of lesion requiring surgery
Roberson [12]	Non-randomised, prospective	107 patients acute TBI, coma	Serial CTS from day 1 to 12 months	Delayed intracranial lesions	18% of patients with normal CTS at admission present delayed intracranial lesion requiring surgical decompression

GCS: Glasgow Coma Scale; CTS: Computed Tomographic Scan; ICP: Intracranial Pressure; ICU: Intensive Care Unit; ASDH: Acute Subdural Haematoma; TBI: Traumatic Brain Injury; DI: diffuse injury.

mass effect and improving the final outcome. All patients had the initial CTS less than 24 h after injury, several control CTS within the first days of the trauma and ICP monitoring after admission. The mean GCS was 5, 57.1% of the patients showed CTS changes: new contusion (26.8% of the cases), growth of previous contusion (68.2%), previous extra axial haematoma (10.7%), and generalized brain swelling (10.7%). 64.9% of the patients had a favourable outcome and 35.1% an unfavourable outcome. Overall, 27 (48.9%) patients developed clinical deterioration, 21 (37.5%) with concurrent CTS changes and 6 (10.7%) without new pathology. The remaining 29 (51.7%) patients did not develop deterioration in spite of 11(19.6%) showing CTS changes. The presence of contusion at the initial CTS ($P = 0.01$) and the presence of generalized brain swelling ($P = 0.003$) in posterior CTS significantly correlated with the risk of deterioration. This worsening in neurological status increased the risk of death by a factor of 10 (OR = 9.8). Eight (14.2%) patients requiring surgery showed simultaneous ICP deterioration and CTS changes, but another 11 patients in a similar condition were able to be managed without surgery. Over 50% of the patients with initial DI I–II lesions developed new CTS

changes and nearly 50% showed intracranial hypertension. The discordances between ICP and CTS deterioration were seen in 30.3% of patients. Therefore, the authors recommend ICP monitoring in all patients and serial CTS at 2–4, 12, 24, 48, and 72 h after injury with additional controls as indicated by clinical or ICP changes in all cases.

Brown et al. [6] reported a prospective analysis of 100 patients with GSC <14. The study intended to examine the value of routine serial CTS after TBI in a single Level I trauma centre. Repeated CTS was ordered at the discretion of the trauma team or the neurosurgical consultant with no protocol in place. Only patients who showed abnormalities subsequent to the initial CTS scan were included. Patents that died within 24 h were excluded. Patients with moderate TBI were also included. Sixty eight patients who underwent a repeat CTS (Repeat Group, RG) were compared with 32 patients who had CTS only at admission (No Repeat Group, NRG) to evaluate the effect of repeat CTS on patient outcome. Primary outcome was the need for TBI-related intervention. The 68 patients in the RG underwent 90 repeat CTS. Repeat scan were mainly done 34 ± 32 h after admission. This group had a higher incidence of extradural haematoma

(EDH), and a trend towards more SDH. Of those undergoing repeat CTS, 90% (*n* = 81) were performed on a routine basis without neurological changes. Of those routine CTS, 26%, 52%, and 22% were classified as 'better', 'the same', and 'worse', respectively. No patient had any neurosurgical intervention after having a routine repeated CTS. In the RG, every patient (100% of cases) with EDH, intraventricular haemorrhage (IVH) underwent sequential CTS, but only in 70% of the cases of patients with SDH, Intraparenchymal haemorrhage (IPH), contusion, MLS, or multiple injuries. 83% of patients GCS ≤8 underwent repeat CTS scan and showed a trend towards a higher injury severly scane (ISS) and lower GCS. The authors concluded that the use of routine serial CTS in patients without neurological deterioration was not supported.

In a prospective study Oertel et al. [9] looked at patients who underwent two CTS within 24 h after acute TBI to determine the incidence, risks factors, and clinical significance of progressive haemorrhagic injury (PHI). One single Level I Trauma centre, 142 patients with mild, moderate, and severe, closed and penetrating TBI were included. The diagnosis of PHI was determined by comparing the first and second CTS and defined as an unambiguous increase in the full film appearance of lesion size; this amounted to a ≥25% increase in at least one dimension of ≥1 lesion seen on the first post-injury CTS. The mean GCS was 8. Potential risk factors, coagulation status, temperature, ethanol, ICP, and CPP were analysed. Increased MLS, hemispheric swelling, or progressive loss of basilar cisterns on the second CTS was defined as 'progressive shift and swelling'. Similarly, 'progressive brain shift and swelling' was present in 23% of patients with PHI but in only 4% of patients without PHI (*P* = 0.003). The second CTS scan was performed earlier in patients 'with progressive brain shift and swelling' than in patients without this finding (6.4 ± 4.2 h post injury versus 9.3 ± 3.9 h post injury; *P* = 0.01). Of the 17 patients with progressive shift and swelling, eight underwent craniotomy after the second CTS. Male sex (*P* = 0.01), older age (*P* = 0.01), time from injury to first CTS (*P* = 0.02), and initial partial thromboplastin time (*P* = 0.02) were the best predictors of PHI. Of the 46 patients who underwent craniotomy for haematoma evacuation, 24% present the haematoma after the second CTS. Early CTS after moderate or severe TBI did not reveal the full extent of haemorrhagic injury in 45% of patients. PHI approached 50% in patients undergoing scanning within 2 h of injury. Parenchymal lesions in the frontal and temporal lobes are the most likely to progress. Patients with PHI had a greater degree of subsequent ICP elevations, and 25% required a craniotomy. The neurological outcome at 6 months post injury was similar in both groups. The authors recommended early repeated CTS in patients with no surgically treated haemorrhage revealed on the first CTS.

In a prospective study Servadei et al. [5] intended to establish the frequency of deterioration in CTS appearance from an admission scan to subsequent scans and the prognostic significance of such deterioration. Data has been gathered prospectively for 206 patients with moderate and severe head injury. The findings of the initial and the final ('worst') CTS were classified according to the Traumatic Coma Data Bank (TCDB) system and were related to outcome using the GOS at 6 months after injury. The initial CTS findings were classified as a DI for 53% of the cohort, with 16% of these DI demonstrating deterioration on a subsequent scan. In 56(74%) of 76 deteriorations, the change was from a DI to a mass lesion. Patients with normal CTS or with a DI I at admission showed a low rate of evolution (4%). Patients with DI II, III, and IV showed high rates of progression to mass lesion (13–14 for DI II and III and 20% for type IV). A third CTS may be scheduled on the third day post trauma. When the initial CTS demonstrated a DI without swelling or shift, evolution to a mass lesion was associated with a significant increase in the risk of an unfavourable outcome (62% versus 38%). The author recommended follow-up scans when admission CTS demonstrates evidence of a DI, because approximately 1/6 of patients will demonstrate significant CT evolution of this lesions. The CTS may be repeated within 12 h whenever the first scan is obtained within the 3 h after injury and within 24 h in all other situations. A third scan was also recommended on the third day after trauma, even though the author accepted that this recommendation is empiric.

Lubillo et al. [10] prospectively studied 82 patients with isolated, severe TBI (GCS ≤8), all of whom had intracranial haematoma. The author analysed the CTS appearance after evacuation of a mass lesion in relation to outcome. The CTS was performed within 2–12 h after craniotomy; continuous monitoring of the ICP and CPP were also done after the surgery. The mortality rate during the hospital stay was 37%; 50% of the patients achieved a favourable outcome. The postoperative scan revealed DI III–IV in 53 patients and DI I–II in 29 patients. The percentage of time presenting an ICP >20 mmHg and CPP <70 mmHg were higher in the group of patients with DI III–IV (*P* < 0.001); these patients also revealed an unfavourable neurological outcome. Patients with a motor (m) GCS ≤3, bilateral unreactive pupils, associated intracranial injuries, and hypotension demonstrate high incidence of raised ICP, CPP <70 mmHg, DI III–IV, and unfavourable outcome (*P* < 0.001). The author concluded that the features on CTS obtained shortly after craniotomy constitute an independent predictor of outcome in patients with traumatic haematoma.

Cope et al. [11] reported a prospective study looking at routine serial CTS in 47 patients with TBI. This study analysed patients who were admitted to a rehabilitation unit after initial hospitalization. Under a prospective protocol of routine scans (admission, 1 month and 3 months), 22% of patients required neurosurgical intervention for a variety of findings. Most patients had chronic manifestations of TBI not applicable to acutely head injured patients. Though there is no reference regarding exact neurological disability before routine repeat CTS, the patients who underwent neurosurgical intervention had a higher disability rating score. This would imply that the clinical status of the patient, not scan findings alone, played a major role in determining the need for surgical intervention versus observation. These authors concluded that routine serial scanning may allow earlier diagnosis of a progressive intracranial lesion and thereby minimize further brain injury in the rehabilitation setting.

In a prospective study, Servadei et al. [4] looked at patients with large ASDH. Of 65 comatose patients, 15 patients were initially managed conservatively according to a protocol based on clinical, CTS and ICP parameters. Two patients failed non-operative management and underwent a craniotomy after sequential scan. When comparing the different parameters between the surgical group and the patients initially managed conservative, haematoma thickness and shift of the midline structures were predictive of the need of surgery. The authors concluded that GCS scoring at the scene and in the emergency room combined with early and subsequent CTS is crucial when making the decision for non-operative management for selected cases with ASDH with a thickness ≤10 mm and with a shift of the midline structures ≤5 mm.

Roberson et al. [12] reported a prospective study of comatose TBI patients who had routine CTS (on days 1, 3, 5, 7, 14, and at 3 and 12 months). The author compared the value of sequential scans, neurological status, and ICP in 107 patients. Thirty eight (40%) of 95 patients had a normal CTS on admission. Seven (18%) of these 38 patients had scans demonstrating a delayed intracranial lesion requiring surgical decompression. It is important to note that all seven patients had neurological deterioration before the intervention and were not treated based on CTS results alone. They gave a confirmatory value to CTS regarding the changes in ICP monitoring and clinical examination. The author concluded that it is useful to get a control CTS on days 3 and 7 after injury if the patient shows no clinical improvement.

In summary, there is insufficient information and conflicting data on the value of repetitive routinely head CT in adult severe closed head injury patients. Some subgroups of patients with SAH, epidural haematoma, SDH, contusions, and intraparenchymal haematoma with initially conservative management would benefit from serial CTS. More studies are needed to address this issue. Wherever possible, uncertain about the convenience of doing a second CTS in absence of clinical manifestations, for example impaired GCS, ICP elevation, must evaluate the risks/benefits of transporting patients out of the monitoring and controlled ICU environment. Prospective trials including adult patients with moderate/severe blunt head injury admitted to the ICU, first CTS classified according TCDB categories and including confounding variables, worsening GCS and/or clinical examination, elevations of ICP, hypotension, and coagulopathy represent the next step in defining guidelines for obtaining repeat CTS.

3. Anticonvulsive therapy for acute brain injury patients

Among patients with acute TBI, how does the early treatment with antiepileptic drugs affect the risk of early seizure, late seizure, and the probability of long-term death or disabled condition? What are the side effects?

The incidence of post-traumatic seizures (PTS) in patients with acute TBI is between 10–30%. According to some reports between 20–25% of patients with severe head injury (GCS <9) might be expected to have at least one PTS during hospital stay. Depending on the time of occurrence, the PTS can be classified in:

1 immediate seizures, occurring within the first few hours of trauma;

2 early seizures, occurring with in one week;

3 late seizures, after 1 week of the initial trauma; only recurrent 'late seizures' make up the clinical syndrome which can be labelled as 'post-traumatic epilepsy' and can be defined as a disorder characterized by recurrent seizures, not referable to another obvious cause ('unprovoked seizures'), in patients following TBI.

'Prevention' simply means to hinder the occurrence of the attacks without any attempt to block the pathogenetic mechanism. To evaluate the efficacy of prevention it is sufficient to control the number of seizures, if any, in patients to whom antiepileptic drugs in the therapeutic range are given and compare this number to the number of patients presenting or not presenting attacks during drug administration. To evaluate the prophylactic effect of treatment upon late seizures, it is necessary to collect series with a long follow-up after discontinuation of treatment to verify if seizures occur. In fact late seizures may occur years after injury.

One must firstly question if there is any justification for prevention in PTS or epilepsy. Apart from early PTS, partial (especially if recurrent) and generalized attacks, none of the other types of PTS contribute to secondary damage of the injured brain. Prevention and prophylaxis of 'late seizures' can prevent further accidental injuries, cognitive impairment, loss of a driver's licence, job, etc.

A systematic review of the use of drugs to prevent seizures after head injury [13] identified 10 RCTs, which provided data from 2036 patients. Four were unpublished studies, which turned to be unavailable. Therefore, only six trials were reviewed, which included 1218 randomized patients. Four trials randomized 890 patients in order to address prevention of early seizures. They found consistent evidence that the early treatment with antiepileptic drugs, most commonly phenytoin, but also carbamazepine and phenobarbitone, decreased the relative risk (RR) of early seizures (0.34 (95%

Table 15.3 Antiepileptic drugs for acute TBI.

Types of studies (reference)	Intervention	Outcome	Number of patients (number of trials)	Control group risk (range)	Relative risk (95% CI)	Absolute risk reduction (95% CI)	Comment
SR [13]	Antiepileptic versus standard care	Early seizure	890 (4)	15% (4–29)	0.34 (0.21–0.54)	10% (6–13)	Antiepileptic better
		Late seizure	1218 (6)	15% (7–42)	0.92 (0.69–1.23)	1% (ns)	Antiepileptic better Heterogeneity between trials
		Death or disability	555 (2)	35% (34–39)	1.12 (0.80–1.39)	+4% (ns)	Antiepileptic worse Heterogeneity between trials
		Skin rush	568 (2)	7% (1–9)	1.57 (0.90–2.75)	+4% (ns)	Antiepileptic worse

SR: systematic review; CI: confidence intervals; ns: not statistically significant.

CI 0.21–0.54)). For late seizures, six trials were analysed; there was significant heterogeneity between trials, and therefore a summary RR could not be calculated. A reduction in late seizures was not demonstrated. Mortality data were available from five trials (1054 randomized patients), showing no beneficial effect of antiepileptics (pooled RR 1.15; 95% CI 0.89–1.51); or death and severe neurological disability [14], RR 1.49, 95% CI 1.06–2.08 [15]; RR 0.96; 95% CI 0.72–1.39). Skin rashes: based on the pooled RR, for every 100 patients treated, 4 will develop skin rashes. Table 15.3 shows the characteristics of systematic reviews addressing the issue of seizure prevention in head trauma.

A trial by Temkin et al. [16] of patients at high risk for seizures assigned 132 head injured patients to receive phenytoin, 120 to receive a 1-month course of valproate, and 127 to receive a 6-month course of valproate. The cases were followed up to 2 years. The rates of late seizures did not differ among treatment groups. The mortality rates were not significantly different between treatment groups, but there was a trend towards a higher mortality rate in patients treated with valproate. The lack of additional benefit and the potentially higher mortality rate suggest that valproate should not be routinely used for the prevention of early or late PTS.

Based on these findings, antiepileptic drugs seem to control early seizures in patients with TBI. They do not seem to prevent the subsequent development of post-traumatic epilepsy, nor change mortality nor improve disability.

Therefore, as early seizures may contribute to secondary damage to the injured brain, preventive treatment with phenytoin should be initiated as soon a possible after injury among patients with severe TBI. Antiepileptic drugs should not be used after the first 7 days of injury to decrease the risk of PTS occurring beyond that time.

4. Monitoring intracranial hypertension

Among patients with severe acute TBI, how does the ICP monitoring policy affect the probability of death or the severity of neurological impairment?

Many investigators have studied the relationship between increased ICP and patient outcome. Miller et al. [17], were among the first; Marshall et al. [18], Gaab and Haubitz [19], McGraw et al. [20], Narayan et al. [21], and Fearnside et al. [22] have demonstrated significantly worse outcomes in patients with increased ICP. Marmarou et al. [23] reviewed the experience of the TCDB with regard to ICP instability and hypotension. By measuring the percentage of time that ICP was >20 mmHg, they were able to demonstrate that elevated ICP was a highly significant predictor of poor outcome. Unterberg et al. [24] found that patients with late (day 3–5) increases in ICP had significantly worse outcomes than patients without such an increase. The prospective analysis of 394 head injury patients obtained from the database provided by the Selfotel trial [25] showed an important decrease in neurological outcome in those patients with alterations of the ICP.

Controlling and preventing high ICP and aggressive treatment of ICP elevation plus avoiding cerebral ischaemia maintaining the cerebral blood flow (CBF), and the cerebral perfusion pressure is actually the standard of treatment in acute TBI. Unfortunately there is no consensus on the best way to achieve these goals. A systematic review about the effects of ICP monitoring in severe traumatic acute head injury on mortality and severe neurological disability was published by the Cochrane Database. The inclusion criteria were RCTs comparing any kind of ICP monitoring versus no monitoring at all. To the date of publishing there were no RCTs according to the inclusion criteria. In our opinion it is not possible to get any result comparing only a monitoring system. The

Table 15.4 Interventions for lowering ICP.

Type of study (Reference)	Intervention	Outcome	Number of patients (number of trials)	Control group risk (range)	Relative risk (95% CI)	Absolute risk reduction (95% CI)	Comment
SR [27]	Hyperventilation versus control	Death	77 (1)	34%	0.73 (0.36–1.49)	9% (ns)	Hyperventilation better
		Death or disability	77 (1)	61%	1.14 (0.82–1.58)	+8% (ns)	Hyperventilation worse
SR [29]	Barbiturate versus control	Death	208 (3)	42% (27–53)	1.09 (0.81–1.47)	+4% (ns)	Barbiturate worse
		Death or disability	135 (2)	43% (32–61)	1.15 (0.81–1.64)	+7% (ns)	Barbiturate worse
SR [30]	Mannitol versus placebo	Death	41 (1)	14%	1.75 (0.48–6.38)	+11% (ns)	Mannitol worse
		Death	363 (3)	34% (25–66)	0.56 (0.39–0.79)	15% (7–24)	High dose mannitol better
		Death or disability	363 (3)	63% (54–90)	0.58 (0.47–0.72)	26% (17–36)	High dose mannitol better
RCT [37]	Corticosteroid versus control	Death	9673 (1)	22%	1.15 (1.07–1.24)	+3% (2–5)	Corticosteroid worse
		Death or disability	9554 (1)	36%	1.05 (0.99–1.10)	+2% (ns)	Corticosteroid worse

SR: systematic review; RCT: randomized controlled trial; CI: confidence intervals; ns: not statistically significant.

neurological outcome of the patient depends not only on the monitoring technique but also the interpretation of the results obtained from the monitor and the clinical therapeutic decision. Conceptually, a blinded treatment of intracranial hypertension, according to many authors, will give the same result as the one obtained from the blinded treatment of systemic hypertensive emergency.

5. Management of ICP

Among patients with severe acute TBI, how do ICP-lowering interventions affect the probability of death or the severity of neurological impairment?

A systematic review done by Roberts et al. [26], analysed the effectiveness of five medical interventions routinely used in the medical management of severe acute TBI patients. The specific interventions were hyperventilation, mannitol, cerebrospinal fluid (CSF) drainage, barbiturates, and corticosteroids. On the basis of the available randomized evidence, it is not possible to support or refute the existence of a real benefit on mortality and neurological disability from the use of these therapeutic interventions (Table 15.4).

Hyperventilation is often associated with a rapid fall in ICP, therefore, it has been assumed to be effective in the treatment of severe head injury patients. Hyperventilation reduces raised ICP by causing cerebral vasoconstriction and a reduction in cerebral blood volume. A Cochrane Systematic Review was

performed and published in 2000 [27]; only one trial was which randomized 113 patients [28]. Possible disadvantages of hyperventilation include cerebral vasoconstriction to such an extent that cerebral ischaemia ensues. These investigators hypothesized that the short effect of hyperventilation could be related to the CSF pH decrease, with a loss of HCO_3-buffer. The latter disadvantage might be overcome by the addition of the buffer tromethamine (THAM). Accordingly, a trial was performed with patients randomly assigned to receive normal ventilation, hyperventilation ($PaCO_2$ 25 ± 2 mmHg), or hyperventilation plus THAM ($PaCO_2$ 25 ± 2 mmHg). Stratification into subgroups of patients with motor scores of 1–3 and 4–5 took place. Outcome was assessed according to the Glasgow Outcome Scale at 3, 6, and 12 months. There were 41, 36, and 36 patients, respectively. A 100% follow-up was obtained. At 3 and 6 months after injury the number of patients with a favourable outcome was significantly lower in the hyperventilated patients than in the other two groups. This occurred only in patients with a motor score of 4–5. At 12 months post-trauma this difference was not significant ($P = 0.13$). Biochemical data indicated that hyperventilation could not sustain alkalinization in the CSF, although THAM could. Accordingly, CBF was lower in the HV + THAM group than in the control and HV groups, but neither CBF nor arteriovenous difference of oxygen data indicated the occurrence of cerebral ischaemia in any of the three groups. Although mean ICP could be kept well below 25 mmHg in all three groups, the course of ICP was most stable in the HV + THAM group. It is concluded that prophylactic hyperventilation is deleterious in head-injured patients with motor scores of 4–5. Hyperventilation alone, as well as in conjunction with the buffer THAM showed a beneficial effect on mortality at 1 year after injury, although the effect measure was imprecise (RR = 0.73; 95% CI 0.36–1.49 and RR = 0.89; 95% CI 0.47–1.72, respectively). This improvement in outcome was not supported by an improvement in neurological recovery. For hyperventilation alone, the RR for death or severe disability was 1.14 (95% CI 0.82–1.58). In the hyperventilation plus THAM group, the RR for death or severe disability, was 0.87 (95% CI 0.58–1.28). The data available are inadequate to assess any potential benefit or harm that might result from hyperventilation in severe head injury. RCTs to assess the effectiveness of hyperventilation therapy following severe head injury are needed.

Mannitol may sometimes dramatically effective in reversing acute brain swelling, but its effectiveness in the on-going management of severe head injury remains open to question. There is evidence that, in prolonged dosage, mannitol may pass from the blood into the brain, where it might cause reverse osmotic shifts that increase ICP. A Cochrane Systematic Review was performed on this topic [30]. They included 5 RCTs [31–35]. The authors concluded that high-dose mannitol (fast intravenous mannitol in a dose of 1.4 g/kg followed by rapid normal saline infusion 14 mL/kg) appears to be preferable to conventional-dose mannitol in the pre-operative management of patients with acute traumatic intracranial haematomas. However, there is little evidence about the use of mannitol as continuous infusion in patients with raised ICP in patients who do not have an operable intracranial haematoma. Mannitol therapy for raised ICP may have a beneficial effect on mortality when compared to pentobarbital treatment. ICP-directed treatment shows a small beneficial effect compared to treatment directed by neurological signs and physiological indicators. There are insufficient data on the effectiveness of pre-hospital administration of mannitol to preclude either a harmful or a beneficial effect on mortality. It has to be stressed that three of these five trials did not measure ICP, because the patients were examined in the emergency room, and therefore, mannitol was administered for the treatment of clinical signs of severity.

Cortisteroids have been widely used in treating people with TBI. However the increase in mortality with steroids demonstrated by the Cochrane Systematic Review [36] and the CRASH trial [37] suggest that steroids should no longer be routinely used in people with traumatic head injury.

References

1 The Brain Trauma Foundation. The American Association of Neurological Surgeons. The Joint Section on Neurotrauma and Critical Care. Trauma systems. *J. Neurotrauma.* 2000; **17**(6–7): 457–62.

2 Marshall LF, Gautile T, Klauber MR, et al. The outcome of severe closed head injury. *J. Neurosurg.* 1991; **75**: S28–36.

3 Dent DL, Croce MA, Menke PG, et al. Prognostic factors after acute subdural hematoma. *J. Trauma.* 1995; **39**: 36–42.

4 Servadei F, Nasi MT, Cremonini AM, Giuliani G, Cenni P, Nanni A. Importance of a reliable admission Glasgow Coma Score for determining the need for evacuation of posttraumatic subdural hematomas: a prospective study of 65 patients. *J. Trauma.* 1998; **44**: 868–73.

5 Servadei F, Nasi MT, Giuliani G, et al. CT prognostic factors in acute subdural haematomas: the value of the worst CT scan. *Br. J. Neurosurg.* 2000; **14**: 110–6.

6 Brown CV, Weng J, Oh D, et al. Does routine serial computed tomography of the head influence management of traumatic brain injury? A prospective evaluation. *J. Trauma.* 2004; **57**: 939–43.

7 Kaups KL, Davis JW, Parks SN. Routinely repeated tomography after blunt head trauma: does it benefit patients? *J. Trauma.* 2004; **56**: 475–80.

8 Lobato RD, Alen JF, Perez-Nunez A, et al. Value of serial CT scanning and intracranial pressure monitoring for detecting new intracranial mass effect in severe head injury patients showing lesions type I-II in the initial CT scan. *Neurocirugia. (Astur).* 2005; **16**: 217–34 (in Spanish).

9 Oertel M, Kelly DF, McArthur D, et al. Progressive hemorrhage after head trauma: predictors and consequences of evolving injury. *J. Neurosurg.* 2002; **96**: 109–16.

10 Lubillo S, Bolanos J, Carreira L, Cardenosa J, Arroyo J, Manzano J. Prognostic value of early computerized tomography scanning following craniotomy for traumatic hematomas. *J. Neurosurg.* 1999; **91**: 581–7.

11 Cope DN, Date ES, Mar EY. Serial computed tomographic evaluations in traumatic head injury. *Arch. Phys. Med. Rehabil.* 1988; **69**: 483–6.

12 Roberson FC, Kishore PR, Miller JD, Lipper MH, Becker DP. The value of serial computerized tomography in the management of severe head injury. *Surg. Neurol.* 1979; **12**: 161–7.

13 Schierhout G, Roberts I. Prophylactic antiepileptic agents after head injury: a systematic review *J. Neurol. Neurosurg. Psychiatr.* 1998; **64**: 108–12.

14 Glotzner FL, Haubitz I, Miltner F, Kapp G, Pflughaupt KW. Seizure prevention using carbamazepine following severe brain injuries. *Flortschritte Der Neurologie und Psychiarie* (Suppl.) 1983; 66–79.

15 Temkin NR, Dikmen SS, Wilensky AJ, Keihm J, Chabal S, Winn HR. A randomized, double-blind study of phenytoin for the prevention of post-traumatic seizures. *N. Engl. J. Med.* 1990; **323**: 497–502.

16 Temkin N, Dikmen SS, Anderson GD, et al. Valproate therapy for prevention of posttraumatic seizures: a randomized trial. *J. Neurosurg.* 1999; **91**: 593–600.

17 Miller JD, Becker DP, Ward JD, Sullivan HG, Adams WE, Rosner MJ. Significance of intracranial hypertension in severe head injury. *J. Neurosurg.* 1977; **47**(4): 503–16.

18 Marshall LF, Smith RW, Shapiro HM. The outcome with aggressive treatment in severe head injuries. Part I. The significance of intracranial pressure monitoring. *J. Neurosurg.* 1979; **50**: 20–5.

19 Gaab MR, Haubitz I. Intracranial pressure, primary/secondary brain stem injury and prognosis in cerebral trauma. In: Ishii S, Nagai H & Brock M, eds., *Intracranial Pressure V.* Springer-Verlag, Berlin, Germany, 1983: pp. 501–31.

20 McGraw CP, Howard G, O'Connor C. Outcome associated with management based on ICP monitoring. In: Ishii S, Nagai H & Brock M, eds., *Intracranial Pressure V.* Springer-Verlag, Berlin, Germany, 1983: pp. 558–61.

21 Narayan RK, Greenberg RP, Miller JD, et al. Improved confidence of outcome prediction in severe head injury. *J. Neurosurg.* 1981; **54**: 751–62.

22 Fearnside MR, Cook RJ, McDougall P, et al. The Westmead Head Injury Project outcome in severe head injury. A comparative analysis of pre-hospital, clinical and CT variables. *Br. J. Neurosurg.* 1993; **7**(3): 267–79.

23 Marmarou A, Anderson RL, Ward J, et al. Impact of ICP instability and hypotension on outcome in patients with severe head trauma. *J. Neurosurg.* 1991; **75**: S59–66.

24 Unterberg A, Kiening K, Schmiedeck P, et al. Long-term observations of intracranial pressure after severe head injury. The phenomenon of secondary rise of intracranial pressure. *Neurosurgery.* 1993; **32**: 17–24.

25 Juul N, Morris GF, Marshall LF. Intracraneal hypertension and cerebral perfusion pressure: influence on neurological deterioration and outcome in severehead injury. The Executive committee of the international Selfotel Trial. *J. Neurosurg.* 2000; **92**(1): 1.

26 Roberts I, Schierhout G, Alderson P. Absence of evidence for the effectiveness of five interventions routinely used in the intensive care management of severe head injury: a systematic review. *J. Neurol. Neurosurg. Psychiatr.* 1998; **65**: 729–33.

27 Schierhout G, Roberts I. Hyperventilation therapy for acute traumatic brain injury. *Cochrane Database Syst. Rev.* 2000; 2.

28 Muizelaar JP, Marmarou A, Ward A, et al. Adverse effects of prolonged hyperventilation in patients with severe head injury: a randomized clinical trial. *J. Neurosurg.* 1991; **75**: 731–39.

29 Roberts I. Barbiturates for acute traumatic brain injury. *Cochrane Database Syst. Rev.* 1999; 3: CD000033; DOI: 10.1002/14651858. CD000033.

30 Wakai A, Roberts I, Schierhout G. Mannitol for acute traumatic brain injury. *Cochrane Database Syst. Rev.* 2005; 4: CD001049.pub2; DOI: 10.1002/14651858.CD001049.pub2.

31 Smith HP, Kelly Jr DL, McWhorter JM, et al. Comparison of mannitol regimens in patients with severe head injury undergoing intracranial monitoring. *J. Neurosurg.* 1986; **65**(6): 820–4.

32 Schwartz ML, Tator CH, Rowed DW, Reid SR, Meguro K, Andrews DF. The University of Toronto head injury treatment study: a prospective, randomized comparison of pentobarbital and mannitol. *Can. J. Neurol. Sci.* 1984; **11**(4): 434–40.

33 Sayre MR, Daily SW, Stern SA, Storer DL, Van Loveren HR, Hurst JM. Out-of-hospital administration of mannitol to head-injured patients does not change systolic blood pressure. *Acad. Emerg. Med.* 1996; **3**(9): 840–8.

34 Cruz J, Minoja G, Okuchi K. Improving clinical outcomes from acute subdural hematomas with the emergency preoperative administration of high doses of mannitol: a randomized trial. *Neurosurgery* 2001; **49**(4): 864–71.

35 Cruz J, Minoja G, Okuchi K. Major clinical and physiological benefits of early high doses of mannitol for intraparenchymal temporal lobe hemorrhages with abnormal pupillary widening: a randomized trial. *Neurosurgery* 2002; **51**(3): 628–37; discussion 637–8.

36 Alderson P, Roberts I. Corticosteroids for acute traumatic brain injury. *Cochrane Database Syst. Rev.* 2005; 1: CD000196.pub2; DOI: 10.1002/14651858.CD000196.pub2.

37 CRASH trial collaborators. Effect of intravenous corticosteroids on death within 14 days in 10008 adults with clinically significant head injury (MRC CRASH trial): randomised placebo-controlled trial. *Lancet* 2004; **364**: 1321–28.

16

CHAPTER 16

Corticosteroids in central nervous system infections

Anu Jacob, Tom Solomon, Paul Garner

Background

Whether to prescribe corticosteroids for central nervous system infections is a thorny topic for the physician and, as many of these conditions are often fatal and cause long-term neurological deficit in the survivors, is important to get right. Many organisms that infect the central nervous system cause inflammation. This can cause further local damage through compression of the brain parenchyma. In addition, the associated cerebral oedema can cause raised intracranial pressure, leading to reduced cerebral perfusion and ischaemia which results in further oedema. Ultimately this can lead to brainstem herniation and death. Corticosteroids may reduce the inflammation in the parenchyma, subarachnoid space, and blood vessels, reduce cerebral and spinal cord oedema, thus reducing this damage [1–4]. On the other hand, corticosteroids suppress the immune system and this could make the illness worse by allowing the infective organism to proliferate. In addition, adverse effects of steroids (such as gastrointestinal haemorrhage, electrolyte changes, hyperglycaemia, psychosis, and opportunistic infections) can contribute to illness and death. In addition, steroids may reduce inflammation of the meninges which could decrease the penetration of drugs used to treat the infection, across the blood brain barrier.

Framing answerable clinical questions and general approach to search evidence

Despite at least 50 years of physicians using steroids in neurological infections, there remains considerable debate as to which if any diseases should be treated this way [5]. In the light of these debates, and after discussion with acknowledged experts in the field, we have therefore drawn together the best available evidence on this question for six serious neurological infections important globally: (1) tuberculous meningitis, (2) bacterial meningitis, (3) herpes simplex encephalitis, (4) Japanese encephalitis, (5) neurocysticercosis, and (6) cerebral malaria. We drew primarily on existing systematic reviews and randomized controlled trials (RCTs), identified by the search strategy outlined in Table 16.1.

Critical review of the evidence for each question

1. Tuberculous meningitis

Does the use of adjunctive corticosteroids improve mortality or disability in adults or children with tuberculous meningitis?

Tuberculous meningitis (TBM) is caused by *Mycobacterium tuberculosis*, and results in death or severe neurological deficits in more than half of those affected, despite antituberculosis (anti-TB) chemotherapy [6,7]. Clinical features include

Table 16.1 Search strategy.

Search strategy for identification of studies
We attempted to identify all relevant studies regardless of language or publication status (published, unpublished, in press, and in progress).

Databases
We searched the following databases:
• Cochrane Infectious Diseases Group Specialized Register (September 2005).
• Cochrane Central Register of Controlled Trials (CENTRAL), published in *The Cochrane Library* (Issue 3, 2005).
• MEDLINE (1966 to September 2005).
• EMBASE (1974 to September 2005).
• LILACS (1982 to September 2005).

The following strategy was used to search all databases:
(meningitis OR encephalitis OR cerebral OR brain malaria OR neurocysticerc*) AND (steroid* OR corticosteroid* OR hydrocortisone OR dexamethasone OR prednisolone OR glucocorticoid* OR methylpredniso*).

To identify RCTs, this search was combined with the Cochrane Highly Sensitive Search Strategy as contained in the Cochrane Reviewers' Handbook (Higgins 2005).

headache, fever, vomiting, photophobia, anorexia, neck stiffness; sometimes patients are confused, have limb weakness, cranial nerve palsies, seizures or coma [8]. The modified British Medical Research Council clinical criteria allow grading for TBM severity [9]. (Grade I: Alert and orientated without focal neurological deficit. Grade II: Glasgow coma score (GCS) 14–10 with or without focal neurological deficit or GCS 15 with focal neurological deficit. Grade III: GCS less than 10, with or without focal neurological deficit.)

Most clinicians would follow a pragmatic model of TB treatment based on short course chemotherapy for pulmonary TB with an 'intensive phase' four drug phase, followed by two drug 'continuation phase' [10,11]. The first 2 months of treatment should be with isoniazid, rifampicin, pyrazinamide, and either streptomycin, ethambutol, or ethionamide. Pyridoxine should be given with isoniazid. In general 9–12 months of treatment is required. Isoniazid and rifampicin with or without pyrazinamide are continued in the continuation phase. Use of adjunctive corticosteroids was suggested since 1953 but has remained controversial and its use restricted to more severe stage of illness [5].

We found one Cochrane Review conducted in 2000 (with six RCTs) and one recent large RCT [12–19]. The recent trial meets the inclusion criteria of the Cochrane Review so we have therefore added the recent trial [19] to the meta-analysis. Seven trials of 1140 patients met the inclusion criteria. Most trials were recent [13–17,19] but one older study conducted in the 1960s also qualified for inclusion [12]. Trials assessed the effects of steroids in young children [16], adults [14,15,17,19], or both [12,13]. All studies used the British Medical Research Council staging system to assess baseline severity [9,16,17]. Two studies included only patients with stage II and III disease while the rest included patients with all stages of severity [16,17]. The anti-TB drug regimen varied. One study was conducted before the advent of rifampicin and pyrazinamide [12]. A four drug regimen was used in only four studies [15–17,19]. The corticosteroid used in the different studies was dexamethasone [8,12–14,17] and prednisolone [15,16]. The dosages of the corticosteroids varied. For dexamethasone the initial starting doses were around 0.4 mg/kg. This was then tapered gradually. Prednisolone was used in two studies in doses ranging from 60 mg/day to 4 mg/kg/day in divided doses .The duration of steroid usage varied from 4 to 8 weeks. Most studies used a gradually reducing dosage to completely stop the steroids. Death was reported in all six trials and residual neurological deficit in all studies except two [12,17].

Death: Across all trials steroids appeared to be protective in both children and adults (relative risk (RR) 0.78, 95% confidence interval (CI) 0.67–0.91, seven trials, $n = 1140$; Figure 16.1). This appeared to be similar in both adults and children (trials with mostly children: RR 0.77, 95% CI 0.62–0.96; trials of adults: RR 0.79, 95% CI 0.64–0.98). We explored whether the effect varied with disease severity. As data available for stage I patients were sparse, data for stages I and II (mild and moderately severe disease, respectively) were combined for comparison with stage III (severe) disease. One trial [17] was excluded as it did not stratify by stage. Steroids were associated with fewer deaths in both categories, and the effect was significant in both mild–moderate disease, and severe disease (Figure 16.2). For patients with HIV, there is the potential that steroids could do more harm than good. Only one trial addressed this [19]; none of the patients were on antiretroviral drugs, with a trend towards improvement, which was not statistically significant. The numbers of HIV-infected patients were small, and so there is insufficient

Comparison: Any steroid vs control
Outcome: Death

Study or sub-category	Treatment n/N	Control n/N	RR (fixed) 95% CI	Weight %	RR (fixed) 95% CI
O'Toole 1969	6/11	9/12		3.73	0.73 [0.39, 1.37]
Girgis 1991	72/145	79/135		35.44	0.85 [0.68, 1.05]
Kumarvelu 1994	5/20	7/21		2.96	0.75 [0.28, 1.98]
Chotmongkol 1996	5/29	2/30		0.85	2.59 [0.54, 12.29]
Schoeman 1997	4/67	13/67		5.63	0.31 [0.11, 0.90]
Lardizabal 1998	4/29	6/29		2.60	0.67 [0.21, 2.12]
Thwaites 2004	87/274	112/271		48.79	0.77 [0.61, 0.96]
Total (95% CI)	575	565		100.00	0.78 [0.67, 0.91]

Total events: 183 (Treatment), 228 (Control)
Test for heterogeneity: Chi^2 = 5.89, df = 6 (P = 0.44), I^2 = 0%
Test for overall effect: Z = 3.24 (P = 0.001)

0.01 01 1 10 100

Figure 16.1 Meta-analysis of seven RCTs including 1140 patients comparing any corticosteroids + antituberculous treatment versus control + antituberculous treatment with death as the outcome. The overall results show a beneficial effect of steroids. From [18] © Cochrane Collaboration, with permission.

Comparison: Any steroid vs control stratified by severity
Outcome: Death

Study or sub-category	Treatment n/N	Control n/N	RR (fixed) 95% CI	Weight %	RR (fixed) 95% CI
Stage I (mild) or stage II (moderately severe)					
O'Toole 1969	3/7	5/8		2.05	0.69 [0.25, 1.88]
Girgis 1991	10/48	20/50		8.61	0.52 [0.27, 1.00]
Kumarvelu 1994	5/21	5/18		2.87	0.86 [0.29, 2.49]
Chotmongkol 1996	1/23	0/26		0.21	3.38 [0.14, 79.00]
Schoeman 1997	1/30	1/31		0.48	1.03 [0.07, 15.78]
Thwaites 2004	53/213	76/211		33.56	0.69 [0.51, 0.93]
Subtotal 95% CI	342	344		47.22	0.68 [0.53, 0.88]
Total events: 73 (Treatment), 107 (Control)					
Test for heterogeneity: Chi² = 1.93, df = 5 (P = 0.86), I² = 0%					
Test for overall effect: Z = 2.99 (P = 0.003)					
03 Stage III (severe)					
O'Toole 1969	3/4	4/4		1.76	0.76 [0.45, 1.32]
Girgis 1991	62/97	59/85		27.64	0.92 [0.76, 1.13]
Kumarvelu 1994	0/3	2/4		0.98	0.26 [0.02, 3.86]
Chotmongkol 1996	4/6	2/4		1.06	1.33 [0.45, 4.13]
Schoeman 1997	3/24	12/24		5.27	0.26 [0.08, 0.78]
Thwaites 2004	34/62	36/60		16.08	0.91 [0.67, 1.24]
Subtotal (95% CI)	196	181		52.78	0.84 [0.71, 0.99]
Total events: 108 (Treatment), 115 (control)					
Test for heterogeneity Chi² = 6.98, df = 5 (P = 0.22), I² = 28.4%					
Test for overall effect: Z = 2.02 (P = 0.04)					
Total (95% CI)	538	525		100.00	0.77 [0.66, 0.89]
Total events: 179 (Treatment), 222 (control)					
Test for heterogeneity: Chi² = 12.48, df = 11 (P = 0.33), I² = 11.9%					
Test for overall effect: Z = 3.60 (P = 0.0003)					

0.001 0.01 0.1 1 10 100 1000

Figure 16.2 Meta-analysis of seven RCTs comparing any corticosteroids + antituberculous treatment versus control + antituberculous treatment with death as the outcome, stratified according to stage of disease. From [18] © Cochrane Collaboration, with permission.

information to confirm or reject confidently a treatment effect. These results may not be generalizable to populations with access to antiretroviral drugs.

Death combined with long-term disability: Three trials measured residual neurological disability as an outcome. The effect of steroids on number of patients dying combined with the number with long-term disability suggested benefit, but significance was marginal (pooled RR 0.82, 95% CI 0.70–0.97, three trials, $n = 720$). In the largest study no benefit was seen (RR 0.89, 95% CI 0.75–1.07) [19].

Our interpretation

Adjunctive treatment with dexamethasone improves survival in TBM in adults and children at any stage of disease. The impact on long-term disability is less clear. So it is unclear whether survivors are more likely to be severely disabled. The benefits of treatment with steroids in those infected with HIV are not clearly established.

2. Acute bacterial meningitis

Do corticosteroids improve mortality or disability in adults with acute bacterial meningitis?

Acute bacterial meningitis (ABM) is a dangerous illness and an important cause of death and disability worldwide, even

when the best antibiotic therapy is given. The common microbes in ABM in adulthood are *Neisseria meningitides* and *Streptococcus pneumoniae*, which cause 80–85% of all cases [20,21]. *Haemophilus influenzae* is also important in developing countries, but less so in countries where there is routine vaccination. Fatality rates in patients with meningitis caused by these are 10% and 26%, respectively [20]. Those adults with good recovery after pneumococcal meningitis are at substantial risk for cognitive deficits [22]. The clinical features and management are outlined elsewhere and is beyond the scope of this chapter [23–25].

The role of steroids in the treatment of ABM is controversial. In animals, disease outcome is correlated with severity of the inflammatory response in the subarachnoid space. In animals, treatment with steroids reduces inflammation in the subarachnoid space, and this provides the rationale for trials of steroids in humans [3,4]. Research in children suggests some protective effect: In children, two different meta-analyses or RCTs suggest benefit of steroids on severe hearing loss in *Haemophilus influenzae* type b meningitis [26,27]. A third meta-analysis showed dexamethasone to be protective for severe hearing loss in children with pneumococcal meningitis in the subgroup of children who received corticosteroids before or with the first dose of antibiotics; no beneficial effect was found for patients with meningococcal meningitis [28]. The role in adults has been less clear and has only recently been summarized [21].

Two systematic reviews were identified [21,29], one a Cochrane Review in 2003, the second by the same authors published in 2004 with an additional recent trial [30]. We identified no further relevant trials, and have used the 2004 review here [21]. Five eligible trials involving 623 patients [11,30–33] were included in the meta-analysis. Two trials were neither placebo controlled nor double blinded [11,32]. In one study, patients older than 12 years were considered adults [32]. Dexamethasone was used in five trials in 3–7-day regimens and dosages ranged from 16 to 40 mg daily; one study used hydrocortisone [31]. The study medication was started before or with the first dose of antibiotics in two studies [30,32]; in two other studies it was given after the first dose [11,33]. For one study the protocol required that therapy with steroids or placebo be instituted at the time that antibacterial agents were first instituted, or at the time that a major change in antibacterial therapy occurred [31]. Several antibiotic regimens were used. In two studies a sample size calculation was given [30,33] but an intention-to-treat analysis was available for only one study [30]. For the remaining studies only per-protocol data could be ascertained. Mortality rates in the studies ranged from 11% to 45%. Definitions of adverse events varied and the numbers of events were calculated for each study. There could have been selection bias and patient withdrawal in some studies which might affect the results [21]. The results are summarized in Table 16.1.

Death: Fewer patients died in the steroid group (12%) compared with placebo (22%) (RR 0.6, 95% CI 0.4–0.8, five trials, 623 patients) (Table 16.1). The absolute reduction in risk of a fatal outcome was 10%. Stratifying the analysis by causative organism (pneumococcal, meningococcal, and other) was associated in different baseline mortality but effect sizes for steroids were similar.

Neurological disability: Neurological sequelae (defined as one or more focal neurological deficits including hearing loss and epilepsy not present before meningitis onset) could be analysed in three studies, including 340 patients [11,30,33]. The proportion of patients with neurological sequelae was smaller in the steroid group (26 of 184) (14%) than in the placebo group (35 of 156) (22%), bordering on statistical significance (RR 0.6, 95% CI 0.4–1.0, $P = 0.05$) (Table 16.2). Subgroup analysis by causative organisms did not show a significant benefit for patients treated with steroids.

Adverse events: Adverse events were reported in 391 patients and occurred similarly in the treatment and placebo group (RR 1.0, 95% CI 0.5–2, $P = 0.9$). Gastrointestinal bleeding occurred in 2 of 202 (1%) patients in the steroid group and 7 of 189 (4%) in the placebo group.

Our interpretation

Use or not? Steroids appear to be of benefit in bacterial meningitis. Though methodological and design flaws of some studies included in the analysis diminished the reliability of results, the consistency and degree of benefit identified and the presence of one large well-performed clinical trial merit early steroid therapy in most adults with suspected ABM.

Trials have been in selected patients. It may be that the benefits seen in people with meningitis uncomplicated by other

Table 16.2 Summary of outcomes in trials of corticosteroids in tuberculous meningitis and in acute bacterial meningitis.

Types of study (reference)	Intervention	Outcome	Number of patients (number of trials)	Control group risk (range)	Relative risk (95% CI)	Absolute risk reduction	Comment
SR [18] RCT [19]	**Corticosteroids with ATT** (DM 4 mg/kg or prednisolone 20–60 mg/day from 4 to 8 weeks) versus	Death	1140 (7)	40% (19–75)	0.78 (0.67–0.91)	8%	Corticosteroids better NNT = 12
	ATT (with or without placebo)	Death or disability	720 (3)		0.82 (0.70–0.97)		Corticosteroids better Marginal significance
SR [21]	**Corticosteroids with antibiotics** (DM 16–40 mg/day from 3 to 7 days) versus	Death	623 (5)	22% (15–46)	0.6 (0.4–0.81)	10%	Corticosteroids better NNT = 10
	Antibiotics (with or without placebo)	Neurological disability	340 (3)	22%	0.6 (0.4–1.0)	8%	Corticosteroids better Marginal significance

ATT: antituberculous treatment; DM: dexamethasone; NNT: numbers needed to treat; ns: not statistically significant; SR: systematic review.

medical conditions will be modified in other settings, and so policies for the following groups of patients are uncertain and potentially harmful: those who have already received parenteral antimicrobial therapy, those in septic shock, post-neurosurgical meningitis, immunosuppressed patients, haematological malignancy, and those on immunosuppressive therapy.

Duration: It is unclear what the minimum duration of steroid therapy should be. Although one study has shown a 2- and 4-day regimen of dexamethasone to be similarly effective in childhood bacterial meningitis, the 4-day regimen has been used in most clinical trials [34].

Timing: Starting steroids before or with the first dose of parenteral antibiotics appear more effective than starting after the first dose of antibiotics [28,29]. Although it is possible that benefit may still occur, the maximum allowable delay after parenteral antibiotics is not clear. For patients admitted in a late stage of disease adjuvant steroids are less protective and might even be harmful [35]. Also a large controlled trial in children with bacterial meningitis that included mainly children who began treatment late showed no beneficial effect of adjunctive steroid therapy [36].

3. Herpes simplex encephalitis
Do corticosteroids reduce mortality or disability in HSE?

Herpes simplex encephalitis(HSE) is the most commonly diagnosed cause of severe sporadic encephalitis in the Western world with an estimated incidence of about 1 person in 250,000 to 500,000 people per year [37]. Ninety per cent of HSE is due to herpes simplex virus-1 (HSV-1) the rest is mainly due to HSV-2 [38]. The majority of HSV-1, encephalitis cases result from reactivation of latent infection [39]. Untreated the mortality is in excess of 70%, and only about 2.5% of patients overall regain normal neurological function [37]. The prognosis is better when antiviral therapy is initiated relatively early in the course of disease. A recent study showed a favourable outcome in 65% of patients (55 of 85) and complete recovery in 14% (12 of 85) [40]. Young patients (<30 years old) also have a more favourable outcome than older patients. Treatment initiated after consciousness is severely impaired is unlikely to result in a good clinical outcome [41]. Even with appropriate aciclovir therapy, only 38% of patients had mild or no neurological impairment [42]. Persistent cognitive and memory impairment, aphasia, and motor deficits are common sequelae. Aciclovir is the standard treatment for HSE. With aciclovir therapy (10 mg/kg every 8h) the mortality of HSE was reduced from 70% to 28% [41,42]. Therapy with aciclovir was continued for 10 days in this study. However, because of subsequent recognition of recurrent (or relapse) HSE, there has been a trend to extend therapy for a total of 14–21 days. The role of corticosteroids is much less certain. The benefit of combining aciclovir with methylprednisolone as opposed to aciclovir alone has been suggested by mice models [43].

No systematic reviews or RCTs were found. A multivariate analysis of a case series of 45 patients showed that a poor outcome was associated with older age group, duration to initiation of aciclovir, and no administration of corticosteroids [44]; 22/45 patients had been given steroids. Corticosteroids were administered at the same time as the initiation of aciclovir treatment. Dexamethasone was given to 82% of patients and prednisolone to 18%. The initial dosage of corticosteroid, converted to the dosage of prednisolone, ranged from 40 to 96 mg/day (mean 64.6 mg/day; median 64 mg/day). The duration of corticosteroid treatment ranged from 2 days to 6 weeks (mean 13.6 days; median 6.0 days), during which time the corticosteroid dosage was tapered off gradually when it had been administered for more than 7 days.

Our interpretation
There is insufficient data to support the routine use of steroids in HSE outside of the context of a randomized comparison against placebo.

4. Japanese encephalitis
Do corticosteroids improve disability or mortality in adults or children with Japanese encephalitis?

Japanese encephalitis (JE) is caused by the flavivirus JE virus. JE has grown as a problem in the last 50 years because of its geographical spread and increased incidence. There are approximately 50,000 cases and 15,000 deaths annually [45]. The clinical features of JE virus infection range from a nonspecific flu-like illness to a severe and often fatal meningoencephalomyelitis. JE typically presents after a few days of febrile illness, followed by headache, vomiting, and drowsiness often accompanied seizures. Extrapyramidal features may then set in [46]. Convulsions occur frequently in JE and are reported in up to 85% of children and 10% of adults [47]. Multiple or prolonged seizures and status epilepticus (especially subtle motor status epilepticus) are also associated with a poor prognosis [48]. A subgroup of JE patients presented with a polio-like acute flaccid paralysis presentation [49]. About 30% of hospitalized patients with JE die. Half the survivors have disabling neurological sequelae. Improvement in medical care may improve mortality rates but increase the number of patients with sequale [45] which include mixture of upper and lower motor neurone weakness, and cerebellar and extrapyramidal signs [50]. There is no specific antiviral treatment for JE. Nitric oxide, ribavirin, and interferon alpha have been effective in vitro or in animal models [51,52]. Interferon alpha has also been assessed in a randomized placebo controlled trial in humans but it did not improve the outcome [53]. Nursing care and physiotherapy are needed to reduce the risk of bedsores, malnutrition, and contractures. Symptomatic management of seizures and raised intracranial pressure are often needed.

No systematic review was identified. One RCT was identified [54]. Sixty-five patients presenting in Thailand to four hospitals with a diagnosis of acute JE were randomized in a double-masked fashion and stratified by initial mental status into a placebo group (saline) or a treatment group (dexamethasone 0.6 mg/kg intravenously as a loading dose followed by 0.2 mg/kg every 6 h for 5 days). Fifty-five of the 65 had confirmed JE as demonstrated by detection of virus or by JE virus-specific immunoglobulin M (IgM) antibody. The number of deaths were similar (24%, treatment group; 27%, control group), as were other outcomes: days to alert mental status (3.9 versus 6.2), and neurological status 3 months after discharge (45% abnormal in each group). No statistically significant benefit of high-dose dexamethasone could be detected.

Our interpretation

In one small RCT no obvious effect was detected, but the trial was too small to exclude moderate effects (beneficial or harmful) of steroids in this condition.

5. Cerebral malaria

Do corticosteroids reduce illness and death in children or adults or children with cerebral malaria?

Malaria is the most important of the parasitic diseases of humans affecting about 5% of the world's population at any time and causes between 0.5 and 2.5 million deaths each year [55]. There are four species of human malaria, but *Plasmodium falciparum* which causes cerebral malaria accounts for most of the deaths and neurological complications [55,56]. Cerebral malaria is a diffuse febrile encephalopathy in which focal neurological signs are relatively unusual. There may be coma, signs of meningeal irritation, and seizures. Multi-system dysfunction, with anaemia, jaundice, metabolic acidosis, hypoglycaemia, renal failure, pulmonary acidosis, retinal haemorrhages, and shock may occur [56,57]. Mortality of adult cerebral malaria is about 20%. Mortality is correlated with complications, such as acute renal failure and metabolic acidosis. Good intensive care appears to reduce mortality [56,58]. Drug therapy is summarized elsewhere and is based on parenteral artemesinin derivatives where available, or quinine [59,56].

One Cochrane Review containing two RCTs was identified [60–62]; no additional RCTs were identified; the two trials were in children and adults, with a total of 143 patients [60]. One was conducted in Thailand [62]. The second study was done in Indonesia [61]. Quality of allocation concealment was unclear in the Thai study, but both were reported as double blind. Both arms were treated with the same antimalarial regimen, which was IV infusion of quinine given 8 hourly. One study used a loading dose of quinine [61]. IV dexamethasone was the corticosteroid used in both studies. Steroid treatment was given only for the first 48 h. The doses given were different. In the Thai study, the intended total dose was 2 mg/kg, compared with 11.4 mg/kg in the Indonesia study.

Death: No difference in the number of deaths was detected between steroid and control groups in both studies (RR 0.89; 95% CI 0.48–1.68) (Figure 16.3).

Disability: neither study followed up beyond discharge from hospital, so effects of steroids on residual deficits at 3–6 months are unknown.

Life-threatening complications: the occurrence of complications was higher in the steroid group than in the control (steroid group, 27/50; control group, 17/50) with a RR of 1.59 (95% CI 1.0–2.52). More specifically gastrointestinal bleeding and seizures were significantly more in the steroid-treated groups in both studies. In one study pneumonia occurred

Review: Corticosteroids for treating cerebral malaria
Comparison: Dexamethasone vs placebo
Outcome: Death in hospital

Study or sub-category	Corticosteroid n/N	Placebo n/N	RR (fixed) 95% CI	Weight (%)	RR (fixed) 95% CI
Warrell 1982	8/50	9/50		56.83	0.89 [0.37, 2.12]
Hoffman 1988	6/21	7/22		43.17	0.90 [0.36, 2.23]
Total (95% CI)	71	72		100.00	0.89 [0.48, 1.68]

Total events: 14 (Corticosteroid), 16 (Placebo)
Test for heterogeneity: Chi^2 = 0.00, df = 1 (P = 0.99), I^2 = 0%
Test for overall effect: Z = 0.35 (P = 0.72)

0.1 0.2 0.5 1 2 5 10

Favours steroid   Favours placebo

Figure 16.3 Meta-analysis of two RCTs comparing any corticosteroids + quinine versus control + quinine with death as the outcome. From Prasad et al. [60] © Cochrane Collaboration, with permission.

more in the intervention group (7/50 compared with 1/50) [62]. However the authors of the systematic review accept that interpreting data of side effects from the studies was difficult.

Our interpretation

There is insufficient evidence for the use of corticosteroids in cerebral malaria. From the incomplete data available it seems to do more harm than good.

6. Neurocysticercosis

Do corticosteroids improve seizures or lesion resolution in adults or children with neurocysticercosis?

Neurocysticercosis (NCC) remains endemic in most low-income countries, where it is one of the most common causes of acquired epilepsy [63]. WHO has calculated that over 50,000 deaths are due to NCC each year, and many times this number of people have active epilepsy [64]. A seroprevalence of 8–12% of the population in some regions of Latin America indicates systemic contact with the parasite at some time [65]. Human NCC is caused by ingestion of eggs of the tapeworm *Taenia solium*, excreted in the faeces of an individual carrying the parasite. NCC can be categorized broadly into parenchymal (inside brain substance) or extraparenchymal (outside the brain substance, e.g. in the subarachnoid space). These two groups differ in modes of presentation and treatment [66]. Seizures occur in up to 70% of patients [67]. Patients may also present with intracranial hypertension due to hydrocephalus, related to arachnoiditis, granular ependymitis, ventricular cysts, or cysticercotic encephalitis [68]. The treatment of NCC should be individualized based on the location, stage, number and size of the lesions [66,69].

Therapy when needed is with antiepileptic, antiparasitic drugs, steroids, and neurosurgical interventions and is summarized elsewhere [66,69]. The roles of antiparasitic drugs and steroids are controversial. A Cochrane Systematic Review (2000) that aimed to assess the effect of drug treatment concluded that there was insufficient evidence to assess whether treatment with antihelmintic drugs is associated with beneficial results in NCC [70]. Several randomized trials have since been published that suggest benefit from antiparasitic treatment in parenchymal NCC and has been summarized recently [66]. Steroids are commonly administered in NCC on the premise that they reduce inflammation and oedema around dying cysts (either spontaneously or with treatment) and are also recommended for treatment of large subarachnoid cysts, arachnoiditis, angitis, ependymiitis, and cysticercotic encephalitis [66,67,71]. However, the dose, duration, forms, mode, and, most importantly, timing of administration of corticosteroids are not clear.

Extraparenchymal neurocysticercosis: We found no trials that looked specifically at the effect of steroids on extraparenchymal NCC.

Parenchymal neurocystercosis: Several trials examined albendazole in combination with steroids compared with placebo [72–74] but only two trials randomized patients to receive or not receive steroids [73,75].

One open-label trial by Mall et al. randomized 97 patients with new-onset seizures and a single enhancing computed tomography (CT) detected lesion of cysticercosis into two groups: one to receive antiepileptic monotherapy alone (*n* = 48); and the second to receive antiepileptic monotherapy with prednisolone (*n* = 49). No antiparasitic drugs were given; 50% of those enrolled were less than 20 years old. The patients in the steroid group received prednisolone, 1 mg/kg/day for 10 days, followed by tapering over next 4 days. The patients were followed up for 6 months. Repeated CT scans were performed after 1 and 6 months. Simple partial seizure, with or without secondary generalization, was the commonest seizure type encountered. For incidence of seizures up to 6 months, results given in the article are presented ostensibly as a Kaplan–Meier curve, but do not report cumulative incidence, and is therefore difficult to interpret. Follow-up CT scans at 1 and 6 months demonstrated better resolution of CT lesion in the steroid group.

In a second trial in 133 children [73] with focal seizures of recent onset (<3 months) and single small enhancing CT lesions were randomly assigned to receive corticosteroids, albendazole, or both corticosteroids and albendazole for 28 days. CT was done at 3 and 6 months after enrolment in the study. Of the 133 patients enrolled, 23 were lost to follow up. We consider the comparison between albendazole and albendazole plus corticosteroids. At 3 months follow-up disappearance of the lesion on CT scan was noted in 60% in albendazole alone compared with 63% in albendazole plus steroid (*P* > 0.1). At 6 months there again was little change (76% compared with 74% (*P* > 0.1)). Differences in seizure recurrence were not significant.

Our interpretation

If clinicians decide to treat neurocystercosis, they are likely to give an antiparasitic drug and then the question is whether steroids provide additional benefit. Thus the clinical relevance of the first trial, treating only with steroids, is unclear. The second trial does not show an effect of steroids, but was small, so it is not possible to exclude a beneficial or harmful effect. These studies have dealt with parenchymal disease with single CT enhancing lesions. Future randomized trials with antiparasitic treatment given to all patients who are then randomized to steroids or placebo will be needed.

Summary

Over the last 10 years the role of corticosteroids in neurological infection has become clearer beneficial in tubercular meningitis, acute bacterial meningitis, and harmful in cerebral malaria. But it is still early days for its role in neurocysticer-cosis, Japanese encephalitis and herpes simplex encephalitis. Future randomized and blinded trials with antimicrobial treatment given to all patients who are then randomized to steroids or placebo will provide clinically relevant results.

Acknowledgements

We wish to thank Vittoria Lutje for conducting the searches and Katharine Jones for assisting in the meta-analysis. We would also like to thank Peter Kennedy, Richard Johnson, Richard Whitely, and Avindra Nath who have given valuable suggestions.

Disclosures and conflicts of interest

Anu Jacob, Tom Solomon, and Paul Garner have nothing to disclose.

References

1 Feldman S, Behar AJ, Weber D. Experimental tuberculous meningitis in rabbits. 1: Results of treatment with antituberculous drugs separately and in combination with cortisone. *AMA Arch. Pathol.* 1958; **65**(3): 343–54.

2 van der Flier M, Hoppenreijs S, van Rensburg AJ, et al. Vascular endothelial growth factor and blood–brain barrier disruption in tuberculous meningitis. *Pediatr. Infect. Dis. J.* 2004; **23**(7): 608–13.

3 Tauber MG, Khayam-Bashi H, Sande MA. Effects of ampicillin and corticosteroids on brain water content, cerebrospinal fluid pressure, and cerebrospinal fluid lactate levels in experimental pneumococcal meningitis. *J. Infect. Dis.* 1985; **151**(3): 528–34.

4 Scheld WM, Dacey RG, Winn HR, Welsh JE, Jane JA, Sande MA. Cerebrospinal fluid outflow resistance in rabbits with experimental meningitis. Alterations with penicillin and methylprednisolone. *J. Clin. Invest.* 1980; **66**(2): 243–53.

5 Shane SJ, Riley C. Tuberculous meningitis: combined therapy with cortisone and antimicrobial agents. *N. Engl. J. Med.* 1953; **249**(21): 829–34.

6 Girgis NI, Sultan Y, Farid Z, et al. Tuberculosis meningitis, Abbassia Fever Hospital-Naval Medical Research Unit No. 3-Cairo, Egypt, from 1976 to 1996. *Am. J. Trop. Med. Hyg.* 1998; **58**(1): 28–34.

7 Hosoglu S, Geyik MF, Balik I, et al. Predictors of outcome in patients with tuberculous meningitis. *Int. J. Tuberc. Lung. Dis.* 2002; **6**(1): 64–70.

8 Thwaites GE, Tran TH. Tuberculous meningitis: many questions, too few answers. *Lancet Neurol.* 2005; **4**(3): 160–70.

9 British Medical Research Council: Streptomycin treatment of tuberculous meningitis. *BMJ* 1948; (I): 582–97.

10 Centers for Disease Control. Treatment of tuberculosis. *MMWR Recomm. Rep.* 2003; **52**: 1–77.

11 Bhaumik S, Behari M. Role of dexamethasone as adjunctive therapy in acute bacterial meningitis in adults. *Neurol. India* 1998; **46**: 225–8.

12 Otoole RD, GF T, MK M, LH N. Dexamethasone in tuberculous meningitis. *Ann. Int. Med.* 1969; **70** :39–47.

13 Girgis NI, Farid Z, Kilpatrick ME, Sultan Y, Mikhail IA. Dexamethasone adjunctive treatment for tuberculous meningitis. *Pediatr. Infect. Dis. J.* 1991; **10**(3): 179–83.

14 Kumarvelu S, Prasad K, Khosla A, Behari M, Ahuja GK. Randomized controlled trial of dexamethasone in tuberculous meningitis. *Tuber. Lung. Dis.* 1994; **75**(3): 203–7.

15 Chotmongkol V, Jitpimolmard S, Thavornpitak Y. Corticosteroid in tuberculous meningitis. *J. Med. Assoc. Thai.* 1996; **79**(2): 83–90.

16 Schoeman JF, Van Zyl LE, Laubscher JA, Donald PR. Effect of corticosteroids on intracranial pressure, computed tomographic findings, and clinical outcome in young children with tuberculous meningitis. *Pediatrics* 1997; **99**(2): 226–31.

17 Lardizabal D, Roxas A. Dexamethasone as adjunctive therapy in adult patients with probable tuberculous meningitis stage II and III: an open randomised controlled trial. *Philip. J. Neurol.* 1998; **4**: 4–11.

18 Prasad K, Volmink J, Menon G. Steroids for treating tuberculous meningitis. *Cochrane Database Syst. Rev.* 2000; 3: CD00224.

19 Thwaites GE, Nguyen DB, Nguyen HD, et al. Dexamethasone for the treatment of tuberculous meningitis in adolescents and adults. *N. Engl. J. Med.* 2004; **351**(17): 1741–51.

20 Durand ML, Calderwood SB, Weber DJ, et al. Acute bacterial meningitis in adults. A review of 493 episodes. *N. Engl. J. Med.* 1993; **328**(1): 21–8.

21 van de Beek D, de Gans J, McIntyre P, Prasad K. Steroids in adults with acute bacterial meningitis: a systematic review. *Lancet Infect. Dis.* 2004; **4**(3): 139–43.

22 van de Beek D, Schmand B, de Gans J, et al. Cognitive impairment in adults with good recovery after bacterial meningitis. *J. Infect. Dis.* 2002; **186**(7): 1047–52.

23 Heyderman RS. Early management of suspected bacterial meningitis and meningococcal septicaemia in immunocompetent adults – second edition. *J. Infect.* 2005; **50**(5): 373–4.

24 Heyderman RS, Lambert HP, O'Sullivan I, Stuart JM, Taylor BL, Wall RA. Early management of suspected bacterial meningitis and meningococcal septicaemia in adults. *J. Infect.* 2003; **46**(2): 75–7.

25 British, Infection, Society. Early Management of Suspected Bacterial Meningitis and Meningococcal Septicaemia in Immunocompetent adults. http://www.britishinfectionsociety.org/meningitis.html. Second edition ed, 2005.

26 Geiman BJ, Smith AL. Dexamethasone and bacterial meningitis. A meta-analysis of randomized controlled trials. *West J. Med.* 1992; **157**(1): 27–31.

27 Havens PL, Wendelberger KJ, Hoffman GM, Lee MB, Chusid MJ. Orticosteroids as adjunctive therapy in bacterial meningitis. A meta-analysis of clinical trials. *Am. J. Dis. Child.* 1989; **143**(9): 1051–5.

28 McIntyre PB, Berkey CS, King SM, et al. Dexamethasone as adjunctive therapy in bacterial meningitis. A meta-analysis of randomized clinical trials since 1988. *JAMA* 1997; **278**(11): 925–31.

29 van de Beek D, de Gans J, McIntyre P, Prasad K. Corticosteroids in acute bacterial meningitis. *Cochrane Database Syst. Rev.* 2003; 3: CD004305.

30 de Gans J, van de Beek D. Dexamethasone in adults with bacterial meningitis. *N. Engl. J. Med.* 2002; **347**(20): 1549–56.

31 Bennett IL, Finland M, Hamburger M, Kass EH, Lepper M, Waisbren BA. The effectiveness of hydrocortisone in the management of severe infections. *JAMA* 1963; **183**: 462–5.

32 Girgis NI, Farid Z, Mikhail IA, Farrag I, Sultan Y, Kilpatrick ME. Dexamethasone treatment for bacterial meningitis in children and adults. *Pediatr. Infect. Dis. J.* 1989; **8**(12): 848–51.

33 Thomas R, Le Tulzo Y, Bouget J, et al. Trial of dexamethasone treatment for severe bacterial meningitis in adults. Adult Meningitis Steroid Group. *Intens. Care Med.* 1999; **25**(5): 475–80.

34 Syrogiannopoulos GA, Lourida AN, Theodoridou MC, et al. Dexamethasone therapy for bacterial meningitis in children: 2- versus 4-day regimen. *J. Infect. Dis.* 1994; **169**(4): 853–8.

35 Prasad K, Haines T. Dexamethasone treatment for acute bacterial meningitis: how strong is the evidence for routine use? *J. Neurol. Neurosurg. Psychiatr.* 1995; **59**(1): 31–7.

36 Molyneux EM, Walsh AL, Forsyth H, et al. Dexamethasone treatment in childhood bacterial meningitis in Malawi: a randomised controlled trial. *Lancet* 2002; **360**(9328): 211–8.

37 Whitley RJ, Lakeman F. Herpes simplex virus infections of the central nervous system: therapeutic and diagnostic considerations. *Clin. Infect. Dis.* 1995; **20**(2): 414–20.

38 Aurelius E, Johansson B, Skoldenberg B, Forsgren M. Encephalitis in immunocompetent patients due to herpes simplex virus type 1 or 2 as determined by type-specific polymerase chain reaction and antibody assays of cerebrospinal fluid. *J. Med. Virol.* 1993; **39**(3): 179–86.

39 Whitley R, Lakeman AD, Nahmias A, Roizman B. DNA restriction-enzyme analysis of herpes simplex virus isolates obtained from patients with encephalitis. *N. Engl. J. Med.* 1982; **307**(17): 1060–2.

40 Raschilas F, Wolff M, Delatour F, et al. Outcome of and prognostic factors for herpes simplex encephalitis in adult patients: results of a multicenter study. *Clin. Infect. Dis.* 2002; **35**(3): 254–60.

41 Whitley RJ, Soong SJ, Dolin R, Galasso GJ, Ch'ien LT, Alford CA. Adenine arabinoside therapy of biopsy-proved herpes simplex encephalitis. National Institute of Allergy and Infectious Diseases Collaborative Antiviral Study. *N. Engl. J. Med.* 1977; **297**(6): 289–94.

42 Whitley RJ, Alford CA, Hirsch MS, et al. Vidarabine versus acyclovir therapy in herpes simplex encephalitis. *N. Engl. J. Med.* 1986; **314**(3): 144–9.

43 Meyding-Lamade UK, Oberlinner C, Rau PR, et al. Experimental herpes simplex virus encephalitis: a combination therapy of acyclovir and glucocorticoids reduces long-term magnetic resonance imaging abnormalities. *J. Neurovirol.* 2003; **9**(1): 118–25.

44 Kamei S, Sekizawa T, Shiota H, et al. Evaluation of combination therapy using aciclovir and corticosteroid in adult patients with herpes simplex virus encephalitis. *J. Neurol. Neurosurg. Psychiatr.* 2005; **76**(11): 1544–9.

45 Solomon T. Viral encephalitis in Southeast Asia. *Neurol. Infect. Epidemiol.* 1997; **2**: 191–9.

46 Solomon T, Dung NM, Kneen R, Gainsborough M, Vaughn DW, Khanh VT. Japanese encephalitis. *J. Neurol. Neurosurg. Psychiatr.* 2000; **68**(4): 405–15.

47 Dickerson RB, Newton JR, Hansen JE. Diagnosis and immediate prognosis of Japanese B encephalitis. *Am. J. Med.* 1952; **12**: 277–88.

48 Solomon T, Dung NM, Kneen R, et al. Seizures and raised intracranial pressure in Vietnamese patients with Japanese encephalitis. *Brain* 2002; **125**(Pt 5): 1084–93.

49 Solomon T, Kneen R, Dung NM, et al. Poliomyelitis-like illness due to Japanese encephalitis virus. *Lancet* 1998; **351**(9109): 1094–7.

50 Richter R, Shimojyo S. Neurologic sequelae of Japanese B encephalitis. *Neurology* 1961; **11**: 553–9.

51 Saxena SK, Singh A, Mathur A. Antiviral effect of nitric oxide during Japanese encephalitis virus infection. *Int. J. Exp. Pathol.* 2000; **81**(2): 165–72.

52 Solomon T, Vaughn D. Pathogenesis and clinical features of Japanese encephalitis and West Nile infections. In: Deubel V, ed., *Current Topics in Microbiology and Immunology: Japanese Enecphalitis and West Nile Virus Infections.* Springer-Verlag, 2002: pp. 171–94.

53 Solomon T, Dung NM, Wills B, et al. Interferon alfa-2a in Japanese encephalitis: a randomised double-blind placebo-controlled trial. *Lancet* 2003; **361**(9360): 821–6.

54 Hoke Jr CH, Vaughn DW, Nisalak A, et al. Effect of high-dose dexamethasone on the outcome of acute encephalitis due to Japanese encephalitis virus. *J. Infect. Dis.* 1992; **165**(4): 631–7.

55 Newton CR, Krishna S. Severe falciparum malaria in children: current understanding of pathophysiology and supportive treatment. *Pharmacol. Ther.* 1998; **79**(1): 1–53.

56 Newton CR, Hien TT, White N. Cerebral malaria. *J. Neurol. Neurosurg. Psychiatr.* 2000; **69**(4): 433–41.

57 White NJ, Looareesuwan S. Cerebral malaria. In: Kennedy PGE, Johnson RI, ed. *Infections of the Nervous System.* Butterworths, London, 1987: pp. 118–43.

58 Warrell DA, Molyneux ME, Beales PF. Severe and complicated malaria. *Trans. R. Soc. Trop. Med. Hyg.* 1990; **84**(Suppl. 2): 1–65.

59 World Health Organization. *Guidelines for Treating Uncomplicated and Severe Malaria.* WHO Malaria Technical Guidelines Group. WHO, Geneva, 2006.

60 Prasad K, Garner P. Steroids for treating cerebral malaria. *Cochrane Database Syst. Rev.* 1999; 3: DOI: 10.1002/14651858. CD000972.

61 Hoffman SL, Rustama D, Punjabi NH, et al. High-dose dexamethasone in quinine-treated patients with cerebral malaria: a double-blind, placebo-controlled trial. *J. Infect. Dis.* 1988; **158**(2): 325–31.

62 Warrell DA, Looareesuwan S, Warrell MJ, et al. Dexamethasone proves deleterious in cerebral malaria. A double-blind trial in 100 comatose patients. *N. Engl. J. Med.* 1982; **306**(6): 313–9.

63 Garcia HH, Gonzalez AE, Evans CA, Gilman RH. Taenia solium cysticercosis. *Lancet* 2003; **362**(9383): 547–56.

64 Roman G, Sotelo J, Del Brutto O, et al. A proposal to declare neurocysticercosis an international reportable disease. *Bull. World Health Organ.* 2000; **78**(3): 399–406.

65 Goodman KA, Ballagh SA, Carpio A. Case-control study of seropositivity for cysticercosis in Cuenca, Ecuador. *Am. J. Trop. Med. Hyg.* 1999; **60**(1): 70–4.

66 Garcia HH, Del Brutto OH. Neurocysticercosis: updated concepts about an old disease. *Lancet Neurol.* 2005; **4**(10): 653–61.

67 Del Brutto OH, Santibanez R, Noboa CA, Aguirre R, Diaz E, Alarcon TA. Epilepsy due to neurocysticercosis: analysis of 203 patients. *Neurology* 1992; **42**(2): 389–92.

68 Estanol B, Kleriga E, Loyo M, et al. Mechanisms of hydrocephalus in cerebral cysticercosis: implications for therapy. *Neurosurgery* 1983; **13**(2): 119–23.

69 Carpio A. Neurocysticercosis: an update. *Lancet Infect. Dis.* 2002; **2**(12): 751–62.

70 Salinas R, Prasad K. Drugs for treating neurocysticercosis (tapeworm infection of the brain). *Cochrane Database Syst. Rev.* 2000; 2: Oxford: Update Software, CD000215.

71 Woo E, Yu YL, Huang CY. Cerebral infarct precipitated by praziquantel in neurocysticercosis – a cautionary note. *Trop. Geogr. Med.* 1988; **40**(2): 143–6.

72 Kalra V, Dua T, Kumar V. Efficacy of albendazole and short-course dexamethasone treatment in children with 1 or 2 ring-enhancing lesions of neurocysticercosis: a randomized controlled trial. *J. Pediatr.* 2003; **143**(1): 111–4.

73 Singhi P, Jain V, Khandelwal N. Corticosteroids versus albendazole for treatment of single small enhancing computed tomographic lesions in children with neurocysticercosis. *J. Child. Neurol.* 2004; **19**(5): 323–7.

74 Garcia HH, Pretell EJ, Gilman RH, et al. A trial of antiparasitic treatment to reduce the rate of seizures due to cerebral cysticercosis. *N. Engl. J. Med.* 2004; **350**(3): 249–58.

75 Mall RK, Agarwal A, Garg RK, Kar AM, Shukla R. Short course of prednisolone in Indian patients with solitary cysticercus granuloma and new-onset seizures. *Epilepsia* 2003; **44**(11): 1397–401.

17 CHAPTER 17
Brain tumours

Michael G. Hart, Robin Grant

Background

Brain tumours are a common consideration in the differential diagnosis of many neurological conditions. Their presence often results in a relentless progression of symptoms and disability, often in a young person. They are the most common solid malignancy of childhood, the fourth most common in the under 45 age group, and the eighth most common in the under 65 age group [1]. Overall, brain tumours are the second most common cause of death from neurological disease, after stroke.

Brain tumours can be either primary or secondary. Primary brain tumours are uncommon, and have an incidence of less than 10 per 100,000/year [1]. Gliomas account for the majority of primary brain tumours. Prognosis is determined by clinical and histological criteria. Histological classification and grading are crucial to the understanding of brain tumours and their management, and most commonly follows the World Health Organisation classification [2]. High-grade gliomas (HGG) account for approximately 80% of gliomas and include most commonly glioblastoma multiforme (GBM), anaplastic astrocytoma and anaplastic oligodendrocytoma. They have a poor survival of less than 20% at 5 years, with death usually resulting from expansion of the mass lesion or invasion into vital structures. Low-grade gliomas (LGG) account for approximately 20% of gliomas, and most commonly include astrocytomas, oligodendrocytomas and oligoastrocytomas. Their natural history is to follow a generally more benign course, with between 50% and 80% of patients alive at 5 years. They infiltrate the brain, and usually transform to a higher grade with death resulting from locally aggressive disease [3].

Pre-therapeutic prognostic factors for gliomas are the most important determinants of survival. For HGG, data from three randomized controlled trials (RCTs) identified age over 50 years, GBM on histology, poor performance status (Table 17.1) or abnormal mental status at diagnosis as poor prognostic factors [4]. For LGG two RCTs identified age over 40 years, astrocytoma histology, the presence of clinical neurological deficits, tumour size over 6 cm and tumour crossing the midline (both from computed tomography (CT) scanning) as poor prognostic factors [5]. A subgroup of those patients with LGG who present solely with epilepsy enjoy a much better prognosis [6].

Table 17.1 KPS score (adapted from Karnofsky D, et al. *Cancer* 1948; 1: 634–56).

Score	Description
100	Normal: no complaints; no evidence of disease
90	Able to carry on normal activity; minor symptoms
80	Normal activity with effort; some symptoms
70	Cares for self; unable to carry on normal activities
60	Requires occasional assistance; cares for most needs
50	Requires considerable assistance and frequent care
40	Disabled: requires special care and assistance
30	Severely disabled: hospitalized but death not imminent
20	Very sick: active supportive care needed
10	Moribund: fatal processes are progressing rapidly
0	Dead

Brain metastases are considerably more common than primary brain tumours. Up to 30% of those with systemic cancer will develop brain metastasis [7]. Brain metastases can present either with a confirmed primary tumour, or as the first presentation of disease. The most common primary sites are the lung (50%) and breast (25%), with other primary sites including kidney and melanoma. Previously up to 50% were thought to be single, but with the advent of modern imaging they are now found to be multiple in around three-quarters of patients [8].

Prognostic factors for brain metastasis include age, performance score, the number of brain metastasis, the site of the primary tumour and the activity of any extracranial disease. These variables can be used to stratify patients into prognostic groups, with the best group having a median survival of 13.5 months, and the worst only 2.3 months [9,10].

Patients are usually referred to general physicians or neurologists first. The most common symptom at hospital referral is headache (46.5%) [11]. Further symptoms were present in 86%, and include a mixture of focal signs (hemiparesis, hemisensory symptoms, dysphasia or diplopia) and non-focal symptoms (confusion/memory problems, personality change, visual changes or unsteadiness). Overall, seizures were present in 26.5% of patients, but are much more common in LGG (between 60% and 80% prevalence), where they may also be the sole complaint.

Following the presumptive diagnosis of a brain tumour, management decisions follow an orderly pattern, including the use of:

- *Steroids*: to reduce peri-tumoural oedema and improve symptoms.
- *Surgery*: The first decision is whether surgery should be performed or not, and if the decision is to operate, the second decision is whether diagnostic biopsy or resection should be performed.
- *Radiotherapy*: either as an adjunct to resection or as primary therapy after biopsy.
- *Chemotherapy*: either during primary therapy, either concomitantly or adjuvantly or for recurrence.

The majority of tumours are not curable, and management is geared towards symptomatic relief and increasing survival. With a multitude of treatment options available and almost universally poor results, careful attention to evidence-based practice will result in an optimum balance of symptom relief while avoiding side effects and intensive treatment regimes that may impinge on a vastly shortened life.

An evidence-based medicine approach to management of brain tumours is aided by clear guidelines for grading and interpreting evidence [12]. Phase II studies should simply be considered a step on the way to a well-conducted RCT. With regard to brain tumours, specific questions include whether prognostic stratification was used during randomization: poor prognosis patients do badly regardless of treatment, while it should be no surprise that well-selected good prognosis patients do substantially better, often regardless of treatment. Attention should be paid to the degree of missing data and drop-outs. Outcome measures should pay attention to quality of life outcomes as well as survival. For interpretation to clinical practice, care should be taken in considering how highly selected were the participants, and to what degree they reflect normal clinical practice. Finally, the practicality of the therapeutic approach is also important. Attention to these methodological principles should allow proper interpretation of trials and useful therapeutic application of results.

Formulation of clinical questions

In the management of brain tumours, the application of evidence-based practice required the formulation of specific questions ideally where there is an area of controversy in the management. Literature searching was done using a wide variety of search headings and Boolean operator characteristics. Specific questions were formulated to include the patient, intervention, comparison and outcome:

1 In patients with a clinically suspected brain tumour, what is the best method for diagnosis? [Diagnostic test] Specific outcomes include will sensitivity, specificity, false positives and negatives, predictive value. Trials will be prospective series only.

2 For patients with presumed HGG, should surgery be either biopsy or resection? [Therapy] Lesions will not have been confirmed histologically prior to intervention. Any form of resection or biopsy will be valid. Specific outcomes include survival, symptom relief, quality of life and procedure-related complications. Trials considered will be meta-analyses, RCTs or prospective cohort studies only.

3 In patients with primary or secondary brain tumours, what is the evidence that corticosteroids are more effect than placebo? [Therapy] All lesions must be histologically proven. Interventions are any corticosteroid via any route of administration. Outcomes include survival, quality of life, symptoms and side effects. Trials again will include meta-analyses or RCTs only.

4 For patients with HGG, is radiotherapy an effective treatment, and what should be given? [Therapy] Patients have histologically proven disease. Interventions include radiotherapy of any kind including stereotactic radiosurgery (SRS) and focal techniques. Outcomes include survival, quality of life, symptoms and side effects. Trials again will include meta-analyses or RCTs only.

5 For those with HGG, is chemotherapy an effective treatment? [Therapy] Patients are histologically proven HGG. Interventions include chemotherapy of any nature, including focal techniques. Outcomes include survival, quality of life, symptoms and side effects. Trials again will include meta-analyses or RCTs only.

6 For patients with brain metastasis, what is the optimum regime of therapy, when considering surgery, focal radiotherapy or whose brain radiotherapy (WBRT)? [Therapy] Patients include those with histologically proven or clinically suspected metastasis. Intervention: surgery or radiotherapy (either focal of any kind or WBRT). Outcomes include survival, quality of life, symptoms and side effects. Trials again will include meta-analyses or RCTs only.

Search strategy

A number of different search engines were used to allow the widest range of possible trials to be included, including abstracts and foreign language publications. These databases included Medline, PubMed, Embase, CancerLit, Web of Science and the Cochrane Library.

Search strategies were further specified depending on whether the data sought related to diagnosis (sensitivity, specificity, predictive value) or therapy (randomized, controlled, placebo, blinded).

Critical review of the evidence for each question

1. Diagnosis

What is the best approach to diagnosis of brain tumours?

Diagnosis of a brain tumour will usually be from radiological imaging in the first instance, which may then be followed up by histological confirmation. The accuracy and limitations of radiology in comparison to histology need to be realized in order to determine the best approach to diagnosis for each individual patient. Radiology has the main advantage of being non-invasive, however further specific information from histology may significantly alter treatment and prognosis.

Imaging of a presumed intracranial tumour usually includes CT scanning initially, followed by magnetic resonance imaging (MRI), both with contrast. Neuroradiologists will correctly predict an intracerebral tumour in about 90–95% of cases using CT and MRI [13]. The differential diagnosis of non-contrast enhancing lesions includes demyelination, encephalitis, infarction, vasculitis, post-traumatic and non-specific inflammatory changes. The differential diagnosis in patients with contrast enhancing lesions include demyelination, arterio-venous malformation, haemorrhagic stroke and cerebral abscess. For multiple lesions, the differential diagnosis includes metastases, glioblastoma, primary central nervous system lymphoma or toxoplasmosis.

Radiology may predict tumour grade accurately in up to 74% [14], and algorithms based on contrast enhancement, space occupation, cyst formation, necrosis and oedema to help in predicting the grade of malignancy. Low grade tumours such as astrocytomas and oligodendrogliomas are commonly homogeneous and may be cystic or show areas of calcification and usually do not enhance, whereas high grade tumours such as anaplastic astrocytoma and GBM are generally heterogeneous with cysts or necrosis, commonly demonstrate shift of midline structures with significant oedema and contrast enhancement. In one study, 45% of patients who were suspected of having an astrocytoma had on imaging actually an anaplastic astrocytoma and 5% had a non-malignant histology following biopsy [13]. Grade I astrocytomas; pilocytic astrocytomas, subependymal giant cell astrocytoma and desmoplastic neuro-epithelial tumours can show contrast enhancement and may be misdiagnosed as malignant glioma or metastases. Interpretation of magnetic resonance spectroscopy may fair slightly better but still does not reach the level of diagnostic accuracy as histology [14,15].

Radiological interpretation of suspected tumour type and grade is only moderately reliable. Around 10% of patients will have had a previous image that has been reported as either normal or an alternative pathology (including vascular, abscess or demyelination) [16], with approximately one-third of these false negative scans done without contrast. While this may partly explain the findings, CT scanning without contrast is standard practice for an acute neurological deficit (e.g. transient ischaemic attack, stroke), and up to 30% of anaplastic astrocytomas will not show contrast enhancement [17]. In one study of single brain metastasis, 11% of patients with known systemic malignancy with a solitary brain lesion thought on imaging to be a metastasis turned out to have a different pathology (primary brain tumour or inflammatory tissue) [18]. However, in this study diagnosis involved only CT imaging and

the true incidence of misdiagnosis in current clinical practice with contrast enhanced MRI is likely to be lower. The main areas of difficulty are where tumours have an exophytic extension with involvement of the meninges, intense contrast enhancement or sometimes calcification of meningeal/vascular origin (e.g. meningioma/haemangiopericytoma) or of glial origin (e.g. glioblastoma or oligodendroglioma). In these cases it may be very difficult to say whether the tumour is extracerebral and invading the brain or intrinsic and becoming exophytic. In some cases who present with a stroke-like onset, it may not be evident that the haemorrhage has occurred into an existing mass lesion. The common tumours to present with intratumoural haemorrhage are glioblastoma, metastatic lung cancer, melanoma and choriocarcinoma.

Histology can provide further advantages over imaging. This includes accurate grading and typing of the tumour, and more accurate survival information. Histology also allows genotyping, which may improve accuracy of histological classification (e.g. oligodendroglioma versus astrocytoma), prognostication and management. The diagnosis on histology of certain types of brain tumours, such as germ cell tumours or lymphoma, can lead to specific treatment regimes which may be curative, such as chemotherapy or radiotherapy. In cases where treatment is highly successful requirements for placebo controlled trials are often not appropriate, although RCTs of different modalities of effective therapy may be justified.

Although pathology is the gold standard for diagnosis, there are inter-observer variations in the interpretation of the histology, and surgery can have substantial morbidity and mortality depending on the site of the tumour. Results have to be visually scored or graded and there is inter-observer variation either due to technical or interpretative factors. Concordance rates between experienced neuro-pathologists have been found to be between 81% and 90% [19,20] when histological typing and grading of neuro-epithelial tumours is concerned, and higher when diagnosing other types of brain tumours such as metastasis.

In summary, radiology (especially MRI) is highly accurate in diagnosing a mass or infiltrating lesion as being a tumour. It is less good at defining the nature of the tumour. All patients with adult onset partial epilepsy should have an MRI scan [24]. Histology provides improved accuracy, identification of rare entities requiring specific therapy, as well as further prognostic information and molecular data that can predict response to therapy. Hence surgery should usually be performed. However, radiology is non-invasive, and in poor prognosis patients with severe co-morbidity in which treatment options are limited, this level of accuracy may be considered sufficient.

2. Surgery
Biopsy or resection for HGG?

If it is decided that histology should be pursued, this will involve either sampling through biopsy, or an attempted complete resection of the lesion. In determining the procedure of choice, the potential benefits of resection over biopsy need to be assessed in light of the increased risks of the more invasive resection approach. Hypothesized benefits of resection include improved histological accuracy, improved survival, symptomatic relief and the application of adjuvant therapies. The diffuse infiltrative nature of gliomas decree that resection is rarely complete, and recurrence inevitable; resection therefore is rarely curative. Selection of patients according to prognostic factors may identify groups with median survival ranging from under 5 months to almost 5 years [4].

Previous data from non-randomized retrospective series was used as evidence for the effectiveness of surgery in improving survival. However, these trials are uncontrolled and confounded by selection bias due to their non-randomized nature: they cannot be used to justify the use of surgery over biopsy. A recent Cochrane Review was completed on biopsy versus resection for HGG and found one RCT in the area [21]. In this trial a total of 30 elderly patients were randomized, but due to errors in diagnosis and missing data only 18 patients were assessable. This trial was grossly under-powered to reliably prove an effect, and errors in trial design mean that any conclusions are impossible to apply to clinical practice.

Only prospective analysis with a clear protocol for defining and identifying deficits are valid; you only find what you look for! Analysis from retrospective series is fraught with the hazard of interpreting inadequate recording of results, creating variable definitions of conditions and incomplete data. Due to the aggressive nature of these tumours, many patients will develop new deficits without treatment, and this rate of progression must be controlled for in trials.

Symptomatic relief is a common anecdotal benefit. Only two prospective trials have collected data on symptoms before and after resection. They report that 32% had an improvement in their symptoms, 58–76% were not different, and 9–26% had a worsening [22,23]. Often however such deficits from surgery are temporary. Nevertheless, while neurosurgery can improve some symptoms, it can also create new ones. New operative adjuncts such as functional MRI, intra-operative MRI and intra-operative awake brain mapping are identifying eloquent areas that can be subsequently avoided at operation [24]. None of these techniques have been evaluated in a proper RCT.

Neurological complications following surgery include focal haematoma, abscess and seizures; systemic complications include pneumonia and thromboembolic disease. Morbidity rates range from 11% to 32%, with a mortality rate of 0–20% [22,23].

Biopsy aims to deliver the benefits of tissue diagnosis and allows specific therapies when needed, without the complications associated with more invasive resection. No attempt is made at symptomatic improvement with biopsy. The accuracy of stereotactic biopsy has been confirmed in two prospective series, which have found it provides a diagnosis in 98.5% of patients. However, small samples of tissue risk sampling error due to the heterogenous nature of many brain tumours, containing foci of higher and lower grades. The accuracy of samples from stereotactic biopsy has been analysed in a series of 21 patients who later had open resection. Stereotactic biopsy agreed with the diagnosis in 74% of patients, and correctly guided therapy in 91% [25]. Larger tumours increase this risk of sampling error, which may be reduced by multiple biopsies. Resection provides a larger tissue sample and will allow more complete analysis of the tumour type. The consequences of this are possibly that resection may grade tumours higher than biopsy due to less sampling error. Patients with under-graded tumours may have their treatment deferred which could lead to a poorer outcome. This discrepancy in histological diagnosis between the two techniques can also lead to a confounding variable when assessing survival in any RCT comparing surgery with biopsy for HGG.

Morbidity and mortality are lower with stereotactic biopsy than with resection at craniotomy. The single prospective RCT of biopsy versus resection, although not aimed at assessing morbidity and mortality rates, found no side effects in the 16 patients having biopsy, compared to one post-operative haematoma in the 14 patients undergoing complete resection at craniotomy [26]. A retrospective comparison of 7471 biopsies found a morbidity rate of 3.5% and mortality rate of 0.7% [27].

In practice, biopsy may be the only option for certain deep-seated tumours (thalamic, callosal, brainstem), while small superficially placed frontal tumours can be resected completely with little difficulty. Due to the associated risks of resection, biopsy is currently preferred for those with poor performance status (Karnofsky performance status (KPS) <70), elderly (>60 years), lesions in an eloquent area and diffuse lesions (multi-lobe or multi-focal). In other selected groups of patients the risks of resection may be lower, and there may be a greater likelihood for benefits from surgery. Complete resection is more commonly performed in patients with peripherally situated 'lobar' tumours (frontal), good performance status (KPS > 70), younger (age < 60 years), focal lesions (<3 cm in size).

In summary, histological diagnosis is essential for the management of a suspected brain tumour. There is no good evidence from randomized trials that resection offers any survival advantage over stereotactic biopsy [21]. There is little evidence from prospective trials that resection improves symptoms over that from medical therapy alone (i.e. corticosteroids). While surgery can relieve many symptoms, it can be associated with local or systemic complications. Stereotactic biopsy has a lower risk of focal complications than resection and is an effective tool for histology. However, this procedure is not risk free, and may result in inadequate sampling. The potential benefits and risks of each procedure, which are often not evidence based, need to be considered in determining the most appropriate treatment for an individual. This is best done in the contact of a multi-disciplinary team meeting, where the history, examination, radiology and management plan can be discussed by the complete neuro-oncology team (ref: Nice http://www.nice.org.uk/page.aspx?0=282226). Future trials in this area need to be larger and randomized, with greater attention to symptom profile and quality of life in their outcome analysis.

3. Steroids

Are steroids an effective treatment, and if so how much and for how long?

Most brain tumours are associated with significant surrounding oedema, which is believed to be of vasogenic origin. This is particularly common with HGG and metastasis. This oedema can cause symptoms and have a mass effect with increasing intracranial pressure.

Corticosteroids have a well-documented role in providing control of oedema and symptomatic improvement [28,29], with dexamethasone the preferred option. Although there is a shortage of RCTs for the use of corticosteroids, clinical experience and data from retrospective studies have meant that their role in brain tumours has been established beyond reasonable doubt: it would not be ethically acceptable to randomize symptomatic patients to no steroid treatment in light of the known benefits. In particular, numerous observational studies noted an increase in the average survival for those with brain tumours at the same time as corticosteroids were being introduced in the 1960s. However, side effects are common and a balance needs to be reached with the dose and duration of treatment.

A single RCT found that a dose of 4-mg dexamethasone did not produce statistically significant difference in effect when compared to 8- or 16-mg dexamethasone. The mean improvement in KPS with the 4-mg dose was 6.7 points (SD 11.3), which was present by day 7 and maintained until at least 28 days, when the steroids were tapered off. Up to 50% of patients will show an improvement of 10 points and 17% had an improvement of over 20 points. The baseline KPS for patients entered ranged from 30 to 80.

A dose of 4-mg dexamethasone also had significantly lower rates of proximal myopathy (14% versus 38%) and cushingoid facies (32% versus 69%) than 8 or 16 mg. The prevalence of specific side effects at day 28 with 4-mg dexamethasone were gastric upset 18%, mental changes 14%, infection 9% and hypertension 45%. However, these were not statistically different from day 0, but as only 20 patients were in the 4-mg arm this may be due to a lack of statistical power. Corticosteroids are not commonly given to those without deficits. Deficits that remain following steroid treatment have been suggested to be less likely to improve following surgery, although this has not been convincingly shown in studies. Corticosteroids, enzyme inducing anticonvulsants and chemotherapy agents can affect liver enzyme function and adversely affect the blood levels of each other.

In summary, corticosteroids are an established treatment for symptomatic relief from brain oedema. However, there is a lack of RCTs to prove their effectiveness. Side effects are common and can be significant. Care needs to be taken when withdrawing steroids and in combining them with anticonvulsants or chemotherapy agents. Evidence suggests that a low dose of 4-mg dexamethasone orally for 28 days is as effective as an 8- or 16-mg high-dose regimen in producing symptomatic improvement and also results in fewer side effects.

4. Radiation therapy

Is radiation therapy effective for gliomas and what is the optimum type, dose and schedule?

The overall goal of radiotherapy is to provide adequate radiation to the tumour with minimal damage to the surrounding brain. There is good evidence from two RCTs that radiotherapy improves survival. In the first trial, 303 patients were randomized to receive chemotherapy plus or minus radiotherapy [30]. Those undergoing radiotherapy had a statistically significant survival advantage of 9–10 months compared with 3–4 months with best standard care. A second trial randomized 467 patients and compared chemotherapy, radiotherapy, both or neither following resection [31]. Again a similar survival advantage of around 6 months was found with radiotherapy when compared to best standard care. Subgroup analysis found these effects to be robust throughout prognostic factors. These trials only included patients less than 70 years old, and the application of radiotherapy to those over this age has remained controversial. A recent RCT, presented in abstract form, randomized those over 65 years old with HGG to radiotherapy or best medical care as primary therapy, and found a survival advantage of 2 months with radiotherapy [32].

The dose and schedule characteristics of radiotherapy have also been assessed in RCTs. An RCT comparing whole brain radiotherapy with a coned down boost to the tumour site did not demonstrate a difference in survival over focal radiotherapy [33]. A focal boost of 10 Gy did not confer benefit in further RCT [34]. With the knowledge that the majority of recurrences (80%) occur within 2 cm of the margin of the original lesion [35], radiotherapy focused to the enhancing tumour and a 2–3-cm margin is now the norm to prevent damage to surrounding normal brain. The dose of radiotherapy to be given has been examined in RCTs too. In 474 randomized patients who received surgery, a radiotherapy schedule of 60 Gy in 30 fractions over 6 weeks resulted in a median survival advantage of 3 months (from 9 to 12 months, hazard ratio 0.75) compared with 45 Gy in 20 fractions over 4 weeks without a difference in short-term morbidity; long-term morbidity was not assessed [36]. Variations of dosing schedules have been advocated to increase responsiveness of gliomas to radiotherapy. Hyperfractionation involves multiple small fractions per day for a higher overall dose without increased toxicity, and acceleration involves multiple treatments per day with the same overall dose but reducing overall treatment time. Neither has been robustly shown to improve results, with only one RCT for hyperfractionation. This did not demonstrate any increase in effect from acceleration [37], but the accelerated regime did not show any increase in toxicity and allows treatment to be completed faster [37].

The demonstration that gliomas do respond to radiotherapy led to the development of numerous focal techniques and adjunctive therapies to deliver higher doses to the tumour whilst preserving healthy brain, the tolerance of which is often the limiting factor in treatment. Focal therapies include interstitial brachytherapy [38], neutron therapy [39] and particle (pion) [40] therapy, none of which have found a significant survival advantage. There are no RCTs for Stereotactic Radiosurgery (SRS) in HGG.

Hypoxia within the tumour is believed to limit the efficacy of radiotherapy. Hypoxic radiosensitisers aim to overcome this

Table 17.2 Comparison of RCTs on radiotherapy for high grade gliomas.

Reference	Intervention	No. of patients Histology	Patients characteristics	Median survival time	Comment
Walker et al. [30]	Best conventional care (BCC) versus BCNU versus RT 50–60 Gy in 30 fractions versus BCNU + RT	303 Malignant glioma (Grades III and IV)	Post-operative <65 years	BCC 17 weeks BCNU 25 weeks RT alone 37 weeks BCNU + RT 40 weeks	RT doubles median survival 2-year survival RT alone 1%
Walker et al. [31]	RT versus MeCCNU versus MeCCNU + RT versus BCNU versus BCNU + RT 60 Gy in 30 fractions	467 Malignant glioma (Grades III and IV)	Post-operative <65 years	RT 9 months RT + BCNU 12.3 months RT + MeCCNU 10.8 months	RT more effective than chemotherapy 2-year survival RT 14.1%
Sandberg-Wollheim et al. [65]	PCV alone versus PCV + RT 58 Gy in 27 fractions	171 Malignant glioma (Grades III and IV)	Post-operative	PCV 42 weeks PCV + RT 62 weeks	RT more effective than chemotherapy
Keime-Guibert et al. 2005 [32]	BCC versus RT 50 Gy in 28 fractions	84 Malignant glioma (Grades III and IV)	Post-operative >65 years	BCC 17.8 weeks RT 28.8 weeks Hazard ratio 0.49; $P < 0.001$	Abstract only RT effective even in the elderly
Shapiro et al. [66]	RT 60 Gy versus RT + focal boost (43 + 17 Gy) Multiple chemotherapy arms	571 Malignant glioma (Grades III and IV)	Post-operative	No significant difference in survival	Limit high RT dose to normal brain. Use focal RT rather than WBRT
Bleehen et al. [36]	RT dose 45 Gy (over 4 week) versus 60 Gy (over 6 weeks)	474 Malignant glioma (Grades III and IV)	Post-operative No chemotherapy	45 Gy 9 months versus 60 Gy 12 months Hazard ratio 0.75; $P = 0.007$	2-year survival 28% 60 Gy is now standard
Chang et al. [34]	Focal boost; 60 Gy WBRT + 10 Gy boost to tumour Multiple chemotherapy arms too	626	Post-operative	No significant difference in survival	60 Gy is now standard
Brada et al. [37] RTOG 9006	RT (60 Gy) + BCNU versus hyperfractionated RT (72 Gy) + BCNU	712 Malignant glioma (mainly Grade III)	Post-operative	No significant difference in survival	60 Gy is now standard

RT: radiotherapy; BCC: best conventional care; BCNU: bischloroethylnitrosourea; RT: radiotherapy; CCNU: chloroethylcyclohexylnitrosourea Vincristine; WBRT: whole brain radiotherapy.

difficulty, and although individual RCTs have not demonstrated a benefit, a meta-analysis has demonstrated a 5% better survival for the hypoxic radiosensitiser misonidazole [41]. Hyperbaric oxygen given at time of radiation administration has a similar aim at reducing the resistant effects of hypoxia. A single small pilot RCT did not show a clear effect but was statistically under-powered [42].

Patients with LGG frequently present with epilepsy only and have a good prognosis, and with long-term survival come risks of late radiation toxicity. Therefore radiotherapy schedules are given in a lower total dose (e.g. 54 Gy over 6 weeks) than for HGG. The main question is whether radiotherapy should be given early or later. A single RCT randomized patients to early radiotherapy at surgical diagnosis or at the time of radiological or clinical progression [43]. Early radiotherapy did not improve survival but did lead to a slightly delayed time to progression. The late effects of radiotherapy were not studied. The long-term efficacy study of this trial confirmed that early radiation therapy lengthened the period without progression (5.3 versus 3.4 years), but did not affect median survival (7.4 versus 7.2 years) [49]. Since quality of life was not measured it is not known whether time to progression reflects clinical deterioration. The late effects of radiotherapy were not measured. The issue of early or late radiotherapy remains controversial, but radiotherapy can be deferred for patients with LGG who are in a good condition, provided that they are carefully followed up.

In summary, radiotherapy is an effective primary therapy for HGG (Table 17.2). There is good evidence for a clinically significant improvement in survival, and the specifics of radiotherapy schedules and doses have also been tested. The best evidence in HGG is for a dose of 60 Gy in 30 daily fractions to a localized volume. Side effects from radiotherapy include local scalp irritation, hair loss, somnolence and fatigue in the short term. Late side effects include radiation leuco-encephalopathy (comprising of dementia, incontinence and gait disturbance), although survival is seldom so long in HGG that this becomes an issue. Its effectiveness, ease of administration and acceptable short-term side effects profile make it a standard treatment for most with HGG, however the risk of late damage makes the early use of radiotherapy in LGG less certain.

5. Chemotherapy

Does chemotherapy confer an advantage in HGG when used as primary adjunctive therapy?

The role of chemotherapy in gliomas can be either as part of primary treatment or for palliation after relapse, by which point the maximum tolerable dose of radiotherapy will have already been given. When deciding on the use of chemotherapy, the likelihood of response, choice of agent and route of administration need to be considered. While gliomas can show some clinical and radiological response to chemotherapy,

the role of chemotherapy in the adjuvant setting is not agreed upon.

Selection of chemotherapeutic agents has focused on those that are lipid soluble and can cross the blood brain barrier. Nitrosoureas are the most favoured agent for these reasons, although the alkylating agent temozolomide also reaches high concentrations in the brain. More recently, locally administered chemotherapy to the resection bed has become available to bypass these problems. There is no consistent evidence that polytherapy has any advantage over monotherapy. Procarbazine, chloroethylcyclohexylnitrosourea (CCNU) and vincristine together (PCV) is preferred in many European and North American centres although intravenous bischloroethyl-nitrosourea (BCNU) (Carmustine) is preferred in others. Recently these agents have been challenged by oral temozolomide concomitantly or adjuvantly either with radiation therapy.

Chemotherapy causes a partial response (reduction in tumour size by 50%) in 30% of patients with malignant glioma. Certain factors are indicative of a greater response to chemotherapy. Patients aged less than 40 years old are more likely to respond to chemotherapy (40%) than those 40–60 years (17%) or over 60 years (<5%) [44]. Histology can also predict response. Patients with Grade III tumours are more likely to respond than patients with Grade IV (GBM). Patients with oligodendrogliomas are more likely to respond to chemotherapy than patients with astrocytic tumours. Oligodendrogliomas, either low or high grade, with a deletion of chromosome 1p19q are more likely to respond [45,46]. In GBM, methylation at the promoter site of O_6 methylguanine methyltransferase (MGMT) that inactivates a DNA repair enzyme is associated with a greater likelihood of response to chemotherapy with the alkylating agent temozolomide [47].

A Cochrane Review has been conducted on the use of chemotherapy for adult HGG [48]. A meta-analysis used individual patient data to allow a complete and robust analysis. Data was available from 12 published and 1 unpublished trial out of the 24 RCTs identified from literature searching. All patients received surgery and radiotherapy first. Radiotherapy schedules of included trials varied between doses of 40–60 Gy, and volumes ranged from local including tumour and a surrounding margin to whole brain therapy. Chemotherapy included a nitrosourea in all cases, either alone or in combination.

The results found that although only one individual trial reached statistical significance, when trials were combined there was a significant increase in survival. The benefit was an increase in median survival from 10 to 12 months for chemotherapy, with an increase in 1-year survival from 40% to 46% and 2-year survival from 10% to 15%. The hazard ratio was 0.85 (95% confidence intervals (CI) 0.78–0.92), equating to a 15% risk reduction of death for each patient randomized. This improvement occurred after the first 6 months of survival. There was a 17% reduction in

Table 17.3 Recent meta-analysis/RCTs on chemotherapy for malignant glioma.

Type of study (reference)	Intervention	No. of patients (no. of trials)	Patients characteristics	Outcome	Comment
SR GMTG [48]	Nitrosourea alone or in combination + surgery and RT versus surgery and RT alone	3004 (12)	Post-surgery RT 40–60 Gy focal or WBRT	Hazard ratio 0.85 (95% CI 0.78–0.91) $P < 0.0001$	Individual patient data analysis
RCT Double-blinded placebo control Westphal et al. [51]	Gliadel (BCNU impregnated wafers) + RT versus RT	240 (1)	First operation GBM Age 18–65 years KPS ⩾ 60	Median survival RT 11.6 months Gliadel + RT 13.9 months	Multi-institution Expensive treatment
RCT Stupp et al. [53]	Temozolomide (concomitant and adjuvant) + RT versus RT alone (chemotherapy on relapse if indicated)	573 (1)	Post-operative GBM (mainly) Age 18–70 WHO ⩽ 2 Exclusions: unstable or increasing steroid dose	Hazard ratio 0.63 (95% CI 0.52–0.75) $P < 0.001$ Median survival RT 12.1 months RT + temozolomide 14.6 months 2-year survival RT 10.4% RT + temozolomide 26.5%	16% grade III/IV Haematologic toxicity Only 37% completed concomitant + six courses adjuvant

BCNU: bischloroethylnitrosourea; RT: radiotherapy; WBRT: whole brain radiotherapy; GBM: Glioblastoma Multiforme.

progression free survival also. Subgroup analysis confirmed that this effect held true when stratified for primary tumour, prognostic factors or radiotherapy regime, indicating that the improvement in survival was unlikely to be due to patient stratification or inadequate radiotherapy. However there were very few patients aged greater than 70 years enrolled in the studies and re-analysis of cases older than 70 years showed a non-significant deleterious effect of chemotherapy (personal communication with L. Stewart).

The increased statistical power of meta-analysis and robustness of individual patient data analysis mean that this review provides the most authoritative evidence for the effect of chemotherapy in HGG. Two previous reviews for chemotherapy in HGG were flawed in their selection of trials, and did not have the advantages of individual patient data analysis [49,50].

Two recent studies have confirmed the findings of this meta-analysis. The first has shown that BCNU impregnated wafers (Gliadel) inserted at the time of initial resective surgery improves survival by 2 months [51]. However, only approximately 20% of patients will be eligible for this based on study entry criteria [52]. An RCT of concomitant and adjuvant temozolomide in addition to standard radiation therapy versus standard radiation therapy in patients with glioblastoma has demonstrated a 2.5-month survival benefit and significant difference in 2-year survivors favouring temozolomide (26.5% versus 10.4%) [53]. There is an ongoing trial comparing temozolomide versus PCV in malignant glioma.

In summary, there is now clear evidence that chemotherapy can improve survival in those with HGG (Table 17.3). Debates have continued over whether this increase in survival is clinically significant. Nitrosoureas are the most studied agents, while the newer agents such as Gliadel wafers and temozolomide are also effective and may have fewer side effects. Attention to prognostic factors and thorough consultation with the patient over risks and side effects of chemotherapy are necessary to make the best decision for each patient: concomitant or adjuvant chemotherapy is not yet standard care. Further trials need to consider the quality of life as well as survival benefit.

6. Treatment of brain metastasis

What is the most effective treatment for brain metastasis?

Brain metastasis are usually multiple and occur most often in the setting of active disease elsewhere. In this instance, the management is mainly palliative, since the prognosis is poor. A small subgroup of those with a single brain metastasis may enjoy longer survival, particularly if it is the only site of metastatic disease (solitary metastasis). Treatment options for brain metastases can involve surgical resection or radiotherapy [54,55]. The later can be in the form of WBRT, or as a focal technique (SRS or stereotactic radiotherapy). Chemotherapy is seldom used as primary therapy alone.

WBRT has long been considered the palliative treatment of choice. Historical retrospective series have demonstrated survival beyond which was encountered from palliative therapy, for instance from 3 months with steroids alone to up to 7 months with WBRT [56]. It provides symptomatic relief and can prevent neurological deterioration. Neurological side effects can occur early or later in long-term survivors. The most common late neurological side effect of radiation is leuco-encephalopathy and is characterized by dementia, ataxia and incontinence. However, these rarely become relevant due to the poor survival and their incidence is likely to be less than 11%, which was found in one retrospective series using inordinately high doses of radiation [57]. Although the benefits have not been thoroughly assessed in RCTs, clinical experience and ease of administration have led WBRT to become the standard palliative treatment. This has only recently been challenged by focal therapies, for example surgery or SRS plus or minus WBRT.

Surgery has been proposed for lesions that are usually well demarcated and superficial, suggesting resection can be complete and with minimal damage to surrounding neural tissue. It may also relieve symptoms, prevent death from neurological deterioration due to the metastasis, and even increase survival. Three RCTs from the 1990s have compared surgery followed by WBRT versus WBRT alone (standard palliative treatment) [18,58,59]. These trials have recently been analysed in a Cochrane Review, which did not demonstrate a significant survival advantage from surgery, or in reducing death from neurological cause [60]. Only one trial provided information on functionally independent survival for the complete sample population, and although this did suggest an improvement with surgery, the small sample size was very small. At best very few highly selected patients may benefit from surgery.

Before this meta-analysis, the results of the three RCTs for surgery in single brain metastasis had generally been interpreted as evidence in favour of resection and a survival benefit. The first two trials generally found an increase in survival for surgery, although for the later this was only in those with stable extracranial disease. The final trial did not report a significant difference in survival, and many were quick to highlight the main reason for this being the less strict entry criteria and a poorer prognosis of patients. However, only a minority of patients were actually of poorer performance status than in the first two trials, and this alone is unlikely to account for the difference in results. Meta-analysis provides the most reliable results, particularly when faced with small conflicting studies, as in this case. The overall results for surgery in single brain metastasis hence suggest no clear improvement in outcomes from resection, other than in a few very highly selected cases.

SRS has received increased attention recently as a means of delivering a high dose of radiation to a tumour. It avoids damage to surrounding brain, and as it avoids craniotomy it should afford fewer side effects and allow treatment of a greater range of patients, including those with multiple metastases. Numerous phase II studies have suggested a survival time on a par with the best achieved from current best therapy.

Due to selection bias, these results have to be disregarded in favour of RCTs. There are three published trials and two presently under way.

Unfortunately the first two RCTs of SRS are not interpretable due to serious methodological shortcomings [61,62]. The only analysable RCT stratified patients into two groups depending on the presence of single or up to three metastases who had WBRT with or without SRS first [63]. Those with single brain metastasis treated by SRS had an increase in median survival from 4.9 to 6.5 months which was statistically significant, and they were also more likely to maintain or improve their KPS at 6 months follow-up. There was no change in the proportion of patients dying from neurological disease. For two or three metastases no improvement was found for SRS in terms of survival, local control or death from neurological disease. A trial is currently ongoing to compare the use of surgery or SRS, both followed by WBRT, for single brain metastasis; this should help decide the optimum treatment for these patients.

Following focal therapy of a single lesion by either surgery or SRS, there is debate as to whether WBRT is necessary. Previously radiology was less accurate in detecting the presence of multiple metastases, and WBRT had the advantage of treating undetected micrometastases. However, better imaging now detects more multiple metastases, and theoretically a single metastasis should be able to be definitively treated. It has been suggested from some phase II studies that WBRT does not improve outcomes after successful SRS.

If surgery is completed, then a single RCT of 95 patients has demonstrated advantages for post-operative WBRT [64]. This found that although overall survival was not increased, there was a decrease in death from neurological disease from 44% to 14% and a decrease in recurrence rates both locally (46–10%) and throughout the brain (37–14%). For SRS, an RCT currently in progress will hopefully allow evidence-based guidelines on the use of WBRT following SRS.

The main cause of death in patients with brain metastases is the activity of extracranial disease. There is good evidence that surgery does not afford any advantage over WBRT in single brain metastasis other than in very highly selected patients (Table 17.4). The results of these RCTs were all in a highly selected group of those of good prognosis which will be the minority of those with brain metastases in clinical practice, and are not applicable to other patient groups. Further trials are underway to fully define the role of SRS in the management of brain metastases. The management for the majority of those with brain metastases will be palliative.

Summary

It must be remembered in neuro-oncology as in other specialities, large numbers of uncontrolled phase II studies pointing in the direction of benefit for an intervention do not necessarily strengthen proof that the therapy is effective (it just

Table 17.4 Comparison of RCTs on surgery and WBRT for single brain metastasis.

Type of study (reference)	Intervention	No. of patients	Patient characteristics	Outcomes hazard ratio (95% CI)	Comment
RCT Patchell [18]	Surgery + WBRT (36 Gy, 3 fractions/day over 12 days) versus WBRT alone	56 met inclusion criteria, 2 patients declined, 6 excluded because histology not metastasis	Stratified by primary site, supra/infratentorial metastasis, active systemic disease KPS ≤ 70; supratentorial lesions biopsied first	0.50 (0.26–0.95)	Patients mainly with lung primary tumours
RCT Vecht [58]	Surgery + WBRT (40 Gy, 2 fractions/day over 14 days) versus WBRT alone	66 met inclusion criteria, 2 excluded due to challenge of their diagnosis, 1 excluded due to delay in treatment initiation	Block stratification by primary site and active systemic disease KPS ≤ 70 Life expectancy over 6 months Lesion on CT only, no biopsy	0.57 (0.30–1.06)	No use of biopsy before treatment
RCT Mintz [59]	Surgery + WBRT (3000 cGy, 1 fraction/day over 14 days) versus WBRT alone	143 met inclusion criteria, 84 randomized	Stratified by primary site, metastasis size, active systemic disease KPS ≤ 50	1.39 (0.76–2.55)	Minimum survival not an inclusion criteria

magnifies the same errors in design, compounded by publication bias and 'gearing'). Good outcomes in good prognosis patients are to be expected!

With an increasing evidence basis for practice in neuro-oncology, it is important to remember some important principles when interpreting trials. The fact that a study is a RCT trial is not by itself an indication of quality or that the results are valid. Statistical significance must not be confused with clinical significance. Although survival is an important endpoint, quality of life is as important. The study power, method of randomization, blinding, selection and stratification criteria are each important and can confound results. For example, if studies are not blinded, patients who realize that they are receiving the 'standard' rather than 'novel' arm may wish to switch after randomization and find a reason for coming out of the standard limb of the study (such as side effects or toxicity). If studies are not double blinded, doctors can have an influence, whether intentional or not on further interventions. Blinding of doctors can also affect the reporting of quality of life data and disease progression. Very few RCTs in gliomas are able to report on quality of life, and where they have attempted to do so, studies are fraught with missing data and attrition of return of questionnaires due to illness or death.

There are small but growing number of good quality trials in neuro-oncology with which to base evidence-based practice. With chemotherapy for gliomas and surgery for single metastasis, excellent quality Cochrane Reviews have provided results that have challenged previously held beliefs and breathed new air into treatment areas. Furthermore, thorough literature searches have identified clear areas of

weakness in our knowledge, for example for surgery in HGG. Continuing this growth of evidence-based research will no doubt lead to changes and hopefully improvements in the way these devastating conditions are managed.

References

1 Counsell CE, Grant R. Incidence studies of primary and secondary intracranial tumors: a systematic review of their methodology and results. *J. Neurooncol.* 1998; **37**(3): 241–50.

2 Kleihues P, Burger PC, Scheithauer BW. The new WHO classification of brain tumours. *Brain Pathol.* 1993; **3**(3): 255–68.

3 Piepmeier J, Christopher S, Spencer D, Byrne T, Kim J, Knisel JP, et al. Variations in the natural history and survival of patients with supratentorial low-grade astrocytomas. *Neurosurgery* 1996; **38**(5): 872–8.

4 Curran Jr WJ, Scott CB, Horton J, Nelson JS, Weinstein AS, Fischbach AJ, et al. Recursive partitioning analysis of prognostic factors in three Radiation Therapy Oncology Group malignant glioma trials. *J. Natl. Cancer Inst.* 1993; **85**(9): 704–10.

5 Pignatti F, van den Bent M, Curran D, Debruyne C, Sylvester R, Therasse P, et al. European Organization for Research and Treatment of Cancer Brain Tumor Cooperative Group. European Organization for Research and Treatment of Cancer Radiotherapy Cooperative Group. Prognostic factors for survival in adult patients with cerebral low-grade glioma. *J. Clin. Oncol.* 2002; **20**(8): 2076–84.

6 van Veelen ML, Avezaat CJ, Kros JM, van Putten W, Vecht C. Supratentorial low grade astrocytoma: prognostic factors, dedifferentiation, and the issue of early versus late surgery. *J. Neurol. Neurosurg. Psychiatr.* 1998; **64**(5): 581–7.

7 Cairncross JG, Posner JB. The management of brain metastases. In: Walker MD, ed., *Oncology of the Nervous System*. Matinus Nijhoff, Boston, 1983: pp. 341–77.

8 Sze G, Milano E, Johnson C, Heier L. Detection of brain metastases: comparison of contrast-enhanced MR with unenhanced MR and enhanced CT. *Am. J. Neuroradiol.* 1990; **11**(4): 785–91.

9 Gaspar L, Scott C, Rotman M, Asbell S, Phillips T, Wasserman T, et al. Recursive partitioning analysis (RPA) of prognostic factors in three Radiation Therapy Oncology Group (RTOG) brain metastases trials. *Int. J. Radiat. Oncol. Biol. Phys.* 1997; **37**(4): 745–51.

10 Gaspar LE, Scott C, Murray K, Curran W. Validation of the RTOG recursive partitioning analysis (RPA) classification for brain metastases. *Int. J. Radiat. Oncol. Biol. Phys.* 2000; **47**(4): 1001–6.

11 Grant R, Whittle IR, Collie DA, Gregor A, Ironside JW. Referral pattern and management of patients with malignant brain tumours in south east Scotland. *Health Bull.* 1996; **54**(3): 212–22.

12 Brainin M, Barnes M, Baron J-C, Gilhus NE, Hughes R, Selmaj K, et al. Guidance for the preparation of neurological management guidelines by EFNS scientific task forces – revised recommendations 2004. *Eur. J. Neurol.* 2004; **11**(9): 577–81.

13 Kondziolka D, Lunsford LD, Martinez AJ. Unreliability of contemporary neurodiagnostic imaging in evaluating suspected adult supratentorial (low-grade) astrocytoma. *J. Neurosurg.* 1993; **79**(4): 533–6.

14 Murpy M, Loosemore A, Clifton AG, Howe FA, Tate AR, Cudlip SA, et al. The contribution of proton magnetic resonance spectroscopy (1HMRS) to clinical brain tumour diagnosis. *Br. J. Neurosurg.* 2002; **16**(4): 329–34.

15 Moller-Hartmann W, Herminghaus S, Krings T, Marquardt G, Lanfermann H, Pilatus U, et al. Clinical application of proton magnetic resonance spectroscopy in the diagnosis of intracranial mass lesions. *Neuroradiology* 2002; **44**(5): 371–81.

16 Bell D, Grant R, Collie D, Walker M, Whittle IR. How well do radiologists diagnose intracerebral tumour histology on CT? Findings from a prospective multicentre study. *Br. J. Neurosurg.* 2002; **16**(6): 573–7.

17 Chamberlain MC, Murovic JA, Levin VA. Absence of contrast enhancement on CT brain scans of patients with supratentorial malignant gliomas. *Neurology* 1988; **38**(9): 1371–4.

18 Patchell RA, Tibbs PA, Walsh JW, Dempsey RJ, Maruyama Y, Kryscio RJ, et al. A randomized trial of surgery in the treatment of single metastases to the brain. *N. Engl. J. Med.* 1990; **322**(8): 494–500.

19 Castillo MS, FG Davis, Surawicz T, Bruner JM, Bigner S, Coons S, et al. Consistency of Primary Brain Tumor Diagnoses and Codes in Cancer Surveillance Systems. *Neuroepidemiology* 2004; **23**: 85–93.

20 Velasquez-Perez L, Jimenez-Marcial ME. Clinical-Histopathologic Concordance of Tumors of the Nervous System at the Manuel Velasco Suárez National Institute of Neurology and Neurosurgery in Mexico City. *Arch. Pathol. Lab. Med.* 2002; **127**(2): 187–92.

21 Metcalfe SE, Grant R. Biopsy versus resection for malignant glioma. *Cochrane Database Syst. Rev.* 2001; 3: CD002034.

22 Fadul C, Wood J, Thaler H, Galicich J, Patterson Jr RH, Posner JB. Morbidity and mortality of craniotomy for excision of supratentorial gliomas. *Neurology* 1988; **38**(9): 1374–9.

23 Sawaya R, Hammoud M, Schoppa D, Hess KR, Wu SZ, Shi WM, et al. Neurosurgical outcomes in a modern series of 400 craniotomies for treatment of parenchymal tumors. *Neurosurgery* 1998; **42**(5): 1044–55.

24 Whittle IR. Surgery for gliomas. *Curr. Opin. Neurol.* 2002; **15**(6): 663–9.

25 Woodworth G, McGirt MJ, Samdani A, Garonzik I, et al. Accuracy of frameless and frame-based image-guided stereotactic brain biopsy in the diagnosis of glioma: comparison of biopsy and open specimen. *Neurol. Res.* 2005; **27**: 358–62.

26 Vuorinen V, Hinkka S, Farkkila M, Jaaskelainen J. Debulking or biopsy of malignant glioma in elderly people – a randomised study. *Acta Neurochir.* 2003; **145**(1): 5–10.

27 Hall WA. The safety and efficacy of stereotactic biopsy for intracranial lesions. *Cancer* 1998; **82**(9): 1749–55.

28 French LA, Galicich JH. The use of steroids for control of cerebral oedema. *Clin.Neurosurg.* 1962; **10**: 212–23.

29 Kaal ECA, Vecht CJ. The management of brain edema in brain tumours. *Curr. Opin. Oncol.* 2004; **16**: 593–600.

30 Walker MD, Alexander Jr E, Hunt WE, MacCarty CS, Mahaley Jr MS, Mealey Jr J, et al. Evaluation of BCNU and/or radiotherapy in the treatment of anaplastic gliomas. A cooperative clinical trial. *J. Neurosurg.* 1978; **49**(3): 333–43.

31 Walker MD, Green SB, Byar DP, Alexander Jr E, Batzdorf U, Brooks WH, et al. Randomized comparisons of radiotherapy and nitrosoureas for the treatment of malignant glioma after surgery. *N. Engl. J. Med.* 1980; **303**(23): 1323–9.

32 Keime-Guibert F, Chinot O, Taillandier L, et al. Phase 3 study comparing radiotherapy with supportive care in older patients with newly diagnosed anaplastic astrocytomas (AA) or glioblastoma multiforme (GBM): an ANOCEF group trial. *Neurooncology* 2005; **7**(3): 260.

33 Walker MD, Strike TA, Sheline GE. An analysis of dose–effect relationship in the radiotherapy of malignant gliomas. *Int. J. Radiat. Oncol. Biol. Phys.* 1979; **5**(10): 1725–31.

34 Chang CH, Horton J, Schoenfeld D, Salazar O, Perez-Tamayo R, Kramer S, et al. Comparison of postoperative radiotherapy and combined postoperative radiotherapy and chemotherapy in the multidisciplinary management of malignant gliomas. A joint Radiation Therapy Oncology Group and Eastern Cooperative Oncology Group study. *Cancer* 1983; **52**(6): 997–1007.

35 Halperin EC, Herndon J, Schold SC, Brown M, Vick N, Cairncross JG, et al. A phase III randomized prospective trial of external beam radiotherapy, mitomycin C, carmustine, and 6-mercaptopurine for the treatment of adults with anaplastic glioma of the brain. CNS Cancer Consortium. Clinical Trial. Clinical Trial, Phase III. *Int. J. Radiat. Oncol. Biol., Phys.* 1996; **34**(4): 793–802.

36 Bleehen NM, Stenning SP. A Medical Research Council trial of two radiotherapy doses in the treatment of grades 3 and 4 astrocytoma. The Medical Research Council Brain Tumour Working Party. *Br. J. Cancer* 1991; **64**(4): 769–74.

37 Brada M, Sharpe G, Rajan B, Britton J, Wilkins PR, Guerro D, et al. Modifying radical radiotherapy in high grade gliomas; shortening the treatment time through acceleration. *Int. J. Radiat. Oncol. Biol. Phys.* 1999; **43**(2): 287–92.

38 Laperriere NJ, Leung PM, McKenzie S, Milosevic M, Wong S, Glen J, et al. Randomized study of brachytherapy in the initial management of patients with malignant astrocytoma. *Int. J. Radiat. Oncol. Biol. Phys.* 1998; **41**(5): 1005–11.

39 Duncan W, McLelland J, Jack WJ, Arnott SJ, Gordon A, Kerr GR, et al. Report of a randomised pilot study of the treatment of patients with supratentorial gliomas using neutron irradiation. *Br. J. Radiol.* 1986; **59**(700): 373–7.

40 Pickles T, Goodman GB, Rheaume DE, Duncan GG, Fryer CJ, Bhimji S, et al. Pion radiation for high grade astrocytoma: results of a randomized study. *Int. J. Radiat. Oncol. Biol. Phys.* 1997; **37**(3): 491–7.

41 Huncharek M. Meta-analytic re-evaluation of misonidazole in the treatment of high grade astrocytoma. *Anticancer Res.* 1998; **18**(3B): 1935–9.

42 Chang CH. Hyperbaric oxygen and radiation therapy in the management of glioblastoma. *Natl. Cancer Inst. Mongr.* 1977; **46**: 163–9.

43 Karim AB, Maat B, Hatlevoll R, Menten J, Rutten EH, Thomas DG, et al. A randomized trial on dose–response in radiation therapy of low-grade cerebral glioma: European Organization for Research and Treatment of Cancer (EORTC) Study 22844. *Int. J. Radiat. Oncol. Biol. Phys.* 1996; **36**(3): 549–56.

44 Grant R, Liang BC, Page MA, Crane DL, Greenberg HS, Junck L. Age influences chemotherapy response in astrocytomas. *Neurology* 1995; **45**(5): 929–33.

45 Reifenberger J, Reifenberger G, Liu L, James CD, Wechsler W, Collins VP. Molecular genetic analysis of oligodendroglial tumors shows preferential allelic deletions on 19q and 1p. *Am. J. Pathol.* 1994; **145**(5): 1175–90.

46 Cairncross JG, Ueki K, Zlatescu MC, Lisle DK, Finkelstein DM, Hammond RR, et al. Specific genetic predictors of chemotherapeutic response and survival in patients with anaplastic oligodendrogliomas. *J. Natl. Cancer Inst.* 1998; **90**(19): 1473–9.

47 Hegi ME, Diserens AC, Gorlia T, Hamou MF, de Tribolet N, Weller M, et al. MGMT gene silencing and benefit from temozolomide in glioblastoma. *N. Engl. J. Med.* 2005; **352**(10): 997–1003.

48 Glioma Meta-analysts Trialists (GMT) Group. Chemotherapy for high grade glioma. *Cochrane Database Syst. Rev.* 2002; 3: CD003913.

49 Stenning SP, Freedman LS, Bleehen NM. An overview of published results from randomized studies of nitrosoureas in primary high grade malignant glioma. *Br. J. Cancer* 1987; **56**(1): 89–90.

50 Fine HA, Dear KB, Loeffler JS, Black PM, Canellos GP. Meta-analysis of radiation therapy with and without adjuvant chemotherapy for malignant gliomas in adults. *Cancer* 1993; **1**(8): 2585–97.

51 Westphal M, Hilt DC, Bortey E, Delavault P, Olivares R, Warnke PC, et al. A phase 3 trial of local chemotherapy with biodegradable carmustine (BCNU) wafers (Gliadel wafers) in patients with primary malignant glioma. *Neurooncology* 2003; **5**(2): 79–88.

52 Whittle IR, Lyles S, Walker M. Gliadel therapy given for first resection of malignant glioma: a single centre study of the potential use of Gliadel. *J. Neurosurg.* 2003; **17**(4): 352–4.

53 Stupp R, Mason WP, van den Bent MJ, Weller M, Fisher B, Taphoorn MJ, et al. European Organisation for Research and Treatment of Cancer Brain Tumor and Radiotherapy Groups. National Cancer Institute of Canada Clinical Trials Group. Radiotherapy plus concomitant and adjuvant temozolomide for glioblastoma. *N. Engl. J. Med.* 2005; **352**(10): 987–96.

54 Patchell RA. The management of brain metastases. *Cancer Treat. Rev.* 2003; **29**(6): 533–40 (Abstract).

55 Kaal EC, Niel CG, Vecht CJ. Therapeutic management of brain metastasis. *Lancet Neurol.* 2005; **4**(5): 289–98 (Abstract).

56 Diener-West M, Dobbins TW, Phillips TL, Nelson DF. Identification of an optimal subgroup for treatment evaluation of patients with brain metastases using RTOG study 7916. *Int. J. Radiat. Oncol. Biol. Phys.* 1989; **16**(3): 669–73.

57 DeAngelis LM, Delattre JY, Posner JB. Radiation-induced dementia in patients cured of brain metastases. *Neurology* 1989; **39**(6): 789–96.

58 Vecht CJ, Haaxma-Reiche H, Noordijik EM, Padberg GW, Voormolen JH, Hoekstra FH, et al. Treatment of single brain metastasis: radiotherapy alone or combined with neurosurgery? *Ann. Neurol.* 1993; **33**(6): 583–90.

59 Mintz AH, Kestle J, Rathbone MP, Gaspar L, Hugenholtz H, Fisher B, et al. A randomized trial to assess the efficacy of surgery in addition to radiotherapy in patients with a single cerebral metastasis. *Cancer* 1996; **78**(7): 1470–6.

60 Hart MG, Grant R, Walker M, Dickinson H. Surgical resection and whole brain radiation therapy versus whole brain radiation therapy alone for single brain metastases. *Cochrane Database Syst. Rev.* 2005; CD003292.

61 Flickinger JC, Kondziolka D, Lunsford LD, Coffey RJ, Goodman ML, Shaw EG, et al. A multi-institutional experience with stereotactic radiosurgery for solitary brain metastasis. *Int. J. Radiat. Oncol. Biol. Phys.* 1994; **28**(4): 797–802.

62 Chougule PB, Burton-Williams M, Saris S, Zheng Z, Ponte B, Alderson NL, et al. Randomized treatment of brain metastasis with gamma knife radiosurgery, whole brain radiotherapy or both. *Int. J. Radiat. Oncol. Biol. Phys.* 2000; **48**(3 Suppl.): 114 (Abstract).

63 Andrews DW, Scott CB, Sperduto PW, Flanders AE, Gaspar LE, Schell MC, et al. Whole brain radiation therapy with or without stereotactic radiosurgery boost for patients with one to three brain metastases: phase III results of the RTOG 9508 randomised trial. *Lancet* 2004; **363**(9422): 1665–72 (Abstract).

64 Patchell RA, Tibbs PA, Regine WF, Dempsey RJ, Mohiuddin M, Kryscio RJ, et al. Postoperative radiotherapy in the treatment of single metastases to the brain: a randomized trial. *JAMA* 1998; **280**(17): 1485–9.

65 Sandberg-Wollheim M. Malmstrom P. Stromblad LG. Anderson H. Borgstrom S. Brun A. Cronqvist S. Hougaard K. Salford LG. A randomized study of chemotherapy with procarbazine, vincristine, and lomustine with and without radiation therapy for astrocytoma grades 3 and/or 4. *Cancer* 1991; **68**: 22–9.

66 Shapiro WR. Green SB. Burger PC. Mahaley Jr MS, Selker RG, VanGilder JC, Robertson JT, Ransohoff J, Mealey Jr J, Strike TA, et al. Randomized trial of three chemotherapy regimens and two radiotherapy regimens and two radiotherapy regimens in postoperative treatment of malignant glioma. Brain Tumor Cooperative Group Trial 8001. *J. Neurosurg.* 1989; **71**: 1–9.

CHAPTER 18
Epilepsy

Sridharan Ramaratnam, Anthony Marson

Background

Epilepsy is characterized by recurrent unprovoked seizures of cerebral origin, with motor, sensory or autonomic disturbance with or without loss of consciousness. The epilepsies are a group of disorders rather than a single disease. Seizures can be classified by type as partial (categorized as simple partial, complex partial, and secondary generalized tonic clonic seizures) or generalized (categorized as generalized tonic clonic, absence, myoclonic, tonic, and atonic seizures) [1].

Epilepsy is common, with an estimated prevalence in the developed world of 5–10/1000, and an annual incidence of 50/100,000 people [2]. About 3% of people will be given a diagnosis of epilepsy at some time in their lives [3].

Seizures are essentially a symptom, rather than a disease, and may be caused by various disorders involving the brain. The causes/risk factors include birth/neonatal injuries, congenital or metabolic disorders, head injuries, tumours, infections of the brain or meninges, drug or alcohol abuse, genetic defects, degenerative disease of the brain, cerebrovascular disease, or demyelinating disease.

Epilepsy can be classified by aetiology [1]. Idiopathic generalized epilepsies (such as juvenile myoclonic epilepsy or childhood absence epilepsy) are genetic. Symptomatic epilepsies result from a known cerebral abnormality; for example, temporal lobe epilepsy may result from a congenital defect, mesial temporal sclerosis, or a tumour. Cryptogenic epilepsies are those thought to be symptomatic, but the causative factor has not been identified.

About 60% of untreated people have no further seizures in the 2 years after their first seizure [4]. A diagnosis of epilepsy is usually made following two or more unprovoked seizures, and for most people with epilepsy the prognosis is good. About 70% go into remission, defined as being seizure free for 5 years on or off treatment. This leaves 20–30% who develop chronic epilepsy, which is often treated with multiple antiepileptic drugs (AEDs) [5].

Framing clinical questions and search for evidence

The aims of the intervention are:
- To reduce the risk of subsequent seizures.
- To improve the prognosis of the seizure disorder.
- To minimize adverse effects of treatment.
- For people in remission, to withdraw AEDs without causing seizure recurrence.
- To improve of quality of life.

We searched the Cochrane Epilepsy Group Trial Register, Cochrane Systematic Reviews (Cochrane Library Issue I, 2006), and Medline in November 2005.

We investigated the following outcomes:
- *For treatment after a single seizure*: Proportion of people having recurrence of seizure after 1, 2, or 5 years after the first seizure, time to subsequent seizures, time to achieve a 12-month or 2-year remission, proportion of people achieving 12-month or 2-year remission 2 or 5 years after their first seizure.
- *For treatment of newly diagnosed epilepsy*: Retention on allocated treatment or time to withdrawal of allocated treatment, time to remission, time to first seizure after treatment, recurrence rates.
- *For treatment of drug-resistant epilepsy*: Percentage reduction in seizure frequency, proportion of responders (response defined as 50% or greater reduction in seizure frequency), withdrawal from treatment and side effects.
- *For drug withdrawal*: Time to seizure recurrence, improvement in quality of life.
- *For epilepsy surgery*: Seizure freedom 1 or 2 years after surgery, improvement in quality of life, mortality/morbidity.

Critical review of the evidence for each question

1. Treatment of first seizure

In persons with the first unprovoked seizure (single seizure), does AED treatment, started immediately, affect the probability of seizure recurrence and long-term prognosis?

We found no systematic review. We found six randomized-controlled trials (RCTs).

The Multicentre Study of Early Epilepsy and Single Seizures (MESS study) [6] was an unmasked, multicentre, randomized study of immediate and deferred AED treatment in 1443 patients (children and adults) with single seizures or early epilepsy. Outcomes comprised time to first, second, and fifth seizures; time to 2-year remission; no seizures between years 1 and 3 and between years 3 and 5 after randomization;

and quality of life. Seven hundred and twenty-two were assigned to immediate treatment with AEDs and 721 were assigned deferred treatment. Immediate treatment increased time to first, second, and first tonic clonic seizures. It also reduced the time to achieve 2-year remission of seizures ($P = 0.023$). At 5-year follow-up, 76% of patients in the immediate treatment group and 77% of those in the deferred treatment group were seizure free between 3 and 5 years after randomization (difference − 0.2% [95% CI (confidence interval) −5.8 to 5.5%]). The two policies did not differ with respect to quality of life outcomes or serious complications. Immediate AED treatment reduced the occurrence of seizures in the next 1–2 years, but did not affect long-term remission in individuals with single or infrequent seizures. Quality of life outcomes found no advantage for either treatment policy and indicate that the benefits of preventing seizures is balanced by the adverse effects and stigma of taking AEDs.

The FIRST Group [7] randomized 419 people (42% women, 28% aged <16 years, 66% aged 16–60 years, 6%

aged >60 years), and compared immediate treatment after a first unprovoked seizure versus no immediate treatment. People were randomized within 7 days of their first tonic clonic seizure. Longer-term follow-up of the RCT [8] found that there were half as many second seizures with immediate treatment compared with no immediate treatment at 2 years (hazard ratio (HR) 0.4, 95% CI 0.2–0.5). However, no significant difference was found in the proportion of people achieving a 2-year remission in seizures (absolute risk (AR) 60% with immediate treatment versus 68% with no treatment; relative risk (RR) 0.82, 95% CI 0.64–1.03; RR adjusted for time of starting treatment 0.96, 95% CI 0.77–1.22). Forty-one patients discontinued AEDs – 14 citing adverse effects.

Gilad [9] randomized 91 patients aged 18–50 years, presenting to the hospital within 24 h of the first unprovoked seizure: 46 patients were treated with carbamazepine (CBZ) and 45 with no medication Nine subjects who did not tolerate carbamazepine were changed over to treatment with

Table 18.1 Treatment of single seizure (immediate versus no immediate treatment).

Study (reference)	Number of patients	Recurrence % (follow-up time)	Time to recurrence HR (95% CI)	Remission % (follow-up time)	Remission RR (95% CI)	Comments
FIRST [7,8]	436	Control 51% Treatment 25% (2 years)	0.40 (0.2–0.5)	Control 61% Treatment 68% (2 years)*	0.82 (0.64–1.03) 0.96 (0.77–1.22)*	Children and adults, randomized within 7 days of seizure, 65 had previous uncertain seizures *Adjusted for time of starting treatment
MESS [6]	812	Control 39% Treatment 32% (2 years) Control 44% Treatment 35% (5 years)	0.82 (0.68–0.99)	Control 61% Treatment 69% (2 years) Control 92% Treatment 92% (5 years)	Proportional hazards model not valid	Children and adults, 30% randomized within a week, 55% within 1 month
Gilad [9]	91	Control 59% Treatment 13% (1 year) Control 68% Treatment 20% (2 years) Control 71% Treatment 22% (3 years)				Not blinded, adults, randomized within 24 h after the first seizure, 20% changed from CBZ to VPA due to side effects
Camfield [11]	31	Control 53% Treatment 14% (1 year)				Children randomized within 1 month of seizure, unblinded, four discontinued CBZ due to side effects
Chandra [10]	228	Control 56% Treatment 4% (1 year)				Adults, randomized within 2 weeks of seizure, double blind

sodium valproate (VPA). They were followed up for 36 months. Seizures recurred in 29 of the untreated and 10 in the treatment group. The number of subjects having seizure recurrences in the treatment and control groups were 6 versus 24 at the end of 1 year, 9 versus 28 at the end of 2 years, 10 versus 29 at the end of 3 years. The risk rates for relapse (AR) at the end of 1, 2, and 3 years in the treatment group was 0.1, 0.2, and 0.4 compared to 0.33, 0.62, and 0.77 in untreated $P = 0.001$; 95% CI not given.

Chandra [10] performed a double-blind RCT of 228 adult (16–79) patients presenting within 2 weeks after the first seizure to treatment with sodium valproate or placebo in a double-blind manner. The follow-up was for 12 months. One hundred and fifteen patients received VPA and 113 placebo. Seizures recurred in 5 of the VPA treated and 63 of placebo group. Side effects were noted in 10 on VPA and 2 on placebo but were not considered serious.

Camfield [11] randomized 31 children with first afebrile seizure to treatment with carbamazepine or no immediate treatment. At the end of 1 year, afebrile seizures recurred in two of the 14 randomized to CBZ and nine of 17 with no medication. Four discontinued CBZ due to side effects and two on CBZ had febrile recurrences. Thus six of the 14 taking CBZ and seven of 17 on no medication were free of seizures and without adverse effects, 1 year after their initial seizure.

Pauranik [12] randomized 84 adults presenting within 1 week of a single unprovoked cerebral seizure into two groups, one receiving phenytoin and other placebo. This was a double-blind study. The follow-up ranged from 8 to 18 months (mean 12.3). About a third of patients had their second attack within 1 month and 80% within 1 year. The study has been published only as a conference abstract and further details of this study are not available. The results of the RCTs are summarized in Table 18.1.

Summary

RCTs found that AED treatment following a single seizure reduces seizure recurrence compared with no treatment. However, we found no evidence that treatment alters long-term prognosis. Quality of life outcomes from the MESS study indicate that the benefits of preventing seizure are balanced by the adverse effects and stigma of taking AEDs.

2. AED for partial epilepsy

In patients with partial epilepsy, which AED is most effective and safe?

Carbamazepine

We found no placebo-controlled RCTs of carbamazepine used as monotherapy in people with partial epilepsy, but widespread consensus holds that it is effective. Placebo-controlled trials of carbamazepine would now be considered unethical. We found three systematic reviews comparing carbamazepine versus sodium valproate, phenobarbital, and phenytoin.

The first systematic review (5 RCTs, 1265 people, of whom 830 had partial epilepsy and 395 had generalized epilepsy, aged 3–83 years, follow-up <5 years) compared sodium valproate versus carbamazepine [13]. The systematic review included a meta-analysis of the subgroup of people with partial epilepsy. Sodium valproate had decreased 12-month remission compared with carbamazepine and significantly increased risk of first seizure. A test for statistical interaction was performed and was significant for time to first seizure but not for time to 12-month remission. These subgroup analyses must therefore be treated with caution. The review found no significant difference for treatment withdrawal between sodium valproate and carbamazepine. The meta-analysis provides weak evidence in support of the consensus view to use carbamazepine as the drug of choice in people with partial epilepsy.

The second systematic review (4 RCTs, 680 people, of whom 523 had partial epilepsy) compared carbamazepine versus phenobarbital [14]. For people with partial epilepsy it found no significant difference in remission during the next 12 months. However, it found that phenobarbital significantly increased time to first seizure compared with carbamazepine. The review found that phenobarbital was significantly more likely to be withdrawn than carbamazepine.

The third systematic review (3 RCTs, 552 adults and children, of whom 431 had partial epilepsy) compared carbamazepine versus phenytoin [15]. The review did not present results separately for people with partial and generalized epilepsy. Overall, however, it found no significant difference between carbamazepine and phenytoin for treatment withdrawal, first seizure, or 12-month remission.

Phenobarbital

We found no placebo-controlled RCTs of phenobarbital used as monotherapy in people with partial epilepsy, but widespread consensus holds that it is effective. Placebo-controlled trials of phenobarbital would now be considered unethical. We found two systematic reviews comparing phenobarbital versus carbamazepine and phenytoin.

The first systematic review (3 RCTs, 599 people with partial or generalized epilepsy, aged 3–77 years) compared phenobarbital versus phenytoin [16], but it did not undertake subgroup analyses for people with partial or generalized epilepsy. Overall, it found no significant difference in 12-month remission or first seizure. The review found that treatment withdrawal was greater with phenobarbital than with phenytoin, presumably because it was less well tolerated.

The second systematic review (4 RCTs, 680 people, of whom 523 had partial epilepsy) compared carbamazepine versus phenobarbital [14]. For people with partial epilepsy it found no significant difference in remission during the next 12 months. However, it found that phenobarbital significantly increased time to first seizure compared with carbamazepine but was significantly more likely to be withdrawn than carbamazepine.

Phenytoin

We found no placebo-controlled RCTs of phenytoin used as monotherapy in people with partial epilepsy, but widespread consensus holds that it is effective. Placebo-controlled trials of phenytoin would now be considered unethical. We found three systematic reviews comparing phenytoin versus sodium valproate, phenobarbital, and carbamazepine.

The first systematic review (5 RCTs, 250 people with partial epilepsy and 395 with generalized epilepsy, aged 3–95 years, follow-up < 5 years) compared sodium valproate versus phenytoin [17]. It included a meta-analysis in people with partial epilepsy. It found no significant difference in 12-month remission, or first seizure or in treatment withdrawal between phenytoin and sodium valproate.

The second systematic review (3 RCTs, 599 people with partial or generalized epilepsy, aged 3–77 years) compared phenobarbital versus phenytoin [16], but it did not undertake subgroup analyses for people with partial or generalized epilepsy. Overall, it found no significant difference in 12-month remission or first seizure. The review found that treatment withdrawal was greater with phenobarbital than with phenytoin, presumably because it was less well tolerated.

The third systematic review (3 RCTs, 552 adults and children, of whom 431 had partial epilepsy) compared carbamazepine versus phenytoin [15]. The review did not present results separately for people with generalized epilepsy and people with partial epilepsy. Overall, however, it found no significant difference between carbamazepine and phenytoin for treatment withdrawal, first seizure, or 12-month remission.

Sodium valproate

We found no placebo-controlled RCTs of sodium valproate used as monotherapy in people with partial epilepsy, but widespread consensus holds that it is effective. Placebo-controlled trials of sodium valproate would now be considered unethical.

We found two systematic reviews comparing sodium valproate versus carbamazapine and phenytoin. The first systematic review (5 RCTs, 1265 people, of whom 830 had partial epilepsy and 395 had generalized epilepsy, aged 3–83 years, follow-up <5 years) compared sodium valproate versus carbamazepine [13]. The systematic review included a meta-analysis of the subgroup of people with partial epilepsy. Sodium valproate had decreased 12-month remission compared with carbamazepine and significantly increased risk

of first seizure. A test for statistical interaction was performed and was significant for time to first seizure but not for time to 12-month remission. These subgroup analyses must therefore be treated with caution. The review found no significant difference for treatment withdrawal between sodium valproate and carbamazepine.

The second systematic review (5 RCTs, 250 people with partial epilepsy and 395 with generalized epilepsy, aged 3–95 years, follow-up <5 years) compared sodium valproate versus phenytoin [17]. It included a meta-analysis in people with partial epilepsy. It found no significant difference in 12-month remission or first seizure. The review found no significant difference in treatment withdrawal between sodium valproate and phenytoin.

Other AEDs

We found no placebo-controlled RCTs of other AEDs used as monotherapy in people with partial epilepsy.

The details of the results of the systematic reviews are given in Table 18.2.

Summary

We found no placebo-controlled RCTs of carbamazepine, phenobarbital, phenytoin, or sodium valproate used as monotherapy in people with partial epilepsy, but widespread consensus holds that they are effective. Systematic reviews found that phenobarbital was more likely to be withdrawn than phenytoin or carbamazepine. The systematic review comparing carbamazepine and valproate provides weak evidence to support carbamazepine as a drug of first choice. We found no RCTs of other AEDs used as monotherapy in people with partial epilepsy. Systematic reviews found no reliable evidence on which to base a choice among AEDs in terms of seizure control.

3. AED for generalized epilepsy

In patients with generalized epilepsy (tonic clonic type), which AED is most effective and safe?

Carbamazepine

We found no placebo-controlled trials of carbamazepine used as monotherapy in people with generalized epilepsy (tonic clonic type), but widespread consensus holds that these drugs are effective. We found three systematic reviews comparing carbamazepine versus sodium valproate, phenobarbital, and phenytoin.

The first systematic review compared carbamazepine versus sodium valproate [13] (5 RCTs, 4 of the RCTs included 395 people with generalized epilepsy, aged 3–79 years, follow-up <5 years). RCTs included in the review recruited people if they had generalized onset tonic clonic seizures with or without other generalized seizure types (e.g. absence or myoclonus). A meta-analysis of the generalized epilepsy

Table 18.2 Comparisons of first-line AEDs in partial and generalized epilepsy.

SR (reference)	Outcome (time to event)	Partial HR (95% CI)	Generalized HR (95% CI)	Both HR (95% CI)	Comment
PHB versus CBZ [14]	12-month remission	1.03 (0.72–1.49)	0.61 (0.36–1.03)		Non-statistical significant difference
	First seizure	0.71 (0.55–0.91) PHB better	1.50 (0.95–2.35)		Non-statistical significant difference for generalized epilepsy Advantage to PHB for partial seizures
	Withdrawal	1.60 (1.18–2.17) PHB worse	1.78 (0.87–3.62)		**More withdrawals on PHB**. Statistically significant difference only for partial onset but with significant heterogeneity
VPA versus CBZ [13]	12-month remission	0.82 (0.67–1.00) VPA worse	0.96 (0.75 to 1.24)		Non-statistical significant difference
	First seizure	1.22 (1.04–1.44) VPA worse	0.86 (0.68–1.09)		Statistically significant difference only for partial onset with **advantage for CBZ**
	Withdrawal	1.00 (0.79–1.26)	0.89 (0.62–1.29)		Non-statistical significant difference
PHT versus VPA [17]	12-month remission	1.02 (0.68–1.54)	1.06 (0.71–1.57)		Non-statistical significant difference
	First seizure	0.81 (0.59–1.10)	1.03 (0.77–1.39)		Non-statistical significant difference
	Withdrawal	1.23 (0.77–1.98)	0.98 (0.60–1.58)		Non-statistical significant difference
PHB versus PHT [16]	12-month remission			0.93 (0.70–1.23)	Non-statistical significant difference
	First seizure			0.84 (0.68–1.05)	Non-statistical significant difference
	Withdrawal			1.62 (1.22–2.14)	Statistically significant difference PHB worse
PHT versus CBZ [15]	12-month remission			1.0 (0.78–1.29)	Non-difference
	First seizure			0.91 (0.74–1.12)	Non-statistical significant difference
	Withdrawal			0.97 (0.74–1.28)	Non-statistical significant difference

12 month remission: HR > 1 indicates first drug is better or more remission with first drug. First seizure < 1 indicates first drug is better or less seizure recurrence with first drug. Withdrawals > 1 worse for the first drug more withdrawals with the first drug.
PHT: phenytoin; PHB: phenobarbital; CBZ: carbamazepine; VDA: valproate.

subgroup found no significant difference between sodium valproate and carbamazepine for 12-month remission or first seizure. The review found no significant difference between sodium valproate and carbamazepine for treatment withdrawal. Although no difference was found in the systematic review between sodium valproate and carbamazepine, the CI is wide and this result does not establish equivalence of sodium valproate and carbamazepine. Also, the age distribution of people classified as having generalized epilepsy suggests errors in the classification of epilepsy type. Failure of the RCTs to document generalized seizures other than tonic clonic seizures is an important limitation.

The second systematic review (4 RCTs, 680 people, of whom 157 had generalized epilepsy) compared carbamazepine versus phenobarbital [14]. Subgroup analysis in people with a generalized epilepsy found no significant differences for first seizure or 12-month remission. The review found no significant differences in treatment withdrawal between carbamazepine and phenobarbital.

The third systematic review (3 RCTs, 552 people, of whom 121 had generalized epilepsy) compared carbamazepine versus phenytoin [15]. It did not present results separately for people with generalized epilepsy. Overall, however, it found no significant difference between carbamazepine and phenytoin for treatment withdrawal, first seizure, or 12-month remission.

Phenobarbital

We found no placebo-controlled trials of phenobarbital used as monotherapy in people with generalized epilepsy, but widespread consensus holds that it is effective.

We found one systematic review (4 RCTs, 680 people, of whom 157 had generalized epilepsy), which compared carbamazepine versus phenobarbital [14]. Subgroup analysis in people with a generalized epilepsy found no significant differences for first seizure, or 12-month remission. The review found no significant difference for treatment withdrawal between carbamazepine and phenobarbital.

Phenytoin

We found no placebo-controlled trials of phenytoin used as monotherapy in people with generalized epilepsy, but widespread consensus holds that it is effective. We found two reviews comparing phenytoin versus carbamazepine and sodium valproate.

The first systematic review compared phenytoin and sodium valproate [17] (5 RCTs, 395 people aged 3–95 years with generalized epilepsy). RCTs included in the review recruited people if they had generalized onset tonic clonic seizures with or without other generalized seizure types (e.g. absence or myoclonus). A meta-analysis of the generalized epilepsy subgroup found no significant difference between sodium valproate and phenytoin for 12-month remission or first seizure. The review found no significant difference between sodium valproate and phenytoin for time to treatment withdrawal. Although no difference was found in the systematic reviews between sodium valproate and phenytoin, the CI is wide and this result does not establish equivalence of sodium valproate and phenytoin.

The second systematic review (3 RCTs, 552 people, of whom 121 had generalized epilepsy) compared carbamazepine versus phenytoin [15]. It did not present results separately for people with generalized epilepsy. Overall, it found no significant difference between carbamazepine and phenytoin for treatment withdrawal, first seizure, or 12-month remission.

Sodium valproate

We found no placebo-controlled trials of sodium valproate used as monotherapy in people with generalized epilepsy, but widespread consensus holds that it is effective. We found two systematic reviews comparing sodium valproate versus carbamazepine and phenytoin. The reviews were of RCTs that recruited people if they had generalized onset tonic clonic seizures with or without other generalized seizure types (e.g. absence or myoclonus).

The first systematic review compared carbamazepine versus sodium valproate [13] (5 RCTs, 4 of the RCTs included 395 people with generalized epilepsy, aged 3–79 years, follow-up <5 years). A meta-analysis of the generalized epilepsy subgroup found no significant difference between sodium valproate and carbamazepine for 12-month remission or first seizure. The review found no significant difference between sodium valproate and carbamazepine for treatment withdrawal.

The second systematic review compared phenytoin and sodium valproate [17] (5 RCTs, 395 people aged 3–95 years with generalized epilepsy). A meta-analysis of the generalized epilepsy subgroup found no significant difference between sodium valproate and phenytoin for 12-month remission or first seizure. The review found no significant difference between sodium valproate and phenytoin for time to treatment withdrawal.

Although no difference was found in the systematic reviews between sodium valproate and either carbamazepine or phenytoin, the CI are wide and these results do not establish equivalence of sodium valproate and carbamazepine or phenytoin. Also, the age distribution of people classified as having generalized epilepsy suggests errors in the classification of epilepsy type. Failure of the RCTs to document generalized seizures other than tonic clonic seizures is an important limitation. The meta-analysis does not provide evidence to support or refute the use of sodium valproate for people with generalized tonic clonic seizures as part of generalized epilepsy.

Other AEDs

We found no placebo-controlled RCTs of other AEDs used as monotherapy in people with generalized epilepsy.

The details of the results of systematic reviews are given in Table 18.2.

Summary

We found no placebo-controlled trials of carbamazepine, phenobarbital, phenytoin, and sodium valproate used as monotherapy in people with generalized epilepsy (tonic clonic type), but widespread consensus holds that these drugs are effective. Systematic reviews found insufficient evidence on which to base a choice among AEDs in terms of seizure control. We found no RCTs of other AEDs used as monotherapy in people with generalized epilepsy.

4. AED for absence seizure
In patients with generalized epilepsy (absence seizures), which AED is most effective and safe?

One systematic review [18] found four small trials, which were of poor methodological quality. One trial (29 participants) compared lamotrigine with placebo using a response conditional design. Individuals taking lamotrigine were significantly more likely to be seizure free than participants taking placebo during this short trial. Three studies compared ethosuximide and valproate, but because of diverse study designs and populations studied, the results could not be pooled. None of these studies found a difference between valproate and ethosuximide with respect to seizure control, but CI were wide and the existence of important differences could not be excluded. Although ethosuximide, lamotrigine, and valproate are commonly used to treat people with absence seizures we have insufficient evidence to inform clinical practice, since the few trials available were of poor methodological quality.

5. Addition of second-line AEDs
What are the effects of adding newer AED in people with partial epilepsy not responding to the first-line AED?

We found eight systematic reviews that compared the addition of second-line drugs (gabapentin, levetiracetam, lamotrigine, oxcarbazepine, tiagabine, topiramate, vigabatrin, or zonisamide) versus placebo in people who had not responded to usual drug treatment:

1 *Gabapentin versus placebo*: One systematic review [19] (5 RCTs, 997 people) found that adding gabapentin to usual treatment significantly reduced seizure frequency compared with adding placebo, and that efficacy increased with increasing dose.

2 *Levetiracetam versus placebo*: One systematic review [20] (4 RCTs, 1023 people) found that adding levetiracetam to usual treatment significantly reduced seizure frequency compared with adding placebo.

3 *Lamotrigine versus placebo*: One systematic review [21] (11 RCTs, 1243 people) found that adding lamotrigine to usual treatment significantly reduced seizure frequency compared with adding placebo. Lamotrigine is associated with a rash, which may be avoided by slower titration of the drug.

4 *Oxcarbazepine versus placebo*: One systematic review [22] (2 RCTs, 961 adults and children) found that adding oxcarbazepine to usual treatment significantly reduced seizure frequency compared with adding placebo.

5 *Tiagabine versus placebo*: One systematic review [23] (3 RCTs, 769 people) found that adding tiagabine to usual

treatment significantly reduced seizure frequency compared with adding placebo (see Table 18.3).

6 *Topiramate versus placebo*: One systematic review [24] (9 RCTs, 1049 people) found that adding topiramate to usual treatment significantly reduced seizure frequency compared with adding placebo.

7 *Vigabatrin versus placebo*: One systematic review [25] (search date 1995, 4 RCTs, 495 people) found that adding vigabatrin to usual treatment significantly reduced seizure frequency compared with adding placebo. Vigabatrin causes concentric visual field abnormalities in about 40% of people, which are probably irreversible [26]. Because of the irreversible visual field abnormalities associated with vigabatrin, the consensus view among neurologists is not to recommend this drug.

8 *Zonisamide versus placebo*: One systematic review [27] (3 RCTs, 499 people) found that adding zonisamide to usual treatment significantly reduced seizure frequency compared with adding placebo.

Adverse effects and treatment withdrawal were more frequent with additional treatment than with placebo. The results of these systematic reviews are tabulated (Table 18.3).

Summary

Systematic reviews in people with drug-resistant partial epilepsy found that adding gabapentin, levetiracetam, lamotrigine, oxcarbazepine, tiagabine, topiramate, vigabatrin, or zonisamide to usual treatment reduced seizure frequency in the short term compared with adding placebo. The reviews found that adding any of the drugs increased the frequency of adverse effects compared with adding placebo. Few RCTs have compared second-line drugs directly with each other, and no trials have examined longer term outcomes. We found no good evidence from RCTs on which to base a choice among drugs.

6. AED withdrawal for people in remission
How does the withdrawal of AEDs in persons with epilepsy who are seizure free with medication, affect the probability of seizure recurrence?

Withdrawal versus continued treatment
One large RCT (1013 people who had been seizure free for >2 years) compared continued antiepileptic treatment with slow AED withdrawal [28,29]. At 2 years, 78% of people who continued treatment remained seizure free compared with 59% in the withdrawal group. There were no significant differences in psychosocial outcomes between groups. Risk reductions with 95% CI for the main factors predicting recurrence of seizures are tabulated (Table 18.4). Sixteen people died during the trial, 10 in the continued treatment group and 6 in the withdrawal group. Only two deaths were attributed to epilepsy, and both of these occurred

Table 18.3 Effects of additional drug versus placebo treatment and dose response in people not responding to usual treatment: results of systematic reviews.

Intervention	Responders* percentage (unless specified otherwise) or RR (95% CI)	RR treatment withdrawal (95% CI)	RR adverse effects with CI (99% CI) for any dose	Comments
Gabapentin (adults only) 0 mg Placebo	9.9 (7.2–13.5)	1.4 (0.8–2.5)		5 RCTs (1 in children, 4 in adults); Efficacy increased with increasing dose. No plateauing of response; so doses tested may not have been optimal.
Gabapentin 600 mg	14.4 (12.0–17.3)			
Gabapentin 900 mg	17.3 (14.6–20.3)			
Gabapentin 1200 mg	20.6 (17.1–24.6)			
Gabapentin 1800 mg	28.5 (21.5–36.7)			
Gabapentin (adults and children) 600–1800 mg	RR 1.81 (1.32–2.49)	1.04 (0.71–1.52)	Dizziness 2.19 (1.24–3.89) Fatigue 2.30 (1.11–4.75) Somnolence 1.91 (1.20–3.05)	
Topiramate 0 mg Placebo	11.7 (8.7–15.7)			9 RCTs
Topiramate 200 mg	26.8 (15.8–41.3)	2.06 (1.38–3.08)	Dizziness 1.55 (1.07–2.24) Fatigue 2.21 (1.42–3.45) Somnolence 2.26 (1.48–3.46) Ataxia 1.95 (1.04–3.65) Difficulty thinking 5.54 (2.34–13.12)	
Topiramate 400–1000 mg	46.5 (42.5–50.5)			
Topiramate 200–1000 mg	RR 3.32 (2.52–4.39)			
Vigabatrin (adults) 0 mg Placebo	13.8 (9.7–19.2)			3 RCTs
Vigabatrin 1000 or 2000 mg	22.8 (14.5–34.9)	2.95 (1.25–7.00)	No adverse effects significantly more frequent but 40% develop concentric visual field abnormalities.	
Vigabatrin 3000 or 6000 mg	45.9 (39.5–52.5)			
Levetiracetam (adults) 1000–3000 mg	RR 3.53 (2.48–5.03)	1.21 (0.88–1.66)	Dizziness 2.50 (1.16–5.41) Infection 1.76 (1.03–3.02)	4 RCTs. Results of regression models with CI (95% unless otherwise stated) do not provide reliable estimates for a response to individual doses.
Lamotrigine (adults) 200–500 mg	RR 2.32 (1.67–3.23)	1.10 (0.81–1.50)	Dizziness 2.05 (1.52–2.78) Ataxia 3.23 (1.93–5.42) Diplopia 3.47 (1.91–6.31) Nausea 1.76 (1.18–2.64)	11 RCTs

(Continued)

Table 18.3 (*Continued.*)

Intervention	Responders* percentage (unless specified otherwise) or RR (95% CI)	RR treatment withdrawal (95% CI)	RR adverse effects with CI (99% CI) for any dose	Comments
Oxcarbazepine (adults and children) 600–2400 mg	RR 2.51 (1.88–3.33)	1.72 (1.35–2.18)	Dizziness 2.87 (1.82–4.52) Fatigue 1.81 (1.00–3.29) Somnolence 2.36 (1.54–3.62) Nausea 3.09 (1.74–5.49) Ataxia 3.54 (1.75–7.13) Diplopia 7.25 (3.12–16.80)	2 RCTs
Tiagabine 16–56 mg	RR 3.16 (1.97–5.07)	1.81 (1.25–2.62)	Dizziness 1.69 (1.13–2.51)	3 RCTs. Results of regression models do not provide accurate estimates for a response to individual doses.
Zonisamide 300–500 mg	RR 2.44 (1.81–3.31)	1.64 (1.2–2.26)	Ataxia 4.50 (1.05–19.22) Somnolence 1.91 (1.08–3.38) Agitation/irritability 2.37 (1.00–5.64)	3 RCTs
Zonisamide 100–500 mg	RR 2.35 (1.74–3.17)	1.47 (1.07–2.02)	Anorexia 3.00 (1.31–6.88)	

Results show percentage responding at particular daily doses, but results for treatment withdrawal and adverse effects are calculated for all doses.
* >50% reduction in seizure frequency. RR (95%) CI for responders calculated for all doses.

Table 18.4 RR of seizure recurrence within 2 years of treatment withdrawal, according to prognostic variable.

Prognostic variable	RR (95% CI) of seizure recurrence within 2 years
Age < 16 years	1.8 (1.3–2.4)
Tonic clonic seizures	1.6 (1.1–2.2)
Myoclonus	1.8 (1.1–3.0)
Treatment with more than one AED	1.9 (1.4–2.4)
Seizures since AEDs were started	1.6 (1.2–2.1)
Any EEG abnormality	1.3 (1.0–1.8)

Risk of recurrence also declined as the seizure-free period increased, but in a complex manner. From Marson AG, et al. *BMJ Clinical Evidence* 2005; **14**: 1576–97 with permission.

in people randomized to continued treatment. People with a seizure recurrence were less likely to be in paid employment at 2 years. One systematic review of observational studies (search date not reported) found that, at 2 years, 29% (95% CI 24–34%) of people in remission from all types of epilepsy would relapse if AEDs were withdrawn.

Early versus late discontinuation

One systematic review [30] investigated seizure relapse risk after early (less than two seizure-free years) versus late (more than two seizure free years) AED withdrawal in epilepsy patients. Seven eligible controlled trials were included in the analysis representing 924 randomized children. There were no eligible trials evaluating seizure-free adults. The pooled

RR for seizure relapse in early versus late AED withdrawal was 1.32 (95% CI 1.02–1.70). On the basis of this estimate, the number needed to harm, that is expose an individual to a higher risk of seizure relapse because of early withdrawal of AED, is 10. Early discontinuation was associated with greater relapse rates in people with partial seizures (pooled RR 1.52, 95% CI 0.95–2.41) or an abnormal electroencephalograph (EEG) (pooled RR 1.67, 95% CI 0.93–3.00).

Rapid versus slow withdrawal of AED

One systematic review [31] found one quasi-randomized trial assigned 149 children to either a 6-week or a 9-month period of drug tapering, after which therapy was discontinued. Each group was composed of patients who had been seizure free for either 2 or 4 years before drug tapering was begun. The majority were receiving one or two AEDs. Sixteen patients were lost to follow up before the beginning of the taper period. Seizures recurred in 53 patients (40%). The mean duration of follow-up was 39 months (range 11–105) for the patients who did not have a recurrence of seizures. Neither the length of the taper period (6 weeks versus 9 months, $P = 0.38$) nor the length of time the patients were free of seizures before the taper period was begun (2 years versus 4 years, $P = 0.20$) significantly influenced the risk of seizure recurrence. The presence of mental retardation (RR 3.1, 95% CI 1.5–6.2) or spikes in the EEG at the time of tapering (RR 1.9, 95% CI 1.0–3.4) increased the risk of seizure recurrence. This small quasi-randomized study with four arms may not have had the power to detect important differences in the effects of treatment policies.

Summary

One RCT in people who had been seizure free for at least 2 years found that further seizures were more likely if people stopped treatment than if they continued antiepileptic medication. Clinical predictors of relapse after drug withdrawal included age, seizure type, number of AEDs being taken, whether seizures had occurred since AEDs were started, and the period of remission before drug withdrawal. There is a need to trade off between benefits and harms while attempting to withdraw AEDs in seizure free individuals.

There is evidence to support waiting for at least two or more seizure free years before discontinuing AEDs in children, particularly if individuals have an abnormal EEG and partial seizures. There is insufficient evidence to establish when to withdraw AEDs in children with generalized seizures. There is no evidence to guide the timing of withdrawal of AEDs in seizure-free adults. The ideal duration over which the drugs should be tapered is not known.

7. Surgery

For people with drug-resistant temporal lobe epilepsy, what is the probability that temporal lobe surgery will render them seizure free after 1 year? Is surgical treatment safe?

Temporal lobectomy

We found one systematic review [32] (1 RCT, 80 people with poorly controlled temporal lobe epilepsy). The RCT [33] compared temporal lobectomy versus medical treatment for 1 year.

Benefits
• *Seizure outcome*: After 1 year, temporal lobectomy significantly increased the proportion of people who were completely free of seizures and the proportion who were free of seizures with or without auras compared with medical treatment (seizure free: 38.0% with surgery versus 2.5% with control; number needed to treat (NNT) 3, 95% CI 2–5; seizure free with or without auras: 58.0% with surgery versus 7.5% with control; NNT 2, 95% CI 2–3).
• *Quality of life*: The RCT found that surgery improved quality of life at 1 year compared with medical treatment (quality of life in epilepsy inventory-89, range 0 to maximum quality of 100: 73.8 with surgery versus 64.3 with medical treatment; $P < 0.001$ after adjusting for baseline differences).
• *Employment status*: The RCT found that surgery increased the proportion of people who were employed or attending school at 1 year compared with medical treatment, but the increase was not significant (56.4% with surgery versus 38.5% with medical treatment; $P = 0.11$).

Harms
• *Mortality*: The RCT found no deaths at 1 year after surgery and one death, of unknown cause, with medical treatment.

• *Other adverse effects*: The RCT found that neurological adverse effects were more common with surgery than with medical treatment at 1 year (4/40 [10%] with surgery [1 small thalamic infarct causing thigh dysaesthesia, 1 infected wound, 2 people with decline in verbal memory affecting occupation for 1 year] versus 0/40 with medical treatment; *P*-value not reported). It found that 22/40 (55%) people had asymptomatic superior subquadrantic visual field defects after surgery. The RCT found similar rates of depression with surgical and medical treatment (18% with surgery versus 20% with medical treatment; *P*-value not reported).
• *Psychosis*: The RCT found transient psychosis in one person (1/40 [2.5%]) in each treatment group.

Amygdalohippocampectomy

We found no systematic review and no RCTs that examined the effect of amygdalohippocampectomy in people with drug-resistant temporal lobe epilepsy. However, there is consensus that amygdalohippocampectomy is likely to be beneficial for people with drug-resistant temporal lobe epilepsy.

Lesionectomy

We found one systematic review of observational studies and no RCTs that examined the effects of lesionectomy in people with drug-resistant temporal lobe epilepsy thought to be caused by a known cerebral lesion. The systematic review of observational studies [34] (8 studies, 131 people with lesions) found that between 1 and 4 years, 63% of the 131 people who had lesionectomy were free of disabling seizures.

Summary

One RCT identified by a systematic review found that temporal lobectomy improved seizure control and quality of life after 1 year compared with continued medical treatment in people with poorly controlled temporal lobe epilepsy. There is consensus that temporal lobectomy is beneficial for people with drug-resistant temporal lobe epilepsy. There is consensus that amygdalohippocampectomy is likely to be beneficial for people with drug-resistant temporal lobe epilepsy. The effect of lesionectomy for seizure control is not known. However, surgical removal of tumours and vascular lesions may be indicated to prevent bleeding, herniation, or paralysis.

References

1 Commission on Classification and Terminology of the International League against Epilepsy. Proposal for revised classification of epilepsies and epileptic syndromes. *Epilepsia* 1989; **30**: 389–99.

2 Hauser AW, Annegers JF, Kurland LT. Incidence of epilepsy and unprovoked seizures in Rochester, Minnesota 1935–84. *Epilepsia* 1993; **34**: 453–68.

3 Hauser WA, Kurland LT. The epidemiology of epilepsy in Rochester, Minnesota, 1935 through 1967. *Epilepsia* 1975; **16**: 1–66.

4 Berg AT, Shinnar S. The risk of seizure recurrence following a first unprovoked seizure: a quantitative review. *Neurology* 1991; **41**: 965–72.

5 Cockerell OC, Johnson AL, Sander JW, et al. Remission of epilepsy: results from the national general practice study of epilepsy. *Lancet* 1995; **346**: 140–4.

6 Marson A, Jacoby A, Johnson A, Kim L, Gamble C, Chadwick D. on behalf of the Medical Research Council MESS Study Group. Immediate versus deferred antiepileptic drug treatment for early epilepsy and single seizures: a randomized controlled trial. *Lancet* 2005; **365**: 2007–13.

7 First Seizure Trial Group (FIRST Group). Randomized clinical trial on the efficacy of antiepileptic drugs in reducing the risk of relapse after a first unprovoked tonic clonic seizure. *Neurology* 1993; **43**: 478–83.

8 Musicco M, Beghi E, Solari A, et al., for the FIRST Group. Treatment of first tonic clonic seizure does not improve the prognosis of epilepsy. *Neurology* 1997; **49**: 991–8.

9 Gilad R, Lampl Y, Gabbay U, Eshel Y, Sarova-Pinhas I. Early treatment of a single generalized tonic-clonic seizure to prevent recurrence. *Arch. Neurol.* 1996; **53**: 1149–52.

10 Chandra B. First seizure in adults: to treat or not to treat. *Clin. Neurol. Neurosurg.* 1992; **94**(Suppl.): S61–3.

11 Camfield P, Camfield C, Dooley J, Smith E, Garner B. A randomized study of carbamazepine versus no medication after a first unprovoked seizure in childhood. *Neurology* 1989; **39**: 851–2.

12 Pauranik A. Short-term anti-epileptic therapy for single seizure cases. *Epilepsia* 1997; **38**(Suppl. 3): 88.

13 Marson AG, Williamson PR, Hutton JL, et al. on behalf of the Epilepsy Monotherapy Trialists. Carbamazepine versus valproate monotherapy for epilepsy (Cochrane Review). *The Cochrane Library*, Issue 4. John Wiley & Sons, Ltd., Chichester, UK, 2003.

14 Tudur Smith C, Marson AG, Williamson PR. Carbamazepine versus phenobarbitone monotherapy for epilepsy (Cochrane Review). *The Cochrane Library*, Issue 4. John Wiley & Sons, Ltd., Chichester, UK, 2003.

15 Tudur Smith C, Marson AG, Clough HE, et al. Carbamazepine versus phenytoin monotherapy for epilepsy (Cochrane Review). *The Cochrane Library*, Issue 4. John Wiley & Sons, Ltd., Chichester, UK, 2003.

16 Taylor S, Tudur Smith C, Williamson PR, et al. Phenobarbitone versus phenytoin monotherapy for partial onset seizures and generalized onset tonic-clonic seizures (Cochrane Review). *The Cochrane Library*, Issue 4. John Wiley & Sons, Ltd., Chichester, UK, 2003.

17 Tudur Smith C, Marson AG, Williamson PR. Phenytoin versus valproate monotherapy for partial onset seizures and generalized onset tonic-clonic seizures (Cochrane Review). *The Cochrane Library*, Issue 4. John Wiley & Sons, Ltd., Chichester, UK, 2003.

18 Posner EB, Mohamed K, Marson AG. Ethosuximide, sodium valproate or lamotrigine for absence seizures in children and adolescents (Cochrane Review). *The Cochrane Library*, Issue 1. John Wiley & Sons, Ltd., Chichester, UK, 2006.

19 Marson AG, Kadir ZA, Hutton JL, et al. Gabapentin add-on for drug-resistant partial epilepsy (Cochrane Review). *The Cochrane Library*, Issue 4. John Wiley & Sons, Ltd., Chichester, UK, 2003.

20 Chaisewikul R, Privitera MD, Hutton JL, et al. Levetiracetam add-on for drug-resistant localization related (partial) epilepsy (Cochrane Review). *The Cochrane Library*, Issue 4. John Wiley & Sons, Ltd., Chichester, UK, 2003.

21 Ramaratnam S, Marson AG, Baker GA. Lamotrigine add-on for drug-resistant partial epilepsy (Cochrane Review). *The Cochrane Library*, Issue 4. John Wiley & Sons, Ltd., Chichester, UK, 2003.

22 Castillo S, Schmidt DB, White S. Oxcarbazepine add-on for drug-resistant partial epilepsy (Cochrane Review). *The Cochrane Library*, Issue 4. John Wiley & Sons, Ltd., Chichester, UK, 2003.

23 Pereira J, Marson AG, Hutton JL. Tiagabine add-on for drug-resistant partial epilepsy (Cochrane Review). *The Cochrane Library*, Issue 4. John Wiley & Sons, Ltd., Chichester, UK, 2003.

24 Jette NJ, Marson AG, Hutton JL. Topiramate add-on for drug-resistant partial epilepsy (Cochrane Review). *The Cochrane Library*, Issue 4. John Wiley & Sons, Ltd., Chichester, UK, 2003.

25 Marson AG, Kadir ZA, Hutton JL, et al. The new antiepileptic drugs: a systematic review of their efficacy and tolerability. *Epilepsia* 1997; **38**: 859–80.

26 Kalviainen R, Nousiainen I, Mantyjarvi M, et al. Vigabatrin, a gabaergic antiepileptic drug, causes concentric visual field defects. *Neurology* 1999; **53**: 922–6.

27 Chadwick DW, Marson AG. Zonisamide add-on for drug-resistant partial epilepsy (Cochrane Review). *The Cochrane Library*, Issue 4. John Wiley & Sons, Ltd., Chichester, UK, 2003.

28 Medical Research Council Antiepileptic Drug Withdrawal Study Group. Randomised study of antiepileptic drug withdrawal in patients in remission. *Lancet* 1991; **337**: 1175–80.

29 Medical Research Council Antiepileptic Drug Withdrawal Study Group. Prognostic index for recurrence of seizures after remission of epilepsy. *BMJ* 1993; **306**: 1374–8.

30 Sirven JI, Sperling M, Wingerchuk DM. Early versus late antiepileptic drug withdrawal for people with epilepsy in remission (Cochrane Review). *The Cochrane Library*, Issue 1. John Wiley & Sons, Ltd., Chichester, UK, 2006.

31 Ranganathan LN, Ramaratnam S. Rapid versus slow withdrawal of antiepileptic drugs (Cochrane Review). *The Cochrane Library*, Issue 2. John Wiley & Sons, Ltd., Chichester, UK, 2006.

32 Cucherat M. [Meta-analysis of surgery trials in refractory epilepsy] *Rev. Neurol. (Paris)* 2004; **160**(Spec. No. 1): 5S232–40 (in French).

33 Wiebe S, Blume WT, Girvin JP, et al. A randomized, controlled trial of surgery for temporal lobe epilepsy. *N. Engl. J. Med.* 2001; **345**: 311–18.

34 Engel Jr J, Wiebe S, French J, et al. Practice parameter: temporal lobe and localized neocortical resections for epilepsy: report of the Quality Standards Subcommittee of the American Academy of Neurology, in association with the American Epilepsy Society and the American Association of Neurological Surgeons. *Neurology* 2003; **60**: 538–47. [Erratum in: *Neurology* 2003; **60**: 1396].

19

CHAPTER 19

Dementia treatment: let the evidence lead us

Bart M. Demaerschalk, Bryan K. Woodruff, Richard J. Caselli

Background

Alzheimer disease (AD) is a degenerative brain disease that is the most common cause of dementia. Incidence and prevalence increase exponentially with age through at least the ninth decade, with little evidence of a plateau at higher ages. The prevalence of severe dementia in all persons older than age 60 is estimated to be 5%, and in those older than age 85 it is estimated to be 20% to 50%. The lifetime risk of AD is estimated at 12% to 17% [1]. With more people living longer, the prevalence of AD is increasing. Since 1980, the number of Americans with AD has doubled to 4.5 million and may triple by 2050 [2]. Prevalence estimates of the co-occurrence of dementia and Parkinsonism vary widely among studies but average 20% to 30%; annual incidence rates of dementia in established Parkinsonism also vary but average 5% to 6% [3]. Statistics for other forms of dementia are less precise, but frontotemporal dementia is probably about one-tenth as common as AD. Vascular changes are common in dementia patients, but the frequency of mixed vascular-degenerative dementia – especially AD – is much more common than 'pure' vascular dementia (VaD).

Although most cases of AD occur after age 60, about 5% are early-onset familial cases related to one of three autosomal dominant mutations. Early-onset familial AD typically strikes young persons ranging in age from the mid-thirties to the mid-fifties. To date, three separate genetic mutations have been identified that may cause early-onset familial AD, and all three are inherited in an autosomal dominant pattern. The most common mutation thought to account for most of the autosomal dominant kindreds is presenilin-1 [4], and it is the only one of the three for which there is currently a commercially available genetic test. The other two include the amyloid precursor protein gene on chromosome 21 [5] and presenilin-2 on chromosome 1 [6]. All result in increased concentrations of abeta-amyloid, which underscores the pathogenic importance of abeta-amyloid in the evolution of AD [7]. The genetic risk factor that accounts for more cases of AD than any other, however, is the apolipoprotein E e4 allele located on chromosome 19. The apolipoprotein E e4 allele is associated with late-onset familial and 'sporadic' AD, not autosomal dominant early-onset familial AD [8]. The prevalence of the apolipoprotein E e4 allele varies worldwide but is about 20% in North America [9].

Dementia imposes an immense burden on families, because 70% of these patients are cared for at home [10]. The cost of care averages $42,000 annually [11], so reducing the financial as well as the medical burden of AD is a major goal of medical diagnosis and management. Parkinsonism further adds to the cost of care. These statistics primarily reflect that most AD patients are retirees and do not account for the few patients who lose years of work productivity because of early-onset AD. The statistics also do not account for potentially reversible conditions mistaken for AD or for the increased medical burden of stress-related illness in caregivers.

Treatment of AD and other forms of dementia primarily focuses on symptoms. Nearly all therapeutic trials have been conducted in patients with AD, with results extrapolated, correctly or not, to other etiologic categories. There is little evidence-based support for any putative prevention therapy; approaches that have shown disappointing results in controlled clinical trials include oestrogen replacement [12], nonsteroidal anti-inflammatory drugs [13], and vitamin E [14]. Intellectual impairment benefits modestly from cholinesterase inhibitor therapy [15] in mild to moderate AD and memantine hydrochloride therapy in moderate to severe AD [16]. Behavioural management includes the control of psychosis and agitation. Although atypical antipsychotic drugs have gained widespread use in this regard, they lack approval from the US Food and Drug Administration for this specific use. In 2005, the Food and Drug Administration required a black box warning label on atypical antipsychotics used to treat elderly patients with dementia because of unpublished data suggesting an increased risk of mortality (http://www.fda.gov/cder/drug/advisory/antipsychotics.htm). Other important aspects of management are lifestyle changes (e.g. driving restrictions [17]), caregiver burnout [18], and assisted living, legal guardianship, and related interventions.

Many controversies and uncertainties about the pathogenesis, diagnosis, and treatment of AD confront the clinician and scientist and will continue to do so until mechanistic insights translate into more effective clinical therapeutics. Evidence will always be an important cornerstone of therapy, but it is especially vital as long as therapeutic inefficacy fosters the proliferation of witch doctors and snake-oil purveyors.

Framing of clinical questions

This chapter on evidence-based management of dementia addresses five main clinical topics: (1) treatment of mild to moderate dementia due to AD, (2) treatment of moderate to severe dementia due to AD, (3) treatment of agitation in dementia, (4) treatment of VaD and vascular cognitive impairment (VCI), and (5) complementary therapy in dementia. The topics are similarly structured, with a clinical patient scenario that has been converted into a focused answerable PICO (patient or problem, intervention, comparison intervention, and outcomes) model question. For each question, a critically appraised topic review is presented. The review outlines the clinical bottom-line or take-home summary message, then delves into the evidence itself, a short summary of the results, and a commentary.

Search strategy

Given that all five main clinical topics concern therapy, the general search strategy was to look first for systematic reviews and meta-analyses of randomized-controlled trials in the Cochrane Library, the Cochrane Database of Reviews of Effectiveness, and MEDLINE. When necessary, individual randomized-controlled trials in the Cochrane Registry and MEDLINE were sought next.

Critical review of the evidence for each question

1. Treatment of mild to moderate dementia due to AD

Is pharmacological treatment effective for mild to moderate dementia due to AD?

Cholinesterase inhibitors (e.g. donepezil hydrochloride, rivastigmine tartrate, and galantamine hydrobromide) and, more recently, memantine have been approved for treatment of cognitive deterioration in patients with dementia due to AD. Numerous studies have evaluated the efficacy of these agents, and a recent systematic review allows detailed analysis of the efficacy of the different available therapies (Table 19.1).

Clinical scenario

A 69-year-old woman presents with her daughter for evaluation of progressive memory loss identified during the past year. She has forgotten several social engagements and appointments and frequently repeats herself, according to her daughter. She is also bothered by word-finding difficulties. Her daughter also notes that she has made several errors managing her household finances. She is having increasing difficulty finding her way around her community when driving. Her neurologic examination is unremarkable aside from memory and orientation difficulties on an office mental status assessment. Magnetic resonance imaging of the brain shows mild generalized cerebral atrophy, and routine laboratory studies are unrevealing. Formal neuropsychologic assessment shows severe deficits with learning and recall of verbal and nonverbal material. She also demonstrates moderate anomia and deficits in cognitive flexibility consistent with early-onset dementia. You diagnose her with AD, and she and her daughter ask what treatments are available.

Donepezil
Clinical bottom line
- *Global assessment*: Donepezil (10 mg/d) benefits the global clinical state compared with placebo, as measured by the 7-point Clinician's Interview-Based Impression of Change, plus caregiver input (CIBIC-Plus) scale (number needed to treat (NNT), 8; 95% confidence interval (CI), 6–15).
- *Cognition*: Donepezil (10 mg/d) produces benefit in cognitive function compared with placebo, as shown by improvement in the Alzheimer Disease Assessment Scale–Cognitive Subscale (ADAS-Cog) (weighted mean difference (WMD), −2.92; 95% CI, −3.74 to −2.1) at 24 weeks.
- *Activities of daily living*: Donepezil (10 mg/d) shows benefit in activities of daily living (ADL) compared with placebo, as shown by improvement in the Progressive Deterioration Scale (mean difference, 3.8; 95% CI, 1.7–5.9) at 12, 24, and 52 weeks.
- *Side effects*: More adverse events were observed in the treatment groups compared with the placebo group (number needed to harm (NNH), 20; 95% CI, 10–163). The highest frequencies were in the groups receiving donepezil 10 mg per day. Withdrawals at 12 weeks were also more common in treatment groups (NNH, 12; 95% CI, 7–52).

Evidence
In 13 included studies [19], patients with AD were treated with donepezil (5–10 mg/d) for 12–52 weeks. Their outcomes were compared with those of patients receiving placebo.

Study design
Seven studies were multicentre, randomized, double-blind parallel-group studies. One study was a crossover study. Primary outcomes were changes in global clinical state, cognition, or ADL. Secondary outcomes were adverse events.

Summary of results
The results of 13 trials demonstrated the apparently dose-related beneficial effect of donepezil versus placebo on

Table 19.1 Efficacy and harm of cholinesterase inhibitors for mild to moderate dementia due to AD (Refs [19–21])*.

Intervention (dosage)	Outcome	Follow-up time	Treatment number/ total (%)	Placebo number/ total (%)	WMD (95% CI)	Relative risk (95% CI)	Absolute risk reduction % (95% CI)	NNT or NNH (95% CI)	Comment
Donepezil (10 mg/d)	Global rating‡	6 months	97/390 (25)	53/409 (13)	–	1.92 (1.42–2.61)	12% (7–17)	8 (6–15)	Donezepil better
	ADAS-Cog§	6 months	404	417	2.9 (3.7–2.1)	–	–	–	Donezepil better
	ADL score**	12 months	136	140	3.8 (1.7–5.9)	–	–	–	Donezepil better
	Withdrawals†	6 months	171/725 (23)	146/735 (20)	–	1.19 (0.98–1.44)	4% (ns)	25 (ns)	Donezepil worse
	Adverse events††	6 months	99/711 (14)	67/721 (9)	–	1.50 (1.12–2.00)	5% (1–8)	20 (12–100)	Donezepil worse
Galantamine (24 mg/d)	Global rating^	3–6 months	770/1110 (69)	526/959 (55)	–	1.17 (1.26–1.35)	14% (10–18)	7 (5–10)	Galantamine better
	ADAS-Cog#§	6 months	170/498 (34)	96/553 (17)	3.1 (2.6–3.7)	1.96 (1.58–2.44)	17% (12–22)	6 (5–9)	Galantamine better
	ADL score**	6 months	212	235	2.3 (0.6–4.0)	–	–	–	Galantamine better
	Withdrawals†	6 months	173/705 (25)	116/714 (16)	–	1.51 (1.22–1.17)	8% (4–12)	12 (8–25)	Galantamine worse
	Adverse events††	6 months	107/705 (15)	55/714 (8)	–	1.96 (1.44–2.67)	7% (4–11)	14 (9–25)	Galantamine worse Mostly gastrointestinal
Rivastigmine (6–12 mg/d)	Global rating‡	6.5 months	258/973 (27)	164/839 (20)	–	1.09 (1.04–1.15)	7% (3–11)	14 (9.2–32.2)	Rivastigmine better
	ADAS-Cog#§	6.5 months	176/1054 (17)	76/863 (9)	–	1.07 (1.04–1.12)	8% (3–10)	12 (9–20)	Rivastigmine better
	ADL score**	6.5 months	1048	864	2.2 (1.1–3.2)	–	–	–	Rivastigmine worse
	Withdrawals†	6.5 months	367/1052 (34)	145/868 (16)	–	1.97 (1.66–2.33)	18% (13–20)	5.5 (4.5–7.0)	Rivastigmine worse
	Adverse events††	6.5 months	257/1052 (24)	74/868 (8)	–	2.75 (2.16–3.50)	16% (12–19)	6 (5–8)	Rivastigmine worse

CI: confidence interval; WMD: weighted mean difference; NNT: number needed to treat; NNH: number needed to harm; ns: not statistically significant. *Non-head-to-head comparison among agents. ‡Those showing improvement or ^no change or improvement on Clinician's Interview-Based Impression of Change, plus caregiver input (CIBIC-Plus); §ADAS Cog Alzheimer's Disease Assessment Scale–Cognitive Subscale (ADAS-Cog) scores for treatment compared with placebo; #Less than 4 points improvement on ADAS-Cog; **ADL, activities of daily living; Progressive Deterioration Scale scores for treatment compared with placebo; †Withdrawals any raisons; ††Withdrawals due to adverse events cognitive function and measures of global clinical state at 12, 24, and 52 weeks. For treatment lasting longer than 12 weeks, there is no difference between donepezil and placebo in the number of patients leaving the trials. There are more adverse events overall in the donepezil groups.

Galantamine

Clinical bottom line

• *Global assessment*: Review of seven trials favour treatment (24 mg/d) in observed case and intent-to-treat (ITT) analyses at 3 months and 6 months. Outcome measures were CIBIC-plus and Alzheimer Disease Cooperative Study–Clinical Global Impression of Change (NNT, 7; 95% CI, 5–10).

• *Cognition*: The analyses favour treatment (24 mg/d) in observed case and ITT analyses at 6 months. Outcome measures were the ADAS-Cog, the European ADAS-Cog, or the expanded ADAS-Cog (NNT, 6; 95% CI, 5–9).

• *Activities of daily living*: A significantly smaller decrease in the Alzheimer Disease Cooperative Study – ADL score was reported for galantamine 16 mg/d compared with placebo (3.1 points; 95% CI, 1.6–4.6) and 24 mg/d (2.3 points; 95% CI, 0.6–4.0).

• *Side effects*: In general, galantamine appeared to be well tolerated. As expected, gastrointestinal side effects were more common in the treatment groups and in a dose-related fashion. For example, the odds ratio for nausea ranged from 2.9 (95% CI, 1.7–5.3) for 16 mg per day to 4.6 (95% CI, 3.0–7.0) for 32 mg per day.

Evidence

In seven included studies [20], patients with AD were treated with galantamine (>8 mg/d) for 3, 5, or 6 months compared with patients treated with placebo.

Study design

All included trials were parallel group designs. Primary outcomes were change in global clinical state, cognition, and ADL. Secondary outcomes were adverse events.

Summary of results

The results of seven trials demonstrated the beneficial effect of galantamine, with subjects showing efficacy on global ratings, cognitive tests, and assessments of ADL. The adverse event profile of galantamine resembles that of other cholinesterase inhibitors with respect to cholinergically mediated gastrointestinal tract symptoms. There appears to be a dose-response relationship for these adverse events, with doses of 32 mg per day associated with an increased incidence of withdrawal from the study.

Rivastigmine

Clinical bottom line

• *Global assessment*: A review of eight included trials [21] favoured treatment by ITT analyses for rivastigmine (6–12 mg/d

for 12–26 weeks). Treatment benefit was demonstrated at 6 months on the CIBIC-Plus (NNT, 14; 95% CI, 9–32).

• *Cognition*: The analyses favoured 6-month treatment. The outcome measure was the ADAS-Cog (NNT, 13; 95% CI, 9–20).

• *Activities of daily living*: Improvement was noted in the Progressive Deterioration Scale score at 26 weeks (WMD, −2.2; 95% CI, −3 to −1).

• *Adverse effects or withdrawals*: Increased adverse effects (NNH, 8; 95% CI, 7–11) and withdrawals (NNH, 6; 95% CI, 5–7) in the treatment group (rivastigmine 6–12 mg).

Evidence

AD patients were treated with rivastigmine (6–12 mg) for 12–26 weeks and compared with patients treated with placebo.

Study design

All trials were randomized, double-blind, parallel-group, placebo-controlled studies. Primary outcomes were change in global clinical state, cognition, and ADL. Secondary outcomes were adverse events and withdrawals.

Summary of results

Results demonstrated the beneficial effect of rivastigmine on global ratings, cognitive tests, and ADL. The adverse event profile of rivastigmine is similar to that of other cholinesterase inhibitors, with an increase in adverse events at 6 months compared with placebo. Dropouts were also more common in the treatment group at 6 months.

2. Treatment of moderate to severe dementia due to AD

Is pharmacological treatment effective in treating moderate to severe dementia due to AD?

Cholinesterase inhibitors have been the mainstay of dementia therapy for years but were approved only for treatment of mild to moderate dementia. Memantine hydrochloride, an *N*-methyl-D-aspartate (NMDA) receptor antagonist, has been approved more recently for moderate to severe dementia due to AD (Table 19.2).

Clinical scenario

An 85-year-old man with a 5-year history of progressive cognitive decline was diagnosed with AD about 3 years ago and is being treated with a stable dose of a cholinesterase inhibitor. He is generally pleasant and cooperative but requires constant supervision because of a tendency to wander. He requires prompting for bathing and toileting. His wife would like to continue caring for him at home but finds that she is having difficulty keeping up with all the household and caregiver responsibilities. She asks if there is any other treatment available for his dementia.

Table 19.2 Efficacy and harm of memantine for severe dementia due to AD.

Outcome	Placebo, number of patients	Memantine, number of patients	Difference			
			Weighted mean (95% CI)	Absolute, % (95% CI)	NNT or NNH (95% CI)	P value
CIBIC-Plus	477	487	0.28 (0.15 to 0.41)	NA	NA	<0.001
SIB	484	492	2.97 (1.68 to 4.26)	NA	NA	<0.001
ADCS-ADLsev	485	493	1.27 (0.44 to 2.09)	NA	NA	0.003
NPI	462	474	2.76 (−0.88 to −4.63)	NA	NA	0.004
Adverse events (agitation)	88/499 (18)*	58/506 (11)*	NA	6 (1.8–10.5)	16.2 (9.5–54.6)	0.005
Dropout rate	139/499 (28)*	103/507 (20)*	NA	7.5 (2.3–12.8)	13.3 (7.8–43.9)	0.005

ADCS-ADLsev: Alzheimer Disease Cooperative Study–Activities of Daily Living, adapted to assess severe impairment; CI: confidence interval; CIBIC-Plus: Clinician's Interview-Based Impression of Change, plus caregiver input; NA: not applicable; NNH: number needed to harm; NNT: number needed to treat; NPI: Neuropsychiatric Inventory; SIB: Severe Impairment Battery; WMD: weighted mean difference.
*Values are number/total (%).

Memantine

Clinical bottom line

• *Global assessment*: A review of three trials favoured treatment at 6 months. Outcome was measured by the CIBIC-Plus (WMD, 0.28 points improvement; 95% CI, 0.15–0.41).
• *Cognition*: The analyses favour treatment at 6 months. The outcome measure was the Severe Impairment Battery (WMD, 2.97 points improvement; 95% CI, 1.68–4.26).
• *Activities of daily living*: A smaller decrease in the Alzheimer Disease Cooperative Study – ADL score was reported for patients treated with memantine versus placebo (WMD, 1.27 points; 95% CI, 0.44–2.09).
• *Behaviour*: Patients taking memantine had significantly less worsening of mood and behaviour at 6 months. The outcome measure was the Neuropsychiatric Inventory (WMD, −2.76 points; 95% CI, −0.88 to −4.63).
• *Side effects*: Aside from fewer reports of agitation with memantine (NNT, 16.2; 95% CI, 9.5–54.6), there were no significant differences in adverse effects between memantine and placebo. Memantine was well tolerated, with fewer dropouts (NNT, 13; 95% CI, 8–44).

Evidence

Patients with moderate to severe AD were treated with memantine for 6 months and compared with patients treated with placebo.

Study design

All trials were parallel-group designs lasting 6 months. Primary outcomes were change in global clinical state, cognition, ADL, and behaviour. Secondary outcomes were adverse events.

Summary of results

Three trials studying different doses of memantine (10–30 mg/d) demonstrated beneficial effects on global ratings, cognition, ADL, and behaviour.

3. Treatment of agitation in dementia

Which pharmacological treatment effective in controlling agitated behaviour in patients with dementia?

Agitated behaviour in patients with AD or other forms of dementia is a common problem that often determines the timing of a transition to a skilled care facility as caregivers become overwhelmed with attempting to cope with the behaviour. Behavioural problems may include delusions, restlessness, aggression (verbal and physical), and anger. Several medications have been used to manage agitated behaviour in dementia. This section reviews the data available about the efficacy of some common therapies.

Clinical scenario

A 78-year-old man with a 2-year history of progressive decline in memory and other cognitive functions has a diagnosis of AD. In recent months, he has become increasingly agitated, with episodes of verbally aggressive behaviour directed at his wife. He accuses her of infidelity when she leaves the house for any length of time, and he is convinced that his family is conspiring against him. Although there have been no physical altercations, he has thrown objects during his more agitated episodes. The patient has no history of psychiatric illness and was previously considered to be pleasant and soft-spoken. Routine laboratory tests demonstrated no major abnormalities, and repeat imaging of the brain is notable only for its identification of generalized cerebral atrophy. The patient's wife and children are concerned about the sustainability of his current living situation and ask how to deal with these behavioural problems.

Haloperidol

Clinical bottom line

• No benefit was found for haloperidol for behavioural symptoms (Behaviour Pathology in Alzheimer Disease Rating Scale, Brief Psychiatric Rating Scale, or Behavioural Syndromes Scale for Dementia) or for agitation (Cohen–Mansfield Agitation Inventory or Behavioural Syndromes Scale for Dementia) in four trials [22,23]. In three trials, benefits (standardized mean difference, −0.31; 95% CI, −0.49 to −0.13) were noted for treatment of aggression (irritability or aggressiveness subscore on the Multidimensional Observation Scale for Elderly Subjects, physical aggression item on the Behavioural Syndromes Scale for Dementia, and aggressiveness subscore on the Behaviour Pathology in Alzheimer Disease Rating Scale – AD).

• In trials providing data, no benefit was noted in global clinical state (Clinician's Global Impression of Change) or ADL (physical or instrumental ADL).

• An increase in the adverse event rate and dropouts (NNH, 10.2; 95% CI, 5.7–45) was noted in the treatment groups compared with placebo.

Evidence

The studies reviewed outcomes in outpatients, hospitalized patients, and institutionalized patients with AD dementia being treated for behavioural problems with varying doses of haloperidol compared with outcomes for placebo, trazodone hydrochloride, risperidone, tiapride, or fluoxetine hydrochloride. The studies were of different durations.

Study design

The five trials included three multicentre, randomized, double-blind, placebo-controlled, parallel-group studies of differing duration; one randomized, double-blind, placebo-controlled, crossover study; and one randomized, double-blind, placebo-controlled, parallel-group study. Primary outcomes were global improvement (Clinical Global Improvement Scale), control of behavioural symptoms (Behaviour Pathology in Alzheimer Disease Rating Scale, Brief Psychiatric Rating Scale, and Behavioural Syndromes Scale for Dementia), reduced agitation (Consortium to Establish a Registry for Alzheimer Disease, Behavioural Rating Scale for Dementia, Cohen–Mansfield Agitation Inventory, Agitated Behaviour Inventory for Dementia, Schedule for Affective Disorders and Schizophrenia, Brief Psychiatric Rating Scale, and Multidimensional Observation Scale for Elderly Subjects irritability or aggressiveness subscores), and functional status (the Physical Self-Maintenance Scale and the instrumental ADL scale). Secondary outcomes were adverse events and dropout rates.

Trazodone

Clinical bottom line

• *Global assessment*: Thirty-four percent of participants [24] improved relative to baseline (Alzheimer Disease Cooperative Study–Clinician's Global Impression of Change). There were no significant differences between treatment and placebo groups.

• *Behavioural disturbance*: Behavioural disturbance was measured by the Agitated Behaviour Inventory for Dementia, the Consortium to Establish a Registry for Alzheimer Disease–Behavioural Rating Scale for Dementia, and the Cohen–Mansfield Agitation Inventory. There were no statistically significant differences between treatment (trazodone, mean dose 200 mg/d) and placebo groups from baseline to 16 weeks.

• *Function*: Measures of the Physical Self-Maintenance Scale and the instrumental ADL showed no statistically significant differences between trazodone and placebo.

• *Caregiver burden*: There were no statistically significant differences between trazodone and placebo in either of the two scales (Screen for Caregiver Burden–objective and Screen for Caregiver Burden–subjective and Revised Memory and Behaviour Problems Checklist).

• *Cognition*: Analyses revealed worsening of cognitive function, as measured by change from baseline in Mini-Mental State Examination score (WMD, −1.69; 95% CI, −3.18 to −0.20), for trazodone compared with placebo at 16 weeks.

• *Adverse events*: Analysis of individual adverse symptoms showed no significant differences between the trazodone and placebo groups.

Evidence

Outpatients with probable AD and agitated behaviour who lived at home were treated either with trazodone or placebo.

Study design

Multicentre, double-blind, randomized studies compared trazodone with placebo. The trials varied by inclusion and exclusion criteria. Primary outcomes were global assessment, behavioural disturbance, functional status, caregiver burden, and cognitive function. Secondary outcomes were adverse events and dropouts.

Summary of results

There was no statistically significant difference between the placebo and treatment groups on any outcome measure, aside from lower MMSE scores in the treatment group at 16 weeks.

Valproic acid

Clinical bottom line

• *Global assessment (Clinical Global Improvement Scale)*: The results of two studies [23] could not be interpreted, and the third showed no benefit relative to placebo.

• Behavioural Disturbance (Agitation and Aggression) (Cohen–Mansfield Agitation Inventory, Social Dysfunction and Aggression Scale – 9, Clinical Global Improvement Scale, Nurses' Observation Scale). For agitation, the results of two studies [23] could not be interpreted, and the third showed no benefit relative to placebo. No study showed benefit of treatment versus placebo for aggression.

• *Tolerability or adverse events*: In one study [23], 54% of treated patients versus 29% of control patients dropped out because of adverse effects, prompting discontinuation of the study. In another study [23], no significant difference in adverse effects was noted between treatment and placebo groups. In the third study [23], 68% of treated patients experienced adverse effects compared with 33% of the placebo group, although no adverse effects prompted withdrawal. Overall, high-dose divalproex sodium (median dose, 1000 mg/d) was associated with an unacceptable frequency of adverse effects.

Evidence

Institutionalized patients with dementia and agitated behaviour were treated either with valproic acid or placebo.

Study design

One study [22,23] involved delayed-release divalproex sodium tablets versus placebo titrated over 6 weeks. Another study involved administration of a fixed dose of sodium valproate over 3 weeks. The last study [23] involved rapid-acting divalproex sodium titrated over 6 weeks by a nonblinded physician with results reviewed by blinded reviewers. Outcome measures were effects on behavioural disturbance (agitation, aggression, and mania), overall functional status, adverse events, tolerability, and safety.

Summary of results

High-dose divalproex sodium (median dose, 1000 mg/d) is not tolerated in this patient population, and low-dose divalproex sodium (480 mg/d) is ineffective for agitation. Meta-analysis of efficacy in treating agitation and aggression was not feasible given variations in methods, type of valproic acid, duration of treatment, and patient assessment methods.

Others

Although atypical antipsychotics such as risperidone, olanzapine, and quetiapine fumarate have been used in clinical practice to manage behavioural symptoms of dementia, there are insufficient data in the medical literature to evaluate its efficacy of these medications. Although atypical antipsychotics are generally viewed as better tolerated than typical neuroleptics such as haloperidol, they lack safety and tolerability and their use in a dementia population mandates further study. There is an active protocol in the Cochrane Database of Systematic Reviews to evaluate the efficacy of such medications for dementia-related agitation.

4. Treatment of VaD and vascular cognitive impairment

Is pharmacological treatment effective for patients with VaD?

Stroke and dementia increase exponentially with the aging of the population [25]. How they relate is less well understood. Stroke may result in VCI and VaD, but brain ischaemia may also worsen the cognitive effects of AD [26–28]. As longevity increases, the damaging effects of cerebrovascular disease on cognition are expected to become the main cause of dementia in elderly persons [29].

VaD (formerly multi-infarct dementia) is defined clinically by the sudden onset of cognitive decline, stepwise deterioration, and focal neurologic findings [30]. The concept of VaD has been broadened to encompass all forms of cognitive loss due to cerebrovascular disease under the nosology of VCI [31–33]. VaD is the second most common form of dementia after AD, accounting for approximately 20% of dementia cases worldwide.

The numerous subtypes of VaD include poststroke VaD, which is characterized by abrupt onset of focal neurologic signs and symptoms, along with cortical cognitive impairments such as aphasia, apraxia, or agnosia [30]. Single-infarct dementia occurs when a small but strategically located infarct (e.g. in the thalamus, basal forebrain, or caudate) produces an acute VaD [34]. Subcortical ischaemic VaD is a common form of VaD resulting from small-vessel disease, lacunar infarctions, and white matter ischaemia [35]. Mixed AD with cerebrovascular disease is termed mixed dementia [36].

Secondary stroke prevention strategies are indicated for patients with a VaD diagnosis. These strategies should include early diagnosis of cerebral infarction, determination of mechanism (large-artery atherosclerosis, cardioembolism, small-vessel disease, or any combination of the three, or other), carotid endarterectomy, angioplasty or stenting or both (when indicated), anticoagulation with warfarin (when indicated), antiplatelet therapy, and management of hyperlipidaemia, hypertension, diabetes mellitus, smoking, elevated homocysteine, obesity, diet, and exercise.

Cholinergic deficits are well documented in VaD, independent of any concomitant AD pathology [37]. Cholinergic structures (e.g. basal forebrain cholinergic nuclei and hippocampal CA1 neurons) are vulnerable to ischaemic damage [38]. Forty percent of VaD patients examined neuropathologically have a loss of cholinergic neurons with reduced acetylcholine activity in the cortex, hippocampus, striatum, and cerebrospinal fluid [39]. Therefore, it is not surprising that three of the acetylcholinesterase inhibitors approved for AD (donepezil, galantamine, and rivastigmine), have also been used for VaD [40,41].

Glutamate is the principal excitatory amino acid neurotransmitter in cortical and hippocampal neurons. Accumulating evidence suggests that the cortical neuronal loss underlying dementia may be related to an increased sensitivity to glutamate or to sustained increases in glutamate levels [42]. Glutamate exposure leads to a cumulative influx of calcium into neurons, impaired homeostasis, and, eventually, neurodegeneration resulting in cell death. One receptor activated by glutamate is the NMDA receptor, which is involved physiologically in learning and memory [43]. Because excessive NMDA stimulation induced by ischaemia leads to excitotoxicity, agents that block pathologic stimulation of NMDA receptors might protect against further cortical neurodegeneration in patients with VaD while the physiologic function of the remaining neurons could be restored, resulting in symptomatic improvement [44]. Memantine is an NMDA receptor antagonist with few side effects that has therapeutic potential in numerous central nervous system disorders. Memantine also appears to reduce neuronal damage in global and focal animal models of brain ischemia [45].

Clinical scenario

A 78-year-old, right-handed, white woman presents with stepwise cognitive decline over the previous 2 years and a history of stroke, coronary artery disease, hypertension, and hyperlipidaemia. Brain imaging discloses multiple chronic cerebral infarctions. You diagnose VaD. She has difficulties with ADL. Her family asks what can be done for cognitive complaints beyond secondary stroke prevention.

Donepezil

Clinical bottom line

Donepezil demonstrated statistically significant improvement in cognitive function, clinical global impression, and ADL compared with placebo. Compared with placebo, donepezil 5 mg/d resulted in a greater proportion of patients improving on the CIBIC-Plus measure (NNT, 10; 95% CI, 6–32). In other words, 100 of 1000 patients treated for 6 months will demonstrate improvement in global function. Compared with placebo, donepezil 10 mg/d resulted in a greater proportion of patients having adverse events (NNH, 20; 95% CI, 10–65) but donepezil 5 mg/d appeared to be well tolerated.

Evidence

Two large-scale clinical trials, donepezil 307 and 308, were parallel-group, 24-week, double-blind, randomized placebo-controlled multicentre trials with 603 and 616 subjects, respectively (total, 1219) [46–48]. Patients with mild to moderate cognitive decline due to probable VaD were recruited and randomized to donepezil (5–10 mg) or to placebo. Vascular risk factors were treated medically but not standardized. Approximately 80% of patients completed each study. A systematic review was conducted to assess the clinical efficacy and tolerability of donepezil on cognitive function, clinical global impression, ADL, and social functioning of people with VCI [49]. Relevant randomized-controlled trials were

identified from a search of the Cochrane Dementia and Cognitive Impairment Improvement Group Specialized Register. Unpublished trial data were requested from pharmaceutical companies. Only unconfounded, randomized, double-blind trials comparing donepezil with placebo were eligible. Two reviewers applied inclusion and exclusion criteria and extracted data, which were pooled where appropriate; WMD or Peto odds ratios with 95% confidence intervals were calculated. ITT analysis was undertaken whenever possible.

Summary of results

Proportion data were available for the CIBIC-Plus measure. Calculations of relative risk increase, absolute risk increase, and NNT were performed by combining data from studies 307 and 308. The outcome measure was the proportion of patients experiencing mild, moderate, or marked improvement on the CIBIC-Plus measure at the primary outcome evaluation (24 weeks). In terms of cognitive function, the donepezil groups showed statistically significantly better performance than the placebo groups on the ADAS-Cog at 24 weeks. In terms of global function, participants taking a 5-mg/d dose showed improvement on the CIBIC-Plus (NNT, 10), but this improvement was not observed in the higher-dose group. The sum of the boxes of the Clinical Dementia Rating showed a statistically significant benefit of 10 mg/d over both placebo and the lower dose. On the instrumental ADL scale, there was no statistically significant difference between the groups taking donepezil 5 mg/d and placebo, but the 10-mg group showed benefit. A broad range of adverse events was reported. In general, donepezil 5 mg/d was well tolerated but the 10-mg dose resulted in significantly more adverse events (especially gastrointestinal) compared with placebo (NNH, 20) (Table 19.3).

Commentary

These two studies are the largest cholinesterase inhibitor clinical trials thus far for VaD. Both studies were well designed. Analysis was conducted of both the objective clinical and the functional or quality-of-life factors. However, the studies were relatively brief (24 weeks). The outcome measures considered relatively small increments of improvement as statistically significant. Their clinical significance is uncertain. Outcome measures were not VaD-specific but instead were geared towards AD. Enrolled patients were required to have stabilization of cerebrovascular disease and other comorbid conditions before entering the study. These studies were not powered for subgroup analysis (i.e. the ability to differentiate between probable versus possible VaD and outcomes of treatment. Most patients remained on the study medication but adverse events (especially nausea) were more common in the donepezil 10-mg group. The dropout rate was similar between the groups: 84% of patients completed the studies.

Table 19.3 Treatments of vascular dementia (Refs [49–55])*.

Intervention (dosage)	Outcome	Follow-up time	Treatment number/ total (%)	Placebo number/ total (%)	WMD (95% CI)	Relative risk (95%CI)	Absolute risk reduction % (95% CI)	NNT or NNH (95% CI)	Comment
Donepezil (5 mg/d)	Global rating improvement	6 months	148/398 (37)	105/382 (27)	–	1.35 (1.10–1.67)	10% (3–15)	10 (6–33)	Donezepil better
	ADAS-Cog§	6 months	384	368	1.66 (2.40–0.92)	–	–	–	Donezepil better
	One or more adverse events	6 months	366/406 (90)	343/392 (87)	–	1.02 (0.97–1.08)	+2% (ns)	50 (ns)	Donezepil worse
Donepezil (10 mg/d)	Global rating improvement	6 months	119/397 (30)	105/382 (27)	–	1.09 (0.87–1.36)	7% (ns)	14 (ns)	Donezepil better
	ADAS-Cog§	6 months	380	368	2.17 (2.97–1.37)	–	–	–	Donezepil better
	One or more adverse events	6 months	392/421 (93)	343/392 (87)	–	1.06 (1.02–1.11)	+6% (2–10)	17 (10–50)	Donezepil worse
Galantamine (16–24mg/d)	Global rating‡	6 months	213/288 (74)	95/161 (59)	–	1.25 (1.08–1.45)	+15% (6–24)	7 (4–16)	Galantamine better; Not statistically significant on sub-group with pure VaD
	ADAS-Cog§	6 months	357	186	2.29 (3.46–1.12)	–	–	–	Galantamine better
	Withdrawals†	6 months	102/396 (26)	33/196 (17)	–	1.53 (1.07–2.18)	+9% (2–16)	11 (5–6)	Galantamine worse
	One or more adverse events	6 months	330/396 (83)	133/196 (68)	–	1.23 (1.10–1.37)	+15% (8–23)	7 (4–12)	Galantamine worse
Rivastigmine	Insufficient evidence								
Memantine 20 mg/d	NNT 13 (NS); NNH Safe and well tolerated								

CI: confidence interval; WMD: weighted mean difference; NNT: number needed to treat; NNH: number needed to harm; ns: not statistically significant.

*Non-head-to-head comparison among agents. ‡Those showing no change or improvement on Clinician's Interview-Based Impression of Change, plus caregiver input (CIBIC-Plus); §ADAS Cog, Alzheimer's Disease Assessment Scale–Cognitive Subscale (ADAS-Cog) scores for treatment compared with placebo; †Withdrawals any raisons.

Galantamine

Clinical bottom line

Galantamine (24 mg/d) significantly improved cognition (by ADAS-Cog), disability (by Disability Assessment for Dementia), and neuropsychiatric symptoms (by Neuropsychiatric Inventory) compared with placebo. Compared with placebo, galantamine (24 mg/d) resulted in a greater proportion of patients remaining stable or improving on the CIBIC-Plus measure (NNT, 7; 95% CI, 4–20). In other words, if 1000 patients are treated for 6 months, 140 fewer will suffer a deterioration in cognition. Compared with placebo, galantamine treatment resulted in a greater proportion of patients having adverse events (NNH, 7; 95% CI, 4–13). NNH for nausea and vomiting was 4 (95% CI, 3–6), and NNH for subsequent withdrawal was 8 (95% CI, 6–11).

Evidence

Patients with probable VaD or with AD combined with cerebrovascular disease were randomly assigned (2:1 ratio) to galantamine 24 mg/d ($N = 396$) or placebo ($N = 396$) in an international, multicentre, double-blind, 6-month trial [50]. Primary outcomes were cognition (ADAS-Cog) and global functioning (CIBIC-Plus), and secondary outcomes were assessments of ADL, behavioural symptoms, and adverse events. A Cochrane Systematic Review protocol, Galantamine for Vascular Cognitive Impairment, is not yet complete [51].

Commentary

The spectrum of patients and the diagnosis of disease were well defined. Eligibility criteria appeared appropriate. Treatment allocation was random and the randomization method was explained. Not all patients were accounted for after randomization, with 23% lost to follow-up (17% taking placebo, 26% taking galantamine). The two treatment groups had similar baseline demographic characteristics. Patients, care providers, and investigators were blinded and outcomes assessed in a blinded fashion. Side effects and adverse events were explicitly sought and estimates of their frequency and severity presented. The main analysis was stated as ITT but efficacy outcomes appeared to be calculated and presented only for those patients completing 6 months of therapy. CIBIC-Plus results have been presented as they were in the paper but also recalculated and presented as if all those lost to follow-up had the worst possible outcome (deterioration). The reanalysed CIBIC-Plus results are no longer statistically significant. The magnitude of the treatment effect and its precision were given. A key concern is the high proportion of patients lost to follow-up with disproportionate representation of the two groups (treatment and placebo). The ITT analysis appeared not to take into account the lost patients (Table 19.3).

Rivastigmine

Clinical bottom line

There may be some benefit of rivastigmine for VCI; however, this conclusion is based on small studies comparing rivastigmine to other treatments (not placebo) or using data extrapolated from trials involving AD patients with vascular risk factors of unclear significance.

Evidence

A Cochrane Systematic Review was conducted to assess the efficacy of rivastigmine in the treatment of patients with VCI, VaD, or mixed dementia [52]. Unfortunately, no suitable unconfounded randomized double-blind trials were identified.

Summary of results

Placebo-controlled trials of VaD patients are not yet complete. Post hoc data from large placebo-controlled trials in AD patients with arbitrarily defined vascular risks showed that patients who possessed additional vascular risks responded better cognitively to high-dose rivastigmine compared with patients without vascular risks. Small, open-label studies of patients with subcortical dementia comparing rivastigmine to aspirin or to aspirin and nimpodipine showed significant benefits with rivastigmine in measures of executive functioning, verbal fluency, ADL, behaviour, and depression.

Commentary

Using markers of vascular risk, such as hypertension, in AD patients as a surrogate for VCI is simplistic and invalid. Available studies of VCI patients are small, unblinded, and not placebo controlled. Further trials are required before rivastigmine can be recommended for treatment of VaD.

Memantine

Clinical bottom line

Two 6-month studies of patients with mild to moderate VaD showed that memantine improved cognition (ADAS-Cog, 1.85 points; 95% CI, 0.88–2.83; $P < .001$) and behaviour (0.48 points, 95% CI, 0.06–0.91; $P = 0.03$). However, these findings were not supported by clinical global measures or assessments of ADL. There was significantly less agitation with memantine than with placebo (odds ratio, 0.54 (95% CI, 0.31–0.96); $P = 0.04$; NNT, 30 (95% CI, 15–377)). Memantine is well tolerated.

Evidence

A Cochrane Systematic Review was conducted to determine the efficacy and safety of memantine for patients with AD, VaD, and mixed dementia [53]. Two large, multicentre, 28-week trials compared memantine (20 mg/d) with placebo: MMM 300 (609 patients) and MMM 500 (1127 patients) [54,55].

Summary of results

Compared with placebo, memantine produced no difference in clinical global impression (WMD, 0.03; 95% CI, −0.13–0.19; $P = 0.72$). Both studies provided ADAS-Cog data, and the change at 28 weeks from baseline showed statistically significant improvement with memantine (ADAS-Cog, 1.85 points;

95% CI, 0.88–2.83; $P < 0.001$). There were no differences in ADL on the self-care subscale of the Nurse Observation Scale for Geriatric Patients (0.12 points; 95% CI, −0.43–0.67; $P = 0.66$). There was significantly less agitation with memantine than with placebo (odds ratio, 0.54 (95% CI, 0.31–0.96); $P = 0.04$; NNT, 30 (95% CI, 15–377)). The disturbing behaviour subscale of the Nurse Observation Scale for Geriatric Patients identified less disturbed behaviour in the memantine group (0.48 points compared with placebo; 95% CI, 0.06–0.91; $P = 0.03$). The dropout rates and numbers of patients with adverse events, dizziness, or confusion were similar for the treatment and placebo groups.

Commentary
The two available trials appear to be of high quality. Unfortunately, the beneficial effect of memantine on cognition in patients with mild to moderate VaD was not clinically discernible at 6 months.

Aspirin
Clinical bottom line
A Cochrane Systematic Review reported that there were no randomized-controlled trials investigating aspirin for VaD [56]. As yet, there is still no evidence that aspirin is effective for VaD. Generally, though, these patients already have an approved indication for aspirin (or other antiplatelet agent).

5. Complementary therapy in dementia
Is complementary therapy efficacious and safe for treatment of patients with dementia or cognitive decline?

Complementary and alternative medicine may help treat certain forms of dementia and related symptoms or slow disease progression by ameliorating disturbances in cognition, mood, sleep, and ADL. Suggested mechanisms of action include modifications in neurotransmitter synthesis, inhibition of neurotransmitter reuptake and enzyme-induced breakdown, antioxidants, antiplatelet activity, enhanced blood flow, and glucose metabolism. Many inconclusive studies of complementary and alternative medicines are characterized by methodologic deficiencies such as small sample size, inadequate controls that are not randomized or blinded, short follow-up, and poor measurement strategies. If complementary interventions can be shown to be efficacious by using more rigorous experimental designs, both patients and clinicians alike could avail themselves of a wider range of pharmacologic and nonpharmacologic therapies that may be better tolerated and safer than some allopathic medicines [57–59].

Clinical scenario
A 72-year-old retired pharmacist presents with his daughter for progressive memory loss identified in the preceding 2 years. He is forgetful, repeats himself frequently, and has difficulty managing the household finances. His neurologic examination is unremarkable aside from cognitive impairment on mental status assessment. Magnetic resonance imaging of his brain simply demonstrates mild generalized atrophy, and the findings of routine laboratory studies are within normal ranges. He refuses to acknowledge his cognitive decline. You diagnose dementia and explore treatment options. He will not accept 'dementia drugs,' but is receptive to an over-the-counter medication to assist with memory. What might be available for him to try?

Ginkgo biloba
Ginkgo biloba is an extract of the maidenhair tree that has long been used in China as a traditional medicine for various health conditions. In many European nations, a standardized extract is widely available for a broad range of conditions (e.g. memory and concentration problems, depression, anxiety, dizziness, tinnitus, and headache). The proposed mechanisms of action are increased blood supply by dilation of blood vessels, modification of neurotransmitter systems, and reductions in blood viscosity and the density of oxygen-free radicals.

Clinical bottom line
Compared with placebo, ginkgo biloba appears to be safe with no excess side effects. Ginkgo biloba <200 mg/d and >200 mg/d resulted in clinical global improvement in patients with acquired cognitive impairment at 12 weeks (NNT, 2; 95% CI, 1–3) and at 24 weeks (NNT, 6; 95% CI, 3–37), respectively. Cognition, ADL, and measures of mood and emotion also showed statistically significant benefit for ginkgo biloba compared with placebo at 12 to 52 weeks.

Evidence
A Cochrane Systematic Review assembled all the relevant, unconfounded, double-blind, placebo-controlled studies of ginkgo biloba (of any strength) over any time period, in patients with acquired cognitive impairment, including dementia, of any severity [60]. For the meta-analyses, data were based on reported summary statistics for each study. Efficacy and safety results were presented.

Summary of results
Overall, there were no significant differences between ginkgo biloba and placebo in the proportion of patients experiencing adverse events. Clinical global improvement (Clinical Global Improvement Scale) was associated with a dose of ginkgo that was less than 200 mg/d versus placebo at 12 weeks and a dose greater than 200 mg/d at 24 weeks. Cognition, ADL, and measures of mood and emotion also showed statistically significant benefit for ginkgo compared with placebo at 12 to 52 weeks.

Commentary
Most of the studies reported the analyses of data from participants who completed treatment. There were few attempts at ITT analysis and no data on quality of life, measures of depression, or dependency. Many early trials were

small and used unsatisfactory methods. The possibility of publication bias in the systematic review could not be excluded. Thus, there is still need for a large modern trial that would permit ITT analysis to provide robust estimates of the magnitude and precision of any treatment effects.

Homeopathy

Clinical bottom line

A Cochrane Systematic Review reported that no randomized-controlled trials with a sample size of more than 20 existed [61]. Since no studies were found that fulfilled criteria for inclusion, no data were presented. This absence of evidence makes it impossible to comment on the use of homeopathy for dementia.

Folic acid and vitamin B_{12}

Mild degrees of folate inadequacy, not severe enough to cause anaemia, are associated with increased homocysteine. Increased homocysteine is linked to an increased risk of arterial diseases, dementia in general, and AD. Folate inadequacy might arise because of insufficient folates in the diet, inefficient absorption, or deranged metabolic utilization of folates because of genetic variations. There is an interest in whether or not dietary supplements of folic acid can improve cognitive function of people with cognitive decline associated with aging or dementia. There is some risk that folic acid given to patients with an undiagnosed vitamin B_{12} deficiency may lead to neurologic damage. The administration of folate would correct the anaemia, resulting in a delay in diagnosis while neurologic effects progress. Thus, trials of folic acid supplementation may involve simultaneous administration of vitamin B_{12}.

Clinical bottom line

A Cochrane Systematic Review identified four small, limited, randomized, placebo-controlled, double-blind trials fulfilling inclusion criteria [62]. Analysis of the trials found no benefit from folic acid, with or without vitamin B_{12}, compared with placebo on any measures of cognition or mood for healthy elderly persons, cognitively impaired persons, or persons with dementia. Folic acid plus vitamin B_{12} was effective in reducing serum homocysteine concentrations and was well tolerated with no reported adverse effects.

Dehydroepiandrosterone

Clinical bottom line

Four randomized trials met inclusion criteria. Three trials studied cognition in normal elderly people, and one studied cognition in perimenopausal women. There were no studies in persons with dementia. Overall, the data offered no support for improvement in memory or other aspects of cognition after dehydroepiandrosterone treatment in healthy older people. Because of the growing public enthusiasm for dehydroepiandrosterone supplementation and the theoretical possibility of a neuroprotective effect, high-quality trials are needed [63].

Aroma therapy

Aroma therapy has been used, especially in the UK, for persons with dementia for whom verbal interaction may be difficult and conventional medicine of marginal value. Other reported uses are for dementia patients with behavioural disturbances, sleep disorders, and amotivation.

Clinical bottom line

A Cochrane Systematic Review identified two randomized-controlled trials of aroma therapy for dementia but usable data could be extracted only from one of the two [64]. There was, indeed, a statistically significant treatment effect in favour of aroma therapy on measures of agitation and neuropsychiatric symptoms.

Acetyl-L-carnitine

Acetyl-L-carnitine (ALC) is described as having several properties that may be beneficial in dementia. These include activity affecting cholinergic neurons, membrane stabilization, and mitochondrial function. Early studies suggested a beneficial effect of ALC on cognition in aging patients, but later larger studies did not support these findings. ALC is not currently in routine clinical use.

Clinical bottom line

A Cochrane Systematic Review identified 16 double-blind, randomized trials that compared ALC with placebo in persons with mild to moderate dementia [65]. ALC showed some benefit as evidenced on clinical global impression and on MMSE at 24 weeks, but there was no supportive evidence from any other objective assessments in any other realm of cognition or behaviour. Given the large number of statistical comparisons, the significant results might be due to chance alone. There is no current evidence to recommend routine use of ALC in clinical practice.

Nicotine

Nicotine is a cholinergic agonist that also releases acetylcholine presynaptically. Observational studies have suggested a protective effect of smoking against AD, but more recent studies have called this conclusion into question.

Clinical bottom line

A Cochrane Systematic Review identified only a single unconfounded, double-blind, randomized trial that met inclusion criteria, but the results were not presented in a way that allowed further analysis [66]. Therefore, the review provided no evidence that nicotine is either an effective or safe treatment for AD.

Music therapy

Clinical bottom line

A Cochrane Systematic Review identified randomized-controlled trials but the methodologic quality was generally poor and the study results could not be validated or pooled for further analysis [67]. No useful conclusions could be drawn.

Phototherapy

Sleep-wake cycles are controlled by the endogenous circadian rhythm generated by the suprachiasmatic nuclei of the hypothalamus. In patients with dementia, degenerative changes in the suprachiasmatic nuclei may be a biological basis for circadian disturbances, which may be reversible by light stimulation.

Clinical bottom line

A Cochrane Systematic Review identified five randomized-controlled studies that met inclusion criteria, but the necessary data could be extracted from only three of them [68]. The review found no adequate evidence of effectiveness of bright-light therapy for managing sleep, behaviour, mood, or cognitive disturbances associated with dementia.

Lecithin

AD patients may lack the enzyme responsible for converting choline into acetylcholine within the brain. Lecithin is a major dietary source of choline, and extra consumption of it may reduce disease progression.

Clinical bottom line

A Cochrane Systematic Review identified 12 randomized trials involving a total of 376 patients with AD, Parkinsonian dementia, or subjective memory decline [69]. No clinical trials reported any clear benefit of lecithin for AD or dementia associated with Parkinsonism. Lecithin had a dramatic result in a single trial of patients with subjective memory decline. Overall, however, the evidence does not support the use of lecithin for treatment of patients with dementia.

Conclusion

Beginning, as always, with familiar clinical scenarios and vignettes, this evidence-based review of therapies for dementia has carefully outlined the central clinical questions related to treatment of dementia due to AD, treatment of agitation in dementia, treatment of VaD and VCI, and complementary therapies. We have emphasized the clinical bottom-line messages to better equip clinicians to combine this best evidence with their own clinical experience and the wishes of their patients for sensible answers during the clinical decision-making process.

Acknowledgment

Editing, proofreading, and reference verification were provided by the Section of Scientific Publications, Mayo Clinic.

References

1 Kokmen E, Beard CM, O'Brien PC, Kurland LT. Epidemiology of dementia in Rochester, Minnesota. *Mayo. Clin. Proc.* 1996; **71**: 275–82.

2 Hebert LE, Scherr PA, Bienias JL, Bennett DA, Evans DA. Alzheimer disease in the US population: prevalence estimates using the 2000 census. *Arch. Neurol.* 2003; **60**: 1119–22.

3 Bower JH, Maraganore DM, McDonnell SK, Rocca WA. Incidence and distribution of Parkinsonism in Olmsted County, Minnesota, 1976–1990. *Neurology* 1999; **52**: 1214–20.

4 Sherrington R, Rogaev EI, Liang Y, Rogaeva EA, Levesque G, Ikeda M, et al. Cloning of a gene bearing missense mutations in early-onset familial Alzheimer's disease. *Nature* 1995; **375**: 754–60.

5 Wisniewski KE, Wisniewski HM, Wen GY. Occurrence of neuropathological changes and dementia of Alzheimer's disease in Down's syndrome. *Ann. Neurol.* 1985; **17**: 278–82.

6 Levy-Lahad E, Wasco W, Poorkaj P, Romano DM, Oshima J, Pettingell WH, et al. Candidate gene for the chromosome 1 familial Alzheimer's disease locus. *Science* 1995; **269**: 973–7.

7 Hardy JA, Higgins GA. Alzheimer's disease: the amyloid cascade hypothesis. *Science* 1992; **256**:184–5.

8 Corder EH, Saunders AM, Strittmatter WJ, Schmechel DE, Gaskell PC, Small GW, et al. Gene dose of apolipoprotein E type 4 allele and the risk of Alzheimer's disease in late onset families. *Science* 1993; **261**: 921–3.

9 Corbo RM, Scacchi R. Apolipoprotein E (APOE) allele distribution in the world: is APOE4 a 'thrifty' allele? *Ann. Hum. Genet.* 1999; **63** (Part 4): 301–10.

10 US Congress, Office of Technology Assessment. Losing a million minds: confronting the tragedy of Alzheimer's disease and other dementias, OTA-BA-323. US Government Printing Office, Washington, DC, 1987.

11 Rice DP, Fillit HM, Max W, Knopman DS, Lloyd JR, Duttagupta S. Prevalence, costs, and treatment of Alzheimer's disease and related dementia: a managed care perspective. *Am. J. Manag. Care* 2001; **7**: 809–18.

12 Shumaker SA, Legault C, Rapp SR, Thal L, Wallace RB, Ockene JK, et al, WHIMS Investigators. Estrogen plus progestin and the incidence of dementia and mild cognitive impairment in postmenopausal women: the Women's Health Initiative Memory Study: a randomized controlled trial. *JAMA.* 2003; **289**: 2651–62.

13 Aisen PS, Schafer KA, Grundman M, Pfeiffer E, Sano M, Davis KL, et al, Alzheimer's Disease Cooperative Study. Effects of rofecoxib or naproxen vs placebo on Alzheimer disease progression: a randomized controlled trial. *JAMA.* 2003; **289**: 2819–26.

14 Petersen RC, Thomas RG, Grundman M, Bennett D, Doody R, Ferris S, et al. Alzheimer's Disease Cooperative Study Group. Vitamin E and donepezil for the treatment of mild cognitive impairment. *N. Engl. J. Med.* 2005 June 9; **352**: 2379–88. Epub 2005 April 13.

15 Rogers SL, Farlow MR, Doody RS, Mohs R, Friedhoff LT, Donepezil Study Group. A 24-week, double-blind, placebo-controlled trial of donepezil in patients with Alzheimer's disease. *Neurology* 1998; **50**: 136–45.

16 Reisberg B, Doody R, Stoffler A, Schmitt F, Ferris S, Mobius HJ, Memantine Study Group. Memantine in moderate-to-severe Alzheimer's disease. *N. Engl. J. Med.* 2003; **348**: 1333–41.

17 Dubinsky RM, Stein AC, Lyons K. Practice parameter: risk of driving and Alzheimer's disease (an evidence-based review): report of the quality standards subcommittee of the American Academy of Neurology. *Neurology* 2000; **54**: 2205–11.

18 Mittelman MS, Roth DL, Coon DW, Haley WE. Sustained benefit of supportive intervention for depressive symptoms in caregivers of patients with Alzheimer's disease. *Am. J. Psychiatr.* 2004; **161**: 850–6.

19 Birks J, Harvey RJ. Donepezil for dementia due to Alzheimer's disease. *Cochrane Database Syst. Rev.,* 2006; **1**: CD001190.

20 Loy C, Schneider L. Galantamine for Alzheimer's disease. *Cochrane Database Syst. Rev.,* 2004; **4**: CD001747.

21 Birks J, Grimley Evans J, Iakovidou V, Tsolaki M. Rivastigmine for Alzheimer's disease. *Cochrane Database Syst. Rev.,* 2000; **4**: CD001191.

22 Lonergan E, Luxenberg J, Colford J. Haloperidol for agitation in dementia. *Cochrane Database Syst. Rev.,* 2001: CD002852.

23 Lonergan ET, Luxenberg J. Valproate preparations for agitation in dementia. *Cochrane Database Syst. Rev.,* 2004; **2**: CD003945.

24 Martinon-Torres G, Fioravanti M, Grimley EJ. Trazodone for agitation in dementia. *Cochrane Database Syst. Rev.,* 2004; **4**: CD004990.

25 Launer LJ, Hofman A. Frequency and impact of neurologic diseases in the elderly of Europe: a collaborative study of population-based cohorts. *Neurology* 2000; **54**(11 Suppl. 5): S1–8.

26 Snowdon DA, Greiner LH, Mortimer JA, Riley KP, Greiner PA, Markesbery WR. Brain infarction and the clinical expression of Alzheimer disease: The Nun Study. *JAMA* 1997; **277**: 813–7.

27 Esiri MM, Nagy Z, Smith MZ, Barnetson L, Smith AD. Cerebrovascular disease and threshold for dementia in the early stages of Alzheimer's disease. *Lancet* 1999; **354**: 919–20.

28 Neuropathology Group of the Medical Research Council Cognitive Function and Aging Study (MRC CFAS). Pathological correlates of late-onset dementia in a multicentre, community-based population in England and Wales. *Lancet* 2001; **357**: 169–75.

29 Roman GC. Stroke, cognitive decline and vascular dementia: the silent epidemic of the 21st century. *Neuroepidemiology* 2003; **22**: 161–4.

30 Erkinjuntti T. Cerebrovascular dementia: pathophysiology, diagnosis and treatment. *CNS Drugs* 1999; **12**: 35–48.

31 Rockwood K, Howard K, MacKnight C, Darvesh S. Spectrum of disease in vascular cognitive impairment. *Neuroepidemiology* 1999; **18**: 248–54.

32 Wentzel C, Rockwood K, MacKnight C, Hachinski V, Hogan DB, Feldman H, et al. Progression of impairment in patients with vascular cognitive impairment without dementia. *Neurology* 2001; **57**: 714–6.

33 Rockwood K, Davis H, MacKnight C, Vandorpe R, Gauthier S, Guzman A, et al. The consortium to investigate vascular impairment of cognition: methods and first findings. *Can. J. Neurol. Sci.* 2003; **30**: 237–43.

34 O'Brien JT, Erkinjuntti T, Reisberg B, Roman G, Sawada T, Pantoni L, et al. Vascular cognitive impairment. *Lancet Neurol.* 2003; **2**: 89–98.

35 Roman GC, Erkinjuntti T, Wallin A, Pantoni L, Chui HC. Subcortical ischaemic vascular dementia. *Lancet Neurol.* 2002; **1**: 426–36.

36 Zekry D, Hauw JJ, Gold G. Mixed dementia: epidemiology, diagnosis, and treatment. *J. Am. Geriatr. Soc.* 2002; **50**: 1431–8.

37 Gottfries CG, Blennow K, Karlsson I, Wallin A. The neurochemistry of vascular dementia. *Dementia* 1994; **5**: 163–7.

38 Vinters HV, Ellis WG, Zarow C, Zaias BW, Jagust WJ, Mack WJ, et al. Neuropathologic substrates of ischemic vascular dementia. *J. Neuropathol. Exp. Neurol.* 2000; **59**: 931–45.

39 Court JA, Perry EK, Kalaria RN. Neurotransmitter control of the cerebral vasculature and abnormalities in vascular dementia. In: Erkinjuntti T & Gauthier S, eds., *Vascular Cognitive Impairment*. Martin Duniz Ltd, London, UK, 2002: pp. 167–85.

40 Roman GC. Cholinergic dysfunction in vascular dementia. *Curr. Psychiatr. Rep.* 2005; **7**: 18–26.

41 Erkinjuntti T, Roman G, Gauthier S, Feldman H, Rockwood K. Emerging therapies for vascular dementia and vascular cognitive impairment. *Stroke* 2004 April; **35**: 1010–7. Epub 2004 March 4.

42 Cacabelos R, Takeda M, Winblad B. The glutamatergic system and neurodegeneration in dementia: preventive strategies in Alzheimer's disease. *Int. J. Geriatr. Psychiatr.* 1999; **14**: 3–47.

43 Danysz W, Parsons AC. Glycine and N-methyl-D-aspartate receptors: physiological significance and possible therapeutic applications. *Pharmacol. Rev.* 1998; **50**: 597–664.

44 Kornhuber J, Weller M, Schoppmeyer K, Riederer P. Amantadine and memantine are NMDA receptor antagonists with neuroprotective properties. *J. Neural. Transm. Suppl.* 1994; **43**: 91–104.

45 Heim C, Sontag KH. Memantine prevents progressive functional neurodegeneration in rats. *J. Neural. Transm. Suppl.* 1995; **46**: 117–30.

46 Black S, Roman GC, Geldmacher DS, Salloway S, Hecker J, Burns A, et al. Donepezil 307 Vascular Dementia Study Group. Efficacy and tolerability of donepezil in vascular dementia: positive results of a 24-week, multicenter, international, randomized, placebo-controlled clinical trial. *Stroke* 2003 October; **34**: 2323–30. Epub 2003 September 11.

47 Wilkinson D, Doody R, Helme R, Taubman K, Mintzer J, Kertesz A, et al. Donepezil 308 Study Group. Donepezil in vascular dementia: a randomized, placebo-controlled study. *Neurology* 2003; **61**: 479–86.

48 Mayo Clinic Scottsdale Evidence-Based Clinical Practice, Research, Information, and Training (MERIT) Center [homepage on the Internet]. One in 10 patients with vascular dementia experiences at least mild cognitive improvement with oral donepezil (5 mg/d) therapy [cited 2006 June 12]. Available from: http://mcsweb.mayo.edu/Dept/MERIT%5FCenter/CATS/Documents/2004-04-13-EBNP-DonepezilVaD.doc

49 Malouf R, Birks J. Donepezil for vascular cognitive impairment. *Cochrane Database Syst. Rev.,* 2004; **1**: CD004395.

50 Erkinjuntti T, Kurz A, Gauthier S, Bullock R, Lilienfeld S, Damaraju CV. Efficacy of galantamine in probable vascular

dementia and Alzheimer's disease combined with cerebrovascular disease: a randomised trial. *Lancet* 2002; **359**: 1283–90.

51 Craig D, Birks J. Galantamine for vascular cognitive impairment. *Cochrane Database Syst. Rev.*, 2006; **1**: CD004746.

52 Craig D, Birks J. Rivastigmine for vascular cognitive impairment. *Cochrane Database Syst. Rev.*, 2005; **2**: CD004744.

53 Areosa SA, Sherriff F, McShane R. Memantine for dementia. *Cochrane Database Syst. Rev.*, 2005; **3**: CD003154.

54 Wilcock G, Mobius HJ, Stoffler A, MMM 500 group. A double-blind, placebo-controlled multicentre study of memantine in mild to moderate vascular dementia (MMM500). *Int. Clin. Psychopharmacol.* 2002; **17**: 297–305.

55 Orgogozo JM, Rigaud AS, Stoffler A, Mobius HJ, Forette F. Efficacy and safety of memantine in patients with mild to moderate vascular dementia: a randomized, placebo-controlled trial (MMM 300). *Stroke* 2002; **33**: 1834–9.

56 Williams PS, Rands G, Orrel M, Spector A. Aspirin for vascular dementia. *Cochrane Database Syst. Rev.*, 2000; **4**: CD001296.

57 Diamond B, Johnson S, Torsney K, Morodan J, Prokop B, Davidek D, et al. Complementary and alternative medicines in the treatment of dementia: an evidence-based review. *Drugs Aging* 2003; **20**: 981–98.

58 Sierpina VS, Sierpina M, Loera JA, Grumbles L. Complementary and integrative approaches to dementia. *South Med. J.* 2005; **98**: 636–45.

59 Kidd PM. A review of nutrients and botanicals in the integrative management of cognitive dysfunction. *Altern. Med. Rev.* 1999; **4**: 144–61.

60 Birks J, Grimley EV, Van Dongen M. Ginkgo biloba for cognitive impairment and dementia. *Cochrane Database Syst. Rev.*, 2002; **4**: CD003120.

61 McCarney R, Warner J, Fisher P, Van Haselen R. Homeopathy for dementia. *Cochrane Database Syst. Rev.*, 2003; **1**: CD003803.

62 Malouf M, Grimley EJ, Areosa SA. Folic acid with or without vitamin B_{12} for cognition and dementia. *Cochrane Database Syst. Rev.*, 2003; **4**: CD004514.

63 Huppert FA, Van Niekerk JK. Dehydroepiandrosterone (DHEA) supplementation for cognitive function. *Cochrane Database Syst. Rev.*, 2001; **2**: CD000304.

64 Thorgrimsen L, Spector A, Wiles A, Orrell M. Aroma therapy for dementia. *Cochrane Database Syst. Rev.*, 2003; **3**: CD003150.

65 Hudson S, Tabet N. Acetyl-L-carnitine for dementia. *Cochrane Database Syst. Rev.*, 2003; **2**: CD003158.

66 Lopez-Arrieta JM, Rodriguez JL, Sanz F. Nicotine for Alzheimer's disease. *Cochrane Database Syst. Rev.*, 2000; **2**: CD001749.

67 Vink AC, Birks JS, Bruinsma MS, Scholten RJ. Music therapy for people with dementia. *Cochrane Database Syst. Rev.*, 2004; **3**: CD003477.

68 Forbes D, Morgan DG, Bangma J, Peacock S, Pelletier N, Adamson J. Light therapy for managing sleep, behaviour, and mood disturbances in dementia. *Cochrane Database Syst. Rev.*, 2004; **2**: CD003946.

69 Higgins JP, Flicker L. Lecithin for dementia and cognitive impairment. *Cochrane Database Syst. Rev.*, 2003; **3**: CD001015.

20 CHAPTER 20

Parkinson's disease

Miguel Coelho, Joaquim Ferreira, Cristina Sampaio

Background

Parkinson's disease (PD) is a neurodegenerative disorder of the central nervous system resulting from neuronal loss in the dopaminergic neurons of the substancia nigra pars compacta, and subsequent loss of dopaminergic input to the striatum. It is characterized clinically by the cardinal signs of asymmetrical bradykinesia, rest tremor, rigidity, and postural instability [1], though non-motor symptoms such as dementia, depression, pain, sleep disorders, and dysautonomia occur frequently, mainly with advanced stages of disease [1,2].

PD is one of the most common neurodegenerative disorders, its prevalence increasing with age. Age adjusted prevalence is 1%, rising to 3.5% at age 85–89 years [3,4]. It occurs worldwide with equal incidence in male and female, and the mean age of onset is 65 years [3,4]. It is more common in whites than in those of Asian or African descent though interracial variability remains to be established [5].

The cause is unknown and actually PD is not regarded as a single disease and may represent different conditions with a common final pathway [1]. No clear environmental risk factors have been identified and 10–15% of PD patients will have an affected first-degree or second-degree relative [6,7]. First-degree relatives of patients may have twice the risk of developing the disease compared to the general population [8,9].

Although the diagnosis can be straightforward in patients with typical presentation and excellent response to levodopa, the differential diagnosis with other forms of Parkinsonism and essential tremor can be very difficult [1], and error rates of 24% have been found in some studies [10]. The use of clinical criteria (ex: UK Parkinson's Disease Brain Bank criteria) greatly improves diagnosis, but even then the diagnosis of 10% of patients will be changed after necropsy [11].

Available treatment for PD is only symptomatic, and disability from PD is progressive. There is an increased risk of mortality when compared to matched controls (relative risk (RR) ranging from 1.6 to 3.0) [12], and in an Italian cohort study, age at initial census was the main predictor of death [13].

Framing answerable clinical questions

1 In patients with early PD, how do the pharmacological treatments change the UPDRS motor score and affect the probability of motor fluctuations or dyskinesias? And which is the risk for treatment withdrawal?

2 Among patients with PD and levodopa-induced motor complications, how does the pharmacological treatments affect the probability of improvement of motor fluctuations and dyskinesias? Which is the risk of withdrawals?

3 Among patients with PD and levodopa-induced motor complications, how does functional surgery affect the probability of improvement of motor fluctuations and dyskinesias? Which is the risk of withdrawals?

4 In patients with PD and psychosis, what is the benefit and safety of clozapine, quetiapine and olanzapine for the treatment of psychosis?

5 In patients with Parkinson's disease dementia (PDD), what is the benefit and safety of rivastigmine and donepezil for the treatment of cognitive or behavioural disturbances? Which is the risk of withdrawal?

Search strategy

Search strategy for finding evidence was done using electronic databases including Medline (1966–2005), EMBASE (1974–2005) and The Cochrane Database of Systematic Reviews, and checking of reference lists from three evidenced-based review reports [14–16].

Papers were selected for review if they met the following inclusion/exclusion criteria: Inclusion criteria: (1) randomized study; (2) non-randomized controlled or non-controlled, prospective or retrospective study; (3) patients with a diagnosis of PD; (4) established scales for evaluating symptoms; (5) ⩾20 patients; (6) ⩾4-week treatment period; (7) report published in English language; (8) full paper citation; and (9) original research. Exclusion criteria: (1) outcome measures non-validated or unconventional; (2) duplicated reports; (3) incomplete or uncertain length of follow-up; (4) non-English publication; (5) report in the form of abstract or review; and (6) patients with a diagnosis of Parkinsonism other than PD.

Some exceptions to these rules were applied:

1 When assessing the effect of dopamine agonists in treating motor complications, we excluded trials comparing different dopamine agonists head-to-head.

2 For surgical techniques, only studies concerning deep brain stimulation (DBS) of the globus pallidus pars interna

(GPi)or the subthalamic nucleus (STN), or pallidotomy were included.

3 For surgical studies no sample size constraint was applied for Level-I studies, but a minimum of 20 patients was maintained for Level-II and Level-III trials, and a period >3 months after surgery was required; studies were excluded if levodopa was started for the first time during follow-up after surgery.

4 For dementia studies, we excluded trials allowing for a concomitant reduction of anti-Parkinsonian drugs dosage, and we allowed to include a trial with <20 patients because of premature stoppage.

Critical review of the evidence

1. Early PD

In patients with early PD, how do the pharmacological treatments (MAO-B inhibitors, dopamine agonists, controlled-released levodopa, and standard levodopa), compared to no treatment, placebo or standard levodopa, change the UPDRS motor score and affect the probability of occurrence of motor fluctuations or dyskinesias? And which is the risk for treatment withdrawal?

The results of some studies are summarized in Table 20.1.

MAO-B inhibitors

The systematic review by Macleod et al. [17] included randomized-controlled trials (RCTs) with treatment and follow-up for at least 1 year. They identified nine trials for selegiline and one for lazabemide compared with no treatment or placebo, which comprised a total of 2422 patients (mean Hoehn and Yahr scale 2) with a mean follow-up of 5.8 years, and with reasonable methodological quality. Previous treatment with levodopa or agonists varied among studies. To distinguish between a symptomatic effect and an effect on disease progression, six studies included a washout period. Data on deaths at the end of follow-up was available for 2389 patients: results showed a non-significant increase in deaths with MAO-B inhibitors (OR, 1.15; 95% CI, 0.92–1.44, $P = 0.21$). Analysis of UPDRS motor score change in five trials showed a highly statistical significant decrease in favour of MAO-B inhibitors, although not clinically relevant, with a weighted mean difference (WMD) of −3.81 (95% CI, −5.36 to −2.27, $P = 0.00001$). Analysis of UPDRS ADL score change in five trials favoured treatment with MAO-B inhibitors (WMD, −1.50; 95% CI, −2.53 to −0.48, $P = 0.004$), though not clinically relevant. Fewer patients on MAO-B inhibitors initiated levodopa at 1 year (combined OR from three studies 0.53; 95% CI, 0.36–0.79, $P = 0.01$). Analysis of data from five trials (all using selegiline, comprising 1319 patients) showed a statistical significant lower occurrence of motor fluctuations with MAO-B inhibitors compared to control (OR, 0.75; 95% CI, 0.59–0.94, $P = 0.01$), although this significance was lost when using raw data from one of

the studies and when performing a modified worst-case analysis. Data on dyskinesias from four trials (all using selegiline, comprising 1228 patients) showed no difference between selegiline and control in the development of dyskinesias (OR, 0.98; 95% CI, 0.76–1.26). There was a reporting bias between trials concerning adverse events. Overall, results showed a non-significant increase in adverse events with MAO-B inhibitors (OR, 1.38; 95% CI, 0.92–2.06, $P = 0.12$); studies did not find lower mean blood pressure nor consistent data on more cardiac arrhythmias or other ECG abnormalities with MAO-B inhibitors; two studies reported significantly elevated liver enzymes with MAO-B inhibitors (not clinically relevant). Total number of withdrawals did not differ between MAO-B inhibitors and control in all 10 trials (OR, 0.93; 95% CI, 0.74–1.16). Six trials showed significantly more withdrawals due to adverse events with MAO-B inhibitors (OR, 2.36; 95% CI, 1.32–4.20, $P = 0.004$).

Caraceni and Musicco [18] randomized 473 untreated early PD patients to monotherapy of levodopa ($n = 156$), bromocriptine or lisuride ($n = 172$), or selegiline ($n = 155$). At median follow-up of 34 months, results showed a reduced RR of motor fluctuations and dyskinesias with selegiline and agonists compared to levodopa (RR for fluctuations: 0.5 and 0.6, respectively; RR for dyskinesias: 0.8 and 0.6, respectively). These differences lose significance when a multivariate analysis was performed.

The Tempo [19] study assessed the efficacy of monotherapy with rasagiline in 404 early PD patients, in a randomized double-blind placebo-controlled trial comparing rasagiline 1 or 2 mg/day with placebo, during 26 weeks. Adjusted mean difference in change on total UPDRS scores were −4.2 comparing rasagiline 1 mg to placebo ($P < 0.001$) and −3.56 comparing rasagiline 2 mg to placebo ($P < 0.001$). There was no statistically significant difference in the time to need levodopa. Adverse events were not significantly different between rasagiline and placebo, except for supine systolic blood pressure that was significantly higher on rasagiline 2 mg. The Parkinson Study Group extended the Tempo trial for another 6 months ('active treatment phase') using a delayed-start design [20]: patients initially allocated to placebo in the Tempo trial were started on rasagiline 2 mg/day for another 6 months ('delayed rasagiline 2 mg/d arm') while the patients allocated to 1 and 2 mg/d at baseline continued to receive that dosage for the next 6 months. This design tried to overcome the distinction between a symptomatic effect and a disease-modifying effect. The intention-to-treat cohort were 371 patients (delayed rasagiline arm: 130, rasagiline: 1 mg/d arm: 122, and rasagiline 2 mg/d arm: 199); at the end of follow-up, 259 subjects did not start additional dopaminergic therapy, with no significant differences between treatment arms. Adjusted mean difference on total UPDRS comparing rasagiline 1 mg/d with delayed rasagiline 2 mg/d was −1.82 points (95% CI, −3.64 to 0.01 points, $P = 0.05$), and −2.29 points (95% CI, −4.11 to −0.48 points,

Table 20.1 Monotheraphy compared to levodopa for early Parkinson's disease.

Type of study (reference)	Intervention (dosage)	Follow-up time	Outcome	Number of patients (number of trials)	Control group value	Relative risk (95% CI)	Absolute risk reduction or WMD (95% CI)	Comment
RCT [18]	Selegiline (max 10 mg) versus levodopa (max 750 mg)	2.8 years	UPDRS motor*	–	–	–	–	Selegiline worse
			Motor fluctuations	473 (1)	30%	0.63 (0.42–0.95)	11% (1–20)	Selegiline better Not statistically significant at multivariable analysis
			Dyskinesias	473 (1)	27%	0.77 (0.51–1.15)	6% (ns)	Selegiline better
			Withdrawals**	473 (1)	2.6%	0.5 (0.09–2.71)	1% (ns)	Selegiline better
RCT [21]	Ropinirole (mean dose 12.2 mg) versus levodopa (mean dose 558.7 mg)	2 years	UPDRS motor*	162 (1)	5.6	–	6.3 (5.9–6.6)	Ropinirole worse
			Motor fluctuations	–	–	–	–	
			Dyskinesias	162 (1)	27%	0.09^^ (0.02–0.29)	23%	Ropinirole better
			Withdrawals	162 (1)	5.3%	3.12^ (0.97–10.0)	10% (ns)	Ropinirole worse
RCT [22]	Ropinirole (16.5 mg) versus levodopa (753 mg)	5 years	UPDRS motor*	130 (1)	0.08	–	4.0 (0.76–7.24)	Ropinirole worse
			Motor fluctuations	–	–	–	–	
			Dyskinesias	268 (1)	45%	2.82^^ (1.78–4.44)	25%	Ropinirole better
			Withdrawals	268 (1)	33%	–	6% (ns)	Ropinirole worse
RCT [23]	Pramipexole (2.78 mg) versus levodopa (406 mg)	2 years	UPDRS motor*	150 (1)	7.3	–	3.9 (5.7–2.1)	Pramipexole worse
			Motor fluctuations	150 (1)	38%	0.57^^ (0.3 –0.88)	14%	Pramipexole better
			Dyskinesias	150 (1)	30.7%	0.33^^ (0.1–0.6)	21%	Pramipexole better
			Withdrawals	150 (1)	12.7%	–	3% (ns)	Pramipexole worse

(Continued p. 202)

Table 20.1 (Continued.)

Type of study (reference)	Intervention (dosage)	Follow-up time	Outcome	Number of patients (number of trials)	Control group value	Relative risk (95% CI)	Absolute risk reduction or WMD (95% CI)	Comment
SR [33]	Bromocriptine (7–120 mg) versus levodopa (300–600 mg)	3 years	UPDRS motor*	–	–	–	–	–
			Motor fluctuations	512 (1)	33%	0.14 (0.9–0.22)	28% (22–34)	Bromocriptine better
			Dyskinesias	589 (3)	27%	0.09 (0.04–0.11)	25% (20–31)	Bromocriptine better
			Withdrawals **	823 (5)	17%	4.66 (3.41–6.36)	29% (24–35)	Bromocriptine worse
RCT [31]	Bromocriptine (52 mg) versus levodopa (569 mg)	5 years	UPDRS motor*	60 (1)	11	NA	NA	Open-label; no significant difference between groups
			Motor fluctuations	54 (1)	34%	16% (1.32 to 0.42)	6% (20 to 31)	Less on levodopa
			Dyskinesias	54 (1)	48.2%	0.75 (0.23 to 0.92)	36% (14 to 58)	Less on bromocriptine
			Withdrawals**	NA	NA	NA	NA	Less on bromocriptine
RCT [26]	Lisuride (1.2 mg) versus levodopa (300–668 mg)	4 years	UPDRS motor*	–	–	–	–	No significant differences Open label
			Motor fluctuations	60 (1)	52%	–	52%	Lisuride better. Statistical evaluation not available
			Dyskinesias	60 (1)	64%	–	64%	Lisuride better. Statistical evaluation not available
			Withdrawals**	60 (1)	17%	–	66%	Lisuride worse. Statistical evaluation not available
RCT [25]	Cabergoline (2.9 mg) versus levodopa (427 mg)	5 years	UPDRS motor*	419 (1)	9.5	–	1.7 (ns)	Cabergoline worse
			Motor fluctuations	419 (1)	34%	0.56^ (0.37–0.87)	11% (20–30)	Cabergoline better
			Dyskinesias	419 (1)	21%	0.39^ (0.22–0.69)	12% (5–18)	Cabergoline better
			Withdrawals**	419 (1)	14%	1.53^ (0.91–2.57)	6% (1–13)	Cabergoline better

SR: systematic review; RCT: randomized controlled trial; CI: confidence intervals; ns: not statistically significant; SD: standard deviation; SE: standard error.
*Difference of mean change in UPDRS motor score; **due to adverse events; ^OR instead of RR; ^^HR in stead of RR.
C Ramaker, van Hilten JJ. Bromocriptine versus levodopa in early Parkinson's disease. *Cochrane Database Syst. Rev.* 2000, 2: CD002258. DOI: 10.1002/14651858.CD002258.

$P = 0.01$) for comparing rasagiline 2 mg/d versus delayed rasagiline 2 mg/d. Adverse events did not differ significantly between treatments.

Dopamine agonists

Ropinirole

The REAL-PET study [21] assessed the effects of ropinirole or levodopa monotherapy on slowing disease progression in 186 patients with early untreated PD, using as primary outcome measure the decline of the putaminal value of [18]Flurodopa uptake with PET scan, from baseline till 24 months; secondary outcome measures included changes in motor UPDRS scores and the incidence of dyskinesias (UPDRS item 32). Patients with normal scans at baseline were excluded from the final analysis. Final analysis ($N = 162$) showed statistically significant differences in the decline of putaminal Ki values in favour of ropinirole: 13.4% versus 20.3% ($P < 0.022$); a placebo arm was absent from this trial and one cannot exclude the possibility of levodopa or ropinirole influences on striatal decarboxylase activity. Mean UPDRS score change from baseline significantly favoured levodopa compared to ropinirole with an improvement of 5.6 versus a decline of 0.7 points (score difference 6.3 points; 95% CI, 3.54–9.14). Ropinirole was associated with a lower incidence of dyskinesias compared with levodopa (3.4% versus 26.7%; OR, 0.09; 95% CI, 0.02–0.29; $P < 0.001$).

Rascol et al. [22] studied the effect of ropinirole in a randomized, double-blind, parallel, levodopa-controlled, 5-year follow-up study in 268 de novo PD patients. At final follow-up, incidence of dyskinesia was 20% (ropinirole) versus 45% (levodopa), and 'disabling' dyskinesia was less frequent with ropinirole ($P = 0.002$). Difference in 'time to dyskinesia' significantly favoured ropinirole (hazard ratio for remaining free of dyskinesia, 2.82; 95% CI, 1.78–4.44, $P < 0.001$). Incidence of wearing-off favoured ropinirole, although nonsignificant. Motor UPDRS scores significantly favoured levodopa, although considered not to be clinically relevant, and there was no significant difference in ADL scores between treatments. Hallucinations were more frequent with ropinirole (ropinirole 17% versus levodopa 6%), but severe hallucinations were infrequent in either arms, and no difference was observed with other dopaminergic adverse events.

Pramipexole

The CALM-PD trial [23] randomized patients to pramipexole or levodopa monotherapy in 301 early PD patients, and open-label supplementation with levodopa was possible after a titration period of 10 weeks. At 2 years, 28% of patients on pramipexole versus 51% on levodopa developed motor complications ($P < 0.001$). A second report of this study at 4 years showed that 68 (45%) patients dropped-out in the pramipexole group compared with 50 (33%) on levodopa: 12 due to somnolence (pramipexole = 11 versus levodopa = 1), 5 due to oedema and 1 because of both (all with pramipexole);

percentage of patients developing motor complications were 74% (levodopa) versus 52% (pramipexole) (hazard ratio, 0.48; 95% CI, 0.35–0.66; $P < 0.001$); this difference was statistical significant for either dyskinesias (24.5% versus 54%; hazard ratio, 0.37; 95% CI, 0.25–0.56, $P < 0.001$) or wearing-off (47% versus 62.7%; hazard ratio, 0.68; 95% CI, 0.49–0.63, $P = 0.02$) but not for On–Off phenomena (hazard ratio, 0.64; 95% CI, 0.26–1.59, $P = 0.34$); occurrence of disabling dyskinesias was uncommon (pramipexole = 4 versus levodopa = 7); the majority of motor complications occurred after the introduction of levodopa in the pramipexole group and before the introduction of supplemental levodopa in the levodopa group. Patients initially randomized to levodopa had higher mean improvement in total UPDRS (-2, ±15.4 points versus 3.2, ±17.3 points, $P = 0.003$). Levodopa requirement was 72% in patients on pramipexole with 59% in the levodopa group (hazard ratio, 1.64; 95% CI, 1.22–2.21; $P = 0.001$); mean daily dose of pramipexole was 2.78 ± 1.1 mg, and of levodopa was 434 ± 498 mg in the pramipexole arm (supplemental levodopa), and 702 ± 461 mg in the levodopa arm (experimental: 427 ± 112 mg; supplemental: 274 ± 442 mg). A subset of 82 patients underwent β-CIT SPECT evaluation and were followed-up for 46 months [24]. Results showed a statistically significant difference in decline of tracer favouring pramipexole (pramipexole 16.0% versus levodopa 25.5%; $P = 0.01$). 'Off' total and motor UPDRS scores change did not differ significantly between treatments (change in total UPDRS: pramipexole 4.1 versus levodopa 4.0 points, $P = 0.61$; change in motor UPDRS: pramipexole 1.0 versus levodopa 2.1 points, $P = 0.84$).

Cabergoline

A randomized, double-blind, parallel-group trial compared cabergoline with levodopa monotherapy as initial therapy in 419 PD patients [25]. Open-label addition of levodopa was possible, and followed-up was 3–5 years. Drop-out rate was 16% for cabergoline and 13% for levodopa. At 5 years, the incidence of motor complications was 22% with cabergoline versus 34% with levodopa ($P < 0.02$); most complications were end-of-dose failure although the difference between treatments was more prominent for dyskinesias (cabergoline 9.5% versus levodopa 21.2%, $P < 0.001$). The introduction of levodopa more than doubled the risk of motor complications in both groups. Cabergoline RR of developing motor complications was >50% lower than that of levodopa (HR, 0.46; $P < 0.001$). Mean UPDRS motor scores at 5 years favoured levodopa (cabergoline 19.2 versus levodopa 16.3 points, $P < 0.01$); satisfactory clinical improvement (a 30% decrease in UPDRS III from baseline) also favoured levodopa, the difference being statistical significant at 3 (cabergoline 58.9% versus levodopa 75.6% of patients, $P < 0.01$) and 4 years (cabergoline 50% versus levodopa 65% of patients, $P < 0.05$). Peripheral oedema was more frequent with cabergoline than with levodopa (16.1% versus 3.4%, $P < 0.0001$), but no other adverse events (most frequent being nausea and vomiting, dizziness, hypotension, and sleep problems).

Lisuride

Two studies showed conflicting results in the efficacy of lisuride in prevention of motor complications:

In an open-label design, Rinne [26] studied 90 de novo PD patients who were randomized to lisuride, levodopa, or lisuride plus levodopa. Levodopa could be added to lisuride after 3 months if needed. Five patients remained on lisuride monotherapy after 4 years; the risk to develop dyskinesias and wearing-off was: lisuride plus levodopa arms: 13% wearing-off, 19% peak-dose dyskinesia versus levodopa monotherapy arm: 52% wearing-off, 64% peak-dose dyskinesia ($P < 0.01$). Anti-Parkinsonian efficacy measured by the Columbia University Rating Scale was equivalent between treatments.

In other open-label (first year was double-blind), parallel group, 5-year study [27], 82 early PD patients receiving levodopa for less than 6 months were randomized to levodopa or levodopa plus lisuride. The incidence of motor complications was low in both arms and the difference favouring combination therapy was not significant. UPDRS score remained unchanged with combination therapy while it deteriorated with levodopa monotherapy.

Bromocriptine

We identified six trials in which bromocriptine was used as initial monotherapy and levodopa added later as adjunct therapy if needed [28–32], one systematic review [33] and three trials where bromocriptine was used as early combination to levodopa [34–36].

In the bromocriptine monotherapy trials, the comparator was levodopa in three, levodopa and levodopa with selegiline in two and ropinirole in one trial. Two studies are reports of the 10-year follow-up data of two trials (one trial = bromocriptine versus levodopa; other = bromocriptine versus levodopa versus levodopa plus selegiline). These six trials randomized 1326 patients. Both 10-year follow-up trials found no difference in mortality between bromocriptine and levodopa. Overall, bromocriptine reduced the occurrence of motor complications when compared to levodopa; no differences were found between bromocriptine and ropinirole in the incidence of dyskinesias after 3 years (ropinirole: 7.7%; bromocriptine: 7.2%, NS). The three trials using bromocriptine as early combination to levodopa comprise 940 patients. Patients already treated with levodopa were randomized to stay on levodopa monotherapy or receive an adjunct treatment with bromocriptine. All trials reported lower occurrence of motor fluctuations or dyskinesias with a combination of levodopa/bromocriptine.

Levodopa

Standard levodopa

The ELLDOPA trial [37] was a randomized, double-blind, placebo-controlled trial that evaluated the effect of three daily doses of carbidopa–levodopa, 37.5/150 mg, 75/300 mg, or 150/600 mg, or a matching placebo in 361 early PD patients, for 40 weeks followed by a 2-week washout period. Results showed a mean difference on UPDRS total score between baseline and week 42 of 7.8 points in the placebo group, 1.9 points in the levodopa 150 mg group, 1.9 in the levodopa 300 mg group, and 1.4 in 600 mg group ($P < 0.001$). After the washout period, UPDRS scores in all levodopa arms worsened but did not reach the values for the placebo group. The following adverse events were significantly more frequent in the 600 mg arm than in the placebo group: dyskinesias, nausea, infection, hypertonia, and headache. In 116 patients, a [123I] β-CIT evaluation at baseline and week 40 was performed: the mean per cent decline in the [123I] β-CIT uptake was significantly greater with levodopa than placebo (placebo: −1.4; levodopa 150 mg: −6; 300 mg: −4; 600 mg: −7.2, $P = 0.036$).

Controlled-release levodopa formulations

Dupont [38] and colleagues randomized 134 de novo patients to slow release levodopa/benserazide (Madopar HBS®) or standard levodopa/benserazide (Madopar®), in a double-blind parallel group multicentre design, with a follow-up of 5 years; bromocriptine could be added to control motor fluctuations. UPDRS IV section was used to assess motor complications. Number of drop-outs was high in both groups (29 patients in the Madopar® arm and 35 in the Madopar HBS® arm were still in the study at year 5). Twelve patients in each arm developed dyskinesias at year 5 (standard levodopa = 41% versus slow release levodopa = 34%, difference not significant; no statistically significant difference was found in the incidence of motor fluctuations: Madopar standard®, 17 patients (59%) versus Madopar HBS®, 20 patients (57%).

Other 5-year study [39,40] compared sustained-release Sinemet® versus immediate-release Sinemet® in 618 de novo patients. There were no statistical significant difference between the two treatments for the incidence of motor complications: immediate-release = 20.6% versus slow-release = 21.8%.

Conclusion

Both selegiline and rasagiline seem to be efficacious and safe as monotherapy to treat symptoms of PD. Selegiline does not decrease the incidence of dyskinesias compared to control and there is insufficient data regarding incidence of motor fluctuations; there is insufficient data regarding prevention of motor complications by rasagiline. As a group, dopamine agonists are associated with lower incidence of motor complications compared to levodopa though levodopa was associated with better improvements in motor scores; dopaminergic adverse events are more frequent with agonists compared with levodopa; there is insufficient data regarding the efficacy of agonists in slowing disease progression. Standard levodopa is associated with less worsening of Parkinsonism compared to placebo, and there is no clinical evidence that it hastens disease progression; higher doses are associated with greater motor improvement but also more adverse events such as dyskinesias, as compared with lower doses. Controlled-release levodopa is not associated with lower incidence of motor complications compared to standard levodopa.

2. PD patients with levodopa-induced motor complications

Among patients with PD and levodopa-induced motor complications, how does the pharmacological treatments (controlled-release levodopa, amantadine, clozapine, COMT inhibitors, MAO-B inhibitors, and dopamine agonists), compared to placebo, or standard levodopa, affect the probability of improvement of motor fluctuations and dyskinesias? Which is the risk?

The studies' results are summarized in Table 20.2.

Controlled-released levodopa

Wolters et al. [41] compared the efficacy of carbidopa/levodopa CR with standard carbidopa/levodopa in 170 patients, in a Dutch–British multicentre, double-blind, double-dummy, parallel group, 24-week trial preceded by an 8-week open-label phase of dose finding. For patients on standard carbidopa/levodopa, 'On time' averaged 68% of waking day at the end of the open-label period and 64% at week 24, while for patients on carbidopa/levodopa CR, 'On time' averaged 74% at the end of the open-label period and 69% at week 24; direct comparisons between treatments showed a statistically significant increase of 'On-time' favouring Sinemet CR at week 4. The mean daily number of 'Off' periods was significantly less in the carbidopa/levodopa CR group. The decline in NYUPDS scores was significantly greater in the carbidopa/levodopa CR arm; patients' global evaluation of improvement favoured carbidopa/levodopa CR at weeks 12 and 24, while the investigators' rating was not significantly different between treatments. The mean daily number of doses was 5.1 for standard carbidopa/levodopa and 4.9 for carbidopa/levodopa CR. Eighteen patients withdrew from the study, 15 while on car bidopa/levodopa CR.

A double-blind, cross-over trial by The UK Madopar CR Study Group [42] compared the efficacy of bedtime controlled-release to standard Madopar in 103 patients with several nocturnal and early morning motor disabilities; 42 patients had daytime motor fluctuations. Patients received either 125 mg of controlled-release or of standard Madopar at bedtime (possible titration up to 600 mg). Patients were kept on optimized dosing for a 2-week period before crossing-over, and were then restarted at 125 mg on the alternative drug. Fourteen patients dropped out from the trial; the investigator rating favoured Madopar CR, but there were no differences between treatments regarding optimum dosage, motor disability, the percentage of patients improving or wishing to continue each drug, and the percentage of drop-outs.

Hutton et al. [43] compared carbidopa/levodopa CR with standard carbidopa/levodopa in 202 patients, in a randomized, cross-over, double-blind, multicentre, 24-week trial. It included two 8-week cross-over periods preceded by two 4-week phases for drug titration. Forty-four patients withdrew, 19 during the titration period because of a lack of effect (carbidopa/levodopa standard: 11 versus levodopa CR: 8 patients). Results showed a decrease of 'Off' duration with levodopa CR, statistical significant at weeks 4 and 6. The mean daily levodopa dose was greater with levodopa CR (levodopa CR: 1238 mg; standard carbidopa/levodopa: 975 mg). Frequencies of the most common adverse events were similar between treatments.

Jankovic et al. [44] included 20 patients and compared carbidopa/levodopa CR versus standard carbidopa/levodopa, using a similar 24-week trial design to the one described above. Results showed a significant decrease of the 'On without dyskinesias' duration and a non-significant increase of the 'Off' duration in the slow-release levodopa phase, and no difference in the 'On with dyskinesias' time between treatments. Carbidopa/levodopa CR was significantly associated with the lower dose frequency (5.7 versus 3.8) and with an increase in the mean daily dose (685 mg versus 815 mg); there were no differences in UPDRS and Schwab and England scores. An open-label extension with 18 patients showed a significant increase of the 'On with dyskinesias' duration compared to the end of the double-blind phase on standard levodopa, although no differences were observed in the total 'On' and 'Off' time.

Lieberman et al. [45] reported results of a randomized double-blind cross-over study comparing controlled release with standard levodopa, in 24 patients, using the same trial design as previous studies. There were no significant differences between treatments in the mean scores in UPDRS or in the 'On' and 'Off' duration; while on levodopa CR patients took significantly fewer levodopa daily doses (5.0 versus 6.2) but needed a higher levodopa daily dose. During the open-label extension of the study with 35 patients, 9 dropped out during titration of standard levodopa and 2 during levodopa CR titration.

Amantadine

A systematic review by Crosby NJ et al. [46] included RCTs comparing amantadine with placebo in the treatment of dyskinesias. Three trials, all double-blind, cross-over studies, were identified, comprising 53 patients. Due to methodological insufficiency, the results of two trials were not analysed, and the final trial only examined 11 patients. In this trial, the severity of dyskinesia following a levodopa challenge was reduced after oral amantadine (300 mg) treatment by 6.4 points (41%), when compared to the placebo arm. In one study, the authors report no adverse effects; in other study, 4 (22%) patients withdrew because of mild and transient

Table 20.2 Drug treatment for levodopa motor complications.

Type of study (reference)	Intervention	Number of patients (number of trials)	Outcome	Control group risk (range)	Relative risk (95% CI)	Absolute risk reduction or WMD (95% CI)	Comment
RCTs [41–45]	CR levodopa versus levodopa	529 (5)	No SR available. There is insufficient evidence regarding the efficacy and safety.				
SR, RCT [46,47]	Amantadine (300 mg/d) versus placebo	93 (4)	Amantadine seems to reduce dyskinesia compared to placebo, but there is not enough evidence about the safety and effectiveness.				
RCT [48]	Clozapine (39.4 mg/d) versus placebo	50 (1)	Clozapine seems safe and efficacious for dyskinesia. Just one trial.				
SR [49]	COMT inhibitors (entacapone 200 mg per levodopa dose, tolcapone 50–400 mg/d) versus placebo	1584 (14)	Off time minutes	2.4–54		78 (64–93)	COMT inhibitors better
		2537 (19)	Dyskinesia	18% (1–32)	3.09 (2.59–3.69)	22% (19–26)	COMT inhibitors worse
			Adverse event	Fatal hepatic toxicity found during post-marketing surveillance with tolcapone.			
RCTs (51–56)	MAO inhibitors: (selegiline 10 mg/d, zydis selegiline 2.5 mg/d, rasagiline 1 mg/d) versus placebo	1472 (6)	There is not enough evidence to conclude on the efficacy of selegiline; zydis selegiline and rasagiline are possibly useful in reducing off time and increasing on time without dyskinesias.				
			Adverse event				
SR [57]	Ropinirole (24 mg/d) versus placebo	253 (3)	Off time minutes	45–133		29 to +35	No clear effect. Heterogeneity
		195 (2)	Dyskinesia	13–22%	2.90* (1.36–6.19)	21%* (8–34)	Ropinirole worse Just one trial result
			Adverse event	No significant difference for adverse events or withdrawals were observed between treatments.			

Study	Intervention	N (trials)	Outcome				Conclusion
SR [58]	Pergolide (mean 2.94 mg/d) versus placebo	376 (1)	Off time minutes	12		84	Pergolide better. Just one trial
			Dyskinesia	26%	4.64 (3.09–6.97)	38% (29–47)	Pergolide worse
			Adverse event	A growing number of publications reported the occurrence of valvular heart disorders associated with pergolide.			
SR [61]	Pramipexole (8–10 mg/d) versus placebo	611 (4)	Off time minutes	42 to +24		102 (73–140)	Pramipexole better. Heterogeneity
		668 (4)	Dyskinesia	29% (5–41)	2.10 (1.50–2.94)	15% (8–22)	Promipexole worse
			Adverse event	Orthostatic hypotension, nausea, visual hallucination, and dizziness.			
SR [65]	Bromocriptine (maximum 20 mg in 36 weeks to 100 mg in 10 weeks) versus placebo	385 (6)	Off time minutes				No clear effect. Heterogeneity
			Dyskinesia				Bromocriptine worse
			Adverse event	No significant difference in withdrawals due to adverse events was reported.			
SR [67]	Cabergoline (3–5.4 mg/d) versus placebo	61 (2)	Off time minutes	42–148		68 (ns)	Cabergoline better. No statistical significant
		43 (1)	Dyskinesia	0	6.49 (0.13–330)	4% (ns)	Cabergoline worse. No statistical significant
			Adverse event	Autonomic, cardiovascular and neuropsychiatric effects.			
RCT [68]	Apomorphine (subcutaneous) versus placebo	32 (1)	Off time minutes	0		120	Apomorphine better
			Dyskinesia				Apomorphine worse
			Adverse event	Injection site complaints, yawning, somnolence, dyskinesia, and nausea or vomiting.			

SR: systematic review; RCT: randomized controlled trial; CI: confidence intervals; ns: not statistically significant; Off time: time of poor L-dopa response.

adverse events (two with confusion or hallucinations = 2; nausea = 1; recurrence of pre-existing palpitations = 1); and in a third study one patient experienced reversible oedema of both feet during amantadine and other patient withdrew while on placebo due to dizziness. The authors concluded that due to lack of evidence it was impossible to determine whether amantadine is a safe and effective treatment for levodopa-induced dyskinesias.

A randomized, 12 months, double-blind, parallel, placebo-controlled trial [47] evaluated the efficacy of amantadine (300 mg/d) on dyskinesia and motor fluctuations. Amantadine was titrated till 300 mg/d. Forty patients were included and 11 withdrew (placebo 6 versus amantadine 5). Results showed a significant longer treatment effect duration with amantadine of 4.9 versus 1.3 months compared to placebo ($P = 0.001$); at 15 and 30 days, amantadine was significantly associated with reductions in the Dyskinesia Rating Scale by 45% and UPDRS item 32–34 compared to placebo ($P = 0.001$); UPDRS I–III scores were significantly reduced with amantadine compared to placebo (amantadine: -3.2 points; placebo $+0.1$ points; $P = 0.01$); there was a non-significant decrease of 'Off' time and an increase of 'On' time with amantadine compared to placebo. After amantadine discontinuation, 11 patients suffered a rebound of dyskinesias, 1 got severely confused and 2 patients reported hyperthermia.

Clozapine

A double-blind, randomized, parallel, placebo-controlled, 10-week trial [48] assessed the efficacy and safety of clozapine for disabling levodopa-induced dyskinesias in 50 patients. Patients were randomized to either an evening dose of placebo or clozapine (12.5–75 mg/d). Mean dose of clozapine was 39.4 mg/d. Results showed a significant reduction in duration of 'On with dyskinesias' favouring clozapine compared to placebo (placebo: day 0: 4.54 h, SD: 0.53, end: 5.28 h, SD: 0.70; clozapine: day 0: 5.68 h, SD: 0.66, end: 3.98 h, SD: 0.57; $P = 0.003$) and diurnal dyskinesias were reduced by about 2 h with clozapine as compared to placebo; there was no increase in duration of 'Off' time; after levodopa challenge, clozapine was associated with a significant reduction in severity of dyskinesias at rest (placebo: 0.15, SD: 1.01; clozapine: -2.22, SD: 0.52, $P = 0.05$); no significant increase in motor UPDRS was associated with clozapine. Twelve patients withdrew because of adverse events: placebo = 7 versus clozapine = 5; three patients on clozapine withdrew due to transient hipereosinophilia; only diurnal drowsiness and somnolence was significantly more frequent in the clozapine arm, and no significant change in leucocyte count was observed.

COMT inhibitors

Two Cochrane Systematic Reviews [49,50] addressed the efficacy and safety of COMT inhibitors for levodopa-induced

motor complications, both with the last substantive update from June 2004.

Deane et al. [49] included RCTs that compared either oral tolcapone or entacapone versus placebo, and with a minimum duration of 4 weeks. The authors identified 14 trials (entacapone = 8, tolcapone = 6), with a total of 2569 patients; the trials using entacapone comprised a total of 1563 patients while the trials of tolcapone comprised overall 1006 patients; all entacapone trials were double-blind and all but one had a parallel-group design, and the dose of entacapone was 200 mg per levodopa dose up to 10 doses × day, with one exception where dose was not specified. All tolcapone trials had a double-blind parallel-group design, and used a dose ranging from 50 to 400 mg tid. Overall, the methodological quality of entacapone trials was moderate and inferior to the tolcapone trials quality. For several outcome measures, published data was provided in a manner not amenable to meta-analysis. The WMD in levodopa dose reduction between entacapone and placebo was 55 mg/day (95% CI, 37–74 mg/day, $P < 0.00001$); the mean 'Off' state time reduction difference between entacapone and placebo was 41 min (95% CI, 13–68 min, $P = 0.004$), and the mean 'On' state time increase difference was 61 min (95% CI, 37–83 min, $P < 0.00001$); UPDRS evaluation was performed in five trials: difference in UPDRS part II and UPDRS part III was significant in four trials, favouring entacapone. The following adverse events were significantly associated with entacapone with a P-value < 0.01: dyskinesia (Peto OR 2.23, $P < 0.00001$), nausea (Peto OR 1.93, $P = 0.0006$), vomiting (Peto OR 4.16, $P = 0.01$), diarrhoea (Peto OR 2.69, $P = 0.0001$) and constipation (Peto OR 2.27 $P = 0.007$); elevation in transaminase levels were considered to be clinically significant if they raised more than 3 times the upper limit of the normal range, and overall entacapone was not associated with a clinically significant increase in transaminase levels. Tolcapone trials duration ranged from 6 weeks to 3 months although in one study there was a double-blind extension up to 1 year. The WMD in levodopa dose reduction showed a dose response trend with tolcapone dosage and a fall off with the highest dose: from 50 mg tolcapone producing a levodopa dose reduction of 72 mg/day (95% CI, 27–117 mg, $P = 0.001$) till 200 mg producing a 148 mg/day decrease (95% CI, 123–174 mg, $P = 0.00001$) and 400 mg giving a 55 mg/day decrease (95% CI, 18–93 mg, $P = 0.003$). Using the investigator's evaluation of 'Off' duration over a 10-h day, the WMD in 'Off' time reduction showed a similar reduction for all tolcapone doses (90 min compared to placebo) except for the 50 mg/d which was the less effective though statistically significant; overall, the 'On' time increase was similar to the 'Off' time reduction. Out of five studies recording UPDRS motor part, one found a significant difference for tolcapone 200 mg/d (tolcapone reduction of 6.5 versus placebo reduction of 2.1 points, $P < 0.01$). The following adverse events were associated with tolcapone at a $P < 0.01$: dyskinesia, nausea, vomiting, and diarrhoea and hallucinations at the 200 mg dose; transaminases levels beyond $3 \times$ the reference range were observed in two reports: four patients under 100 mg and four under 200 mg; two patients on 200 mg withdrew; one study reported a transitory elevation of mean transaminases levels in the 200 mg arm. There was no significant increase in drop-outs in patients on tolcapone.

The second systematic review by Deane et al. [50] included RCTs that compared either oral entacapone or tolcapone with any dopamine agonist, MAO inhibitor, anticholinergic or amantadine, with a minimum duration of 4 weeks. They included two trials, with a total of 349 patients, one comparing tolcapone with pergolide (203 patients) and other comparing tolcapone with bromocriptine (146 patients), and both using a randomized, open-label, parallel-group design, though one used a blinded rater. In the pergolide study, tolcapone dose was 100 mg tid with a optional increase to 200 mg tid, and pergolide titrated to a maximum of 5 mg/d (mean final dose 2.2 mg), while in the bromocriptine trial tolcapone dose was 200 mg tid with bromocriptine dose titrated to a maximum of 30 mg/d (mean final dose 22.4 mg/d). The methodological quality of included studies was good. The pergolide trial was 12 weeks long while the bromocriptine trial had a duration of 8 weeks; efficacy data of pergolide trial was not amenable to meta-analysis. Levodopa mean reduction difference was only statistically significant for tolcapone versus bromocriptine (124 mg versus 30 mg, $P < 0.01$); total 'On' and 'Off' times was only available in bromocriptine trial, and no significant difference was observed between treatments; differences in motor UPDRS were not significant (tolcapone 3.3 points improve versus pergolide 2.7 points; tolcapone 3.1 points improve versus bromocriptine 3.3 points); in the pergolide trial, results on quality of life assessed by the PD Questionnaire 39 were statistically significant in PDQ-39 favouring tolcapone ($P = 0.005$). The following adverse events were statistically significant at a $P = 0.01$: more nausea (OR = 0.42, $P = 0.0003$), constipation (OR = 0.26, $P = 0.00007$) and orthostatic complaints (OR = 0.24, $P = 0.0002$) with dopamine agonists than tolcapone; abnormalities in liver function, only reported in one trial, showed rise in aspartate aminotransferase levels greater than $3 \times$ normal range in one patient, that subside after drug discontinuation; withdrawals due to adverse events, also reported in one trial only, were more frequent in the pergolide arm (OR 0.34, $P = 0.02$).

MAO-B inhibitors

Selegiline

Nine RCTs were identified and a Cochrane Collaboration Systematic Review will be completed very soon.

Lees et al. [51] studied the effect of adding selegiline (10 mg/d) or placebo to levodopa in 41 patients with motor fluctuations, in a double-blind, placebo-controlled trial. The authors reported that selegiline improved 'wearing-off' disability in 65% of patients; no significant improvement occurred in akinesia or On–Off phenomena. Patients on selegiline had the following adverse events: dyskinesia (14), nausea (9), dry mouth (6), dizziness (3), postural hypotension (2), syncope (1), paraesthesia (1), hallucinations (1) and unpleasant taste (1).

A randomized, double-blind, placebo-controlled, parallel-group, 8-week trial [52] evaluated the effect of adding selegiline to levodopa in 33 patients. No withdrawals occurred. Patients on selegiline had a significant 22% decrease in Parkinsonian symptoms and 17.4% decrease in Parkinsonian signs, and a significant decrease of 21% in levodopa dose; 'On' time did not differ significantly between both interventions though patients reported a longer duration of levodopa effect, less abrupt transition between 'On' and 'Off' and better 'On' and 'Off' periods quality. Adverse events were similar between treatments.

Other randomized, double-blind, placebo-controlled, parallel-group, 6-weeks trial [53] studied the effect of adding selegiline to levodopa in 99 patients. Results showed a significant improvement on gait and overall symptom control in patients receiving selegiline; objective rating of 'On' period quality did not differ between groups; levodopa dose decrease was 17% for selegiline and 7% for placebo.

One randomized, double-blind, placebo-controlled, parallel-group, 12-week trial [54] evaluated the effect of adding Zydis selegiline (1.25–2.5 mg once daily) to levodopa in 140 patients. Zydis selegiline dissolves on contact with saliva, undergoing pre-gastric absorption, which minimizes first-pass metabolism, provides high plasma concentrations of selegiline and reduces amphetamine metabolites. Ninety-three per cent of patients on selegiline and 92% of patients on placebo completed the trial, the main reason for withdrawal being adverse events; no differences between groups were noted for withdrawal. Patients on selegiline had a significant decrease compared to placebo in percentage of 'Off' time (13.2% versus 3.8% reduction; $P = 0.001$ at weeks 10–12), in the number of 'Off' h/d (2.2 h versus 0.6 h reduction; $P = 0.001$), a significant increase of 'On without dyskinesia' time (12% versus 3% increase, $P = 0.008$) and a non-significant difference in 'On with dyskinesia'; no data was reported on ADL and motor parts of UPDRS. No differences were detected in the occurrence of adverse events between treatment groups; there were no report of drug-related cardiac arrhythmias or hypertensive events and the ECG showed no significant change in QTc duration between treatment arms.

Rasagiline

We identified two large trials [55,56] with a maximum follow-up of 26 weeks. The Largo study [55] consisted of a randomized, double-blind, double-dummy, parallel-group, placebo-controlled (entacapone as a comparator drug), 18-week, multicentre design; 687 patients were randomized either to rasagiline (1 mg once daily), entacapone 200 mg with each levodopa dose, or placebo. The trial was powered to compare one active arm with placebo. Eighty-eight (13%) patients withdrew from study (23 rasagiline, 30 entacapone, and 35 placebo), mainly due to withdrawal of consent (n = 34) and adverse events (n = 34). Both rasagiline and entacapone reduced mean daily 'Off' time (rasagiline −1.18 h, entacapone −1.2 h versus placebo −0.4 h; $P \leqslant 0.0001$) and increased daily duration of 'On without troublesome dyskinesia' (rasagiline and entacapone 0.85 h versus placebo 0.03 h; $P = 0.0005$) compared to placebo, with no difference in 'On with troublesome dyskinesia'; active treatments significantly improved ADL UPDRS during 'Off' time (rasagiline versus placebo −1.71, $P < 0.0001$; entacapone versus placebo −1.38, $P = 0.0006$) and motor UPDRS during 'On' time (rasagiline versus placebo −2.94, $P < 0.0001$; entacapone versus placebo −2.73, $P < 0.0001$). Half of patients reported adverse events, whose frequency was similar between treatment arms.

The Presto trial [56] evaluated the efficacy and safety of rasagiline (0.5 mg/d or 1 mg/d) compared to placebo in levodopa-induced motor complications in a randomized, double-blind, parallel-group, placebo-controlled, 26 weeks and multicentre design. Safety variables included dermatologic examinations due to the reported increased frequency of skin tumours in PD; 472 patients were included and 87.7% completed the trial (withdrawals not differing between groups); patients on rasagiline 1 mg/d decreased total 'Off' time by 1.85 h (29%), those on 0.5 mg/d by 1.41 h (23%) and patients on placebo by 0.91 h (15%); compared to placebo, patients on rasagiline 1.0 mg/d had 0.94 h (95% CI, 0.51–1.36 h; $P < 0.001$), and patients on rasagiline 0.5 mg/d had 0.49 h (95% CI, 0.08–0.91 h; $P = 0.02$) less 'Off' time. Scores in ADL UPDRS during 'Off' and motor UPDRS during 'On' also significantly favoured rasagiline compared to placebo; rasagiline 1 mg/d significantly increased 'On with troublesome dyskinesia' time compared to placebo ($P = 0.048$). Weight loss, anorexia, and vomiting were significantly more frequent in the 1 mg/d arm and balance difficulty was more frequent in the 0.5 mg/d group ($P = 0.03$), compared to placebo. Serious adverse events, including melanoma or cardiovascular abnormalities, had a similar frequency between rasagiline arms and placebo.

Dopamine agonists
Ropinirole
A systematic review by Clarke and Deane [57] identified three trials (1 not published) evaluating the effect of adjuvant ropinirole versus placebo to levodopa in patients with levodopa-induced motor complications. The three trials comprised 263 patients; all had a randomized, double-blind, parallel-group design; two were short-term phase II trials using a maximum dose of ropinirole of 8 mg/d and 10 mg/d,

and one was a large phase III trial using a maximum dose of 24 mg/d. For methodological problems, the phase II trials did not allow for appropriate formal statistical meta-analysis; the phase III trial compared the proportion of patients achieving at least a 20% reduction in levodopa dose and in 'Off' time, and reported that 35% of patients on ropinirole achieved this endpoint compared to 13% of those on placebo ($P = 0.003$); the systematic review authors used additional data to express the change in 'Off' time in hours but it was not possible to draw firm conclusions on this outcome due to a significant difference in 'Off' duration between treatment arms at baseline. Nevertheless the authors conclude that had the trial been larger, the baseline imbalance would not have occurred and therefore an unequivocal benefit in 'Off' duration favouring ropinirole would have been noted. In the phase III trial the occurrence of dyskinesia was significantly more frequent with ropinirole (OR 2.90; 95% CI, 1.36–6.19); in the same trial, motor impairment and disability was significantly more improved with ropinirole than placebo as was the decrease in levodopa dose. No significant adverse events or withdrawals were observed between treatments.

Pergolide
A systematic review by Clarke and Speller [58] assessed the effect of adjuvant pergolide versus placebo to levodopa in patients with levodopa-induced motor complications. They identified one large study that included the results of small studies previously published. The trial may have been subjected to selection and detection bias. It enrolled 376 patients and was conducted for 24 weeks; patients on pergolide decreased 'Off' time by 1.8 h compared with 0.2 h with placebo ($P < 0.001$); dyskinesia developed or deteriorated in 62% of patients on pergolide compared with 25% with placebo; by week 24, the difference in dyskinesia had disappeared due to reduction of levodopa; reduction in levodopa dose was greater with pergolide than with placebo (235 versus 51 mg; $P < 0.001$); patients on pergolide had significant greater improvements than placebo in Hoehn and Yahr stage, and motor and ADL scores. Patients on pergolide had significantly more nausea (24% versus 13%) and hallucinations (14% versus 3%), and more withdrawals due to adverse events (9.5% versus 4.3%).

A growing number of publications reported the occurrence of valvular heart disorders associated with pergolide. Van Camp et al. [59] reported the presence of signs of restrictive valvular heart disease in 26 of 78 (33%) PD patients treated with pergolide, and found no signs of such disease in 18 PD patients never treated with an ergot-derived agonist. Severe valvular heart disease was present in 19% of patients with valvular heart disease, and a correlation was observed between cumulative dose of pergolide and valvular findings. Fibrotic reaction has also been reported associated with other ergot dopamine agonists and with non-ergot agonists [60].

Pramipexole

A Cochrane Collaboration Systematic Review by Clarke et al. [61] included randomized-controlled trials assessing the efficacy and safety of pramipexole versus placebo for the control of levodopa-induced motor complications. They identified four double-blind, parallel-group, multicenter trials in 669 patients (2 phase III studies with a 24-week mainenance period and 2 phase II studies with a 4-week maintenance period). The results showed a highly significant decrease of 'Off' period duration with pramipexole (WMD 1.8 h; 95% CI, 1.2–2.3). No significant changes were noted in a dyskinesia rating scale, although more patients on pramipexole reported dyskinesia as an adverse event. Improvement in UPDRS motor complications sub-score diverged between studies; significant improvement in UPDRS motor score in 'On' state was observed in three trials. Levodopa dose reduction significantly favoured pramipexole (WMD 115 mg; 95% CI, 87–143 mg). Withdrawal rate was significantly less with pramipexole; hallucinations were significantly more frequent with pramipexole, with no difference in other adverse events.

A randomized, parallel-group, three-arm placebo versus pramipexole versus bromocriptine, double-blind, 12-week trial [62] included 325 patients. Both pramipexole and bromocriptine significantly reduced ADL UPDRS (4.0 and 3.25 versus 2.03, $P < 0.001$ and $P < 0.007$, respectively) and 'On' motor UPDRS scores (11.8 and 9.98 versus 5.6, both $P < 0.001$) compared to placebo. This trial was not powered to detect differences between pramipexole and bromocriptine arms.

A randomized, double-blind, placebo-controlled, parallel-group, flexible-dose, 15-week trial [63] included a heterogeneous population of 150 PD patients. Results showed a significant improvement in ADL and 'On' motor UPDRS scores with pramipexole compared to placebo (12.14 points versus 2.45 points $P < 0.001$), and a change in 'Off' duration from 7.07 to 6.15 h/d with pramipexole compared to an increase from 5.59 to 6.87 h/d with placebo.

Carsten Möller et al. [64] performed a randomized, placebo-controlled, parallel-group, 32-week, double-blind trial followed by a 57-month open-label extension in 363 patients. Pramipexole dihydrochloride maximum dose was 4.5 mg/d (corresponding to 3.15 mg of pramipexole); 44% of patients withdrew from trial and the intention-to-treat population were 354 patients; mean dose of pramipexole was 3.7 mg/d. Pramipexole significantly improved ADL UPDRS (4.2 points versus 1.8 points, $P < 0.0001$), motor UPDRS (10.3 points versus 4.5 points, $P < 0.0007$), 'Off' duration by approximately 2.5 h/d ($P < 0.0001$) and decreased levodopa dose ($P = 0.001$) compared to placebo; most frequent adverse events were dyskinesia (pramipexole 30.0% versus placebo 8.7%), asymptomatic orthostatic hypotension (23.3% versus 20.2%), nausea (16.1% versus 12.0%), visual hallucination (11.1% versus 4.4%), and dizziness (10.6% versus 7.1%); 262 patients were enrolled

in the open-label phase and results showed consistency with double-blind phase.

Bromocriptine

A systematic review by Hilten et al. [65] assessed the efficacy and safety of adjunct bromocriptine versus placebo to levodopa in the treatment of levodopa-induced motor complications. They identified 7 RCTs (parallel-group = 5; crossover = 2; all double-blind) that comprised almost 400 patients: trials varied in the description of studied population, mean pre-trial daily dosages of levodopa, ratios of levodopa/decarboxylase inhibitor, bromocriptine titration schemes, trial duration and methods for evaluating motor complications and Parkinsonism. Results showed discrepancy between trials in the occurrence and severity of dyskinesias or dystonia, and in the improvement of motor fluctuations; compared to placebo, bromocriptine improved impairment in all trials (statistically significant in 2); the only trial allowing levodopa reduction reported no difference between groups; adverse events was fully reported in two trials and in one significant level were not reported; the other trial reported no statistically significant differences between the two groups; no significant difference in withdrawals due to adverse events was reported.

Guttman et al. [66] conducted a randomized, parallel-group, double-blind, 36-week trial in 247 patients. Patients were randomized into three arms: placebo, pramipexole (up to 4–5 mg/d), or bromocriptine (up to 30 mg/d). Bromocriptine did not significantly reduce the amount of time spent 'off' compared to placebo (specific data endpoints not reported).

Cabergoline

A systematic review by Clarke and Deane [67] included 3 randomized, multicentre, double-blind, controlled trials. Cabergoline was associated with a nonsignificant decrease in 'off' time duration compared to placebo and a nonsignificant increase in dyskinesia despite inadequate data report. Mean levodopa dose reduction was significantly greater with cabergoline compared to placebo (WMD 149.6 mg/d; 95% CI, 94.1–205.1 mg, $P < 0.00001$). There was a trend for fewer withdrawals with cabergoline.

Subcutaneous apomorphine

Dewey et al. [68] conducted a 4-week, randomized, double-blind, placebo-controlled, parallel-group trial in 32 patients. Apomorphine was administered in individualized subcutaneous injections to correct 'Off' state. Intention-to-treat population were 29 patients. Results showed that apomorphine compared to placebo significantly improved motor UPDRS scores (62% versus 0% improvement, $P < 0.001$), significantly aborted 'Off' states (95% versus 23% of 'Off' periods, $P < 0.01$) and significantly decreased daily 'Off' duration (2-h reduction versus no reduction, $P < 0.02$).

The most frequent adverse events were injection site complaints, yawning, somnolence, dyskinesia, and nausea or vomiting.

Conclusion

There is insufficient evidence regarding the efficacy and safety of controlled-release levodopa in improving levodopa-induced motor complications. Amantadine seems efficacious and safe in reducing dyskinesias compared to placebo, with an estimated duration of effect of 5 months; there is insufficient evidence regarding its effect on motor fluctuations. Clozapine seems safe and efficacious in reducing levodopa-induced dyskinesias compared to placebo. Entacapone is efficacious in reducing 'Off' time and increasing 'On' time duration, and in improving motor scores in fluctuators, compared to placebo; dyskinesia, nausea/vomiting, constipation, and diarrhoea are more frequent with entacapone than with placebo. Tolcapone is efficacious in reducing 'Off' time and increasing 'On' time duration, and in improving motor signs in fluctuators, though its liver toxicity makes its use only acceptable for patients that failed all other treatments and only under specialized monitoring. There is not enough evidence to conclude on the effect of selegiline in improving motor complications; Zydis selegiline is possibly useful and safe in reducing 'Off' time duration and increasing 'On time without dyskinesias' compared to placebo. Rasagiline is efficacious and safe in reducing 'Off' time duration and increasing 'On without troublesome dyskinesias', and in improving motor signs in fluctuators, compared to placebo. The dopamine agonists ropinirole, pramipexole, and pergolide are efficacious in treating motor fluctuations and improving motor scores in fluctuators compared to placebo, while data on bromocriptine and cabergoline is less robust. Intermittent subcutaneous apomorphine is efficacious and safe in correcting 'Off' states, reducing 'Off' duration and improving motor scores. Increase in dyskinesias is more frequent with agonists than with placebo, as other dopaminergic adverse events such as nausea, vomiting, and psychosis; pergolide has been associated with fibrotic reactions such as restrictive valvular heart disease, but reports also concern other ergot and non-ergot agonists.

3. Surgery

Among patients with PD and levodopa-induced motor complications, how does functional surgery (DBS or ablative surgery) affect the probability of improvement of motor fluctuations and dyskinesias? What is the risk of withdrawals?

Stimulation surgery

Pallidal (GPi) stimulation

Burchiel et al. [69] conducted a 12-month, randomized, parallel-group, blind-assessment trial comparing bilateral GPi stimulation to bilateral STN stimulation in 10 patients with severe PD and motor complications. There are some problems with data presentation in the manuscript. Anderson et al. [70] extended this study with the enrolment of 15 patients and reported the combined results of the two studies: the 14 new patients (1 dropped out before randomization) were randomized to immediate surgery or best medical therapy and delayed surgery. Due to premature termination of the study because of logistical reasons, only 2 patients were randomized to delayed surgery. Overall, 23 patients were randomized to either GPi ($N = 11$) or STN stimulation ($N = 12$) and 20 patients were available for 12-month follow-up ($N = 10$ in each group; 3 drop-outs: 1 death due to unrelated causes, 1 rapid progression of Parkinsonism, 1 intraoperative ischaemic stroke). The efficacy analysis included 20 and the safety analysis 23 patients. At 12 months, 'Off' medication motor UPDRS scores were improved by 39% in the GPi group and 48% in the STN group, with no significant differences between groups; and with a trend for better improvement of bradykinesia and axial symptoms with STN; 'Off' medication ADL UPDRS scores improved by 23% in either group. 'On' medication UPDRS motor and ADL sub-scores did not improve, and there were no significant cognitive or behavioural changes. Levodopa dose reduction was: STN stimulation 38% and GPi stimulation 3% ($P = 0.08$). At 3 months, STN stimulation reduced dyskinesia severity whether stimulators were 'Off' or 'On' while GPi group required active stimulation for dyskinesia reduction, but at 12 months dyskinesia was improved in both groups with or without stimulator 'On' (GPi: 89%; STN: 62%, no significant difference). Surgical complications included intraoperative ischaemic stroke (1), infraclavicular haematomas (1), prophylactic antibiotics after difficulty tunnelling of extension wire (1) and extracranial lead fracture (1); perioperative complications were frequent with STN stimulation: mild delirium (3), transient anxiety (2), hallucinations (1), short-term memory deficits associated with decrease concentration and apathetic mood (1), and cognitive function decline with increased Parkinsonism (1); 1 GPi patient had transient mild visual field defect.

The DBS For PD Study Group conducted a prospective, 6-month, multicentre study [71] on bilateral stimulation of the GPi or STN in advanced PD patients with motor complications. The design was double-blind, with a randomized and cross-over assessment of the acute effects of stimulation 3 months after surgery, and an open-label evaluation of the motor effects of stimulation 2 weeks before and 1, 3, and 6 months after surgery. A direct comparison between the two treatments was not conducted; the choice of the target was the responsibility of each centre. The double-blind assessment was performed after overnight withdrawal of both medication and stimulation. Patients were randomly allocated to undergo cross-over assessments in two sequences: sequence 1 – evaluation with stimulation Off then evaluation with stimulation On; sequence 2 – the reversed order. In the open-label assessment, patients were evaluated in four conditions: medication Off, stimulation Off; medication Off, stimulation On; medication On, stimulation On; medication On, stimulation Off. 143 patients were enrolled and 134 (STN = 96, GPi = 38) were implanted bilateral electrodes (efficacy analysis). For STN group, the double-blind evaluation ($N = 91$) showed a significant treatment effect associated with stimulation (sequence 1 – mean motor UPDRS Off: 50 and On: 27; sequence 2 – mean motor UPDRS On: 31 and Off: 52, $P < 0.001$) with no carry-over or period effects; unblinded assessments at 6 months showed a significant improvement in motor UPDRS with stimulation On and medication Off compared to baseline (mean baseline score 54, mean 6 months score 25.7, $P < 0.001$), a significant small benefit with the association of stimulation and medication, a significant improvement in 'On without dyskinesia' (from 27% to 74% of the day, $P < 0.001$) and 'Off' states duration (from 49% to 19% of the day, $P < 0.001$), a significant improvement in the mean ($\pm$SD) dyskinesia score (from 1.9 ± 1.1 to 0.8 ± 0.8, $P < 0.001$), and a reduction in levodopa dose from a mean of 1218.8 mg to 764 mg ($P < 0.001$). For GPi, the double-blind assessment ($N = 35$) showed a significant treatment effect with stimulation (sequence 1 – mean motor UPDRS Off: 44 and On: 28; sequence 2 – mean motor UPDRS On: 34 and Off: 48, $P < 0.001$), with no carry-over or period effects; unblinded assessments at 6 months showed a significant improvement in motor UPDRS with stimulation On and medication Off (mean baseline score 50.8, mean 6 months score 33.9, $P < 0.001$), a significant small improvements with stimulation On and medication On, significant improvement in 'On without dyskinesia' (from 28% to 64% of the day, $P < 0.001$) and 'Off' states duration (from 37% to 24% of the day, $P < 0.001$), a significant improvement in the mean (+SD) dyskinesia score (from 2.1 ± 1.5 to 0.7 ± 0.8, $P < 0.01$), but no change in levodopa dose. Major adverse events were intracranial haemorrhage (7), the number of electrode tracks used to determine target location correlating with the risk of haemorrhage ($P = 0.05$), seizures (4), explanted of device due to infection (2) and stimulation-induced dyskinesias (5). Although not direct comparison was conducted, STN stimulation seemed to induce better improvement and reduction in levodopa dose.

Subthalamic nucleus
Refer to the Burchiel et al. study, Anderson et al. [69,70] and the DBS Study Group trial [71] above ('Pallidal stimulation'). Deuschl et al compared STN stimulation with best medical therapy in a randomized-pairs trial with a 6-month follow-up. The primary end points were the changes from baseline to 6 months in the quality of life (assessed by the Parkinson's Disease Questionnaire – PDQ-39), and the severity of parkinsonism in the 'Off' period (assessed by the UPDRS-III). Secondary end points included a dyskinesia scale, UPDRS-II,

UPDRS-III during 'On' period, the Schwab & England Scale, home diaries, and a neuropsychiatric evaluation. A conservative approach was used regarding missing data, that favoured medical therapy. The trial included 156 patients (78 pairs). The results showed that stimulation compared to medication alone had greater benefit on the quality of life ($P = 0.02$) and on the severity of motor symptoms ($P < 0.01$): the mean change from baseline in the PDQ-39 scale was -9.5 ± 15.3 points (95% CI -13.1 to -5.9) in the stimulation arm compared with 0.2 ± 11.2 points (95% CI -2.4 to 2.9) in the medication alone arm; the mean change from baseline in the UPDRS-III during 'Off' period was -19.5 ± 15.1 points (95% CI -16.1 to -23.1) in the stimulation arm compared with 0.4 ± 9.5 points (95% CI -2.6 to 1.8) in the medication alone arm. 'Off' period duration was reduced by 4.2 hours in the stimulation group and remained unchanged in the medication alone group ($P < 0.001$); the time spent in 'On' with troublesome dyskinesias was reduced by 1 hour in the surgical arm and increased by 1 hour in the medication alone arm ($P = 0.003$). Serious adverse events were more common in the STN arm compared to the medication alone one (13% vs. 4%, $P < 0.04$), including a fatal intracerebral hemorrhage, though the frequency of adverse events was higher in the medication group (64% vs. 50%, $P = 0.08$); 1 patient committed suicide 5 months after surgery.

Limousin et al. [72] addressed the efficacy and safety of bilateral STN stimulation in a series of 24 patients (efficacy analysis population at 12 months: 20 patients); reasons for drop-out were: intracerebral haematoma with persistent paralysis and aphasia (1), infection at the implantation site (1), death of unrelated causes (1) and impossibility to travel to centre (1); adverse events were transient delirium, hallucinations or abulia in eight patients, dyskinesia induced by increasing voltage (18), and eyelid dyspraxia (5). Stimulation significantly improved UPDRS scores in both the medication On and Off conditions: medication Off mean UPDRS motor score before surgery = 55 versus medication Off, stimulation On mean UPDRS motor score = 25; medication On mean UPDRS motor score before surgery = 18 versus medication On, stimulation On mean UPDRS motor score = 14; 10 patients followed-up for 2 years retained improvement compared to pre-surgery. All 16 patients with painful dystonia improved and 12 fully recovered; dyskinesias decreased (not statistical significant) and motor fluctuations (item 39 from UPDRS Part IV) improved (mean score before surgery 2.2 versus 0.6 at 12 months). Levodopa dose was reduced from a mean of 1224 to 615 mg/day.

This study (Deuschl et al. A randomized trial of deep-brain stimulation for Parkinson's disease. *N Engl J Med* 2006;**355**: 896–908) was published after our electronic search date limit, but it was included due to clinical and scientific relevance.

Katayama et al. [73] addressed the efficacy of STN DBS in 14 patients, 6–8 months after surgery, using blinded ratings and a 2-day random-ordered protocol: 1 day with stimulator On and 1 day with stimulator Off. Medication Off UPDRS motor scores improved by 27% ($P < 0.001$) with the stimulator, UPDRS ADL scores by 18% ($P < 0.002$), and 'Off' duration by 33% ($P < 0.02$).

Rodriguez-Oroz et al. [74] assessed the efficacy of STN DBS at 4 years after surgery in 10 patients, using a double-blind, cross-over, randomized evaluation with two treatment sequences and an open-label evaluation in four conditions. Stimulation was associated with a mean reduction of 39.5% in motor UPDRS score (Off stimulation: 43, On stimulation: 26 points, $P < 0.04$); the dyskinesia severity decreased by 53% compared to baseline (absolute decrease) ($P < 0.01$), medication Off ADL UPDRS improved by 61% with stimulation (absolute decrease) ($P < 0.02$), and levodopa dose decreased from 1287.5 to 641 mg (50%) ($P < 0.01$). Adverse events were mild and transient paraesthesia while turning stimulator On (1), dementia (1), other cognitive impairment (2), and severe dysarthria (1).

Ford et al. [75] conducted a prospective, blinded and randomized videotape rating, 1-year study in 30 patients. Two patients could not return to final evaluation and six had undergone other previous surgical intervention for PD. Stimulation was associated with a 29.5% reduction in medication Off motor UPDRS score ($P < 0.0001$), a decrease of 'Off' duration from 7.25 to 2.25 h/d ($P < 0.001$), a significant reduction in dyskinesia severity ($P < 0.001$) and a 30% decrease in dopaminergic therapy ($P < 0.001$); medication On ADL UPDRS worsened by 34.3% ($P = 0.031$) and Hoehn and Yahr and Schwab and England scores kept unchanged. Nine serious adverse events occurred: ischaemic stroke (1), subdural haematoma (2), intracerebral haemorrhage (1), infection (3), and chest wall haematoma (2).

Ablative surgery
Pallidotomy
Vitek et al. [76] conducted a 6-month, blinded ratings, randomized trial comparing unilateral pallidotomy with medical therapy in 36 patients. At 6 months, group differences in UPDRS was statistical significant for pallidotomy ($P < 0.0001$) but not for medical therapy; dyskinesias and fluctuations also significantly favoured surgery. Adverse events occurred in six patients: focal motor seizures during surgery that implicated the arrest of surgery and maintenance of anticonvulsant through follow-up period (1), a 'seizure' consisting of a staring episode with facial grimacing (1), a subcortical haemorrhage in the pallidum causing a transient worsening in speech (1), small asymptomatic cortical haemorrhage (2), and a small asymptomatic subcortical haemorrhage (1).

Kondziolka et al. [77] assessed the efficacy of pallidotomy in an open-label, 1-year, prospective study in 58 patients. Results showed a significant improvement in total 'Off' UPDRS score (mean of 95.8 at baseline versus 77.6 points

after surgery), and in reduction of contralateral dyskinesias (from 1.5 to 0.9 points); reduction in dyskinesias was maintained in the 21 patients followed-up for 18 months. Adverse events were mild and occurred in 9% of the patients including dysarthria (four patients) and delirium (one patient).

Giller et al. [78] reported the effects of pallidotomy, which was unilateral in 49 patients. Mean 'Off' motor UPDRS scores improved from 42.0 to 24.9 at 12 months (12 patients), and dyskinesia improved from a mean 5.5 to 2.1 points. Adverse events included speech problems (8), hemiparesis (3), cognitive deficits (1), infection (1), or confusion (1); speech problems were frequent with bilateral pallidotomies.

Shannon et al. [79] evaluated the effects of pallidotomy at 6 months in 22 patients. 'Off' UPDRS scores improved from mean of 49.0 to 41.7 points at 6 months; UPDRS-based dyskinesia scores improved in both duration (mean baseline 2.2 versus 1.0 points at 6 months) and severity (mean baseline 1.5 points versus 0.5 points at 6 months). Adverse events included death (1), frontal lobe haematomas (3), cognitive and personality changes (2), frontal lobe dysfunction (3), aphasia (1), and hemiparesis (1).

Kishore et al. [80] conducted an evaluation of unilateral pallidotomy on 23 patients (20 were followed-up for 6 months and 11 for 1 year). Total 'Off' UPDRS score significantly improved from a mean of 47.3 to 30.0 (6 months) and 25.5 (1 year); and contralateral dyskinesia significantly decreased from a mean score of 7.5 to 3.8 (6 months) and 4.3 (1 year). Adverse effects included a delayed intracerebral haemorrhage and death (4%), transient hemiparesis and visual field deficit (12.5%) and facial paresis (1 patient).

Krauss et al. [81] assessed the effect of unilateral pallidotomy at 6 months in 36 patients. Significant improvements in motor 'Off' UPDRS scores (from a mean 58.1 to 33.0 points), and decrease in percentage of waking day with dyskinesia (from 37.5 to 18.1%) were documented: Adverse events included transient adverse effects from surgery (6), arterial infarctions (2), and venous infarction (1).

Utti et al. [82] conducted unilateral medial pallidotomy in 20 patients. Results showed an improvement in 'On' and 'Off' motor UPDRS scores and timed tests in the contralateral arm 3 months after surgery, a reduction in dyskinesia severity (mean Goetz Dyskinesia score improved from 1.4 to 1.2 and the Mayo Dyskinesia score from 11.6 to 7.6), and an increase in 'On' time obtained in nine patients (from a mean of 4.1 to 8.8 h). Neuropsychological evaluation showed mild decline in word fluency with no major cognitive deterioration; no significant surgical complications occurred.

The majority of the adverse events from pallidotomy are mild and well tolerated; there is a risk of serious adverse events including intracerebral haemorrhage, speech impairment (especially with bilateral pallidotomy), and visual field defects. Global neuropsychological function is usually preserved after unilateral pallidotomy, especially when performed on the right hemisphere [83–85]. Nevertheless, loss of verbal learning and verbal fluency may follow unilateral left pallidotomy, right hemisphere lesions may lead to transient visuospatial constructional deficits, and frontal behavioural changes were reported in 25% to 30% of patients [86].

Conclusion

There is insufficient evidence regarding the effect of DBS of either GPi or STN, and the effect of unilateral pallidotomy, in improving motor complications.

4. PD and psychosis

In patients with PD and psychosis, what is the benefit and safety of clozapine, quetiapine, olanzapine for the treatment of psychosis?

Clozapine

The Parkinson Study Group randomized 60 patients with idiopathic PD and drug-induced psychosis (DIP), in a parallel group, double-blind 4-week trial, to either placebo or clozapine, with an optional extension phase of 3 months [87]. The mean (±SE) scores on the Clinical Global Impression Scale (CGIS; 1 = normal; 7 = among the most severely psychotic patients ever seen) for psychosis improved by 1.6 ± 0.3 points for patients on clozapine versus 0.5 ± 0.2 point for patients on placebo ($P < 0.001$); all other psychosis outcome measures were highly statistically significant in favour of clozapine; there were no differences in the total and motor UPDRS scores, and actually the tremor item 20 of UPDRS Part III significantly improved with clozapine. There were no significant changes in the Mini-Mental State Examination (MMSE) in either group. Doses of clozapine were less than 25 mg/d, with some patients responding to 6.25 mg/d. Six drop-outs occurred, three in each arm (clozapine: 1 reversible leucopaenia, 1 myocardial infarction and 1 sedation; placebo: 2 increase in psychosis; 1 pneumonia). Mean neutrophile white-cell blood count and orthostatic blood pressure did not differ between treatments, but there was a small but significant increase in the mean heart rate of patients on clozapine. Fifty-three patients entered into the extension phase (patients on clozapine): 1 dropped-out due to reversible low white-cell count, and 6 died (unexpected high death rate) – stroke ($n = 1$), bronchitis ($n = 2$), or unknown ($n = 3$). After the end of extension phase, three other patients died: pneumonia ($n = 2$) and cardiac arrest ($n = 1$).

The French Clozapine Parkinson Study Group enrolled 60 patients with PD, in a multicentre, placebo-controlled trial [88]. The trial was divided in four periods: a screening phase, a 4-week, double-blind period (period II), an open-label period of 12 weeks (period III) and a washout period (period IV). Patients included in the trial had a score in MMSE at least of 20 and the DIP a minimum duration of 2 weeks. Patients were randomized to placebo or clozapine (6.25–50 mg/day). Mean (±SD) scores in the CGI (clozapine:−1.8 ± 1.5; placebo:−0.6 ± 1.1, $P = 0.011$) and in the Positive Subscore

of the Positive and Negative Syndrome Scale (clozapine: −5.6 ± 3.9; placebo: −0.8 ± 2.8, $P < 0.001$) significantly favoured clozapine; mean UPDRS motor scores did not differ between treatments. Mean dose of clozapine in period II was 35.8 mg/d and in period III 40 mg/d in patients previously on clozapine and 42.5 mg/d in those previously on placebo. At the end of period III, 25 patients fully recovered from delusions and hallucinations; washout of clozapine was tried in these 25 patients, but relapse occurred in 19 patients. Overall, adverse events were more frequent in the placebo arm. Somnolence was more frequent with clozapine; reversible neutropenia was seen in two clozapine patients but no agranulocytosis was observed. Two patients in period III died (sudden death = 1, aspiration pneumonia = 1).

Other than leucopaenia, the use of clozapine has been associated with severe myocarditis and cardiomyopathy in physically healthy young adults, and with acute interstitial nephritis and venous thromboembolism in psychiatric patients.

Quetiapine

Ondo et al. conducted a double-blind, parallel-group, placebo-controlled study to evaluate the efficacy, tolerability, and safety of quetiapine for dopaminergic-induced hallucinations [89]. The study included 31 patients with a MMSE score > 21; patients were randomized to placebo or quetiapine, titrated up to 200 mg/day in two doses. Evaluations took place at 3 and 12 weeks; drop-outs were not included in the analysis if data were not available. Four patients on quetiapine arm dropped-out (serious unrelated illness = 2; lack of efficacy = 2) and two on placebo (death due to serious unrelated illness = 2); Efficacy measures did not differ significantly compared to placebo, neither did UPDRS; tolerability was good; sedation occurred in nine patients taking quetiapine and four patients referred subjective worsening in PD.

Olanzapine

A 9-week RCT [90] compared clozapine with olanzapine in PD patients. The study was prematurely stopped because of unacceptable deterioration of Parkinsonism in the olanzapine group. Patients were initially randomized to either clozapine 6.25 mg/d or olanzapine 2.5 mg/d; mean peak dose for clozapine was 25.8 mg/d while for olanzapine was 11.4 mg/d. Patients on clozapine showed a statistically significant improvement from baseline in the total score of the Assessment of Positive Symptoms Scale (SAPS) for psychotic symptoms (from 13.5 ± 7.7 at baseline to 6.6 ± 6.2 at study end, $P = 0.016$), in the visual hallucination item on SAPS (from 3.9 ± 1.0 at baseline to 1.9 ± 1.2 at study end, $P = 0.013$) and in the BPRS (from 31.4 ± 7.6 at baseline to 23.8 ± 3.9 at study end, $P = 0.031$). Motor and ADL UPDRS subscores improved in clozapine arm but did not reach statistical significance, but the change scores for motor and

ADL UPDRS between clozapine and olanzapine significantly favoured clozapine (mean change of UPDRS motor score from baseline to study end: clozapine -6.0 ± 8.2, olanzapine $+12.3 \pm 11.5$, $P = 0.004$; mean change of UPDRS ADL 'on' score from baseline to study end: clozapine -1.5 ± 4.3, olanzapine $+3.9 \pm 7.2$, $P = 0.017$; mean change of UPDRS ADL 'off' score from baseline to study end: clozapine -4.5 ± 10.4, olanzapine $+2.4 \pm 2.1$, $P = 0.005$). The small number of patients completing the study did not allow for comparison of antipsychotic efficacy; patients on olanzapine did not improve significantly over baseline in total SAPS and SAPS visual hallucination scores. Leucocyte counts did not change significantly in both groups.

Conclusion
Clozapine is efficacious in treating DIP, requiring however weekly blood count monitoring due to the risk of agranulocytosis. There is insufficient data regarding the effect of quetiapine in treating DIP, while olanzapine carries an unacceptable risk of deterioration of Parkinsonism.

5. Parkinson's disease dementia
In patients with PDD, what is the benefit and safety of rivastigmine and donepezil for the treatment of cognitive or behavioural disturbances? What is the risk of withdrawal?

The studies' results are summarized in Table 20.3.

Rivastigmine
A 24-week, randomized, double-blind, parallel-group, placebo-controlled trial [91] tested the efficacy and safety of rivastigmine in 541 patients with mild-to-moderately severe dementia as defined by DSM-IV criteria and a MMSE score of 10–24, and onset of dementia at least 2 years after diagnosis of PD. Patients were randomized to rivastigmine or placebo in a 2:1 ratio. Exclusion criteria included a history of a major depressive episode. Treatment started with 1,5 mg of rivastigmine or placebo twice daily, with doses increases of 3 mg/d at 4-week intervals during a 16-week escalation period. A total of 501 patients were included in the efficacy analysis and 131 patients (24.2%) discontinued the study prematurely (rivastigmine = 27.3%, placebo = 17.9% of patients) mainly due to adverse events (rivastigmine = 17.1%, placebo = 7.8% of patients). At week 24, statistically significant improvements favoured rivastigmine in the Alzheimer's Disease Assessment Scale (ADAS-cog) score (rivastigmine: mean improvement of 2.1 points, placebo: mean worsening of 0.7 point, $P < 0.001$); in the Alzheimer's Disease Cooperative Study-Clinician's Global Impression of Change (ADCS-CGIC) score (rivastigmine: mean score 3.8; placebo: mean score 4.3, $P = 0.007$; moderate or marked improvement in 19.8% of patients in rivastigmine arm and in 14.5% of patients in placebo arm; marked or moderate worsening in 13% of patients in rivastigmine arm and in 23.1% of patients in placebo arm). Patients on rivastigmine reported more aggravation of Parkinsonian symptoms (27.3%

Table 20.3 Drugs treatment for Parkinson's disease dementia.

Type of study (reference)	Intervention (dosage)	Follow-up time	Outcome	Number of patients (Number of trials)	Control group (range)	Relative risk (95% CI)	Absolute risk reduction or WMD	Comment
RCT [91]	Rivastigmine (8.6 mg) versus placebo	6 months	ADAS-cog	490 (1)	0.7 (SD, 7.5)	–	2.8 (4.26–1.34)	Rivastigmine better
			ADCS-CGIC	494 (1)	4.3 (SD, 1.5)	–	0.5 (0.77–0.23)	Rivastigmine better
			Withdrawals *	501 (1)	14	1.19 (2.8–0.26)	9% (ns)	Rivastigmine worse
			Parkinsonian symptoms	Patients on rivastigmine reported more aggravation of Parkinsonian symptoms. Differences in motor UPDRS were not significant.				
RCT Cross-over trial [92]	Donepezil (5–10 mg) versus placebo	6.5 weeks	ADAS-cog	19 (1)	–	–	1.9 (ns)	Donepezil better
			ADCS-CGIC	–	–	–	–	–
			Withdrawals *	22 (1)	1	1.0 (0.79–17.98)	9% (ns)	Donepezil worse
			Parkinsonian symptoms	There was no impact on UPDRS.				

RCT: randomized controlled trial; CI: confidence intervals; ns: not statistically significant; SD: standard deviation; ADAS-cog: Alzheimer`s Disease Assessment Scale; ADCS-CGIC: Alzheimer`s Disease Cooperative Study-Clinician`s Global Impression of Change score. *due to adverse events.

versus 15.6%, $P = 0.002$), mainly tremor (10.2% versus 3.9%, $P = 0.01$). Tremor was the cause of withdrawal in 1.7% of patients in the rivastigmine arm and none in the placebo arm ($P = 0.19$). Bradykinesia, dystonia, or muscle rigidity were the cause for withdrawal in <0.6% of patients in both groups. Differences in motor UPDRS were not significant ($P = 0.83$). The most frequent adverse events were nausea (rivastigmine = 29.0% versus placebo 11.2% of patients, $P < 0.001$), and vomiting (rivastigmine = 16.6% versus placebo 1.7% of patients, $P < 0.001$), and serious adverse events did not differ significantly between groups.

Donepezil

A randomized, double-blind, cross-over, placebo-controlled trial [92] evaluated the efficacy and safety of donepezil. Patients were included if fulfilled DSM-IV criteria for dementia, if had a mild to moderate dementia as defined by a MMSE score between 17 and 26, and if dementia developed $\geqslant 12$ months after Parkinsonism. Each treatment period lasted 10 weeks and a washout open-label period of 6 weeks (17 half lives) occurred between treatment periods. Safety and efficacy were assessed at weeks 7 and 10 for each period. Donepezil or matching placebo was taken at 5 mg/d for 4 weeks and then increased to 5 mg twice-a-day. Only patients with at least one visit in the second period were included in the efficacy analysis. Twenty-two patients were randomized (28 were screened) for either donepezil/placebo or placebo/donepezil; in the first period three patients (donepezil: = 1 worsening psychosis, 1 arrhythmia versus placebo = 1 worsening psychosis) dropped out and were not included in the efficacy analysis; in the second period two patients on donepezil and one on placebo discontinued medication but continued on the trial. Donepezil had a non-significant improvement on ADAS-cog compared to placebo (average score 1.9 points better than placebo, $P = 0.18$); scores on MMSE ($P = 0.004$) and on the Clinical Global Impression of Change scale ($P = 0.0056$) significantly favoured donepezil, and no significant differences were observed on the Mattis Dementing Rating Scale or the Brief Psychiatric Rating Scale. The drug was well tolerated and adverse events occurred in 52% on donepezil and in 45% on placebo: worsening of psychosis and agitation were the most frequent and occurred equally between groups; there was no impact on UPDRS. A carry-over effects test showed a non-significant trend in the same direction as treatment effects in the cognitive domains.

Conclusion

Rivastigmine is efficacious in treating symptoms of mild-to-moderately severe dementia compared with placebo, though it might aggravate Parkinsonism, mainly tremor. There is insufficient data to conclude about the effect of donepezil in the treatment of PDD.

Conclusions

It was not the aim of this chapter to cover all possible answerable questions regarding the treatment of PD neither all therapeutic interventions, and that limitation is an assumed one. We focused on those that were thought to be more important to clinical practice and at the same time less consensual. Sometimes, there is evidence showing both efficacy and safety for different interventions regarding a given question; choice between interventions will depend on different variables such as availability of drug, patient features, cost, and physician preferences.

Until now, no intervention has proved neuroprotective. Agonists are efficacious and safe in reducing the incidence of motor complications, in treating motor fluctuations and in improving motor scores in fluctuators. Both selegiline and rasagiline are efficacious and safe as monotherapy for PD, while rasagiline is beneficial in treating motor fluctuations, as might be Zydis selegiline. Entacapone and tolcapone are efficacious in treating motor fluctuations and improving motor impairment in fluctuators, but use of tolcapone is very limited due to safety. Amantadine and clozapine are both beneficial in reducing levodopa-induced dyskinesias, and clozapine in the only neuroleptic proved to be efficacious and safe to treat LIP. Although DBS and pallidotomy are efficacious as symptomatic adjunct therapy to levodopa to treat Parkinsonism, no good trial has shown evidence regarding the treatment of motor complications. Rivastigmine is efficacious in treating symptoms of mild-to-moderately severe PDD, though it may aggravate Parkinsonism.

References

1 Tolosa E, Wenning G, Poewe W. The diagnosis of Parkinson's disease. *Lancet Neurol.* 2006; **5**: 75–86.

2 Chaudhuri KR, Healy DG, Schapira HVA. Non-motor symptoms of Parkinson's disease: diagnosis and management. *Lancet Neurol.* 2006; **5**: 235–45.

3 Zhang Z, Roman G. Worldwide occurrence of Parkinson's disease: an update review. *Neuroepidemiology* 1993; **12**: 195–208.

4 De Rijk MC, Tzourio C, Breteler MMB, et al. Prevalence of parkinsonism and Parkinson's disease in Europe: the EUROPARKINSON collaborative study. *J. Neurol. Neurosurg. Psychiatr.* 1997; **62**: 10–15.

5 Tanner CM, Hubble JP, Chan P. Epidemiology and genetics of Parkinson's disease: In: Watts RL & Koller WC, eds., *Movement Disorders: Neurologic Principles and Practice* McGraw-Hill, New York, 1997: pp.137–52.

6 Marras C, Tanner CM. Epidemiology of Parkinson's disease. In: Watts RL & Koller WC, eds., *Movement Disorders: Neurologic Principles & Practice,* 2nd edn. McGraw-Hill, New York, 2004: pp. 177–95.

7 Payami H, Larsen K, Bernard S, Nutt J. Increased risk of Parkinson's disease in parents and siblings of patients. *Ann. Neurol.* 1994; **36**: 659–61.

8 Marder K, Tang M, Mejia H, et al. Risk of Parkinson's disease among first degree relatives: a community based study. *Neurology* 1996; **47**: 155–60.

9 Lazzarini A, Myers R, Zimmerman T, et al. Clinical genetic study of Parkinson's disease: evidence for dominant transmission. *Neurology* 1994; **44**: 499–506.

10 Hughes AJ, Daniel SE, Kilford L, Lees AJ. Accuracy of clinical diagnosis of idiopathic Parkinson's disease: a clinico-pathological study of 100 cases. *J. Neurol. Neurosurg. Psychiatr.* 1992; **55**: 181–4.

11 Hughes AJ, Daniel SE, Lees AJ. Improved accuracy of clinical diagnosis of Lewy body Parkinson's disease. *Neurology* 2001; **57**: 1497–9.

12 Parkinson Study Group. Mortality in DATATOP: a multicenter trial in early Parkinson's disease. *Ann. Neurol.* 1998; **43**: 318–25.

13 Morgante L, Salemi G, Meneghini F, et al. Parkinson's disease survival. A population-based study. *Arch. Neurol.* 2000; **57**: 507–12.

14 Clarke C, Moore AP. Parkinson's disease. *Clin. Evid.* 2005 June; (13): 1658–77. (Review).

15 Goetz CG, Koller WC, Poewe W, et al. Management of Parkinson's disease: an evidence-based review. *Mov. Disord.* 2002; **17**(Suppl. 4): S1–166.

16 Goetz CG, Poewe W, Rascol O, Sampaio C. Evidence-based medical review update: pharmacological and surgical treatments of Parkinson's disease: 2001 to 2004. *Mov. Disord.* 2005; **20**(5): 523–39 (review).

17 Macleod AD, Counsell CE, Ives N, Stowe R. Monoamine oxidase B inhibitors for early Parkinson's disease. *Cochrane Database Syst. Rev.* 2005 July; (3): CD004898 (review).

18 Caraceni T, Musicco M. Levodopa or dopamine agonists, or deprenyl as initial treatment for Parkinson's disease. A randomized multicenter study. *Parkinsonism Relat. Disord.* 2001; **7**: 107–14.

19 Parkinson Study Group. A controlled trial of rasagiline in early Parkinson disease: the Tempo Study. *Arch. Neurol.* 2002; **59**: 1937–43.

20 Parkinson Study Group. A controlled randomized, delayed-start study of rasagiline in early Parkinson disease. *Arch. Neurol.* 2004; **61**: 561–6.

21 Whone AL, Watts RL, Stoessl AJ, et al. Slower progression of Parkinson's disease with ropinirole versus levodopa: the REALPET study. *Ann. Neurol.* 2003; **54**: 93–101.

22 Rascol O, Brooks DJ, Korczyn AD, De Deyn PP, Clarke CE, Lang AE, for the 056 Study Group. A five-year study of the incidence of dyskinesia in patients with early Parkinson's disease who were treated with ropinirole or levodopa. *N. Engl. J. Med.* 2000; **342**: 1484–91.

23 Parkinson Study Group. Pramipexole vs levodopa as initial treatment for Parkinson disease: a randomized controlled trial. JAMA. 2000; **284**: 1931–8.

24 Parkinson Study Group. Dopamine transporter brain imaging to assess the effects of pramipexole vs. levodopa on Parkinson disease progression. JAMA. 2002; **287**: 1653–61.

25 Bracco F, Battaglia A, Chouza C, Dupont E, Gershanik O, Marti Masso JF, Montastruc JL and PKDS0098. The Long-Acting Dopamine Receptor Agonist Cabergoline in Early Parkinson's Disease: Final Results of a 5-Year, Double-Blind, Levodopa-Controlled Study. *CNS Drugs* 2004; **18**(11): 733–46.

26 Rinne UK. Lisuride, a dopamine agonist in the treatment of early Parkinson's disease. *Neurology* 1989; **39**: 336–9.

27 Allain H, Destée A, Petit H, et al. Five-year follow-up of early lisuride and levodopa combination therapy versus levodopa monotherapy in de novo Parkinson's disease. The French Lisuride Study Group. *Eur. Neurol.* 2000; **44**: 22–30.

28 Parkinson's Disease Research Group in the United Kingdom. Comparisons of therapeutic effects of levodopa, levodopa and selegiline, and bromocriptine in patients with early, mild Parkinson's disease: three year interim report. *BMJ.* 1993; **307**: 469–72.

29 Lees AJ, Katzenschlager R, Head J, Ben-Shlomo Y, on behalf of the Parkinson's disease research group on the United Kingdom. Ten-year follow-up of three different initial treatments in de-novo PD. A randomized trial. *Neurology* 2001; **57**: 1687–94.

30 Hely MA, Morris JGL, Reid WGJ. The Sydney multicentre study of Parkinson's disease: a randomized, prospective five year study comparing low dose bromocriptine with low dose levodopa–carbidopa. *J. Neurol. Neurosurg. Psychiatr.* 1994; **57**: 903–10.

31 Montastruc JL, Rascol O, Senard JM, Rascol A. A randomized controlled study comparing bromocriptine to which levodopa was later added, with levodopa alone in previously untreated patients with Parkinson's disease: a five year follow-up. *J. Neurol. Neurosurg. Psychiatr.* 1994; **57**: 1034–8.

32 Korczyn AD, Brunt ER, Larsen JP, Nagy Z, Poewe WH, Ruggieri S. A 3-year randomized trial of ropinirole and bromocriptine in early Parkinson's disease. The 053 Study Group. *Neurology* 1999; **53**: 364–70.

33 Ramaker C, van Hilten JJ. Bromocriptine versus levodopa in early Parkinson's disease. *Cochrane Database Syst. Rev.* 2002; **2**: CD002258. DOI: 10.1002/14651858. CD002258.

34 Nakanishi T, Iwata M, Goto I, Kanazawa I, Kowa H, Mannen T, Mizuno Y, Nishitani H, Ogawa N, Takahashi A, Tashiro K, Tohgi H, Yanagisawa N. Nationwide collaborative study on the long-term effects of bromocriptine in the treatment of parkinsonian patients. Final Report. *Eur. Neurol.* 1992; **32**(Suppl. 1): 9–22.

35 Przuntek H, Welzel D, Gerlach M, et al. Early institution of bromocriptine in Parkinson's disease inhibits the emergence of levodopa-associated motor side effects. Long-term results of the PRADO study. *J. Neural Transm.* 1996; **103**: 699–715.

36 Gimenez-Roldan S, Tolosa E, Burguera JA, Chacon J, Liano H, Forcadell F. Early combination of bromocriptine and levodopa in Parkinson's disease: a prospective randomized study of two parallel groups over a total follow-up period of 44 months including an initial 8-month double-blind stage. *Clin. Neuropharmacol.* 1997; **20**: 67–76.

37 The Parkinson Study Group. Levodopa and the Progression of Parkinson's Disease. *N. Engl. J. Med.* 2004; **351**: 2498–508.

38 Dupont E, Anderson A, Boqs J, et al. Sustained-release Madopar HBS compared with standard Madopar in the long-term treatment of de novo parkinsonian patients. *Acta Neurol. Scand.* 1996; **93**: 14–20.

39 Block G, Liss C, Scott R, Irr J, Nibbelink D. Comparison of immediate-release and controlled release carbidopa/levodopa in Parkinson's disease. A multicenter 5-year study. *Eur. Neurol.* 1997; **37**: 23–27.

40 Koller WC, Hutton JT, Tolosa E, Capildeo R, Carbidopa/ Levodopa Study Group. Immediate-release and controlled-release carbidopa/levodopa in PD: a 5-year randomized multicenter study. *Neurology* 1999; **53**: 1012–19.

41 Wolters EC, Tesselaar HJM, International (NL & UK) Sinemet CR Study Group. International (NL-UK) double-blind study of Sinemet CR and standard Sinemet (25/100) in 170 patients with fluctuating Parkinson's disease. *J. Neurol.* 1996; **243**: 235–40.

42 UK Madopar CR Study Group. A comparison of Madopar CR and Standard Madopar in the treatment of nocturnal and early-morning disability in Parkinson's disease. *Clin. Neuropharmacol.* 1989; **12**: 498–505.

43 Hutton JT, Morris JL, Bush DF, Smith ME, Liss CL, Reines S. Multicenter controlled study of Sinemet CR vs Sinemet (25/100) in advanced Parkinson's disease. *Neurology* 1989; **39**: 67–72.

44 Jankovic J, Schwartz K, Vander Linden C. Comparison of Sinemet CR4 and standard Sinemet: Double-blind and long-term open trial in parkinsonian patients with fluctuations. *Mov. Disord.* 1989; **4**: 303–9.

45 Lieberman A, Gopinathan G, Miller E, Neophytides A, Baumann G, Chin L. Randomized double-blind cross-over study of Sinemet-Controlled Release (CR4 50/200) versus Sinemet 25/100 in Parkinson's disease. *Eur. Neurol.* 1990; **30**: 75–8.

46 Crosby NJ, Deane KHO, Clarke CE. Amantadine for dyskinesia in Parkinson's disease. *Cochrane Database Syst. Rev.* 2003; (2):CD003467 (review).

47 Thomas A, Lacono D, Luciano AL, Armellino K, Di Lorio A, Onofri M. Duration of amantadine benefit on dyskinesia of severe Parkinson's disease. *J. Neurol. Neurosurg. Psychiatr.* 2004; **75**: 141–3.

48 Durif F, Debilly D, Galitzki M, Morand D, Viallet F, Borq M, Thobois S, Broussolle E, Rascol O. Clozapine improves dyskinesias in Parkinson's disease: a double-blind, placebo-controlled study. *Neurology* 2004; **62**(3): 381–8.

49 Deane, KHO; Spieker, S; Clarke, CE. Catechol-O-methyltransferase inhibitors for levodopa-induced complications in Parkinson's disease. *Cochrane Database Syst. Rev.* 2004; (4): CD004554 (review).

50 Deane KHO, Spieker S, Clarke CE. Catechol-O-methyltransferase inhibitors versus active comparators for levodopa-induced complications in Parkinson's disease. *Cochrane Database Syst. Rev.* 2004; (4): CD004553 (review).

51 Lees AJ, Shaw KM, Kohout LJ, et al. Deprenyl in Parkinson's disease. *Lancet* 1977; **2**: 791–5.

52 Lieberman AN, Gopinathan G, Neophytides A, Foo SH. Deprenyl versus placebo in Parkinson's disease. A double-blind study. *NY State J. Med.* 1987; **87**: 646–9.

53 Golbe LI, Lieberman AN, Muenter MD, et al. Deprenyl in the treatment of symptom fluctuations in advanced Parkinson's disease. *Clin. Neuropharmacol.* 1988; **11**: 45–55.

54 Waters CH, Sethi KD, Hauser RA, Molho E, Bertoni JM and the Zydis Seleginine Study Group. Zydis Seleginine Reduces Off Time in Parkinson's Disease. Patients With Motor Fluctuations: A 3-Month, Randomized, Placebo-Controlled Study. *Mov. Disord.* 2004; **4**: 426–32.

55 Rascol O, Brooks DJ, Melamed E, Oertel W, Poewe W, Stocchi F, Tolosa E, for the LARGO study group. Rasagiline as an adjunct to levodopa in patients with Parkinson's disease and motor fluctuations (LARGO, Lasting effect in Adjunct therapy with Rasagiline Given Once daily, study): a randomised, double-blind, parallel-group trial. *Lancet* 2005; **365**: 947–54.

56 Parkinson Study Group. A randomized placebo-controlled trial of rasagiline in levodopa-treated patients with Parkinson's disease and motor fluctuations: The PRESTO Study. *Arch. Neurol.* 2005; **62**: 241–8.

57 Clarke CE, Deane KHO. Ropinirole for levodopa-induced complications in Parkinson's disease. *Cochrane Database Syst. Rev.* 2001; (1): CD001516 (review).

58 Clarke CE, Speller JM. Pergolide for levodopa-induced complications in Parkinson's disease. *Cochrane Database Syst. Rev.* 2000; (2): CD000235 (review).

59 Van Camp G, Flamez A, Cosyns B, et al. Treatment of Parkinson's disease with pergolide and relation to restrictive valvular heart disease. *Lancet* 2004; **363**: 1179 –83.

60 Chaudhuri KR, Dhawan V, Basu S, Jackson G, Odin P. Valvular heart disease and fibrotic reactions may be related to ergot dopamine agonists, but non-ergot agonists may also not be spared. *Mov. Disord.* 2004; **12**:1522–3.

61 Clarke CE, Speller JM, Clarke JA. Pramipexole for levodopa-induced complications in Parkinson's disease. *Cochrane Database Syst. Rev.* 2000; (3): CD002261 (review).

62 Mizuno Y, Yanagisawa N, Kuno S, et al. Randomized, double-blind study of pramipexole with placebo and bromocriptine in advanced Parkinson's disease. *Mov. Disord.* 2003; **18**: 1149–56.

63 Wong KS, Lu C-S, Shan D-E, et al. Efficacy, safety, and tolerability of pramipexole in untreated and levodopa-treated patients with Parkinson's disease. *J. Neurol. Sci.* 2003; **216**: 81– 7.

64 Möller JC, Oertel W, Koster J, Pezzoli G, Provinciali L. Long-term efficacy and safety of pramipexole in advanced Parkinson's disease: results from a European multicenter trial. *Mov. Disord.* 2005; **5**: 602–10.

65 Hilten JJ van, Ramaker C, Beek WJT van de, Finken MJJ. Bromocriptine for levodopa-induced motor complications in Parkinson's disease. *Cochrane Database Syst. Rev.* 2000; (2): CD001203 (review).

66 Guttman M, International Pramipexole–Bromocriptine Study Group. Double-blind randomized, placebo controlled study to compare safety, tolerance and efficacy of Pramipexole and Bromocriptine in advanced Parkinson's disease. *Neurology* 1997; **49**: 1060–5.

67 Clarke CE, Deane KH. Cabergoline for levodopa-induced complications in Parkinson's disease. *Cochrane Database Syst. Rev.* 2001; **1**: CD001518. DOI: 10.1002/14651858. CD001518.

68 Dewey Jr RB, Hutton JT, LeWitt PA, Factor SA. A randomized, double-blind, placebo-controlled trial on subcutaneously

injected apomorphine for parkinsonian Off-state events. *Arch. Neurol.* 2001; **58**: 1385–92.

69 Burchiel KJ, Anderson VC, Favre J, Hammerstad JP. Comparison of pallidal and subthalamic nucleus deep brain stimulation for advanced Parkinson's disease: results of a randomized, blinded pilot study. *Neurosurgery* 1999; **45**(6): 1375–82.

70 Anderson VC, Burchiel KJ, Hogarth P, Favre J, Hammerstad JP. Pallidal vs subthalamic nucleus deep brain stimulation in Parkinson's disease. *Arch. Neurol.* 2005; **62**: 554–60.

71 Deep Brain Stimulation for Parkinson's Disease Study Group. Deep-brain stimulation of the subthalamic nucleus or the pars interna of the globus pallidus in Parkinson's disease. *N. Engl. J. Med.* 2001; **345**: 956–63.

72 Limousin P, Pollak P, Hoffmann D, et al. Abnormal involuntary movements induced by subthalamic nuclear stimulation in parkinsonian patients. *Mov. Disord.* 1996; **11**: 231–5.

73 Katayama Y, Kasai M, Oshima H, et al. Subthalamic nucleus stimulation for Parkinson's disease: benefits observed in levodopa intolerant patients. *J. Neurosurg.* 2001; **95**: 213–21.

74 Rodriguez-Oroz MC, Zamarbide I, Guridi J, Palmero MR, Obeso JA. Efficacy of deep brain stimulation of the subthalamic nucleus in Parkinson's disease 4 years after surgery: double-blind and open label evaluation. *J. Neurol. Neurosurg. Psychiatr.* 2004; **75**: 1382–5.

75 Ford B, Winfield L, Pullman SL, Frucht SJ, Du Y, Greene P, Cheringal JH, Yu Q, Cote LJ, Fahn S, McKhann II GM, Goodman RR. Subthalamic nucleus stimulation in advanced Parkinson's disease: blinded assessments at one year follow-up. *J. Neurol. Neurosurg. Psychiatr.* 2004; **75**: 1255–9.

76 Vitek JL, Bakay RAE, Freeman A, et al. Randomized trial of pallidotomy versus medical therapy for Parkinson's disease. *Ann. Neurol.* 2003; **53**: 558–69.

77 Kondziolka D, Bonaroti E, Baser S, Brandt F, Kim YS, Lunsford LD. Outcomes after stereotactically guided pallidotomy for advanced Parkinson's disease. *J. Neurosurg.* 1999; **90**: 197–202.

78 Giller CA, Dewey RB, Ginsburg MI, Mendelsohn DB, Berk AM. Stereotactic pallidotomy and thalamotomy using individual variations of anatomic landmarks for localization. *Neurosurgery* 1998; **42**: 56–65.

79 Shannon KM, Penn RD, Kroin JS, et al. Stereotactic pallidotomy for the treatment of Parkinson's disease. Efficacy and adverse effects at 6 months in 26 patients. *Neurology* 1998; **50**: 434–8.

80 Kishore A, Turnbull IM, Snow BJ, et al. Efficacy, stability and predictors of outcome of pallidotomy for Parkinson's disease. Six-month follow-up with additional 1-year observations. *Brain* 1997; **120**: 729–37.

81 Krauss JK, Desaloms JM, Lai EC, King DE, Jankovic J, Grossman RG. Microelectrode-guided posteroventral pallidotomy for treatment of Parkinson's disease: postoperative magnetic resonance imaging analysis [see comments]. *J. Neurosurg.* 1997; **87**: 358–67.

82 Uitti RJ, Wharen Jr RE, Turk MF, et al. Unilateral pallidotomy for Parkinson's disease: comparison of outcome in younger versus elderly patients. *Neurology* 1997; **49**: 1072–7.

83 Gironell A, Kulisevsky J, Rami L. Effects of pallidotomy and bilateral subthalamic stimulation on cognitive function in Parkinson's disease. *J. Neurol.* 2003; **250**: 917–23.

84 Green J, McDonald WM, Vitek JL, et al. Neuropsychological and psychiatric sequelae of pallidotomy for PD. *Neurology* 2002; **58**: 858–65.

85 Perrine K, Dogali M, Fazzini E, et al. Cognitive functioning after pallidotomy for refractory Parkinson's disease. *J. Neurol. Neurosurg. Psychiatr.* 1998; **65**: 150–4.

86 Trépanier LL, Saint-Cyr JA, Lozano AM, Lang AE. Neuropsychological consequences of posteroventral pallidotomy for the treatment of Parkinson's disease. *Neurology* 1998; **51**: 207–15.

87 The Parkinson Study Group. Low-dose clozapine for the treatment of drug-induced psychosis in Parkinson's disease. The Parkinson Study Group. *N. Engl. J. Med.* 1999; **340**: 757–63.

88 Pollak P, Tison F, Rascol O, Destée A, Péré JJ, Senard JM, Durif F, Bourdeix I, on behalf of the French Clozapine Parkinson Study Group. Clozapine in drug induced psychosis in Parkinson's disease: a randomised, placebo controlled study with open follow-up. *J. Neurol. Neurosurg. Psychiatr.* 2004; **75**: 689–95.

89 Ondo WG, Tintner R, Dat Voung K, Lai D, Ringholz G. Double-blind, placebo-controlled, unforced titration parallel trial of quetiapine for dopaminergic-induced hallucinations in Parkinson's disease. *Mov. Disord.* 2005; **8**: 958–63.

90 Goetz CG, Blasucci LM, Leurgans S, Pappert EJ. Olanzapine and clozapine. Comparative effects on motor function in hallucinating PD patients. *Neurology* 2000; **55**: 748–9.

91 Emre M, Aarsland D, Albanese A, Byrne EJ, Deuschl G, De Deyn PP, Durif F, Kulisevsky J, van Laar T, Lees A, Poewe W, Robillard A, Rosa MM, Wolters E, Quarg P, Tekin S, Lane R. Rivastigmine for dementia associated with Parkinson's disease. *N. Engl. J. Med.* 2004; **351**: 2509–18.

92 Ravina B, Putt M, Siderowf A, Farrar JT, Gillespie M, Crawley A, Fernandez HH, Trieschmann MM, Reichwein S, Simuni T. Donepezil for dementia in Parkinson's disease: a randomized, double-blind, placebo controlled, crossover study. *J. Neurol. Neurosurg. Psychiatr.* 2005; **76**: 934–9.

CHAPTER 21

Multiple sclerosis: critical review of the evidence for each question

Graziella Filippini, George Ebers

Background

Multiple sclerosis (MS) is an autoimmune disease of the central nervous system resulting from the effect between unidentified environmental factors and susceptibility genes. Together, these factors trigger a cascade of events, involving engagement of the immune system, acute inflammatory injury of axons and glia, recovery of function and structural repair, post-inflammatory gliosis, and neurodegeneration. The sequential involvement of these processes influences the clinical course characterized by relapses with recovery, relapses leaving persistent deficits, and secondary progression that causes fixed physical and cognitive disability [1].

MS is among the commonest causes of neurological disability in young people and it has an annual incidence ranging from 2 to 10 cases/100,000 persons/year; a north–south gradient was found, lower incidence being closer to equator. Its clinical manifestations typically occur between 20 and 40 years of age with symptoms and signs involving different CNS regions (optic nerve; brainstem; cerebellum; cerebral hemispheres; spinal cord) [1].

Optic neuritis (ON) is a common first symptom of MS (20%) but ON remains isolated in perhaps 50% of cases. Symptoms may include pain in or around the eye, abnormal visual acuity and fields, reduced colour vision, a relative afferent pupillary defect, and abnormal visual evoked potentials. Many years may elapse between first and second attacks, and not all patients who experience a first attack develop MS. A prospective cohort study of patients with ON followed for up to 31 years found that the 15-year risk of MS was 40% (95% CI 31–52%). Most cases (60%) occurred within 3 years [2]. Another study of patients with ON found that by 10 years 38% (95% CI 33–43%) had developed MS; of these 50% had received their diagnosis within 3 years and 72% within 5 years [3]. In another study of patients presenting with clinically isolated syndromes (CISs) (optic, spinal cord, or brain symptoms) 68% of patients had developed MS by 14 years, the proportions being similar for the different presenting symptoms but half of the original patients had been lost to follow-up, a fact not mentioned in the published article [4].

The diagnosis of MS is made clinically when a patient has experienced two attacks of neurological dysfunction lasting more than 24 h, occurring at different points in time and affecting different parts of the central nervous system (the Poser criteria) [5]. MRI (magnetic resonance imaging) may help in earlier diagnosis by visualizing lesions in the brain that are clinically silent. The McDonald criteria for the diagnosis of MS, published in 2001, encourage a diagnosis of MS to be made following one first clinical attack if the patient also meets criteria for a positive MRI scan although the value of doing this is not universally seen [6].

Expanded disability status scale (EDSS) is the most widely used disability measure in clinical trials of MS. It is based on the results of a neurological examination and the patient's ability to walk. Scores range from 0 (normal), 3 (mild disability), 6 (cane requirement), 7 (wheelchair use), to 10 (death from MS) [7].

MRI measurement has been accepted as an outcome measure for clinical trials and treatment decisions in MS. However, MRI measures are weakly correlated with disability and their long-term predictive value is unknown. Thus, no MRI measure is close to satisfying the Prentiss criteria for surrogate marker validation. Studies to evaluate MRI measures as independent predictors of long-term outcome are lacking and are urgently needed [8]. Therefore, in this chapter, we consider only clinical outcome for the evaluation of treatment efficacy, in accordance with the Cochrane MS Group who stated that in MS trials the primary outcome must be a clinical measure.

MS has a chronic course evolving over 30–40 years. The clinical phenotypes include relapsing-remitting MS (RRMS), secondary-progressive MS (SPMS), primary progressive MS (PPMS), progressive-relapsing MS (PRMS) [9]. Patients remaining fully ambulatory (EDSS score ≤ 3.0) 20 years from onset, without any treatment, accounted for 17% of all patients or 30% of those with RRMS [10,11]. The development of SPMS is by far the major route to permanent long-term disability and it supervenes in about 80% of relapsing-remitting patients by 20–25 years. After 15–18 years, about 50% of patients need assistance to walk, are confined to wheelchair, bed, or have died [12–14]. The criterion for progressive disease is continuing deterioration of disability, without substantial remission or exacerbation, and requires an elapsed year for confirmation in order to avoid spontaneous reversion [12–14]. PPMS (approximately 10% of all patients with MS) is characterized since the beginning by a slow worsening of neurological deficits without experiencing attacks, and PRMS by a progressive course from onset with relapses and continuing progression [9]. The possibility that the incidence and prevalence of MS is changing could require a reworking of outcome expectations from natural history.

Natural history studies provide little support for the concept that progression in MS is related primarily to a succession of relapses, indicating that relapses play no role in longer-term outcome in the following context: (i) no increased rate of progression in patients with primary progressive disease and subsequent relapses; (ii) no increased rate of progression in those with progressive-relapsing MS compared to SPMS; (iii) no increase in progression rates among individuals with single exacerbations and subsequent progression compared to other forms of progression; (iv) no relationship between relapse frequency and long-term outcome [13,14].

Framing clinical questions

Systematic reviews on efficacy and adverse effects of interventions are set up to inform decisions about using or selecting treatments. These decisions are about questions such as, in ON, Does corticosteroid therapy reduce the risk of development of MS? Does treatment of relapses with corticosteroids improve the speed of recovery? Does early treatment with interferon therapy delay or prevent the development of clinically definite MS in patients with a first isolated neurological event? Are interferons superior to other immunomodulatory or immunosuppressive drugs in the prevention of relapses in RRMS? Are immunomodulatory or immunosuppressive medications effective in slowing down at long-term progression of disability?

Well-formulated questions lead to clear decisions about what research to include and how to summarize it.

The Cochrane Collaboration methodology (www. cochrane. org) was applied to all of the reviews for MS that are reported in this chapter. Randomized, placebo-controlled trials that compared active treatment with placebo in patients diagnosed with MS (RRMS, SPMS, PPMS, PRMS) according to accepted criteria were searched [9]. Trials in which the comparisons of interest were confounded by other active treatments were excluded.

General approach to search evidence

The search strategy for trials included the Cochrane controlled trials register, MEDLINE (1966–2005), and EMBASE (1988–2005), and hand-searched references in identified trials and symposia reports (1990–2005) from the major neurological and MS associations. Trials' investigators and sponsor companies were contacted in order to identify any unpublished trials or data missing from articles.

Critical review of the evidence for each question

1. Corticosteroids for ON

In ON, does corticosteroid therapy (1) improve or accelerate recovery of visual function? (2) reduce the risk of development of MS?

The available evidence on the role of steroids in ON include one clinical practice guideline produced by the Quality standards subcommittee of the American Academy of Neurology [15], and a systematic review of three randomized controlled trials, including 566 patients [16] (Table 21.1).

In the guideline, no attempt was made at combining data to determine the effect of steroid therapy on visual recovery, recurrence of ON or development of MS.

The bulk of data regarding steroids in ON comes from the ONTT (Optic Neuritis Treatment Trial), a randomized controlled trial in which 457 patients with acute ON, age 18 to 46 years, received either intravenous methylprednisolone (IV MP) ($n = 151$) or prednisone per os ($n = 156$) or placebo ($n = 150$) within 8 days of symptoms onset. Outcomes were: (i) number of patients with complete recovery of visual acuity at 8 days, 30 days and at longer follow-up (6–36 months), (ii) number of patients with relapse (recurrence of ON or clinically definite MS) at 2 and 5 years.

High-doses (500 mg or more daily) IV MP for several days followed by a taper, or ACTH, accelerated recovery of visual acuity at 1 month with a 9% (95% confidence interval (CI) 3–15%) absolute risk reduction (ARR) of patients who did not improve, but this effect was no longer significant at 6 months follow-up. Oral prednisone in doses of 1 mg/kg/day had no effect in the recovery of visual function. High-doses IV MP therapy reduced the risk of relapse recurrence at 2 years (7%, 1–14%); however, this effect could not be shown to persist at 5 years follow-up.

A few major and minor side effects were reported by the included trials, but the data available did not allow pooled analysis. Major side effects in patients treated with high-doses IV MP were severe depression, acute pancreatitis and maculopapular eruption (rate 1–7%); minor side effects in patients treated with high- or low-doses of IV MP or oral prednisone were weight gain, moon facies, ankle oedema, acne, sleep disturbance, mood change, facial flushing.

Given the lack of evidence of long-term efficacy for steroid therapy for ON, factors such as patient preference, severity of initial symptoms and adverse effects of therapy must be considered in treatment decisions [15,16].

Table 21.1 Steroid treatment for optic neuritis (systematic review of RCTs [16]).

Intervention (dosage)	Outcome (follow-up time)	Number of patients (number of trials)	Control group risk (range)	Relative risk (95% CI)	Absolute risk reduction (95% CI)	Comments
Steroids – IV MP 1000 mg/day for 3 days then tapering dose – Oral prednisone alone 1 mg/kg/day for 14 days then tapering dose – ACTH for 30 days versus Placebo	Visual acuity unimproved (30 days)	566 (3)	74% (43–83%)	0.89 (0.82–0.96)	9% (3–15)	Steroid therapy accelerated recovery of visual acuity at 1 month (NNT = 11). In the ONTT study treatment allocation was not blinded in patients randomized to treatment with IV MP. Heterogeneity between trials.
	Visual acuity unimproved (6–36 months)	566 (3)	36% (11–43%)	0.98 (ns)	1% (ns)	The effect of steroid therapy was no longer significant at 6 months or longer follow-up. Heterogeneity between trials.
	Relapse recurrence (2 years)	457 (1)	14%	0.67 (ns)	5% (ns)	
	Clinical definite MS (5 years)	388 (1)	25%	0.92 (ns)	2% (ns)	This outcome was reported by the ONTT study.
High dose ≥500 mg IV MP/day (or equivalent dose)	Relapse recurrence (2 years)	301 (1)	14%	0.47 (0.23–0.97)	7% (1–14)	High-dose MP therapy reduced the risk of relapse recurrence at 2 years (NNT = 14).
Low dose <500 mg MP/day (or equivalent dose)	Relapse recurrence (2 years)	306 (1)	14%	0.87 (ns)	2% (ns)	Low dose of steroid therapy was no effective.
High dose ≥500 mg IV MP/day (or equivalent dose)	Clinical definite MS (5 years)	259 (1)	25%	0.83 (ns)	4% (ns)	Both high- and low-doses IV MP therapy did not reduce the risk of development of MS at 5 years.
Low dose <500 mg MP/day (or equivalent dose)	Clinical definite MS (5 years)	255 (1)	25%	1.01 (ns)	0%	

The equivalence between methylprednisolone and prednisone or ACTH was calculated considering 100 mg intravenous methylprednisolone (IV MP) equivalent to 80 mg oral prednisone and to 16 ACTH units. MP: methylprednisolone; ACTH: adrenocorticotropic hormone; NNT: number needed to treat; ns: not statistically significant.

2. Corticosteroids for MS

Does treatment of MS relapses with corticosteroids: (1) Improve the speed of recovery? (2) Influence long-term recovery? (3) Prevent subsequent relapses?

One North American [17] and two European guidelines [18,19] and two systematic reviews are available [16,20]. Six randomized, placebo-controlled clinical trials contributed to the Cochrane Review (Table 21.2) in which 377 participants (199 treatment, 178 placebo) had been randomized [20]. The drugs analysed were IV MP (three trials, 89 participants), oral MP (one trial, 51 participants) and ACTH (two trials, 237 participants).

Overall, IV or oral MP or ACTH showed a protective effect against disability getting worse or unimproved within the first 5 weeks of treatment (ARR 25%; 95% CI 14–35%) with some but non-significant greater effect for IV MP (1 g/day, over 5 days). Long-term efficacy data on disability were available from only one trial (51 patients in the oral MP study). The treatment effect was significant at 8 weeks, but only borderline significant effect was observed at 1 year in this study.

One small study reported disability data and recurrence of relapses at 1 year of follow-up, showing no effect of oral MP (500 mg/day for 5 days followed by a tapering for 10 further days) on these long-term outcome [20].

Short (3 days) or long (15 days) duration of treatment with MP did not show any significant difference.

Although MP may be administered orally (avoiding the need for hospital-based care), the side-effect profile of IV MP was better, with less gastrointestinal and psychiatric disorders compared to the oral formulation (Table 21.4) [20].

The optimal dosage, the specific corticosteroid to be used, and whether to use a taper after initial pulse therapy, have not been directly compared in randomized controlled trials. There is insufficient data to clearly define patient subgroups who are more likely to respond to MP treatment [19,20].

Short-term, high-dose IV MP treatment should be considered for the treatment of relapses of MS. The optimal glucocorticoid treatment regimen, in terms of clinical efficacy and adverse events, remains to be established. There is a need for further randomized controlled trials to address the question of the appropriate regimen and whether intermittent steroid therapy can alter the natural history of MS [16–20].

3. Interferon for CISs

Does early treatment with interferon therapy delay or prevent the development of clinically definite MS in patients with a first isolated neurological event?

Interferon beta-1a has been approved for individuals with first CISs who are at relatively high risk to 'convert to MS.' The Therapeutics and Technology Assessment Subcommittee of the American Academy of Neurology and the MS Council for Clinical Practice Guidelines suggested 'it is appropriate to consider' treatment with approved therapies in these patients [17].

Table 21.2 Corticosteroids or ACTH for relapse treatment (systematic review of RCTs [20]).

Intervention (dosage)	Outcome (follow-up time)	Number of patients (number of trials)	Control group risk (range)	Relative risk (95% CI)	Absolute risk reduction (95% CI)	Comments
Steroid – MP (500–1000 mg/day for 3–5 days) – ACTH (40–60 UI per dose twice/day for 7 days) versus Placebo	Unimproved or worsened* (5 week)	330 (5)	61% (52–78%)	0.59 (0.47–0.75)	25% (14–35)	Steroid better No heterogeneity between trials.
	Unimproved or worsened* (8 weeks)	51 (1)	68%	0.51 (0.28–0.92)	33% (8–59)	Steroid better One study of small sample size with oral MP 500 mg.
	Unimproved or worsened* (1 year)	49 (1)	78%	0.64 (0.41–0.99)	28% (3–54)	Steroid better One study of small sample size with oral MP 500 mg; two control patients lost to follow-up.
	Recurrence of relapses (1 year)	51 (1)	52%	1.26 (ns)	13% (ns)	One study of small sample size with oral MP 500 mg.

ns: not statistically significant. *Least 1 point at Kurtzke's EDSS or DSS score.

Systematic reviews helpful to answer the question are not available. Two clinical trials demonstrated that treatment with interferon beta-1a reduced the likelihood of conversion to clinically definite MS within 2 years of a CIS [21,22]. However, there is no evidence that delaying the second attack by 6 months has any long-term effect on disability. Additionally, more than half of placebo-treated patients in both studies did not have a second attack during the 2- to 3-year follow-up, and those who did convert to clinically definite MS usually did so during the first year, suggesting that a brief period of observation could adequately identify the group in most need of treatment. The incomplete benefit from early interferon treatment is shown by the finding that approximately 50% of interferon beta-1a-treated patients still demonstrated clinical or MRI evidence of active disease during the initial 18 months of treatment in one trial [23]. Furthermore the delay to next attack (in IFN study) was no longer than it was in the ONTT methylprednisolone arm.

4. Immunotherapy for relapses prevention

What is the efficacy and safety of interferons in the prevention of relapses in RRMS? Are interferons superior to other immunomodulatory or immunosuppressive drugs?

Of the treatments aimed at prevention of relapses there is regulatory approval for type-1 interferons, and glatiramer acetate. These drugs are recommended as the first-line treatment of MS in North American and European guidelines [17,18,24]. Mitoxantrone has been approved by the United States Food and Drug Administration (FDA) for the treatment of progressive MS, under the indication 'for reducing neurological disability and/or the frequency of clinical relapses in patients with SPMS, PRMS, or worsening RRMS (i.e. patients whose neurologic status is significantly abnormal between relapses)'.

Interferon

The efficacy of type-1 interferons has been evaluated in one Cochrane Review including five randomized, placebo-controlled trials of either interferon beta-1b (two trials), or interferon beta-1a (three trials) involving 1.130 patients [25] (Table 21.3). Interferon beta especially at higher doses reduced the number of patients who had relapses during the first year of treatment. The absolute risk reduction was 22% (95% CI 3–41%). At 2 years' follow-up data were not robust and were difficult to interpret because of the many dropouts. In one trial, only 57% of enrolled patients were followed up for 24 months or more. Although the number of patients who had exacerbations during the first 2 years fell significantly in the protocol analysis (ARR 14%; 95% CI 8–19%), results were inconclusive after sensitivity analyses.

A flu-like reaction was very common in treated patients, and injection-site reactions were common in those who received interferon subcutaneously. Patients treated with interferon beta had higher frequencies of leucopenia, lymphocytopenia, thrombocytopenia, and raised liver enzymes in blood than controls. The side effects were transient and self-limiting (Table 21.4).

Glatiramer acetate

The efficacy of glatiramer acetate has been assessed in two systematic reviews that did not provide the same results [26,27]. Main differences between the two reviews were inclusion criteria, data extraction and analysis. Patients enrolled in the included trials were not homogeneous in their risk profile. The Cochrane Review took heterogeneity across studies into account and when pooled estimates of treatment effect were adjusted for heterogeneity, no significant statistical difference was found between relapse rates for patients taking glatiramer acetate compared with those taking placebo up to 2 years [27] (Table 21.3). Up to 35 months, the relative risk of at least one clinical relapse was not significantly decreased with glatiramer acetate; the results of a small pilot trial were an exception.

Glatiramer seemed to be a safe drug. The incidence of reported adverse events was not consistent with major toxicity. However, a transient and self-limiting patterned reaction of flushing, chest tightness, sweating, palpitations, and anxiety associated with glatiramer acetate dosage was common, as well as local injection-site reactions (e.g. itching, swelling, erythema, or pain) (Table 21.4).

Azathioprine

Azathioprine has probably been the drug most frequently used for chronic immunosuppressive treatment, since the early 1960s, but it has not been approved for MS treatment. Five clinical trials, recent metanalyses and an ongoing Cochrane Review indicated that the efficacy of azathioprine compared to placebo in the prevention of relapses in RRMS and SPMS during the first 2 years of treatment was equivalent by indirect comparisons to that of interferons [28–30] (Tables 21.3 and 21.4). This result was mainly driven by a major study [31], which accounted for 60% of all patients included in the reviews, but all the trials met good quality criteria and there was not heterogeneity between them.

Adverse events were observed mainly at the beginning of the evaluation period and consisted in gastric intolerance, in particular vomiting often leading to discontinuation of therapy, haematological and liver abnormalities more frequent in treated than in control patients usually not requiring stopping therapy. Frequency of infections was not significantly different in treated and controls (Table 21.4). In the longer term there is a risk of malignancy occurring once/1000 patient years attributable to the drug.

Mitoxantrone

Available evidence on treatment with mitoxantrone includes a clinical practice guideline produced by Therapeutics and

Table 21.3 Immunotherapy to prevent relapses or disability progression for MS patients.

Intervention	Type of patients	Outcome (follow-up time)	Number of patients (number of trials)	Control group risk (range)	Relative risk (95% CI) Analysis per protocol	Absolute risk reduction (95% CI) Analysis per protocol	Comments
Interferon beta (IFN) (SR) [25]	RR	Recurrence of relapses (1 year)**	582 (3)	73% (57–78%)	0.78 (ns)	22% (3–41)	Heterogeneity between the trials. The results were inconclusive after sensitivity analyses.
– IFN-1b 8.0 MIU sc every other day for 2 years		Recurrence of relapses (2 years)***	919 (3)	69% (45–84%)	0.80 (0.73–0.88)	14% (8–19)	
– IFN-1b 16.0 MIU sc 3 times week for 3 years		Progression of disability (2 years)***	919 (3)	29% (20–36%)	0.69 (0.55–0.87)	9% (3–14)	
– IFN-1a 6.0 MIU im weekly for 104 weeks							
– IFN-1a 12.0 MIU sc 3 times week for 2 years							
– IFN-1a 12.0 MIU sc once a week for 48 weeks							
versus Placebo							
Glatiramer acetate (SR) [27]	RR	Recurrence of relapses (1 year)	289 (2)	54% (51–68%)	0.64 (ns)	21% (ns)	Heterogeneity between the trials. When pooled estimates were adjusted for heterogeneity, there was no statistical significant difference.
– 20 mg sc daily for 9 to 35 months	CP						
– 30 mg sc twice daily for 24 months		Recurrence of relapses (2 years)	301 (2)	72% (68–73%)	0.84 (ns)	11% (ns)	
versus Placebo		Progression of disability (2 years)	407 (3)	27% (25–44%)	0.75 (ns)	7% (ns)	No better than placebo in preventing clinical progression at 2 years. No heterogeneity between the trials.

Treatment	MS type	Outcome	n (trials)	Event rate (95% CI)	RR (95% CI)	RRR (95% CI)	Comments
Azathioprine (6 RCTs) [28–31] 2.0–4.4 mg/kg/day for 2–3 years versus control	RR, SP, and PP	Recurrence of relapse (1 year)	543 (5)	54% (32–68%)	0.78 (0.66–0.93)	12% (14–20)	One study [31] accounted for 60% of all patients.
		Recurrence of relapses (2 years)	532 (5)	69% (42–80%)	0.77 (0.67–0.88)	16% (8–24)	No heterogeneity between the trials. The sensitivity analysis (worst-case scenario) confirmed a treatment effect at 1 and 2 years.
		Recurrence of relapses (3 years)	416 (3)	80% (68–89%)	0.83 (0.74–0.93)	14% (5–22)	
		Progression of disability (2 years)	87 (2)	40% (32–50%)	0.56 (ns)	17% (ns)	Two trials of small sample sizes reported this outcome.
		Progression of disability (3 years)	87 (2)	60% (46–79%)	0.60 (0.37–0.97)	23% (3–43)	
Mitoxantrone (SR) [33] – 8–12 mg/m² every month for 6–12 months – 12 mg/m² every 3 months for 2–3 years versus Placebo	RR, PR, and SP	Recurrence of relapses (1 year)	93 (2)	71% (67–75%)	0.44 (0.28–0.70)	40% (22–59)	Heterogeneity between the trials. One study [34] accounted for 71% of all patients. In this study, 26% of participants dropped out. Blindness not assessed completely.
		Recurrence of relapses (2 years)	179 (2)	68% (65–79%)	0.61 (0.41–0.91)	29% (6–52)	
		Progression of disability (2 years)	179 (2)	24% (18–37%)	0.28 (0.12–0.65)	17% (7–27)	

RR: relapsing-remitting MS; CP: chronic-progressive MS; SP: secondary progressive MS; PP: primary progressive MS; PR: relapsing-progressive MS; ITT: intention to treat analysis; ns: not statistically significant.

*Protocol analysis.

**Sufficient data were available from three trials (Knobler 1993, the PRISMS 1998 and the OWIMS 1999) to estimate the RRR of recurrence of relapses during the 1st year of treatment.

***Data from three trials (IFNB MS Group 1993, The MSCRG 1996, and the PRISMS 1998) were available to calculate the number of patients who continued to have relapses or progressed during the first 2 years of treatment.

A sustained (3 or 6 months) increase in EDSS of at least one point recorded in a period when the patient had no exacerbation.

Table 21.4 Adverse effects of immunotherapy treatments for MS (Cochrane Systematic Reviews) [20,25,27,30,33].

Adverse effects[*]	Number of participants (number of trials)	Control group risk (Range)	Protocol analysis. Relative risk increase (95% CI)	Comments
Steroids OR ACTH at 5 weeks				
ACTH:				
– Psychic disorders	197 (1)	1%	1.83 (ns)	Adverse events were not reported in all trials included in the Cochrane Reviews.
– Gastrointestinal bleeding	197 (1)	3%	0.33 (ns)	Design to monitor the adverse effects of the treatment, definitions of reported adverse effects and how were data collected were not specified for most of the studies.
IV MP:				
– Psychic disorders	43 (2)	21%	1.06 (ns)	
– Gastrointestinal bleeding	94 (3)	0	not estimable	
Oral MP:				
– Psychic disorders	51 (1)	4%	5.77 (ns)	
Interferon beta (IFN) at 2 years				
Major adverse effects[**]	919 (3)	3% (1–6%)	2.60 (1.37–4.93)	Information on clinical adverse vents and haematological toxic effects was reported for all trials. However, neither the definitions nor methods of quantification were specified for most of the studies.
Injection-site reactions	816 (3)	14% (6–22%)	4.52 (3.54–5.78)	
Flu-like symptoms	1199 (6)	14% (3–34%)	2.01 (1.60–2.52)	
Myalgias/arthralgias	1199 (6)	13% (0–24%)	1.93 (1.51–2.45)	
Fatigue	952 (5)	12% (5–25%)	1.37 (1.01–1.88)	
Headache	952 (5)	45% (12–57%)	1.16 (1.02–1.33)	
Increased AST	919 (3)	1% (0–3%)	2.72 (1.17–6.27)	
Increased ALT	919 (3)	2% (0–6%)	3.59 (2.09–6.18)	
Leucopenia	1004 (5)	0.5% (0–1.5%)	5.55 (2.68–11.46)	
Lymphopenia	618 (2)	14% (4–29%)	2.45 (1.61–3.72)	
Decreased haemoglobin values	383 (3)	1% (0–1%)	2.92 (ns)	
Thrombocytopenia	383 (3)	0.5% (0–3%)	5.87 (1.34–25.61)	

Intervention / Adverse effect	Patients (studies)	% (range)	Value (95% CI or ns)
Glatiramer acetate at 2 years			
Major adverse effects**	538 (3)	1% (0–1%)	2.97 (ns)
Itching	407 (3)	9% (4–20%)	5.17 (3.31–8.08)
Swelling	407 (3)	13% (8–24%)	3.69 (2.56–5.32)
Pain	646 (4)	24% (0–47%)	1.87 (1.54–2.27)
Patterned reactions	646 (4)	7% (0–13%)	3.40 (2.22–5.21)
Azathioprine at 3 years			
Major adverse effects**	87 (2)	8% (0–14%)	3.17 (2.37–7.23)
Gastrointestinal	688 (5)	0.6% (0–1%)	7.26 (2.50–21.12)
Allergic reactions	604 (3)	0	5.43 (ns)
Leucopenia	742 (6)	0	7.55 (1.34–42.51)
Increased AST/ALT	742 (6)	0	6.18 (ns)
Mitoxantrone			
Major adverse effects**	177 (2)	3.5% (3–5%)	2.93 (ns)
Cardiotoxicity (LVEF reduction below 50%)	268 (4)	0	5.72 (ns)
Urinary tract infections	268 (4)	11% (0–24%)	2.81 (1.43–5.53)
Respiratory tract infections	268 (4)	30% (0–51%)	1.33 (0.76–2.33)
Persistent amenorrea	152 (4)	0	8.27 (1.02–67.18)
Nausea/vomiting	268 (4)	15% (0–33%)	13.54 (6.81–26.93)
Alopecia	268 (4)	19% (0–31%)	4.42 (2.45–7.99)
Increased AST/ALT	268 (4)	1.5% (0–3%)	5.26 (1.09–25.44)
Leucopenia	268 (4)	0	17.95 (2.35–137.00)
Anaemia	168 (2)	2% (0–5%)	4.51 (ns)

Glatiramer acetate at 2 years

The number of patients experiencing adverse events of treatment have been counted, by event, in all studies. However, information on how many patients reported at least one adverse event whatsoever was unavailable, so that the overall incidence of adverse events could not be calculated.

The number of patients who dropped out because of adverse effects could be extracted from three studies.

Azathioprine at 3 years

Design to monitor the adverse effects of the treatment, definitions of reported adverse effects and how were data collected were not specified for most of the studies.

Information on how many patients reported at least one adverse event whatsoever was unavailable, so that the overall incidence of side effects could not be calculated.

Mitoxantrone

Design to monitor the adverse effects of the treatment, definitions of reported adverse effects and how were data collected were not specified for most of the studies.

The time of appearance of the adverse event, whether early in the course of therapy or late, was not reported in any of the studies, as well as the time of withdrawn due to the occurrence of adverse events.

The occurrence of an adverse event was reported when present at least once, irrespective of how many times it appeared.

Echocardiography was performed at the baseline and the end of the study [35], at baseline, 6 and 12 months [36], at baseline, and every 6 months [37], before treatment and once a year [34].

Mitoxantrone was interrupted if LVEF decreased of more than 10% from baseline or below 50% [34,37].

A LVEF reduction lower than 50% was observed in 5/138 (3.6%) of treated participants, determining a discontinuation of therapy in 3 of them.

*Adverse effect: an adverse event for which the causal relation between the drug/intervention and the event is at least a reasonable possibility. This term applies to all interventions.

**Patients withdrawn from the study because of major adverse effects of the drug.

Technology Assessment Subcommittee of the American Academy of Neurology and one Cochrane Systematic Review [32,33]. The guideline recommended 'on the basis of several consistent Class II and III studies, mitoxantrone probably reduces the clinical attack rate in patients with relapsing MS. The potential toxicity of mitoxantrone, however, considerably limits its use in patients with relapsing forms of MS' [32]. The Cochrane Review included four randomized, placebo-controlled trials [33] (Table 21.3). The results confirmed a role of mitoxantrone in reduction of proportion of patients who had relapse at 1 (ARR 40%; 95% CI 22–59%) and 2 years (ARR 29%; 95% CI 6–52%) of treatment for RRMS and SPMS.

The frequency of major adverse effects was not significantly different between mitoxantrone and placebo group; however, rare adverse events are unlikely to be observed in clinical trials of short follow-up period. Urinary tract infections, persistent amenorrea, nausea/vomiting, alopecia, haematological and liver abnormalities were significantly more frequent in treated than in control patients. Moreover, given the increased reports in the literature of cardiotoxicity and therapy-related leukaemias events in patients treated with mitoxantrone, the Cochrane Reviewers recommended that the drug should be limited to treat patients with worsening of disability and who do not respond to other treatments (Table 21.4) and who are prepared to accept the risks.

Immunoglobulins

Efficacy of immunoglobulins in MS has been summarized recently in a guideline produced by the Association of British Neurologists [35] and in one Cochrane Review that included two randomized placebo-controlled trials [36]. The authors of both articles concluded that evidence for this treatment in MS is insufficient to warrant its use without clinical trials.

Each trial included in the review found that there were clear differences in the proportions of patients remaining relapse free on intravenous immunoglobulins. In the larger study 53% (40/75) of immunoglobulin recipients remained relapse free during the 2-year study period. In the other included trial, six participants remained relapse free – all were in receipt of intravenous immunoglobulin. Each trial observed an increase in time to first relapse: mean time to first relapse 237 days (range 4 to 659 days) on intravenous immunoglobulins compared to 151 days (range 2 to 719 days on placebo) and median time to first relapse 233 days on intravenous immunoglobulins compared to 82 days on placebo.

Immunoglobulins were well tolerated with a less than 5% risk of adverse effects in participants in included trials. Depression and skin reactions were the principal reasons leading to withdrawal.

In conclusion, of currently available approved treatments, type-1 interferons offer a mild short-term benefit in individuals with active relapsing disease who are most likely to respond; however, long-term efficacy on prevention of relapses is unproven. The evidence supporting the use of glatiramer acetate in patients with MS is modest and there is no consensus. Indirect comparisons indicate that the efficacy of azathioprine on the relapse rate is equivalent to that of interferons. Therefore new trials directly comparing the efficacy of azathioprine with that of interferons are being planned and executed.

5. Immunotherapy for disability progression

Are immunomodulatory or immunosuppressive medications effective in slowing down at long-term progression of disability?

Interferon

Delaying of disability progression is the most important goal of treatment for MS patients. Available evidence on the effect of interferon beta in slowing down progression of disability include guidelines [17,18,24], one Cochrane Review for RRMS [25] and five clinical trials for SPMS [40–44].

From the available data of three trials, the authors of the Cochrane Review calculated a ARR of RRMS patients who progressed in 2 years (ARR 9%; 95% CI 3–14%) [25] (Table 21.3). However, when patients excluded from the trials (overall 20% patients had been excluded after randomization or were lost to follow-up) were re-analysed by sensitivity analysis, statistical significance was lost. Furthermore, the significance of progression of disability in these three short-term clinical trials of RRMS was uncertain, in particular whether it was associated with development of SPMS, the main prognostic determinant in MS. It has been reported that 47% of patients in the placebo group with at least 2 years of follow-up originally considered treatment failures were in fact transient treatment failures, likely a relapse-related phenomenon [45]. All extended trials' observations beyond 2 years were open, hampering an evaluation of long-term effect of interferons in delaying progression of RRMS patients. There are concerns about the validity of the short-term disability measures used in trials as surrogates for long-term unremitting disability.

The American Academy of Neurology practice parameter recommends considering interferons beta in SPMS if the patient is still experiencing relapses, but regards its effectiveness in patients with SPMS without relapses as uncertain [17]. Five randomized, double blind, placebo-controlled trials studied the effect of interferons beta on progression of disability and number of relapses in SPMS [40–44]. The European trial, which included 718 patients treated with either interferon beta-1b or placebo for 3 years, demonstrated a reduction in the proportion of patients who progressed ⩾1 EDSS point at 2 years (−22%) [40]. The other trials with interferon beta-1b in North America [41] or interferon beta-1a [42–44] failed to confirm this. A major factor contributing to the different results may be the higher frequency of relapses studied in the European trial compared with subsequent studies, suggesting that the effect of interferon was limited to the relapsing phase of the illness.

Glatiramer acetate

Glatiramer acetate was no better than placebo in preventing disability progression at 2 years, whatever the disease course, according to the results of the Cochrane Review [27] (Table 21.3). Furthermore, also the trials with glatiramer raised similar concerns with respect to the definition of disability progression as reported for trials with interferons.

Azathioprine

Information on the effect of azathioprine was available from two small trials reporting the proportion of patients whose disability progressed over a 2–3 years period. Their results showed a reduction of the risk of worsening in disability both at 2 and 3 years. The effect was statistically significant at 3 years (ARR 23%; 95% CI 3–43%) [30] (Table 21.3).

Mitoxantrone

The American Academy of Neurology practice parameter suggests a beneficial effect of mitoxantrone on disease progression in patients with MS whose clinical condition is deteriorating. Nevertheless the authors underline that mitoxantrone is of potentially great toxicity and it should be reserved for patients with rapidly advancing disease who have failed other therapies [32]. The Cochrane Review emphasized that only one small randomized placebo-controlled study is available reporting 6 month confirmed disability progression at 2 years in SPMS. The proportion of patients who deteriorated of ⩾1 EDSS point during the first 2 years fell significantly (ARR 17%; 95% CI 7–27%) in the protocol analysis, but the results were inconclusive after sensitivity analysis (Table 21.3). The authors underlined the potential toxicity of this medication [33].

Immunoglobulins

Evidence regarding the effect of immunoglobulins to delay disability progression is lacking in the literature. Neither of the two trials included in the Cochrane Review reported data on sustained disability worsening [39].

In conclusion, evidence supporting benefit of immunomodulatory or immunosuppressive agents in slowing down progression of disability in RRMS and in SPMS remains questionable.

Discussion

New diagnostic criteria allow a diagnosis of MS to be made following one first clinical attack if the patient also meets criteria for a positive MRI scan. Interferon beta-1a has been shown to delay the second attack by 6 months in two clinical trials. Opinions vary about initiation of treatment with interferons in every patients at the first attack [46,47]. We agree with Pittock et al. that not all patients with MS or clinical isolated syndrome should begin treatment at the time of diagnosis [46]. We base this recommendation on the following important lessons provided by natural history studies and clinical trials during the last 15 years: (i) natural history of MS is greatly variable and patients often have a favourable course; therefore treatment should be started after a period of observation; (ii) unremitting disability and conversion to a secondary progressive course are the main outcome against which to test efficacy of treatments; (iii) relationship between relapses frequency and long-term outcome is unproven; (iv) short-term adverse effects of drugs are a concern and their long-term adverse effects are unknown.

The results of all clinical trials on disease-modifying agents approved for treatment of patients with MS are limited to short-term follow-up while their efficacy and safety in longer follow-up are still unknown. Although interferons beta have been licensed in several countries to treat RRMS and PRMS patients, they are only partially effective in the short term, and prevention of relapses and disability in the long term is unproven. Glatiramer acetate seems to have no beneficial effect on disability progression, the main outcome measure in this disease, and it does not substantially affect the risk of clinical relapses over time. Therefore, there is at present insufficient evidence to support its routine use in clinical practice and more data are needed. Effectiveness of azathioprine in the short- and medium-term prevention of relapses seems equivalent to that of interferon beta, but azathioprine has not been approved for MS. Mitoxantrone might be beneficial in reducing disability progression in patients with rapidly advancing disease who have failed other therapies, but its use is hampered by significant great toxicity.

New clinical trials directly comparing the efficacy of different treatment strategies need to be planned. New studies must develop a reliable working definition of progression, concealed assessment methods for patients who have adverse effects associated with treatment, a comprehensive and relevant measure of patient disability over time.

References

1 Compston A, Coles A. Multiple sclerosis. *Lancet* 2002; **359**: 1221–31.

2 Nilsson P, Larsson EM, Maly-Sundgren P, Perfekt R, Sandberg-Wollheim M. Predicting the outcome of optic neuritis: evaluation of risk factors after 30 years of follow-up. *J. Neurol.* 2005; **252**: 396–402.

3 Beck RW, Trobe JD, Moke PS, et al. High- and low-risk profiles for the development of multiple sclerosis within 10 years after optic neuritis: experience of the optic neuritis treatment trial. *Arch. Ophthalmol.* 2003; **121**: 944–9.

4 Brex PA, Ciccarelli O, O'Riordan JI, Sailer M, Thompson AJ, Miller DH. A longitudinal study of abnormalities on MRI and disability from multiple sclerosis. *N. Engl. J. Med.* 2002; **346**: 158–64.

5 Poser CM, Paty DW, Scheinberg L, McDonald WI, Davis FA, Ebers GC, et al. New diagnostic criteria for multiple sclerosis: guidelines for clinical protocol research. *Ann. Neurol.* 1983; **13**: 227–31.

6 McDonald WI, Compston A, Edan G, Goodkin D, Hartung HP, Lublin FD, et al. Recommended diagnostic criteria for multiple sclerosis: guidelines from the international panel on the diagnosis of multiple sclerosis. *Ann. Neurol.* 2001; **50**: 121–7.

7 Kurtzke JF. Rating neurologic impairment in multiple sclerosis: an expanded disability status scale (EDSS). *Neurology* 1983; **33**: 1444–52.

8 Prentice RL. Surrogate endpoints in clinical trials: definition and operational criteria. *Stat. Med.* 1989; **8**: 431–40.

9 Lublin FD, Reingold SC. Defining the clinical course of multiple sclerosis: results of an international survey. National Multiple Sclerosis Society (USA) Advisory Committee on Clinical Trials of New Agents in Multiple Sclerosis. *Neurology* 1996; **46**: 907–11.

10 Pittock SJ, Mayr WT, McClelland RL, Noseworthy JH, Rodriguez M. Clinical implications of benign MS: a 20 year population-based follow up study. *Ann. Neurol.* 2004; **56**: 303–6.

11 Kurtzke JF, Beebe GW, Nagler B, Kurland LT, Auth TL. Studies on the natural history of multiple sclerosis, 8: early prognostic features of the later course of the illness. *J. Chronic. Dis.* 1977; **30**: 819–30.

12 Weinshenker BG, Bass B, Rice GP, Noseworthy J, Carriere W, Baskerville J, Ebers GC. The natural history of multiple sclerosis: a geographically based study. 1. Clinical course and disability. *Brain* 1989; **112**: 133–46.

13 Kremenchutzky M, Cottrell D, Rice G, Hader W, Baskerville J, Koopman W, et al. The natural history of multiple sclerosis: a geographically based study. 7. Progressive-relapsing and relapsing-progressive multiple sclerosis: a re-evaluation. *Brain* 1999; **122**: 1941–50.

14 Kremenchutzky M, Rice GP, Baskerville J, Wingerchuk DM, Ebers GC. The natural history of multiple sclerosis: a geographically based study. 9. Observations on the progressive phase of the disease. *Brain* 2006; **129**: 584–94.

15 Kaufman DI, Trobe JD, Eggenberger ER, Whitaker JN. Practice parameter: The role of corticosteroids in the management of acute monosymptomatic optic neuritis. Report of the Quality Standards Subcommittee of the American Academy of Neurology. *Neurology* 2000; **54**: 2039–44.

16 Brusaferri F, Candelise L. Steroids for multiple sclerosis and optic neuritis: a meta-analysis of randomized controlled clinical trials. *J. Neurol.* 2000; **247**: 435–42.

17 Goodin DS, Frohman EM, Garmany Jr GP, et al. Therapeutics and Technology Assessment Subcommittee of the American Academy of Neurology; MS Council for Clinical Practice Guidelines. Disease modifying therapies in multiple sclerosis: report of the Therapeutics and Technology Assessment Subcommittee of the American Academy of Neurology and the MS Council for Clinical Practice Guidelines. *Neurology* 2002; **58**: 169–78.

18 Multiple Sclerosis Therapy Consensus Group. Escalating immunotherapies of multiple sclerosis. *J. Neurol.* 2004; **251**: 1329–39.

19 Sellebjerg F, Barnes D, Filippini G, Midgard R, Montalban X, Rieckmann P, et al. EFNS Task Force on Treatment of Multiple Sclerosis Relapses. EFNS guideline on treatment of multiple sclerosis relapses: report of an EFNS task force on treatment of multiple sclerosis relapses. *Eur. J. Neurol.* 2005; **12**: 939–46.

20 Filippini G, Brusaferri F, Sibley WA, Citterio A, Ciucci G, Midgard R, Candelise L. Corticosteroids or ACTH for acute exacerbations in multiple sclerosis (Cochrane Review). *The Cochrane Library*, 2003, **2**, Oxford: Update Software: CD001331.

21 Jacobs LD, Beck RW, Simon JH, et al. CHAMPS Study Group. Intramuscular interferon beta-1a therapy initiated during a first demyelinating event in multiple sclerosis. *N. Engl. J. Med.* 2000; **343**: 898–904.

22 Comi G, Filippi M, Barkhof F, et al. Effect of early interferon treatment on conversion to definite multiple sclerosis: a randomized study. *Lancet* 2001; **357**: 1576–82.

23 Beck RW, Chandler DL, Cole SR, et al. Interferon beta-1a for early multiple sclerosis: CHAMPS trial subgroup analyses. *Ann. Neurol.* 2002; **51**: 481–90.

24 Freedman MS, Blumhardt LD, Brochet B, Comi G, Noseworthy JH, Sandberg-Wollheim M, et al. Paris Workshop Group. International consensus statement on the use of disease-modifying agents in multiple sclerosis. *Mult. Scler.* 2002; **8**: 19–23.

25 Filippini G, Munari L, Incorvaia B, Ebers GC, Polman C, D'Amico R, Rice GP. Interferons in relapsing remitting multiple sclerosis: a systematic review. *Lancet* 2003; **361**: 545–52. (Cochrane Review).

26 Martinelli Boneschi F, Rovaris M, Johnson KP, Miller A, Wolinsky JS, Ladkani D, et al. Effects of glatiramer acetate on relapse rate and accumulated disability in multiple sclerosis: meta-analysis of three double-blind, randomized, placebo-controlled clinical trials. *Mult. Scler.* 2003; **9**: 349–55.

27 Munari L, Lovati R, Boiko A. Therapy with glatiramer acetate for multiple sclerosis. (Cochrane Review). *The Cochrane Library*, 2004, 1, Oxford: Update Software: CD004678.

28 Palace J, Rothwell P. New treatments and azathioprine in multiple sclerosis [letter]. *Lancet* 1997; **350**: 261.

29 Sudlow CLM, Counsell CE. Problems with UK government risk sharing scheme for assessing drugs for multiple sclerosis. *BMJ* 2003; **326**: 388–92.

30 Casetta I, Iuliano G. Azathioprine treatment for multiple sclerosis (Protocol). *The Cochrane Database of Sys. Rev.* 2003; 1: CD003982. DOI: 10.1002/14651858.CD003982.

31 British and Dutch Multiple Sclerosis Azathioprine Trial Group. Double-masked trial of azathioprine in multiple sclerosis. *Lancet* 1988; ii: 179–83.

32 Goodin DS, Arnason BG, Coyle PK, Frohman EM, Paty DW. The use of mitoxantrone (Novantrone) for the treatment of multiple sclerosis. Report of the Therapeutics and Technology Assessment Subcommittee of the American Academy of Neurology. *Neurology* 2003; **61**: 1332–8.

33 Martinelli Boneschi F, Rovaris M, Capra R, Comi G. Mitoxantrone for multiple sclerosis. (Cochrane Review). *The Cochrane Library*, 2005; 4, Oxford: Update Software: CD002127.

34 Hartung HP, Gonsette R, Konig N, Kwiecinski H, Guseo A, Morrissey SP, et al. Mitoxantrone in progressive multiple

sclerosis: a placebo-controlled, double-blind, randomised, multi-centre trial. *Lancet* 2002; **360**: 2018–25.

35 Edan G, Miller D, Clanet M, Confavreux C, Lyon-Caen O, Lubetzki C, et al. Therapeutic effect of mitoxantrone combined with methylprednisolone in multiple sclerosis: a randomised multicentre study of active disease using MRI and clinical criteria. *J. Neurol. Neurosurg. Psychiatry* 1997; **62**:112–8.

36 Millefiorini E, Gasperini C, Pozzilli C, D'Andrea F, Bastianello S, Trojano M, et al. Randomized placebo-controlled trial of mitoxantrone in relapsing-remitting multiple sclerosis: 24-month clinical and MRI outcome. *J. Neurol.* 1997; **244**: 153–9.

37 van de Wyngaert FA, Beguin C, D'Hooghe MB, Dooms G, Lissoir F, Carton H, et al. A double-blind clinical trial of mitoxantrone versus methylprednisolone in relapsing, secondary progressive multiple sclerosis. *Acta Neurol Belg.* 2001; **101**: 210–6.

38 Association of British Neurologists. Guidelines for the use of intravenous immunoglobulin in neurological disease. March 2002.

39 Gray O, McDonnell GV, Forbes RB. Intravenous immunoglobulins for multiple sclerosis. *Cochrane Database Syst. Rev.* 2003; 4: CD002936. Review.

40 European Study Group on Interferon β-1b in Secondary Progressive MS. Placebo-controlled multicentre randomised trial of interferon β-1b in treatment of secondary progressive multiple sclerosis. *Lancet* 1998; **352**: 1491–7.

41 The North American Study Group on Interferon beta-1b in Secondary Progressive MS. Interferon beta-1b in secondary progressive MS: results from a 3-year controlled study. *Neurology* 2004; **63**: 1788–95.

42 SPECTRIMS Study Group, Hughes RAC. Randomized controlled trial of interferon beta-1a in secondary progressive MS. Clinical Results. *Neurology* 2001; **56**: 1496–504.

43 Cohen JA, Cutter GR, Fisher JS, Goodman AD, Heidenreich FR, et al. Benefit of IFN beta-1a on MSFC progression in secondary progressive MS. *Neurology* 2002; **59**: 679–86.

44 Andersen O, Elovaara I, Färkkilä M, Hansen HJ, Mellgren SI, Myhr K-M. The Nordic SPMS Study Group. Multicentre, randomised, double blind, placebo controlled, phase III study of weekly, low dose, subcutaneous interferon beta-1a in secondary progressive multiple sclerosis. *J. Neurol. Neurosurg. Psychiatr.* 2004; **75**: 706–10.

45 Liu C, Blumhardt D. Disability outcome measures in therapeutic trials of relapsing-remitting multiple sclerosis: effects of heterogeneity of disease course in placebo cohorts. *J. Neurol. Neurosurg. Psychiatr.* 2000; **68**: 450–7.

46 Pittock SJ, Weinshenker BG, Noseworthy JH, Lucchinetti CF, Keegan M, Wingerchuk DM, et al. Not every patient with multiple sclerosis should be treated at time of diagnosis. *Arch. Neurol.* 2006; **63**: 611–4.

47 Frohman EM, Havrdova E, Lublin F, Barkhof F, Achiron A, Sharief MK, et al. Most patients with multiple sclerosis or a clinically isolated demyelinating syndrome should be treated at the time of diagnosis. *Arch. Neurol.* 2006; **63**: 614–9.

CHAPTER 22

Motor neurone disorders

Douglas Mitchell

Background

Motor neurone diseases (MND) encompass a group of neurodegenerative disorders in which the premature loss of motor neurones (lower and upper) is the essential pathological hallmark. They comprise MND, known as amyotrophic lateral sclerosis (ALS) in North America and many non-English speaking countries, spinal muscular atrophy and the post-polio syndrome. It has additionally been suggested that hereditary spastic paraparesis should be included in this group but this remains a controversial issue.

MND is the commonest of these diseases and has an incidence of 1.5–2.0/100,000 population per year. It is an inexorably progressive disease with a fatal outcome. Over 50% of patients are dead within 3 years of their first symptom. It is characterized by progressive limb paralysis. If not present at the outset, dysphagia and dysarthria develop sooner or later and death occurs due to respiratory failure. MND is arguably one of the most devastating diseases known to medical science. It is generally a disease of the late middle-aged and elderly but can occur in younger age groups. Although most cases of MND are sporadic, familial forms are also important and may give additional insights into potential basic aetiological mechanisms. Between 5% and 10% of MND is familial with up to 20% of familial patients showing mutations in the copper/zinc superoxide dismutase (SOD1) gene. While a host of putative disease modifying therapies have been reported only one, riluzole has so far been licensed. The thrust of the treatment of MND is thus mainly symptomatic and palliative. Other putative disease modifying therapies have included nerve growth factors such as recombinant human insulin-like growth factor 1 (IGF-1), ciliary neurotrophic growth factor (CNTF) and bovine-derived nerve growth factor (BDNF) as well as xaliproden, a drug given orally and thought to enhance nerve growth factor gene expression and ONO2506, a putative astrocyte stabilizing drug. Further potential disease modifying treatments including stem cell therapy are still in their infancy and evidence from randomized clinical trials (RCTs) is not yet available.

Criteria for the diagnosis of MND were initially aimed at providing a tool which could be used to facilitate multicentre international clinical trials and further investigations of familial MND. These were based on the outcome of a Workshop held under the auspices of the World Federation of Neurology

in 1990 and are known as the Escorial Criteria. They were updated following further Workshops at Airlie House in 1994 and 1998 (the 'Revised Criteria for the Diagnosis of Amyotrophic Lateral Sclerosis', www.wfnals.org/guidelines/1998elescorial/elescorial1998). A schema for the use of these criteria is given in Table 22.1 and Figure 22.1.

Framing answerable clinical questions

Major current therapeutic issues in MND can most conveniently be summarized as follows for the purposes of framing the core questions to be addressed in the remainder of this chapter:

1 Do any pharmacological treatments prolong survival in patients with possible or definite MND?

2 How does non-invasive ventilatory support affect probability of survival and quality of life (QoL) in patients with MND? If non-invasive ventilatory support is to be used when is it best to start?

3 How does long-term mechanical ventilation (LTMV) affect survival and QoL in patients with MND with respiratory insufficiency?

4 Does mechanical insufflation–exsufflation (MI-E) alleviate respiratory symptoms in patients with MND who have excessive secretions?

5 How does feeding gastrostomy improve nutritional state and probability of survival in patients with MND with bulbar involvement?

General approach to the search for evidence

High-quality evidence was first sought in the Cochrane Database of Systematic Reviews (CDSR) searching for reviews relating to ALS, MND and motoneurone disease. The Cochrane Central Database of Controlled Trials was also searched for clinical trials relevant to ALS/MND. This was followed by searches on Medline using search strings 'MND' and 'ALS' to identify papers relevant to ALS/MND and 'riluzole', 'IGF-1', 'CNTF', 'BDNF', 'amino acid', 'lamotrigine', 'gabapentin', 'minocycline', 'xaliproden', 'vent*', 'resp*', 'sniff', 'nippv', 'insuffl*', 'exsuffl*', 'cough', 'dysphagia',

Table 22.1 Summary of modified Escorial Criteria (Airlie House Revision) of diagnosis of ALS/MND.

	Category of diagnosis					
	Suspected	Possible	Definite familial, laboratory supported	Probable, laboratory supported	Probable	Definite
Clinical requirements	Lower motor neurone signs only in one or more regions or upper motor neurone signs in one or more regions	Lower + upper motor neurone signs in only one region	Lower + upper motor neurone signs in only one region	Lower + upper motor neurone signs in one region or upper motor neurone signs in one or more regions	Lower + upper motor neurone signs in two regions	Lower + upper motor neurone signs in three regions
Laboratory requirements			Gene identified	Electromyography (EMG) shows acute denervation in two or more limbs		

Adapted from www.wfnals.org/guidelines/1998elescorial/elescorial1998schema.htm.
To make a diagnosis of ALS/MND under any of the above criteria there *must* also be:
1 evidence of progression over time;
2 no objective sensory signs which cannot be explained on the basis of a co-morbidity.

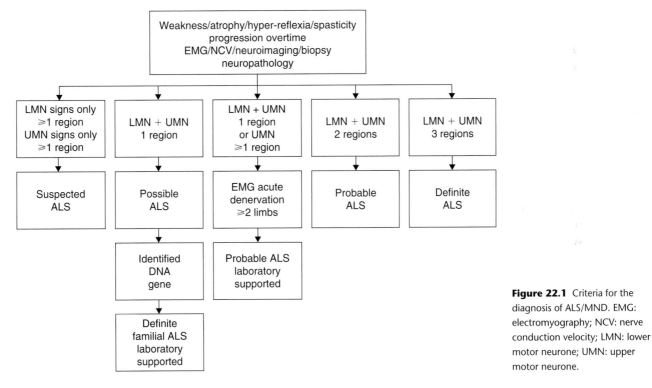

Figure 22.1 Criteria for the diagnosis of ALS/MND. EMG: electromyography; NCV: nerve conduction velocity; LMN: lower motor neurone; UMN: upper motor neurone.

'bulbar', 'peg' and 'gastrost*' to identify papers relevant to the questions asked in this chapter.

Critical review of the evidence for each question

1. Pharmacological treatment

Do any pharmacological treatments prolong survival in patients with possible or definite MND?

A whole host of drugs have been postulated as potential disease modifying therapies in MND. The effectiveness of virtually all these drugs in prolonging survival has not been supported by evidence from RCTs. The glutamate release inhibitor riluzole has however been licensed as a disease modifying treatment in many countries and IGF-1 is undergoing further investigation in North America. The clinical effectiveness of both riluzole and IGF-1 has been examined in Cochrane Systematic Reviews. Cochrane Systematic Reviews have also been undertaken for

Table 22.2 Drugs that could alter the natural history of ALS/MND.

Types of study (reference)	Intervention (dosage)	Outcome (follow-up time)	Number of patients (number of trials)	Control group risk (95% CI)	Relative risk (95% CI)	Absolute risk reduction (95% CI)	Comments
SR [6]	Riluzole (100 mg daily) versus placebo	Death or tracheostomy (12 months)	799 (3)	44% (37–64)	0.78 (0.75–0.92)	10% (3–16)	Riluzole better Heterogeneity between studies
		Nausea	801 (3)	2.2% (1.2–3.4)	1.55 (1.06–2.28)	+5% (1–9)	Riluzole worst Incomplete data
SR [9]	IGF-1 (0.05–0.1 mg/kg/day) versus placebo	Death (12 months)	449 (2)	19% (17–24)	1.11 (1.00–1.23)	+8% (0–16)	IGF-1 worst Methodology of trials unsatisfactory Inconsistent disease progression
		Injection site inflammation	449 (2)	8% (7–10)	3.16 (1.77–5.62)	+17% (11–24)	IGF-1 worst Main adverse effect
SR [10]	CNTF (3.5–90 μg/kg for week) versus placebo	Death (6–9 months)	1300 (2)	25% (17–20)	0.93 (0.71–1.23)	1% (ns)	CNTF better Reactivation of facial herpes as adverse effect
SR [11]	BCAA (valine 6–6.4 g/day, leucine 12 g/day, isoleucine 6–8 g/day) versus control	Death (12 months)	98 (2)	29% (18–31)	1.41 (0.83–2.41)	+12% (ns)	BCAA worst Assessment of outcomes difficult
SR [12]	Antioxidants versus placebo	Death or tracheostomy or ventilatory support (12 months)	426 (3)	31% (34–43)	0.94 (0.83–1.06)	4% (ns)	Antioxidant better Diverse interventions (α-tocopherol, acetylcysteine, L-methionine vitamin E, selenium)

BCAA: branch chain amino acids; SR: systematic review; ns: not statistically significant.

branch-chain amino acids, antioxidants and CNTF. A review of creatine is in progress. Some of the evidence relating to those interventions which have been the subject of Cochrane Systematic Reviews is summarized in Table 22.2.

Riluzole

The first RCT of riluzole demonstrated a modest increase in survival in patients treated with riluzole compared to those given placebo [1]. Many questions were however raised by this study, particularly the apparent disproportionate benefit observed in bulbar as opposed to limb onset patients [2]. A larger dose ranging study also suggested a small prolongation of survival in patients receiving riluzole 100 and 200 mg daily [3]. A third trial in France and Belgium involved patients with advanced MND not included in these studies [4]. This study did not show a significant survival advantage from riluzole. A fourth trial in Japan with multiple outcome measures was also negative [5].

The Cochrane Systematic Review [6] concludes that riluzole 100 mg daily prolongs life by about 2 months in patients with probable and definite MND with symptoms of less than 5 years duration, forced vital capacity (FVC) greater than 60% and age less than 75 years. The most frequent side effects are nausea and asthenia. Alterations of liver function tests sometimes occur and should be monitored with monthly for the first 3 months and 3 monthly thereafter.

IGF-1

RCTs of IGF-1 in MND have so far yielded conflicting results. Two have so far been published. One [7] suggested slowing of progression of functional impairment and QoL, but this was not confirmed in a second, smaller trial [8]. The larger study compared IGF-1 0.05 and 0.1 mg/kg/day with placebo and the smaller IGF-1 0.1 mg/kg/day with placebo. The methodology of both trials was considered unsatisfactory due to a high risk of bias. A substantial number of patients receiving IGF-1 experienced drug-related adverse effects including injection site inflammation which could also have adversely affected blinding. IGF-1 seems otherwise a well-tolerated and safe drug. Its efficacy in MND remains unproven. RCTs to date have been seriously compromised by details of trial design [9]. Maximizing potential efficacy of IGF-1 and other neurotrophins in MND may also depend on effective delivery of the trophin to the site of the pathology. It is possible that such manipulations may be extendable to human studies to achieve an improved treatment effect.

CNTF

A Cochrane Review has also examined the efficacy of CNTF in MND. Two randomized trials were identified including 1300 MND patients treated with CNTF. No significant differences were observed between the CNTF and placebo groups for survival, the primary outcome measure. A significant increase of adverse events occurred in patients given higher doses of CNTF. As with IGF-1, alternative delivery methods might however be usefully evaluated in the future [10].

Amino acids

Amino acid preparations have also been suggested as possible disease modifying treatments for MND. A Cochrane Review addressed the potential efficacy of amino acids in prolonging survival and/or slowing the progression in MND. No benefit could be demonstrated for either branch-chain amino acids or L-threonine in improving survival in MND. There was no evidence of an effect of any of these treatments on muscle strength or disability as measured by functional rating scales [11].

Free radicals

Free radicals and reactive oxygen species have been strongly implicated as potential aetiological vectors in MND. A range of antioxidant medications have been investigated as possible disease modifying treatments. A Cochrane Review (Table 22.1) examined the effects of antioxidant medication in MND. Of 21 studies identified only 8 met the inclusion criteria. There was felt to be insufficient evidence of efficacy of individual antioxidants, or antioxidants in general to justify the use of antioxidant treatment in people with MND. Many were poorly designed, under-powered, of short duration and had low number of participants [12].

BDNF

On the basis that BDNF is a potent survival factor for motor neurones 1135 MND patients were randomized to placebo, 25 or 100 μg/kg BDNF for 9 months. There was no benefit of BDNF treatment for any of the primary end points. Among the 60% of patients with baseline FVC of ≤91% predicted, survival was significantly greater for 100 μg/kg BDNF versus placebo. In the 20% treated with BDNF 100 μg/kg who reported altered bowel function, 9-month survival was significantly better than placebo. Further clinical trials of BDNF using either intrathecal delivery or high-dose subcutaneous administration were suggested [13]. The safety and tolerability of intrathecal BDNF have since been investigated. Twenty-five patients with probable or definite MND received either BDNF (25, 60, 150, 400 or 1000 μg/day) or placebo in a 12-week, randomized, double-blinded, sequential, dose-escalation study. In each dose cohort four patients received BDNF and one received placebo. The majority of patients receiving BDNF reported mild sensory symptoms, including paraesthesiae. Sleep disturbance, dry mouth, agitation and other behavioural

effects were encountered at higher doses (>150 μg/ day). Cerebrospinal fluid (CSF) BDNF levels were directly related to dose. Intrathecal treatment with BDNF in doses of up to 150 μg/day was well tolerated and feasible. The number of patients and study design did not allow conclusions on efficacy to be made [14].

Lamotrigine

The suggestion that glutamate excitotoxicity might be implicated in the pathogenesis of MND lead to a double-blind, placebo-controlled trial of lamotrigine 100 mg/day in which 67 patients were entered. This dose of lamotrigine did not seem to alter the course of MND [15]. A second study examined the effect of lamotrigine 300 mg/day. Thirty patients completed this double-blind, placebo-controlled, crossover study. No effect of lamotrigine on the progression of MND was found [16].

Gabapentin

A randomized, double-blind, placebo-controlled phase II trial was undertaken to evaluate the efficacy of gabapentin 2.4 g/day in slowing the rate of decline of muscle strength in 152 patients with MND. The primary outcome measure was the slope of the arm megascore and the secondary measure FVC. A non-statistically significant trend ($P = 0.057–0.08$) was observed towards slower decline of arm strength in patients taking gabapentin compared with placebo. No effect on FVC was observed [17]. A phase III trial compared gabapentin 3.6 g or placebo daily for 9 months. The mean rate of decline in arm muscle strength was not significantly different between the groups. There was no beneficial effect upon the rate of decline of secondary measures and no symptomatic benefit [18].

Minocycline

A double-blind, randomized, placebo-controlled feasibility trial of minocycline in MND included 19 MND patients who received 200 mg/day or placebo for 6 months. There were no significant differences in adverse events. In a second, 23 MND patients received up to 400 mg/day in an 8-month crossover trial. The mean tolerated dose was 387 mg/day. There was a trend towards more gastrointestinal symptoms ($P = 0.057$), and the urea and liver enzymes became elevated ($P < 0.05$) in the minocycline treated patients. A phase III trial was initiated on the basis of these results [19].

Xaliproden

The safety and functional efficacy of xaliproden was tested in a double-blind, placebo-controlled study which included 54 MND patients treated for up to 32 weeks. The 6-month intent-to-treat analysis showed no statistically significant effect but a trend in favour of 2 mg xaliproden compared to placebo for reduction in the rate of deterioration of FVC, limb functional score and manual muscle testing. These results were thought to suggest a possible disease modifying effect [20]. On the basis of these results two further randomized, double-blind, placebo-controlled, multicentre, multinational studies were undertaken to assess efficacy and safety. Patients were randomly assigned to placebo, 1 or 2 mg xaliproden orally in the first study ($n = 867$ patients); or the same with riluzole 50 mg b.i.d. background therapy in both groups in the second study ($n = 1210$ patients). The two primary endpoints were time to death, tracheostomy or permanent assisted ventilation and time to vital capacity (VC) <50%. Significant results were not obtained in either of these studies [21].

2. Assessment of respiratory function

How does non-invasive ventilatory support affect probability of survival and QoL in patients with MND? If non-invasive ventilatory support is to be used when is it best to start?

The assessment of respiratory function in MND has tended to focus on VC, FVC and forced expiratory volume (FEV1), the usual procedure being to compare readings from individual patients with those predicted for persons of the same age, sex, height and weight. These physiological parameters are thus expressed as percentages of the predicted value (i.e. '% predicted'). More recently novel methods such as sniff pressures have been evaluated.

An early indication that respiratory function monitoring might be valuable in following the course of MND came from a study of 218 patients. Most patients were found to have characteristic abnormalities in pulmonary function, including reduced FVC. FVCs as low as 50% predicted were commonly missed by clinical evaluation [22]. Subsequent experience has confirmed the importance of monitoring respiratory function in the routine care of people with MND and established the vital role of pulmonary function testing in trials of putative disease modifying treatments.

Jackson et al. noted that there was no consensus on the physiological marker of choice to trigger the initiation of non-invasive positive pressure ventilation (NIPPV) in MND. Advice at that time recommended that the decision should be based on FVC. Twenty MND patients with FVC 70–100% predicted were reviewed. Baseline measurements included the ALS functional rating scale-respiratory version (ALSFRS-R), SF-36, FVC%, maximal inspiratory pressure (MIP), maximal expiratory pressure (MEP) and nocturnal oximetry. The patients were randomized to receive NIPPV based on either nocturnal oximetry studies suggesting oxygen desaturation <90% for one cumulative minute ('early intervention') or FVC <50% ('standard of care'). At enrolment, there was no significant correlation between FVC% and the ALSFRS-R, MEP, MIP, or duration of nocturnal desaturation <90%. An increase in the vitality subscale of the SF-36 was demonstrated in 5/6 patients randomized to 'early intervention' with NIPPV. The data indicated that FVC% did not correlate well with respiratory symptoms and suggested that MIP and nocturnal oximetry may be more sensitive measures of early respiratory insufficiency. It was suggested that earlier institution of NIPPV might result in improved QoL [23].

Lyall et al. related physiological measurements to biochemical markers of respiratory failure. Respiratory muscle strength (RMS) was measured in 81 MND patients to evaluate the relationship between RMS and the presence of ventilatory failure, defined as a carbon dioxide tension of 6 kPa or less. Parameters studied included VC, static inspiratory and expiratory mouth pressures (MouthIP, MEP), maximal oesophageal, transdiaphragmatic and nasal sniff (SNP) pressures. No test had significant predictive power for hypercapnia in patients with significant bulbar weakness. It was concluded that in MND patients without significant bulbar involvement, novel tests of RMS have greater predictive power for hypercapnia than conventional tests. In particular, the non-invasive SNP is more sensitive than VC and MouthIP, suggesting that SNP could usefully be included in tests of RMS in MND [24].

The potential utility of SNP in testing RMS in MND was also tested in 16 patients examined monthly over a period of 8–28 months. SNP was recorded in parallel with maximal inspiratory pressure (PI(max)) and maximal expiratory pressure (PE(max)). It was concluded that SNP was the single respiratory test best combining linear decline, sensitivity in mild disease and feasibility of use in advanced disease [25].

Attention has also been drawn to the possible use of respiratory function testing as a predictor of QoL in MND. Most MND patients have evidence of respiratory muscle weakness at diagnosis. Sleep disruption, due to apnoea, hypopnoea, orthopnoea or REM-related desaturation is common. The relative impact of these factors on QoL was studied in 23 people with MND. QoL was assessed using generic and specific instruments, and RMS by measurement of VC, maximum static pressures and SNP. Overall limb and axial muscle strength was estimated using a summated muscle score based on the MRC scale. There were moderate to strong correlations between QoL and all measurements of respiratory muscle function. Multivariate analysis suggested that maximum static inspiratory pressure was the strongest independent predictor of QoL [26].

3. NIPPV

How do we decide when to institute NIPPV?

MND patients with alveolar hypoventilation were reviewed to demonstrate variability in symptoms, physiological status and outcome following the institution of NIPPV. These were 27 consecutive patients who tolerated NIPPV for more than 4 h per 24-h period for more than 2 weeks. All met the El Escorial Criteria for the diagnosis of MND. Spirometry was measured in the sitting and when possible, the supine positions. Resting arterial blood gases were available in 22. Orthopnoea was the most common symptom at the commencement of NIPPV. No correlation existed between age at institution of NIPPV, duration of effective use of NIPPV or VC and duration of effective use of NIPPV. The lack of correlation between VC at the institution of NIPPV and duration of its effectiveness suggest that more sensitive indicators for the onset of alveolar hypoventilation should be defined, particularly since the principal benefit from its use is relief of symptomatic alveolar hypoventilation. No clear guidance was thus given on the optimum timing for the institution of NIPPV [27]. In the absence of clearer pointers attention should be given to the occurrence of orthopnoea in following up patients with MND and the possible need for respiratory support considered when this symptom is reported.

Cognitive dysfunction is present in a proportion of non-demented patients with ALS and respiratory muscle weakness in MND can lead to nocturnal hypoventilation, resulting in sleep disturbance and excessive daytime somnolence. Nocturnal sleep deprivation might contribute to impaired cognitive function. Cognitive function was evaluated in 9 MND patients with sleep disturbance caused by nocturnal hypoventilation (NIPPV group) and 10 similar patients without ventilation problems (control group). The NIPPV group then started nocturnal NIPPV. After about 6 weeks, cognitive function was reassessed. Statistically significant improvement in two of the seven cognitive tests was demonstrated in the NIPPV group, with a trend towards significant improvement in two others. Scores in the control group did not improve significantly. Nocturnal hypoventilation and sleep disturbance may be associated with cognitive dysfunction and this might be helped by NIPPV. These observations have important implications for the investigation of cognitive dysfunction in non-demented patients with MND, and the effect of ventilation on QoL [28].

A further study examined the potential effect of NIPPV on QoL in MND more specifically. QoL was prospectively studied using the SF-36 in 16 ventilated MND patients. NIPPV improved scores in the 'vitality' domain by as much as 25% for up to 15 months. NIPPV was not associated with reduced QoL [29]. Although it is suggested that NIPPV probably improves survival in MND, the magnitude and duration of any improvement in QoL and the optimal criteria for initiating treatment are unclear. QoL was serially evaluated using the SF-36 scale, chronic respiratory disease questionnaire, sleep apnoea QoL index, respiratory function and polysomnography in 22 MND patients. A trial of NIPPV was offered when subjects had orthopnoea, daytime sleepiness, unrefreshing sleep, daytime hypercapnia, nocturnal desaturation or an apnoea–hypopnoea index >10. Of 17 subjects offered NIPPV 15 accepted, and 10 continued treatment subsequently. Outcome was assessed by changes in QoL and NIV (non-invasive ventilation) compliance. Subjects were followed to death or for at least 26 months. QoL domains assessing sleep-related problems and mental health improved. Median survival following successful initiation of NIPPV was 512 days. Survival and duration of improved QoL were strongly related to NIPPV compliance. VC declined more slowly following initiation of NIPPV. Orthopnoea was the

best predictor of benefit from, and compliance with, NIPPV. Moderate or severe bulbar weakness was associated with lower compliance and less improvement in QoL. NIPPV may thus be associated with improved QoL and survival. Subjects with orthopnoea and preserved bulbar function showed the largest benefit [30].

A more recent study by the same group monitored a cohort of 92 patients for orthopnoea, maximum inspiratory pressure <60% predicted or symptomatic hypercapnia. When one of these criteria had been met patients were randomly allocated to NIV or 'standard care' not including NIV. Median survival of the NIV treated patients was 219 days as opposed to 171 days for those given 'standard' care. Primary end points were time to 75% of baseline level for the mental component summary of the SF36 (168 days for NIV treated, 99 days for 'standard' care) and the sleep apnoea, QoL; index symptoms domain (192 days for NIV treated, 46 days for 'standard' care). The authors commented that NIV increased patient survival and QoL, and that the survival advantage was much greater than that from currently available neuroprotective therapy [31].

4. Invasive assisted ventilation

How does LTMV affect probability of survival and QoL in patients with MND with respiratory insufficiency?

This is a controversial issue and considerable differences exist in approach and practice in different countries. Acute respiratory insufficiency (ARI) with alveolar hypoventilation or incapacitating dyspnoea without peripheral muscle involvement can both be early features in MND. It has been suggested that such patients might benefit from more invasive assisted ventilation (LTMV).

Moss et al. examined advance care planning and outcomes of patients with MND receiving LTMV in a population-based study in homes and chronic care facilities. Seventy-five MND patients were identified; 50 of the 58 (86%) who were able to communicate consented to structured interviews, 36 at home and 14 in an institution. Thirty-eight had completed advance directives, and 96% wanted them. Thirty-eight also wished to stop LTMV in certain circumstances. Those who had completed advance directives were more likely to have communicated their preference to stop LTMV to their family and physician than those who had not (76% versus 29%; P = 0.05). Patients living at home rated their QoL as being better than those in an institution (7.2 versus 5.6; P = 0.0052). Their annual expenses were also less ($136,560 versus $366,852; P = 0.0018). Most patients receiving LTMV would want to stop it under certain circumstances, and advance care planning enhances communication of patient preferences to family and physicians. Home-based LTMV is less costly and associated with greater patient satisfaction [32].

A further study made a retrospective analysis of the results of LTMV in 10 MND patients. LTMV outside the intensive care unit (ICU) was found to be possible in these patients and seven of these returned home. Return to the home environment was however found to be very difficult for ventilator-dependent patients lacking family support [33].

Moss et al. conducted a further study to better inform MND patients about home ventilation. They gathered data on the prevalence of MND patients on home ventilation in Northern Illinois and the percentage who chose it, and asked patients, families and physicians about attitudes towards home ventilation. Fewer than 10% of MND patients had chosen home ventilation, and less than 5% remained on it for any length of time. Seventeen (90%) were however glad to have chosen home ventilation and would choose it again. Family caregivers reported major burdens. Only half said they would choose it for themselves. The mean yearly cost of home ventilation was estimated at $153,252. Home ventilation thus seems effective for a small number of MND patients but imposes significant burdens on families [34].

A more recent retrospective study evaluated a protocol for early respiratory assessment of MND patients who might be helped by LTMV in their homes and investigated the effects of the protocol and bulbar involvement on the survival of patients receiving NIPPV. LTMV was indicated in 86 MND patients, 22 of whom presented with bulbar involvement. Treatment with LTMV had been initiated in one group of patients before and in a second group after protocol initiation. The majority of patients in the first group began treatment with LTMV during an acute episode requiring ICU admission ($P = 0.001$) and tracheal ventilation ($P = 0.025$), with a lower percentage of patients beginning LTMV treatment without ARI ($P = 0.013$). No significant differences in survival were found between the groups but greater survival was observed in the second group ($P = 0.03$) when patients with bulbar involvement were excluded. Multivariate analysis showed bulbar involvement to be an independent prognostic factor for survival (relative risk, 1.6; 95% confidence interval, 1.01–2.54; $P = 0.04$). It was concluded that early and systematic respiratory evaluation is necessary to improve the results of LTMV in patients with MND [35].

The implementation of LTMV varies widely in different countries. LTMV appears sometimes to be helpful in small number of MND patients but imposes considerable additional burdens on families and carers. LTMV may also be less useful in patients with substantial bulbar involvement.

5. Cough assist devices (insufflation/exsufflation)
Does MI-E alleviate respiratory symptoms in patients with MND who have excessive secretions?

There has been recent interest in cough assist devices (insufflation/exsufflation) in the alleviation of respiratory symptoms in MND. Elimination of airway secretion is a major issue in the care of patients with MND. Bulbar muscle weakness is often a reason for failure of NIPPV and may lead to tracheostomy.

Expiratory aids may help to overcome these problems, at least for a while. Lahrmann et al. reported a patient with advanced MND, receiving nocturnal NIPPV, who was reported to benefit from regular use of an MI-E device [36]. Other studies have included other disorders associated with excessive secretions and have not focused exclusively on MND. One examined the physiological effects and tolerance of MI-E prospectively in patients with chronic ventilatory failure from various causes in 13 MND patients, 9 with severe COPD and 7 with other neuromuscular disorders. The results suggested good tolerance and physiological improvement in patients with restrictive and obstructive disease, suggesting that MI-E may be a useful complement to NIPPV for patients with a wide variety of neuromuscular diseases [37]. A further investigation focused on 26 consecutive patients with MND, 15 of whom had severe bulbar dysfunction. Although both groups had a similar time from MND symptom onset to diagnosis, differences ($P < 0.05$) were found between non-bulbar and bulbar patients in lung function and cough capacity parameters: MI-E is able to generate clinically effective peak cough flows in stable MND patients except for those with bulbar dysfunction who also have a maximum insufflation capacity >11 and peak cough flow maximum insufflation capacity <2.7 L/s who probably have severe dynamic collapse of the upper airways during the exsufflation cycle. Clinically, stable patients with mild respiratory dysfunction probably only benefit from MI-E except during an acute respiratory illness [38].

6. Feeding gastrostomy
How does feeding gastrostomy improve nutritional state and probability of survival in patients with MND with bulbar involvement?

In the natural progression of MND, a state of malnutrition often develops, associated with reduced oral intake, caused by difficulties with swallowing and/or anorexia. The issue of when and how a feeding tube should be inserted remains controversial.

It is well established that bulbar involvement in MND is an adverse prognostic indicator on account of a higher risk of aspiration and consequences of dysphagia. One study assessed the effects of percutaneous endoscopic gastrostomy (PEG) in 31 MND patients with bulbar involvement at 3-monthly intervals over 2 years following PEG insertion. The data were compared with a control group of 35 MND patients who refused PEG. Mortality did not differ significantly between the two groups during the first 6 months but after this time was lower in the PEG group. In the patients who had had PEG, the body mass index showed a mild but statistically significant improvement while in the controls it decreased significantly. It was suggested that PEG could improve survival in elderly and young MND patients with bulbar involvement, enhance QoL and help integration in social and family surroundings [39].

In a further study, safety and factors related to survival after PEG were reviewed in a series of 50 consecutive MND patients.

No major acute or long-term complications were observed. Stabilization or increase in weight were observed after PEG. Median survival after PEG was 185 days, with a worse outcome in patients with weight loss ≥10% healthy body weight and FVC <65%. It was noted that PEG may be a useful option in the symptomatic treatment of dysphagia in MND [40].

PEG insertion has been considered a reliable route for nutrition and hydration in MND patients with dysphagia. A retrospective analysis of the CNTF and BDNF databases was made to determine the clinical status of MND patients during the 30 days preceding PEG insertion. By comparing the rate of decline pre- and post-PEG, nutritional supplementation via PEG seemed to stabilize the weight loss otherwise experienced. Death within 30 days of PEG was associated with a marked reduction in FVC and identified a group of patients in whom PEG should be inserted with caution. These data were thought to emphasize the importance of sequential measurement of FVC in managing MND patients to guide the timing of PEG insertion [41].

Thirty-three MND patients with erect or supine FVC <50% predicted underwent attempted PEG placement using NIPPV, oxygen support and conscious sedation anaesthesia. Gastrostomy tubes were successfully placed in all patients. Mean survival was 211 days with 67% surviving >180 days. FVC at the time of PEG placement did not predict survival [42].

A retrospective evaluation of gastrostomy placement in 36 MND patients over a 3.5-year period attempted to determine the optimal insertion method. Twenty patients were referred for PEG and 16 for radiologically inserted gastrostomy (RIG). Gastrostomy method, success rate of each technique and reason for procedure failure were reviewed in each patient. Preoperative FVC was recorded. The log-rank test was used to compare survival rates after PRG (percutaneous radiological gastrostomy) and RIG, and the Wilcoxon-rank sum test to evaluate the influence of declining FVC on PEG success. The Kaplan–Meier product limit method was used to estimate survival probabilities. Of 20 patients referred for PEG, 11 were successful. The nine failures resulted from failure to transilluminate the abdominal wall. All 16 patients initially referred for RIG were successful. The nine patients in whom PEG failed subsequently had a successful RIG. In patients with diaphragmatic palsy and a high subcostal stomach, an angled subcostal approach or intercostal approach was recommended for RIG insertion. One aspiration-related death occurred in the PEG group and a second patient from the PEG group required laparotomy for post-operative peritonitis. One death occurred in the RIG group because of inadvertent placement of the tube in the peritoneal cavity. There was no significant difference between PEG and RIG in terms of patient survival and FVC did not have a statistically significant influence on PEG failure. It was however suggested that RIG was the method of choice on the basis of these observations [43].

Data from patients with and without PEG with MND functional rating scale-bulbar subscale (ALSFRSb) scores ≤5 was evaluated to compare characteristics of MND patients with and without PEG. PEG use was markedly increased as ALSFRSb scores declined. PEG patients used significantly more assistive devices, multidisciplinary care, home care nurses and aides, had more frequent physician, emergency department visits and hospital admissions ($P < 0.0001$), as well as lower health status based on the mini-SIP scale ($P = 0.0047$). PEG use varied greatly between centres. PEG was thought to have a positive impact in 79% of patients as a whole but only in 37.5% of patients who received PEG later. Although only a small number of patients were studied, PEG use showed no survival benefit. It was thought that patients generally did not receive PEG until bulbar function was severely reduced. Aggressive proactive nutritional management was considered essential in patients with MND to try and secure better outcomes [44].

As PEG may not be practicable in patients with severe respiratory impairment, the alternative method of RIG was evaluated for safety, effect on survival and respiratory function in 25 MND patients with respiratory failure. These 25 consecutive MND patients with severe dysphagia and FVC <50% were compared with 25 consecutive patients with FVC <50% who underwent PEG. Respiratory function was evaluated before and after each procedure. The two groups were broadly similar. RIG placement was successful in all cases, PEG in 23/25. One patient in each group died after the procedure. The mean survival time after gastrostomy placement was 204 days in the RIG group and 85 days in the PEG group ($P < 0.004$). Respiratory function decreased more in the PEG group than in the RIG group ($P < 0.02$). RIG appeared to be safer than PEG in MND patients with moderate to severe respiratory impairment, and seemed to be associated with longer survival [45].

Data seeking further insights into the frequency, timing and outcomes following PEG insertion from gastrostomy in MND were obtained from the Scottish MND Register. Descriptive statistics of patients undergoing PEG were extracted. Survival analysis used Kaplan–Meier and Cox proportional hazards methods. For patients diagnosed between 1989 and 1998, 142 PEGs were placed in 1226 patients of which 130 were done before the censoring date. Approximately 5% of patients underwent gastrostomy each year but this rate appeared to double between 1989 and 1998. Mean age at insertion was 66.8 years, following a mean disease duration of 24 months. Median survival from PEG insertion was 146 days. The 1-month mortality after PEG was 25%. PEG did not confer a survival advantage compared with no PEG. The authors concluded that PEGs were being inserted more frequently in people with MND. An unexpectedly high early mortality was detected which probably reflected a lack of selection bias compared with previously published data. It was suggested that changes in practice surrounding PEG placement since 1998 might have resulted in better outcomes for patients with MND [46].

Complications after PEG and RIG along with their effects on survival were evaluated in 50 patients having definite or probable MND. RIG was considered first-line therapy when the slow vital capacity (SVC) was less than 50% predicted or when PEG was refused by the patient. Thirty patients had a PEG and 20 an RIG. The two populations were comparable in age, gender ratio and disease duration before gastrostomy. SVC was lower in those patients having RIG than PEG. The frequency of complications at gastrostomy insertion and during the first month was not significantly different between the two groups. Kaplan–Meier survival curves from the date of gastrostomy were not different in univariate or multivariate analysis. The authors suggested that the main benefit of RIG is its utility in patients who have a relatively higher level of ventilatory compromise [47].

Conclusions

Riluzole remains the only licensed disease modifying treatment for MND. RCT evidence suggests only modest effectiveness. NICE suggested further studies were desirable following the dose ranging trial [3], but these have never been done and seem unlikely to happen in the future. In the meantime any further insights are likely to come from observational studies rather than prospective randomized investigations.

Similar sentiments apply to IGF-1. RCTs so far completed have not had the ability to definitively demonstrate the potential efficacy of IGF-1 as a disease modifying treatment for MND. The results of the current trial in North America are keenly awaited and it is also possible that novel delivery methods such as viral vectors may lead to new insights into the possible effectiveness of IGF-1 as well as other neurotrophins in MND.

While stem cell therapy has been identified as having huge potential as a disease modifying treatments for MND and other neurodegenerative diseases it is too early to make further comment. Interest in respiratory interventions as symptomatic treatments for MND has developed considerably in recent years. NIPPV may favourably influence QoL and survival and cough exsufflator/insufflator devices may also be useful. Optimum methods of monitoring of respiratory function during the course of MND remain uncertain. SNP has been suggested as a possible alternative to traditional methods such as FVC.

Whatever the role of respiratory function monitoring in determining the use of respiratory interventions, it seems increasingly clear that such monitoring is important in judging the timing of feeding gastrostomy in MND. The morbidity and mortality of PEG insertion probably increases as FVC% predicted declines. If an endoscopic technique is to be used, FVC should probably be at least 50%, certainly 40% predicted. RIG may however be preferable to PEG when feeding gastrostomies need to be established in patients with more severe levels of respiratory impairment.

References

1 Bensimon G, Lacomblez L, Meininger V, et al. A controlled trial of riluzole in amyotrophic lateral sclerosis. *N. Engl. J. Med.* 1994; **330**: 585–91.

2 Rowland LP. Riluzole for the treatment of amyotrophic lateral sclerosis – too soon to tell? *N. Engl. J. Med.* 1994; **330**: 636–7.

3 Lacomblez L, Bensimon G, Leigh PN, et al. Dose ranging study of riluzole in amyotrophic lateral sclerosis. *Lancet* 1996; **37**: 1425–31.

4 Bensimon G, Lacomblez L, Delumeau JC, et al. A study of riluzole in the treatment of advanced stage or elderly patients with amyotrophic lateral sclerosis. *J. Neurol.* 2002; **249**: 609–15.

5 Yanagisawa N, Tashiro K, Tohgi H, et al. Efficacy and safety of riluzole in patients with amyotrophic lateral sclerosis: double-blind placebo-controlled study in Japan. *Igakuno Ayumi* 1997; **182**: 851–66.

6 Miller RG, Mitchell JD, Lyon M, Moore DH. Riluzole for amyotrophic lateral sclerosis (ALS)/motor neuron disease (MND) (Cochrane Review). *The Cochrane Library*, Issue 2. Update Software, Oxford, 2002.

7 Lai EC, Felice KJ, Festoff BW, et al. Effect of recombinant human insulin-like growth factor-1 on progression of ALS. A placebo-controlled study. *Neurology* 1997; **49**: 1621–30.

8 Borasio GD, Robberecht W, Leigh PN, et al. A placebo controlled trial of insulin-like nerve growth factor-1 in amyotrophic lateral sclerosis. *Neurology* 1998; **51**: 583–6.

9 Mitchell JD, Wokke JHJ, Borasio G. Recombinant human insulin-like growth factor I (rhIGF-I) for amyotrophic lateral sclerosis (review). *The Cochrane Library*, Issue 3. Update Software, Oxford, 2002.

10 Bongioanni P, Reali C, Sogos V. Ciliary neurotrophic factor (CNTF) for amyotrophic lateral sclerosis/motor neuron disease. *Cochrane Database Syst. Rev.* 2004; 3.

11 Parton M, Mitsumoto H, Leigh PN. Amino acids for amyotrophic lateral sclerosis/motor neuron disease. *Cochrane Database Syst. Rev.* 2003; 4.

12 Orrell RW, Lane RJM, Ross M. Antioxidant treatment for amyotrophic lateral sclerosis/motor neuron disease. *Cochrane Database Syst. Rev.* 2005; 1.

13 BDNF Study Group (Phase III). A controlled trial of recombinant methionyl human BDNF in ALS. *Neurology* 1999; **52**: 1427–33.

14 Ochs G, Penn RD, York M, et al. A phase I/II trial of recombinant methionyl human brain derived neurotrophic factor administered by intrathecal infusion to patients with amyotrophic lateral sclerosis. *Amyotroph. Later. Scler. Other Motor Neuron Disord.* 2000; **1**: 201–6.

15 Eisen A, Stewart H, Schulzer M, Cameron D. Anti-glutamate therapy in amyotrophic lateral sclerosis: a trial using lamotrigine. *Can. J. Neurol. Sci.* 1993; **20**: 297–301.

16 Ryberg H, Askmark H, Persson LI. A double-blind randomised clinical trial in amyotrophic lateral sclerosis using lamotrigine: effects on CSF glutamate, aspartate, branched-chain amino acid levels and clinical parameters. *Acta Neurol. Scand.* 2003; **108**: 1–8.

17 Miller RG, Moore D, Young LA, et al. Placebo-controlled trial of gabapentin in patients with amyotrophic lateral sclerosis. *Neurology* 1996; **47**: 1383–8.

18 Miller RG, Moore II DH, Gelinas DF, et al. Phase III randomised trial of gabapentin in patients with amyotrophic lateral sclerosis. *Neurology* 2001; **56**: 843–8.

19 Gordon PH, Moore DH, Gelinas DF, et al. Placebo-controlled phase I/II studies of minocycline in amyotrophic lateral sclerosis. *Neurology* 2004; **62**: 1845–7.

20 Lacomblez L, Bensimon G, Douillet P, Doppler V, Salachas F, Meininger V. Xaliproden in amyotrophic lateral sclerosis: early clinical trials. *Amyotroph. Later. Scler. Other Motor Neuron Disord.* 2004; **5**: 99–106.

21 Meininger V, Bensimon G, Bradley WR, et al. Efficacy and safety of xaliproden in amyotrophic lateral sclerosis: results of two phase III trials. *Amyotroph. Later. Scler. Other Motor Neuron Disord.* 2004; **5**: 107–17.

22 Fallat RJ, Jewitt B, Bass M, Kamm B, Norris Jr FH. Spirometry in amyotrophic lateral sclerosis. *Arch. Neurol.* 1979; **36**: 74–80.

23 Jackson CE, Rosenfeld J, Moore DH, et al. A preliminary evaluation of a prospective study of pulmonary function studies and symptoms of hypoventilation in ALS/MND patients. *J. Neurol. Sci.* 2001; **191**: 75–8.

24 Lyall RA, Donaldson N, Polkey MI, Leigh PN, Moxham J. Respiratory muscle strength and ventilatory failure in amyotrophic lateral sclerosis. *Brain* 2001; **124**: 2000–13.

25 Fitting JW, Paillex R, Hirt L, Aebischer P, Schluep M. Sniff nasal pressure: a sensitive respiratory test to assess progression of amyotrophic lateral sclerosis. *Ann. Neurol.* 1999; **46**: 887–93.

26 Bourke SC, Shaw PJ, Gibson GJ. Respiratory function vs. sleep-disordered breathing as predictors of QOL in ALS. *Neurology* 2001; **57**: 2040–4.

27 Sivak ED, Shefner JM, Mitsumoto H, Taft JM. The use of non-invasive positive pressure ventilation (NIPPV) in ALS patients. A need for improved determination of intervention timing. *Amyotroph. Later. Scler. Other Motor Neuron Disord.* 2001; **2**: 139–45.

28 Newsom-Davis IC, Lyall RA, Leigh PN, Moxham J, Goldstein LH. The effect of non-invasive positive pressure ventilation (NIPPV) on cognitive function in amyotrophic lateral sclerosis (ALS): a prospective study. *J. Neurol. Neurosurg. Psychiatr.* 2001; **71**: 482–7.

29 Lyall RA, Donaldson N, Fleming T, et al. A prospective study of quality of life in ALS patients treated with non-invasive ventilation. *Neurology* 2001; **57**: 153–6.

30 Bourke SC, Bullock RE, Williams TL, Shaw PJ, Gibson GJ. Non-invasive ventilation in ALS: indications and effect on quality of life. *Neurology* 2003; **61**: 171–7.

31 Bourke SC, Tomlinson M, Williams TL, Bullock RE, Shaw PJ, Gibson GJ. Effects of non-invasive ventilation on survival and quality of life in patients with amyotrophic lateral sclerosis: a randomised controlled trial. *Lancet Neurol.* 2006; **5**: 140–7.

32 Moss AH, Oppenheimer EA, Casey P, et al. Patients with amyotrophic lateral sclerosis receiving long-term mechanical ventilation. Advance care planning and outcomes. *Chest* 1996; **110**: 249–55.

33 Escarrabill J, Estopa R, Farrero E, Monasterio C, Manresa F. Long-term mechanical ventilation in amyotrophic lateral sclerosis. *Respir. Med.* 1998; **92**: 438–41.

34 Moss AH, Casey P, Stocking CB, Roos RP, Brooks BR, Siegler M. Home ventilation for amyotrophic lateral sclerosis patients: outcomes, costs, and patient, family, and physician attitudes. *Neurology* 1993; **43**: 438–43.

35 Farrero E, Prats E, Povedano M, Martinez-Matos JA, Manresa F, Escarrabill J. Survival in amyotrophic lateral sclerosis with home mechanical ventilation: the impact of systematic respiratory assessment and bulbar involvement. *Chest* 2005; **127**: 2132–8.

36 Lahrmann H, Wild M, Zdrahal F, Grisold W. Expiratory muscle weakness and assisted cough in ALS. *Amyotroph. Later. Scler. Other Motor Neuron Disord.* 2003; **4**: 49–51.

37 Winck JC, Goncalves MR, Lourenco C, Viana P, Almeida J, Bach JR. Effects of mechanical insufflation–exsufflation on respiratory parameters for patients with chronic airway secretion encumbrance. *Chest* 2004; **126**: 774–80.

38 Sancho J, Servera E, Diaz J, Marin J. Efficacy of mechanical insufflation–exsufflation in medically stable patients with amyotrophic lateral sclerosis. *Chest* 2004; **125**: 1400–5.

39 Mazzini L, Corra T, Zaccala M, Mora G, Del Piano M, Galante M. Percutaneous endoscopic gastrostomy and enteral nutrition in amyotrophic lateral sclerosis. *J. Neurol.* 1995; **242**: 695–8.

40 Chio A, Finocchiaro E, Meineri P, Bottacchi E, Schiffer D. Safety and factors related to survival after percutaneous endoscopic gastrostomy in ALS. *Neurology* 1999; **53**: 1123–5.

41 Kasarskis EJ, Scarlata D, Hill R, Fuller C, Stambler N, Cedarbaum JM. A retrospective study of percutaneous endoscopic gastrostomy in ALS patients during the BDNF and CNTF trials. *J. Neurol. Sci.* 1999; **169**(1–2): 118–25.

42 Gregory S, Siderowf A, Golaszewski AL, McCluskey L. Gastrostomy insertion in ALS patients with low vital capacity: respiratory support and survival. *Neurology* 2002; **58**: 485–7.

43 Thornton FJ, Fotheringham T, Alexander M, Hardiman O, McGrath FP, Lee MJ. Amyotrophic lateral sclerosis: enteral nutrition provision – endoscopic or radiologic gastrostomy? *Radiology* 2002; **224**: 713–17.

44 Mitsumoto H, Davidson M, Moore D, et al. Percutaneous endoscopic gastrostomy (PEG) in patients with ALS and bulbar dysfunction. *Amyotroph. Later. Scler. Other Motor Neuron Disord.* 2003; **4**: 177–85.

45 Chio A, Galletti R, Finocchiaro C, et al. Percutaneous radiological gastrostomy: a safe and effective method of nutritional tube placement in advanced ALS. *J. Neurol. Neurosurg. Psychiatr.* 2004; **75**: 645–7.

46 Forbes RB, Colville S, Swingler RJ. Scottish Motor Neurone Disease Research Group. Frequency, timing and outcome of gastrostomy tubes for amyotrophic lateral sclerosis/motor neurone disease – a record linkage study from the Scottish Motor Neurone Disease Register. *J. Neurol.* 2004; **251**: 813–17.

47 Desport JC, Mabrouk T, Bouillet P, Perna A, Preux PM, Couratier P. Complications and survival following radiologically and endoscopically-guided gastrostomy in patients with amyotrophic lateral sclerosis. *Amyotroph. Later. Scler. Other Motor Neuron Disord.* 2005; **6**: 88–93.

CHAPTER 23
Peripheral nerve disorders

Richard Hughes, Eva L. Feldman, Jeremy D.P. Bland

Background and clinical questions

Peripheral nerve disorders are among the most common neurological diseases and many papers have been written on their treatment. The prevalence of peripheral neuropathy in the community has been estimated as 2000 per 100,000 or 2% [1].

In September 2005 the register of the Cochrane Neuromuscular Disease Review Group contained 1098 references to randomized trials on peripheral nerve disorders within its scope. At the same time 21 reviews of interventions for peripheral nerve disorders had been written, incorporating the results of 300 references to 290 trials. The focus of many of the reviews has been on inflammatory neuropathies, Bell's palsy and carpal tunnel syndrome (CTS) and their conclusions are incorporated in this chapter. The equally or more important problem of diabetic neuropathy (DN) has been addressed in many trials but the task of summarizing them in systematic reviews has only just begun. Because of its importance the evidence about DN has been incorporated here as well.

Critical review of the evidence for each question

1. Treatment for Guillain–Barré syndrome (GBS)

In adults with severe acute GBS, how does the treatment with plasma exchange (PE), intravenous immunoglobulin (IVIg) or corticosteroids affect the probability of accelerated functional improvement and of reduction of long-term disability? What about the acute general medical care?

GBS has an annual incidence of only about 2 per 100,000 throughout the world but has attracted a disproportionate amount of interest from clinical triallists and systematic reviewers. This is presumably because it is a dramatic, life-threatening disease. The mainstay of treatment is excellent intensive care which is considered further in the next section. If death can be avoided during the acute stage, the reparative capacity of the Schwann cell and axon permit substantial recovery in most patients without treatment. This biological fact has in the past led to premature claims of efficacy for all sorts of treatments ranging from Bordeaux wine in the 19th century to corticosteroids in the 20th century.

The disease is defined as an acute, otherwise idiopathic paralysing disorder with progressive weakness and reduced or absent tendon reflexes consistent with a polyradiculoneuropathy. The cerebrospinal fluid protein concentration is usually increased. The nadir of the illness is reached within 4 weeks. About 25% of patients become so weak that they require artificial ventilation. Most patients make a substantial recovery but between 2% and 10% of patients die and 20% are left with significant disability after a year [2]. Persistent deficits and fatigue are not uncommon. In most cases in Europe and North America, the underlying pathology is an acute inflammatory demyelinating polyradiculoneuropathy (AIDP), histologically resembling the experimental autoimmune neuritis induced in animals by immunization with peripheral nerve myelin proteins. The unproven assumption is that the pathogenesis is a T helper cell mediated immune response against myelin proteins, triggered by an immediately preceding infection. In a small percentage of cases in Europe and North America but in a majority of cases in Japan, China and central America, the underlying pathology is an acute motor or motor and sensory axonal neuropathy [2]. The pathogenesis of these axonal cases is different. There is less inflammation and the disease in many cases is due to antibodies directed against ganglioside GM1 that have been generated in response to a cross-reactive epitope in the lipo-oligosaccharide in the wall of the *Campylobacter jejuni* which caused a preceding enteritis [3]. The treatment trials have mostly been conducted in Europe and North America and most participants will have had AIDP so that their conclusions only apply to AIDP. Whether the response of patients with axonal forms of the disease or other variants, such as the Fisher syndrome of ophthalmoplegia, ataxia and areflexia, is the same, is not known.

Plasma exchange

The first treatment to be shown to have a beneficial effect in GBS was PE. A North American trial with 245 participants demonstrated that significantly more patients improved by one grade on the 7-point GBS disability grade scale after 4 weeks with 200–250 mL PE than with supportive care alone [4]. Our Cochrane Review included eight trials comparing PE with supportive treatment or differing amounts of PE [5]. In this review, the primary outcome was improvement in the same disability scale after 4 weeks. For the 585 participants in the four trials with available data, the weighted mean difference in improvement was −0.89 of grade (95% CI −1.14−−0.63) more improvement in those who received PE than those who did not, $P < 0.00001$ (Table 23.1, Figure 23.1a) [4,6–8]. The relative rate of improving one disability grade, median time to recover independent walking and being dead or disabled after 1 year also all significantly favoured the treated participants compared with those who only received supportive care [9]. The mortality was similar, about 5%, in the treated and untreated arms of the studies. These trials established PE as the standard treatment for adults with severe GBS and by extrapolation PE has also been used in children and in some patients with mild disease.

Intravenous immunoglobulin

Following the serendipitous observation that intravenous infusion of large amounts of human immunoglobulin appeared helpful in a patient with chronic inflammatory demyelinating polyradiculoneuropathy (CIPD) and idiopathic thrombocytopenia, a Dutch group pioneered its use in GBS and then demonstrated similar efficacy to PE [10]. This conclusion was confirmed in subsequent trials. The Cochrane Review [11] now includes five trials with 582 participants comparing IVIg with PE [10,12–15]. The improvement in disability was almost identical (Table 23.1, Figure 23.1b) and there was no significant difference in any other outcome measure. On account of this, IVIg has become widely adopted as the first line treatment for adults with severe GBS and by extrapolation is often used in patients with mild disease and in children [16]. Questions remain about the timing and optimal dose, in particular whether the treatment should be repeated in patients who do not improve rapidly [9].

Corticosteroids

Since GBS is an inflammatory disease and is generally considered to have an autoimmune pathogenesis, the expectation was that corticosteroids would be useful in its treatment. It was therefore surprising that the first trial of prednisolone with 40 participants showed a trend towards worse outcome in prednisolone treated patients [17]. Eight trials with altogether 623 participants are now included in the relevant Cochrane Review [18]. In the six trials with 587 participants with available information, there was no significant difference in the mean improvement in disability after 4 weeks between those who received corticosteroids and those who did not (Table 23.1, Figure 23.1c). In the four small trials which used oral corticosteroids [19–21] there were in total 120 participants and there was significantly less improvement with corticosteroids than without. In the two large trials which used intravenous methylprednisolone [22,23], there were 467 participants and there was no significant difference. An analysis taking into account age and initial disability showed a trend towards greater benefit with the combined

treatment equivalent to a relative risk of improving one or more disability grades of 1.16 (95% CI 0.98–1.32, $P = 0.08$) more with corticosteroids than with placebo [9]. There were no significant differences in other outcome measures including the median time to regain independent walking and relative risks of death or death and disability after a year. In conclusion, there is no evidence of benefit from oral corticosteroids and the benefit from intravenous methylprednisolone is at best marginal and does not affect the long-term outcome. More research is needed to identify better treatments.

General medical and nursing care for GBS

Despite modern immunotherapy, the results of treatment are unsatisfactory and excellent intensive and general medical care are the mainstay of management. However practice is largely based on clinical experience and there are few clinical trials and no directly relevant systematic reviews. A recent consensus report does provide guidance from which we will mention briefly some key points but the reader is directed to the original article for the detail [24].

During the acute stage, regard must be had to the danger of respiratory failure and bulbar palsy which together carry the risk of cardio-respiratory arrest and chest infection. To prevent this, regular monitoring of vital capacity is the simplest method, although measurement of peak inspiratory pressure is an alternative which may be even more sensitive for detecting impending crisis [25–27]. There is a debate as to whether it is preferable to place a tracheostomy early to prevent complications or late in the hope that it may be avoided by rapid recovery [24]. Whichever is decided, there is evidence from elective tracheostomy in other situations that a percutaneous procedure has less complications and better cosmetic result than conventional operation [28].

Cardiac arrhythmias are another serious danger and account for about half the mortality. They are more likely in patients with severe disease and respiratory failure but do occur before the onset of respiratory failure and even after restoration of unassisted ventilation. Several methods have been proposed for identifying patients who are at greatest risk. Wide swings, exceeding 85 mmHg, of systolic blood pressure from day to day [29] and increased beat to beat variation in the R–R interval have been observed with increased frequency in patients who later developed severe bradycardia [30].

The third cause of death is pulmonary embolism so that it is accepted practice to use low-dose subcutaneous heparin and graduated compression stockings. There is no direct evidence in GBS that these practices are effective. However, the use of heparin is supported by trials after operation and in acute medical illness [31]. A meta-analysis confirmed that graduated compression stockings reduced the risk of postoperative thromboembolism by almost 70% in patients at moderate risk [32].

For other aspects of supportive care, there is even less direct evidence. Neuropathic and postural musculoskeletal pain are

Table 23.1 Treatment of Guillain-Barré Syndrome.

Type of study (reference)	Intervention (dosage)	Outcome (follow-up time)	Number of patients (no. of trials)	Control group mean change from baseline (range)	SMD or WMD (95% CI)	Control group risk (range)	Relative risk (95% CI)	Absolute risk reduction (95% CI)	Comment
SR [5]	PE (86–275 mL/kg) versus supportive treatment	Improvement in disability grade* (4 weeks)	485 (4)	−0.27 (−0.40 to 0.10)	0.89 (0.63–1.14)				PE better
		Severe sequelae (1 year)	649 (6)			17% (0–29)	0.65 (0.44–0.96)	6% (1–11)	PE better
SR [11]	IVIg (0.4–0.5 g/kg for 4–5 days) versus PE (200–250 mL/kg)	Improvement in disability grade* (4 weeks)	536 (5)	−1.03 (−1.40 to −0.37)	0.02 (ns)				ns difference
		Dead or disabled (1 year)	243 (1)			17%	0.98 (0.55–1.72)	3% (ns)	ns difference
SR [18]	Corticosteroids (prednisolone 45–80 mg for 4–14 days or MTPH 500 mg for 5 days) versus control	Improvement in disability grade* (4 weeks)	587 (6)	−1.33 (−3.97 to −0.73)	0.36 (ns)				Corticosteroids worse ns Heterogeneity
		Dead or disabled (1 year)	491 (3)			9% (8–11)	1.51 (0.91–2.50)	+5% (ns)	Corticosteroids worst ns

IVIg: Immunoglobulins; MD: Mean difference; MTPH: Methylprednisolone; PE: Plasma exchange; SMD: Standard mean difference; SR: Systematic review; WMD: Weighted mean difference; ns: not statistically significant.

*Disability scale: (0) Healthy, (1) Minor symptoms or signs of neuropathy but capable of manual work, (2) Able to walk without support of a stick but incapable of manual work, (3) Able to walk with a stick, appliance or support, (4) Confined to bed or chair bound, (5) Requiring assisted ventilation, (6) Dead.

Review: PE for GBS
Comparison: 01 4 week-endpoints
Outcome: 03 Change in disability grade 4 weeks after randomization

Study or sub-category	N	PE mean (SD)	N	Control mean (SD)	WMD (fixed) 95% CI	WMD (fixed) 95% CI
Greenwood 1984	14	−0.64 (1.35)	15	−0.27 (1.05)		−0.37 (−1.25, 0.51)
McKhann 1985	122	−1.10 (1.93)	123	−0.40 (1.60)		−0.70 (−1.14, −0.26)
Raphaël 1987	109	−1.30 (1.93)	111	−0.29 (1.60)		−1.01 (−1.48, −0.54)
Raphaël 1997	45	−1.00 (1.20)	46	0.10 (1.00)		−1.10 (−1.55, −0.65)
Total (95% CI)	290		295			−0.89 (−1.14, −0.63)

Test for heterogeneity: Chi² = 3.10, df = 3 (P = 0.38), I² = 3.3%
Test for overall effect: Z = 6.89 (P < 0.00001)

Scale: −4 −2 0 2 4
Favours PE   Favours control

(a)

Review: IVIg for GBS
Comparison: 02 IVIg versus PE
Outcome: 01 Change in disability grade 4 weeks after randomization

Study or sub-category	N	IVIg mean (SD)	N	PE mean (SD)	WMD (fixed) 95% CI	WMD (fixed) 95% CI
van der Meché 1992	74	−0.86 (1.32)	73	−0.37 (1.33)		−0.49 (−0.92, −0.06)
Brill 1996	26	−1.00 (1.32)	24	−1.20 (1.50)		0.20 (−0.59, 0.99)
PSGBS Group 1997	130	−0.80 (1.30)	121	−0.90 (1.30)		0.10 (−0.22, 0.42)
Nomura 2000	23	−1.00 (1.00)	24	−1.40 (1.50)		0.40 (−0.33, 1.13)
Diener 2001	20	−1.20 (1.32)	21	−1.30 (1.50)		0.10 (−0.76, 0.96)
Total (95% CI)	273		263			−0.02 (−0.25, 0.20)

Test for heterogeneity: Chi² = 6.82, df = 4 (P = 0.15), I² = 41.3%
Test for overall effect: Z = 0.21 (P = 0.83)

Scale: −4 −2 0 2 4
Favours IVIg   Favours PE

(b)

Review: Corticosteroids for GBS
Comparison: 01 Corticosteroid versus control
Outcome: 01 Disability grade change after 4 weeks

Study or sub-category	N	Corticosteroids mean (SD)	N	Control mean (SD)	WMD (random) 95% CI	WMD (random) 95% CI
01 Oral regimens						
Bansal 1986	10	−2.38 (0.97)	10	−3.97 (0.70)		1.59 (0.85, 2.33)
Hughes 1978	21	−0.24 (0.94)	19	−0.74 (0.81)		0.50 (−0.04, 1.04)
Shukla 1988	6	0.67 (1.75)	8	−0.88 (1.13)		0.21 (−01.39, 1.81)
Singh 1996	24	0.20 (2.00)	22	−0.80 (2.10)		0.60 (−0.59, 1.79)
Subtotal (95% CI)	61		59			0.82 (0.17, 1.47)

Test for heterogeneity: Chi² = 6.16, df = 3 (P = 0.10), I² = 51.3%
Test for overall effect: Z = 2.47 (P = 0.01)

Study or sub-category	N	Corticosteroids mean (SD)	N	Control mean (SD)	WMD (random) 95% CI	WMD (random) 95% CI
02 Intravenous regimens	124	−0.80 (1.14)	118	−0.73 (1.21)		−0.07 (−0.37, 0.23)
GBS Steroid 1993	112	−1.13 (1.30)	113	−0.83 (1.35)		−0.30 (−0.65, 0.05)
van Koningsveld 2004	236		231			−0.17 (−0.39, 0.06)
Subtotal (95% CI)						

Test for heterogeneity: Chi² = 0.98, df = 1 (P = 0.32), I² = 0%
Test for overall effect: Z = 1.46 (P = 0.15)

Total (95% CI)	297		290			0.36 (−0.16, 0.88)

Test for heterogeneity: Chi² = 24.60, df = 5 (P = 0.0002), I² = 79.7%
Test for overall effect: Z = 1.35 (P = 0.18)

Scale: −4 −2 0 2 4
Favours steroid   Favours control

(c)

Figure 23.1 Change in disability grade 4 weeks after randomization. (a), (b) and (c) were included in the relevant Cochrane Reviews [5,11,18] and are reproduced with permission, Copyright Cochrane Library. (a) PE versus no treatment; (b) PE versus IVIg; (c) corticosteroids versus no treatment or placebo.

common in acute and convalescent GBS. Very small trials confirm the benefit from carbamazepine and gabapentin which have been shown in larger trials in other types of painful neuropathy [33,34]. Fatigue is common following recovery from

the acute stage of GBS. No adequate trials have been published of drug treatment. An open trial of an aerobic exercise regime demonstrated benefit in convalescent patients [35] a result which we have confirmed in a similar study of a physiotherapist-supervised aerobic exercise programme (Graham R and Hughes R 2005, unpublished information).

2. Immunotherapy for CIDP and related disorders

In patients with CIDP or related disorders how does treatment with corticosteroids, PE or IVIg affect the short-term outcome?

CIDP is related to GBS by the distribution of the lesions and similarity of the pathology on the active disease stage. Its prevalence is somewhere between 1 and 7 per 100,000 [36].

In patients with the conventional symmetrical sensory and motor form of CIDP, systematic reviews have confirmed the clinical experience that each of corticosteroids, PE and IVIg produces short-term benefit. For corticosteroids, this conclusion is based on one small low quality trial but the clinical experience of benefit is so embedded that further trials are not considered necessary [37]. For PE, there have been two small high quality trials both indicating significant short-term benefit from PE compared with sham exchange [38]. In a meta-analysis of four trials with altogether 113 participants, IVIg 2.0 g/kg produced significant improvement in disability lasting 2–6 weeks [39]. In small trials the effect of IVIg was not significantly different from that of either PE or oral prednisolone starting with a dose of 60 mg daily [40,41]. There have been no high quality trials of a size large enough to test seriously whether immunosuppressive or immunomodulatory drugs are effective in CIDP [42]. There are two trials in progress, one of interferon beta 1a and one of methotrexate.

Many patients with CIDP have an associated paraprotein. There is even less evidence for treating these patients. About half of those with an IgM paraprotein have a characteristic predominantly sensory neuropathy with marked distal slowing of nerve conduction. These patients characteristically have antibodies to myelin-associated glycoprotein which may be responsible for the pathology which differs from the macrophage-associated demyelination characteristic of CIDP. In this form of IgM paraprotein-associated demyelinating neuropathy, there have been few trials and none have shown convincing evidence of benefit from any treatment [43]. More research is needed. For patients with IgG and IgA paraproteins, the clinical picture and treatment responses seem empirically to resemble those of CIDP without a paraprotein and they are commonly treated along similar lines. Of course, an essential preliminary to treatment is to ensure that there is no underlying malignant plasma cell dyscrasia. If there is, then treatment should follow the guidelines for treatment of haemato-oncological malignancies.

There is some evidence concerning the best management of multifocal motor neuropathy, a pure motor disorder which has been distinguished from CIDP. There is no doubt from controlled trials that IVIg has a beneficial effect lasting typically for 4 weeks [44]. Although beneficial the short-term response requires repeated dosing which is very inconvenient and expensive. Observational studies suggest that immunosuppressive drugs, especially cyclophosphamide, may be beneficial but this needs to be confirmed in randomized trials [45].

3. Treatment for Bell's palsy

How does treatment of patients with Bell's palsy with corticosteroids or antiviral agents affect the proportion of patients who have incomplete recovery after 6 months?

Acute idiopathic facial paralysis or Bell's palsy has an annual incidence of about 25 per 100,000 and there is no sound evidence for using any treatment. This is remarkable because corticosteroids have been used for 50 years and antiviral agents for 20. Part of the reason lies in the natural history of the disease which fortunately is towards spontaneous complete recovery in 95% of patients with partial and 61% of those with complete facial paralysis [46].

Table 23.2 Treatment of Bell's Palsy.

Type of study (reference)	Intervention	Outcome (follow-up time)	Number of patients (number of trials)	Control group risk (range)	Relative risk (95% CI)	Absolute risk reduction (95% CI)	Comment
SR [47]	Corticosteroids versus control	Incomplete recovery (6 months)	117 (3)	26% (14–35)	0.86 (0.47–1.59)	4% (ns)	
SR [48]	Aciclovir with steroid versus steroid	Incomplete recovery (4 months)	99 (1)	24%	0.32 (0.11–0.92)	16% (2–31)	Aciclovir better
	Aciclovir versus steroid	Incomplete recovery (3 months)	101 (1)	6%	3.48 (1.05–11.60)	+10% (3–29)	Aciclovir worse
	Aciclovir alone versus aciclovir with steroid versus placebo	Incomplete recovery (4 months)	53 (1)	–	–	–	Heterogeneity between trials (see text)

CI: confidence intervals; ns: not statistically significant; SR: systematic review.

In the Cochrane Systematic Review of three trials of corticosteroids (Table 23.2), 13/59 (22%) corticosteroid patients had incomplete recovery after 6 months compared with 15/58 (26%) control participants (relative risk 0.86, 95% CI 0.47–1.59) [47]. Similarly in the review of antiviral agents, there were only three trials with altogether 240 patients, one suggesting a beneficial effect, one a negative effect and one no difference [48]. Clearly more evidence is needed about both of these treatments and a trial comparing corticosteroids with acyclovir with placebo is now in progress in Scotland.

4. Treatment for DN

How well do glycaemic control or other pharmacological interventions for the treatment of diabetes mellitus improve symptoms, signs and nerve conduction parameters?

Diabetes has reached epidemic proportions in the Western world. In the US in 2005, 20.8 million or 7% of the population has diabetes, an increase of 2.6 million cases since 2003 [49]. An additional 41 million individuals are estimated to have prediabetes and this number also is growing at an exponential rate. The most common complication of diabetes is peripheral DN which occurs in approximately 60% of all diabetic patients [50]. DN is the most common cause of non-traumatic amputation and a diabetic has a lifetime risk of amputation of 15% [51]. In the US, DN is the leading cause of diabetes-related hospital admissions and every 24 h, 230 diabetic patients undergo amputation [52].

Therapies for DN are divided into two groups: treatments targeted against the disease process itself [53–55] and treatments aimed at providing symptom relief [56]. To date, the only certain way to prevent the onset of DN or to slow progression of the disorder is by strict glycaemic control [57]. Several major studies have compared DN onset and progression in the setting of varying levels of glycaemia. An alternative, and to date less successful approach, is to target the downstream targets of hyperglycaemia with pharmacologic intervention.

Glycaemic control

The most frequently cited study targeted at regulating glycaemic control is the Diabetes Control and Complications Trial (DCCT). The DCCT compared intensive treatment (3 or more daily insulin injections or insulin pump) with conventional treatment (1 or 2 insulin daily injections) in 1441 patients with type 1 diabetes. DN was defined by history or physical exam and confirmed by either abnormal nerve conduction studies or $\geqslant 1$ autonomic function test). The prevalence of DN was 64% lower in patients receiving intensive treatment (HbA_{1c} = 7.2%) compared to patients in the conventional treatment group (HbA_{1c} = 9.1%). Data from the DCCT also suggest that strict glycaemic control prevents progression of DN. Even if abnormal at study onset, nerve conduction studies remained unchanged in patients in the

intensive treatment arm but markedly declined in patients on conventional treatment, suggesting that glycaemic control also halts worsening of existing DN [53].

The Epidemiology of Diabetes Interventions and Complications (EDIC) study is an extension of the original DCCT cohort. In EDIC, the HbA_{1c} of the two original DCCT cohorts has converged for the last 8 years, due to the fact that patients in the conventional group gained stricter control while those in the intensive group assumed more relaxed control. Despite this convergence of glycaemic control, the progression rates of nephropathy and retinopathy in patients in the original DCCT intensive treatment remained significantly lower than that of those originally randomized to the conventional treatment arm [49,58]. This benefit is also reported for DN (www.nih.gov). This unexpected finding, known as 'metabolic memory', suggests that early glycaemic control has far-reaching and long-lasting beneficial effects.

The natural history of DN has also been studied in type 1 patients undergoing pancreatic transplant. When comparing DN in patients after successful pancreas transplant to those undergoing unsuccessful pancreas transplant, there was a significant improvement in neuropathic symptoms and nerve conduction studies relative to those patients who underwent an unsuccessful transplant throughout the course of the 10-year study [59].

While the clinical evidence that strict glycaemic control delays or prevents DN in type 1 patients is well established, the data for patients with type 2 diabetes are less convincing. In the United Kingdom Prospective Diabetes Study (UKPDS), 3867 newly diagnosed type 2 patients were randomized into an intensive treatment arm with an oral hypoglycaemic agent or insulin or conventional treatment with diet. After 10 years, patients in the intensive treatment arm had an average HbA_{1c} that was 1% lower than those patients in the conventional treatment arm. This improvement was associated with a 25% risk reduction in a composite measure of microvascular complications (retinopathy, nephropathy and DN) [50]. However, this reduction was strongly driven by the retinopathy component of the composite score. Patients in the intensive treatment arm required less retinal photocoagulation when compared to patients in the intensive treatment arm. While there was a tendency towards a reduction in the prevalence of amputation and sensory loss, this failed to achieve statistical significance after 10 years. A smaller cohort of patients remained in the study for 15 years, where more patients in the intensive treatment arm had preserved sensory perception when compared to patients in the conventional treatment (31.2% versus 51.7%, $P = 0.0052$) [60].

In the feasibility study for the Veterans Administration Cooperative Study on type 2 diabetes (VA CSDM), the effects of 2 years of intensive treatment on DN were examined in 153 men with an average (SD) duration of type 2 diabetes of 7.8 (4) years [61]. Patients in the intensive treatment arm (multiple insulin injections plus glipizide) achieved an

Table 23.3 Pharmacologic interventions in the treatment of DN.

Abnormality	Compound	Aim of treatment	Status of RCTs
Polyol pathway ↑	Aldose reductase inhibitors	Nerve sorbitol ↓	
	Sorbinil		Withdrawn (AE)
	Tolrestat		Withdrawn (AE)
	Ponalrestat		Ineffective
	Zopolrestat		Withdrawn (marginal effects)
	Zenarestat		Withdrawn (AE)
	Lidorestat		Withdrawn (AE)
	Fidarestat		Effective in RCTs, trials ongoing
	AS-3201		Effective in RCTs, trials ongoing
	Epalrestat		Marketed in Japan
Myo-inositol ↓	_Myo_-inositol	Nerve _myo_-inositol ↑	Equivocal
Oxidative stress ↑	α-Lipoic acid	Oxygen free radicals ↓	Effective in RCTs, trials ongoing
Nerve hypoxia ↑	Vasodilators	NBF ↑	
	ACE inhibitors		Effective in one RCT
	Prostaglandin analogues		Effective in one RCT
	phVEGF$_{165}$ gene transfer	Angiogenesis ↑	RCTs ongoing
Protein kinase C ↑	Protein kinase C-β inhibitor (ruboxistaurin)	NBF ↑	RCTs ongoing
C-peptide ↓	C-peptide	NBF ↑	Studies ongoing
Neurotrophism ↓	Nerve growth factor (NGF)	Nerve regeneration, growth ↑	Ineffective
	BDNF	Nerve regeneration, growth ↑	Ineffective
LCFA metabolism ↓	Acetyl-L-carnitine	LCFA accumulation ↓	Ineffective
GLA synthesis ↓	γ-Linolenic acid (GLA)	EFA metabolism ↑	Withdrawn
NEG ↑	Aminoguanidine	AGE accumulation ↓	Withdrawn

AE: adverse event; AGE: advanced glycation end product; BDNF: brain-derived neurotrophic factor; EFA: essential fatty acid; LCFA: long-chain fatty acid; NBF: nerve blood flow; NEG: non-enzymatic glycation; RCT: randomized clinical trial. From Boulton et al. [50].

average HbA$_{1c}$ of 7.3% compared to 9.4% in patients in the conventional arm. At study onset, the baseline prevalence of DN was 50%, and this increased over the 2-year study period equally in both groups, suggesting that a 2-year period is insufficient time to follow the course of DN or in this population or that improved glycaemia did not alter the course of DN [61].

In summary, interventional evidence supports the idea that improved glycaemic control can both prevent DN and halt progression in patients with type 1 diabetes. The data for type 2 diabetes are less overwhelming, but long observational periods (15 years) suggest the same tenet holds in type 2 patients. Thus aggressive treatment aimed at normalizing fasting and postprandial glucose levels remains the mainstay of treating DN [62,63].

Pharmacologic intervention

Exactly how persistent hyperglycaemia results in nerve damage remains an active area of investigation. Multiple aetiologies have been proposed including altered polyol

metabolism, abnormal protein kinase C activity, unchecked oxidative stress, protein glycation, vascular insufficiency and blunted neurotrophic support [64]. It is likely that a confluence of these factors results in the development of DN [65]. Pharmacologic interventions, aimed at specific pathways, have yet to show a definite difference in either the onset or progression of DN when compared to untreated diabetic patients. Table 23.3 lists the most recent pharmacologic interventions and their outcomes [50].

5. Symptomatic treatment of pain associated with DN

How well do pharmacological and other interventions for painful DN control symptoms?

Pain is common in patients with DN, and frequently responds to treatment. A stepwise approach to therapy, carefully monitoring patients for symptom relief while being vigilant for side effects, usually results in a positive patient outcome. Titration is frequently necessary and it is common

Table 23.4 Treatment options for painful neuropathy.

Non-steroidal anti-inflammatory drugs
 Ibuprofen: 600 mg 4 times daily
 Sulindac: 200 mg twice daily

Antidepressants
 Duloxetine: 60 mg daily
 Amitriptyline: 50–150 mg at night
 Nortriptyline: 50–150 mg at night
 Imipramine: 100 mg daily
 Desipramine: 100 mg daily
 Paroxetine: 40 mg daily
 Trazadone: 50–150 mg 3 × daily

Antiepileptic drugs
 Pregabalin 150 mg, 2 or 3 × daily
 Gabapentin: 600–1200 mg 3 × daily
 Carbamazepine: 200 mg 4 × daily

for patients to require two or more agents for pain control. Table 23.4 summarizes treatments reported to be effective in DN in at least one double blind randomized placebo controlled trial. Detailed reviews of this subject can be found in [66–68] and Chapter 7.

6. Treatment for CTS

In patients with CTS how do different treatments reduce symptoms compared with no treatment and with each other?

Entrapment neuropathy of the median nerve at the wrist is the world's commonest peripheral nerve disorder with a point prevalence for symptomatic CTS of 2.7% in Sweden [69] 9.2% in women and 0.5% in men in Holland [70] and an estimated lifetime risk of 10%. Almost all studies show a female predominance with a female to male ratio varying from 20:1 to 2:1. It most typically presents with bilateral, nocturnal hand paraesthesiae. Though associations have been reported with many medical illnesses such as hypothyroidism and acromegaly, the majority of cases are idiopathic and there is evidence of a strong genetic predisposition [71]. The role of occupation in causation remains controversial with strong opinions on both sides but little concrete evidence. Mild symptoms may persist for many years or run a relapsing and remitting course. Many patients with other pathologies thus have CTS as an incidental finding for which treatment may not be required. Twenty-one per cent of patients reported symptomatic improvement without treatment over a period of 1 year [72]. The most useful investigation is nerve conduction studies and most clinical guidelines recommend their use [73] though they have significant false positive and false negative rates and should always be interpreted in the clinical context. Recently imaging of the median nerve in the carpal tunnel, particularly with high resolution ultrasound, has shown promise as an alternative or complementary

diagnostic tool but at present experience with nerve conduction studies remains much more extensive.

A wide range of treatments have been suggested and evidence for these has been analysed in a series of Cochrane Systematic Reviews [74–77]. The major trials have been summarized in Table 23.5. The findings from these and other studies may be summarized thus:
1 Interventions for which evidence suggests they are no better than placebo: vitamin B6, diuretics, non-steroidal anti-inflammatory drugs, ergonomic keyboard use, magnet therapy, laser acupuncture, exercise and chiropractic care.
2 Interventions for which no adequate evidence of efficacy exists: job modification, neurodynamic mobilization, micro-amps TENS, cognitive behavioural therapy, non-invasive laser neurolysis, biofeedback and serratiopeptidase.
3 Interventions with evidence of possible benefit: oral corticosteroids, splinting, ultrasound, yoga, steroid iontophoresis and carpal bone mobilization.
4 Interventions with definite evidence of benefit: local corticosteroid injection, surgical decompression.
It is notable that the use of even some treatments which are recommended in standard textbooks (diuretics, non-steroidal anti-inflammatory drugs) is not supported by trial evidence. Three interventions can be recommended for routine clinical use.

Splinting
Trial evidence in support of splints is limited but they are inexpensive and safe. The splint used should maintain the wrist at a neutral angle and need only be worn at night. The most recent high quality trial to include splinting as one treatment arm showed a 37% response rate to this intervention after 18 months [78].

Local corticosteroid injection
At the time of the Cochrane Review [74], evidence was found that local corticosteroid injection was more effective than placebo for up to 1 month following treatment but symptom relief beyond this had not been demonstrated. Injection was also superior to oral steroids. Since then, three randomized trials comparing steroid injection with surgery have been published [79–81] and one comparing the alternatives of administering local corticosteroids by injection or iontophoresis [82]. The latter suggests that the injection route is more effective. The trials comparing corticosteroid injection with surgery provide evidence that injection is effective beyond 1 month, in one case finding equivalent outcomes between the surgical and injection arms of the trial at 1 year [79]. Pooling the results of five better quality trials which provide data for outcome 6–18 months after injection suggests that 52% of patients obtain satisfactory symptom relief from injection alone. Only one study has compared different corticosteroids and dosages, finding no significant differences in outcome [83]. Methylprednisolone 40 mg has been

Table 23.5 Treatments for Carpal tunnel syndrome.

Author type of study (reference)	Intervention	Outcome	Number of participants (patients/hands)	Group response rate	Comment
Trials of surgery versus steroid injection					
Ly-Pen [79] RCT note 1	Steroid injection (1 or 2 injections 40 mg Methylprednisolone)	20% improvement in visual analogue scale score for nocturnal paresthesias at 3, 6, 12 months follow-up	83 hands	70%	No difference (3-month outcomes better for injection)
	Open carpal tunnel decompression		80 hands	75%	
Hui [80] RCT	Steroid injection	Change on global symptom scale at 20 weeks (GSS)	25/25	24.2-point mean improvement in GSS	Surgery provides better quality of relief
	Open carpal tunnel decompression		25/25	8.7-point mean improvement in GSS	
Demirci [81] CT note 2	Steroid injection × 2 (6.4 mg betamethasone)	Change in Boston scores at 6 months	46/46	change in SSS − 1.6, FSS − 1.3 (36/46 = 78% considered success)	Results of injection comparable to surgery at 3 months but not long-lasting
	Open carpal tunnel decompression		44/44	change in SSS − 2.1, FSS − 1.9 (42/44 = 95% considered success)	
Trials of surgery versus therapy other than steroid injection					
Gerritsen [78] RCT note 3	Splinting	Subjective symptom relief at 18 months	79/79	75% by intention to treat (37% with splints only)	Surgery better
	Open carpal tunnel decompression		68/68	90%	
Trials of steroid injection versus placebo or other rx					
Dammers [86] RCT	Steroid injection × 1 (40 mg methylprednisolone + lignocaine)	Subjective symptom relief at 1 month	30/30	23/30 (77%)	Injection better
	Placebo wrist injection (lignocaine + saline)		30/30	6/30 (20%)	

Ozdogan [87] RCT	Steroid injection × 1 wrist (1.5 mg betamethasone)	Adequate symptom control at 10–12 months	18/18	4/18 (22%)	Injection better
	Intramuscular (deltoid) steroid injection (1.5 mg betamethasone)		19/19	0/19 (0%)	
Girlanda [88] RCT note 4	Local steroid injection × 2 (15 mg methylprednisolone)	Adequate symptom control at 2 months	?/27	25/27 (92%)	Injection better
	Placebo wrist injection (saline)		?/26	?	
Armstrong [89] RCT	Steroid injection × 1 (6 mg betamethasone + lignocaine)	Subjective symptom relief at 2 weeks	43/43	30/43 (70%)	Injection better
	Placebo wrist injection × 1 (lignocaine and saline)		38/38	13/38 (34%)	
Gokoglu [90] RCT note 5	Injection × 1 (40 mg methylprednisolone) to both hands if both symptomatic	Change in Boston scores at 8 weeks (SSS + FSS)	15 patients	Change in SSS − 1.3, FSS − 1.1	Injection better
	Iontophoresis dexamethasone sodium phosphate		15 patients	Change in SSS − 0.9, FSS − 0.4	
Other notable results					
Scholten [74] SR note 6	Endoscopic versus open carpal tunnel decompression	Subjective symptom relief	13 trials	Meta-analysis not possible	No significant difference in outcome
O'gradaigh [82] RCT note 7	Compared 25/100 mg hydrocortisone, 20 mg triamcinolone, no injection	Subjective change in symptoms at 6 months	148 patients		No difference between different steroids/doses

Many of these trials have multiple endpoints and multiple outcome measures. This table reports the primary one selected by the authors or the one most appropriate for this review.

(1) These are the 12-month follow-up results.

(2) Randomization not described.

(3) Patients who failed to improve with splints had surgery but in analysis this was counted as an outcome of splinting.

(4) 91 hands with initial response followed up in an open fashion for 2 years with clinical and NCS assessments only 8% remained improved at 2 years.

(5) 48 hands. It is not explicit in the paper how the 18 patients bilateral CTS were handled.

(6) This Cochrane Review dealt with the issue of open versus endoscopic decompression, which has been the subject of numerous trials, very well. The conclusion – no difference in long-term outcome – remains valid.

(7) At 6 weeks 5% of the 20 control patients had symptomatic improvement compared with 65% of those receiving corticosteroids.

most widely used. There are several case reports of nerve or tendon injury but the risks of injection are clearly small. The reported trials of corticosteroid injection involve a total of over 2200 injections with no instances of such injury.

Surgery

Surgical decompression is generally regarded as the definitive treatment for CTS but is not without problems. Reported 'success' rates vary from 27–100% in different series. Pooling the data from 207 surgical series yields an average success rate worldwide of 75% in 32,761 procedures where success is taken as relief of symptoms to the extent that no further treatment is required. Variations of surgical technique, including the major division between open and endoscopic approaches which has been subject to several randomized trials, do not appear to influence long-term outcome, though post-operative recovery may be faster after endoscopic procedures [76]. Post-operative follow-up of 4265 operations showed that 7% of patients consider the operated hand to be worse after surgery so the procedure carries higher risks than injection. At the same time, and notwithstanding the results of one recent comparative trial [79] surgery offers both a higher chance of response to treatment and greater quantitative symptom relief than non-surgical treatment, but with a greater risk of adverse effects and greater inconvenience to the patient.

The fact that some surgical series report very high success rates suggests that the average figure of 75% can be improved upon. Studies of second operations on the same hand suggest that approximately half the failures result from incomplete section of the transverse carpal ligament [84]. The outcome of surgery is significantly worse in patients with normal pre-operative nerve conduction studies (51% success) and those with extremely severe nerve conduction abnormalities suggesting axonal degeneration (47% success) [85]. More conventional surgical complications are uncommon – deep wound infection in 0.5% and reflex sympathetic dystrophy in 0.5% [73]. It therefore appears that lack of surgical expertise, misdiagnosis and advanced disease with irreversible nerve damage between them account for the greater proportion of the poor outcomes. Other factors consistently associated with poorer outcomes include greater age, longer duration of symptoms, strenuous occupation, renal dialysis and the presence of an industrial injury compensation claim.

References

1 Martyn CN, Hughes RAC. Epidemiology of peripheral neuropathy. *J. Neurol. Neurosurg. Psychiatr.* 1997; **62**: 310–18.

2 Hughes RAC, Cornblath DR. Guillain–Barré syndrome. *Lancet* 2005; **366**: 1653–66.

3 Yuki N, Susuki K, Koga M, Nishimoto Y, Odaka M, Hirata K, et al. Carbohydrate mimicry between human ganglioside GM1 and Campylobacter jejuni lipooligosaccharide causes Guillain– Barré syndrome. *Proc. Natl. Acad. Sci. USA* 2004; **101**: 11404–9.

4 The Guillain–Barré Syndrome Study Group. Plasmapheresis and acute Guillain–Barré syndrome. *Neurology* 1985; **35**: 1096–104.

5 Raphaël JC, Chevret S, Hughes RA, Annane D. Plasma exchange for Guillain–Barré syndrome. *Cochrane Database Syst. Rev.* 2002; **2**: CD001798.

6 Greenwood RJ, Newsom Davis JM, Hughes RAC, Aslan S, Bowden AN, Chadwick DW, et al. Controlled trial of plasma exchange in acute inflammatory polyradiculoneuropathy. *Lancet* 1984; **1**: 877–9.

7 French Cooperative group in plasma exchange in Guillain– Barré syndrome. Efficiency of plasma exchange in Guillain–Barré syndrome: role of replacement fluids. *Ann. Neurol.* 1987; **22**: 753–61.

8 French Cooperative Group on plasma exchange in Guillain–Barré syndrome. Appropriate number of plasma exchanges in Guillain–Barré syndrome. *Ann. Neurol.* 1997; **41**: 298–306.

9 Hughes RAC, Cornblath DR. Guillain–Barré syndrome. *Lancet* 2005; **366**: 1653–66.

10 van der Meché FGA, Schmitz PIM, Dutch Guillain–Barré Study Group. A randomized trial comparing intravenous immune globulin and plasma exchange in Guillain–Barré syndrome. *N. Engl. J. Med.* 1992; **326**: 1123–9.

11 Hughes RA, Raphael JC, Swan AV, van Doorn PA. Intravenous immunoglobulin for Guillain–Barré syndrome. *Cochrane Database Syst. Rev.* 2006; **2**: CD002063.

12 Bril V, Ilse WK, Pearce R, Dhanani A, Sutton D, Kong K. Pilot trial of immunoglobulin versus plasma exchange in patients with Guillain–Barré syndrome. *Neurology* 1996; **46**: 100–3.

13 Diener HC, Haupt WF, Kloss TM, Rosenow F, Philipp T, Koeppen S, et al. A preliminary, randomized, multicenter study comparing intravenous immunoglobulin, plasma exchange, and immune adsorption in Guillain–Barré syndrome. *Eur. Neurol.* 2001; **46**: 107–9.

14 Plasma Exchange/Sandoglobulin Guillain–Barré Syndrome Trial Group. Randomised trial of plasma exchange, intravenous immunoglobulin, and combined treatments in Guillain–Barré syndrome. *Lancet* 1997; **349**: 225–30.

15 Nomura T, Hamaguchi K, Hattori T, Satou T, Mannen T, et al. A randomized controlled trial comparing intravenous immunoglobulin and plasmapheresis in Guillain–Barré syndrome. *Neurological Therap.* 2000; **18**: 69–81.

16 Hughes RAC, Wijdicks E, Barohn RJ, Benson E, Cornblath DR, Hahn AF, et al. Practice parameter: immunotherapy for Guillain–Barré syndrome: Report of the Quality Standards Subcommittee of the American Academy of Neurology. *Neurology* 2003; **61**: 736–40.

17 Hughes RAC, Newsom-Davis JM, Perkin GD, Pierce JM. Controlled trial of prednisolone in acute polyneuropathy. *Lancet* 1978; **2**: 750–3.

18 Hughes RAC, Swan AV, van Koningsveld R, van Doorn PA. Corticosteroids for Guillain–Barré syndrome. *Cochrane Database Syst. Rev.* 2006; **2**: CD001446.

19 Bansal BC, Sood AK, Gupta AK, Yadav P. Role of steroids in the treatment of Guillain–Barré syndrome – a controlled trial. *Neurol. India* 2004; **34**: 329–35.

20 Shukla SK, Agarwal R, Gupta OP, Pande G, Mamta S. Double blind control trial of prednisolone in Guillain–Barré syndrome – a clinical study. *Clin.–India* 1988; **52**: 128–34.

21 Singh NK, Gupta A. Do corticosteroids influence the disease course or mortality in Guillain–Barré syndrome? *J. Assoc. Phys. India* 1996; **44**: 22–4.

22 Van Koningsveld R, Schmitz PIM, van der Meché FGA, Visser LH, Meulstee J, van Doorn PA, et al. Effect of methylprednisolone when added to standard treatment with intravenous immunoglobulin for Guillain–Barré syndrome: randomised trial. *Lancet* 2004; **363**: 192–6.

23 Guillain–Barré Syndrome Steroid Trial Group. Double-blind trial of intravenous methylprednisolone in Guillain–Barré syndrome. *Lancet* 1993; **341**: 586–90.

24 Hughes RAC, Wijdicks E, Barohn RJ, Benson E, Cornblath DR, Hahn AF, et al. Supportive care for Guillain–Barré syndrome. *Arch. Neurol.* 2005; **62**: 1194–8.

25 Ettayapuram V, Sunderrajan M, Davenport J. The Guillain–Barré syndrome: pulmonary-neurologic correlations. *Medicine* 1995; **64**(5): 333–41.

26 Pontoppidan H, Geffin B, Lowenstein E. Acute respiratory failure in the adult. 2. *N. Engl. J. Med.* 1972; **287**: 743–52.

27 McKhann GM, Griffin JW, Cornblath DR, Mellits ED, Fisher RS, Quaskey SA, et al. Plasmapheresis and Guillain–Barré syndrome: analysis of prognostic factors and the effect of plasmapheresis. *Ann. Neurol.* 1988; **23**: 347–53.

28 Holdgaard HO, Pedersen J, Jensen RH, Outzen KE, Midtgaard T, Johansen LV, et al. Percutaneous dilatational tracheostomy versus conventional surgical tracheostomy. A clinical randomised study. *Acta Anaesth. Scand.* 1998; **42**: 545–50.

29 Pfeiffer G, Schiller B, Kruse J, Netzer J. Indicators of dysautonomia in severe Guillain–Barré syndrome. *J. Neurol.* 1999; **246**: 1015–22.

30 Flachenecker P, Hartung HP, Reiners K. Power spectrum analysis of heart rate variability in Guillain–Barré syndrome. A longitudinal study. *Brain* 1997; **120**(Pt 10): 1885–94.

31 Samama MM, Cohen AT, Darmon JY, Desjardins L, Eldor A, Janbon C, et al. A comparison of enoxaparin with placebo for the prevention of venous thromboembolism in acutely ill medical patients. Prophylaxis in Medical Patients with Enoxaparin Study Group [see comments]. *N. Engl. J. Med.* 1999; **341**: 793–800.

32 Clagett GP, Reisch JS. Prevention of venous thromboembolism in general surgical patients. Results of meta-analysis. *Ann. Surg.* 1988; **208**: 227–40.

33 Pandey CK, Bose N, Garg G, Singh N, Baronia A, Agarwal A, et al. Gabapentin for the treatment of pain in Guillain–Barré syndrome: a double-blinded, placebo-controlled, crossover study. *Anesth. Analg.* 2002; **95**: 1719–23.

34 Tripathi M, Kaushik S. Carbamazepine for pain management in Guillain–Barré syndrome patients in the intensive care unit. *Crit. Care. Med.* 2000; **28**: 655–8.

35 Garssen MP, Bussmann JB, Schmitz PI, Zandbergen A, Welter TG, Merkies IS, et al. Physical training and fatigue, fitness, and quality of life in Guillain–Barré syndrome and CIDP. *Neurology* 2004; **63**: 2393–5.

36 Hughes RAC, Bouche P, Cornblath DR, Evers E, Hadden RDM, Hahn A, et al. European Federation of Neurological Societies/Peripheral Nerve Society guideline on management of chronic inflammatory demyelinating polyradiculoneuropathy. Report of a joint task force of the European Federation of Neurological Societies and the Peripheral Nerve Society. *J. Peripher. Nerv. Syst.* 2005; **10**: 220–8.

37 Mehndiratta MM, Hughes RA. Corticosteroids for chronic inflammatory demyelinating polyradiculoneuropathy. *Cochrane Database Syst. Rev.* 2002; **1**: CD002062.

38 Mehndiratta MM, Hughes RA, Agarwal P. Plasma exchange for chronic inflammatory demyelinating polyradiculoneuropathy. *Cochrane Database Syst. Rev.* 2004; **3**: CD003906.

39 van Schaik IN, Winer JB, de Haan R, Vermeulen M. Intravenous immunoglobulin for chronic inflammatory demyelinating polyradiculoneuropathy. *Cochrane Database Syst. Rev.* 2002; **2**: CD001797.

40 Dyck PJ, Litchy WJ, Kratz KM, Suarez GA, Low PA, Pineda AA, et al. A plasma exchange versus immune globulin infusion trial in chronic inflammatory demyelinating polyradiculoneuropathy. *Ann. Neurol.* 1994; **36**: 838–45.

41 Hughes RAC, Bensa S, Willison HJ, van den Bergh P, Comi G, Illa I, et al. Randomized controlled trial of intravenous immunoglobulin versus oral prednisolone in chronic inflammatory demyelinating polyradiculoneuropathy. *Ann. Neurol.* 2001; **50**: 195–201.

42 Hughes RA, Swan AV, van Doorn PA. Cytotoxic drugs and interferons for chronic inflammatory demyelinating polyradiculoneuropathy. *Cochrane Database Syst. Rev.* 2004; **4**: CD003280.

43 Lunn MP, Nobile-Orazio E. Immunotherapy for IgM anti-myelin-associated glycoprotein paraprotein-associated peripheral neuropathies. *Cochrane Database Syst. Rev.* 2006; **2**: CD002827.

44 van Schaik IN, Van den Berg LH, de Haan R. Intravenous immunoglobulin for multifocal motor neuropathy. *Cochrane Database Syst. Rev.* 2005; **2**: CD004429.

45 Umapathi T, Hughes RA, Nobile-Orazio E, Leger JM. Immunosuppressive treatment for multifocal motor neuropathy. *Cochrane Database Syst. Rev.* 2005; **3**: CD003217.

46 Peitersen E. Bell's Palsy: the spontaneous course of 2,500 peripheral facial nerve palsies of different etiologies. *Acta Otolaryngol. (Stockh)* 2002; **549**(Suppl.): 4–30.

47 Salinas RA, Alvarez G, Ferreira J. Corticosteroids for Bell's palsy (idiopathic facial paralysis). *Cochrane Database Syst. Rev.* 2004; **4**: CD001942.

48 Allen D, Dunn L. Aciclovir or valaciclovir for Bell's palsy (idiopathic facial paralysis). *Cochrane Database Syst. Rev.* 2004; **3**: CD001869.

49 National Center for Chronic Disease Prevention and Health Promotion. *Natl. Diab. Surveil. Syst.* www.cdc.gov/diabetes/statistics.

50 Boulton AJM, Vinik AI, Arezzo JC, Bril V, Feldman EL, Freeman R, Malik RA, Maser RE, Sosenko JM, Ziegler D. Diabetic neuropathies. A statement by the American Diabetes Association. *Diabetes Care* 2005; **28**: 956–62.

51 Thomas PK. Diabetic peripheral neuropathies: their cost to patient and society and the value of knowledge of risk factors for

development of interventions. *Eur. Neurol.* 1999; **41**(Suppl. 1): 35–43.

52 Gordois A, Schuffham P, Shearer A, Oglesby A, Tobian JA. The health care costs of diabetic peripheral neuropathy in the US. *Diabetes Care* 2003; **26**: 1790–5.

53 Boulton AJM. The diabetic foot: from art to science. The 18th Camillo Golgi lecture. *Diabetologia* 2004; **47**: 1343–53.

54 Singh N, Armstrong DG, Lipsky BA. Preventing foot ulcers in patients with diabetes. *JAMA* 2005; **293**: 217–28.

55 Trotta D, Verrotti A, Salladini C, Chiarelli F. Diabetic neuropathy in children and adolescents. *Pediatr. Diab.* 2004; **5**: 44–57.

56 Adriaensen H, Plaghki L, Mathieu C, Joffroy A, Vissers K. Critical review of oral drug treatments for diabetic neuropathic pain-clinical outcomes based on efficacy and safety data from placebo-controlled and direct comparative studies. *Diabetes Metab. Res. Rev.* 2005; **21**: 231–40.

57 Tesfaye S, Chaturvedi N, Eaton SEM, Ward JD, Manes C, Ionescu-Tirgoviste C, Witte DR, Fuller JH for the EURODIAB Prospective Complications Study Group. Vascular risk factors and diabetic neuropathy. *N. Engl. J. Med.* 2005; **352**: 341–50.

58 Writing Team for the Diabetes Control Trial. Effect of intensive therapy on the microvascular complications of type 1 diabetes mellitus. *JAMA* 2002; **287**: 2563–2569.

59 Navarro X, Sutherland DE, Kennedy WR. Long-term effects of pancreatic transplantation on diabetic neuropathy. *Ann. Neurol.* 1997; **42**: 727–36.

60 UK Prospective Diabetes Study (UKPDS) Group. Intensive blood-glucose control with sulphonylureas or insulin compared with conventional treatment and risk of complications in patients with type 2 diabetes (UKPDS 33). *Lancet* 1998; **352**: 837–53.

61 Azad N, Emanuele NV, Abraira C, Henderson WG, Colwell J, Levin SR, Nuttall FQ, Comstock JP, Sawin CT, Silbert C, Rubino FA. The effects of intensive glycaemic control on neuropathy in the VA cooperative study on type II diabetes mellitus (VA CSDM). *J. Diab. Complicat.* 1999; **13**: 307–13.

62 Vinik AI, Mehrabyan A. Diabetic neuropathies. *Med. Clin. N. Am.* 2004; **88**: 947–9.

63 Singleton JR, Smith AG, Russell JW, Feldman EL. Microvascular complications of impaired glucose tolerance. *Diabetes* 2003; **52**: 2867–73.

64 Simmons Z, Feldman EL. Treatment of diabetic neuropathy. In: Williams R, Herman W, Kinmonth A-L & Wareham NJ, eds., *The Evidence Base for Diabetes Care*. John Wiley & Sons, West Sussex, England, 2002: pp. 555–76.

65 Vincent AM, Feldman EL. New insights into the mechanisms of diabetic neuropathy. *Rev. Endo. Metab. Dis.* 2004; **5**: 227–36.

66 Saarto T, Wiffen PJ. Antidepressants for neuropathic pain. *Cochrane Database Syst. Rev.* 2005; **20**(3): CD005454 (Review).

67 Wiffen P, Collins S, McQuay H, Carroll D, Jadad A, Moore A. Anticonvulsant drugs for acute and chronic pain. *Cochrane Database Syst. Rev.* 2005; **3**: CD001133 (Review).

68 Vincent AM, Russell JW, Low P, Feldman EL. Oxidative stress in the pathogenesis of diabetic neuropathy. *Endocr. Rev.* 2004; **25**: 612–28.

69 Atroshi I, Gummesson C, Johnsson R, Ornstein E, Ranstam J, Prevalence of carpal tunnel syndrome in a general population. *JAMA* 1999; **282**: 153–8.

70 de Krom MC, Knipschild PG, Kester AD, Thijs CT, Boekkooi PF, Spaans F. Carpal tunnel syndrome, prevalence in the general population. *J. Clin. Epidemiol.* 1992; **45**: 373–6.

71 Hakim AJ, Cherkas L, El Zayat S, MacGregor AJ, Spector TD. The genetic contribution to carpal tunnel syndrome in women: a twin study. *Arthritis Rheum.* 2002; **47**(3): 275–9.

72 Padua L, Padua R, Aprile I, Pasqualetti P, Tonali P. Multi-perspective follow-up of untreated carpal tunnel syndrome: a multicenter study. *Neurology* 2001; **56**(11): 1459–66.

73 Anon. Practice parameter for carpal tunnel syndrome. *Neurology* 1993; **43**: 2406–9.

74 Marshall S, Tardif G, Ashworth N. Local corticosteroid injection for carpal tunnel syndrome. *Cochrane Database Syst. Rev.* 2002; **4**: CD001554.

75 O'Connor D, Marshall S, Massy-Westropp N. Non-surgical treatment (other than steroid injection) for carpal tunnel syndrome. *Cochrane Database Syst. Rev.* 2003; **1**: CD003219.

76 Scholten RJPM, Gerritsen AAM, Uitdehaag BMJ, van Geldere D, de Vet HCW, Bouter LM. Surgical treatment options for carpal tunnel syndrome. *Cochrane Database of Syst. Rev.* 2004; **4**: CD003905.

77 Verdugo RJ, Salinas RS, Castillo J, Cea JG. Surgical versus non-surgical treatment for carpal tunnel syndrome. *Cochrane Database Syst. Rev.* 2002; **2**: CD001552.

78 Gerritsen AAM, de Vet HCW, Scholten RJPM, Bertelsmann FW, de Krom MCTFM, Bouter LM. Splinting vs Surgery in the treatment of carpal tunnel syndrome: a randomised controlled trial. *JAMA* 2002; **288**: 1245–51.

79 Ly-Pen D, Andreu JL, de Blas G, Sanchez-Olaso A, Millan I. Surgical decompression versus local steroid injection in carpal tunnel syndrome: a one-year, prospective, randomized, open, controlled clinical trial. *Arthritis Rheum.* 2005; **52**: 612–19.

80 Hui AC, Wong S, Leung CH, Tong P, Mok V, Poon D, et al. A randomized controlled trial of surgery vs steroid injection for carpal tunnel syndrome. *Neurology* 2005; **64**: 2074–8.

81 Demirci S, Kutluhan S, Koyuncuoglu HR, Kerman M, Heybeli N, Akkus S, et al. Comparison of open carpal tunnel release and local steroid treatment outcomes in idiopathic carpal tunnel syndrome. *Rheumatol. Int.* 2002; **22**: 33–7.

82 Gokoglu F, Fndkoglu G, Yorgancoglu Z, Okumus M, Ceceli E, Kocaoglu S. Evaluation of iontophoresis and local corticosteroid injection in the treatment of carpal tunnel syndrome. *Am. J. Phys. Med. Rehabil.* 2005; **84**: 92–6.

83 O'Gradaigh D, Merry P. Corticosteroid injection for the treatment of carpal tunnel syndrome. *Ann. Rheum. Dis.* 2000; **59**: 918–19.

84 Assmus H. Korrektur und Rezidiveingriffe beim Karpaltunnel-syndrom. Bericht über 185 Nachoperationen. *Nervenarzt* 1996; **67**: 998–1002.

85 Bland JDP. Do nerve conduction studies predict the outcome of carpal tunnel decompression? *Muscle Nerve* 2001; **24**: 935–40.

86 Dammers JWHH, Veering MM, Vermeulen M. Injection with methylprednisolone proximal to the carpal tunnel: randomised double blind trial. *BMJ* 1999; **319**: 884–6.

87 Ozdogan H, Yazici H. The efficacy of local steroid injections in idiopathic carpal tunnel syndrome: a double-blind study. *Br. J. Rheumatol.* 1984; **23**: 272–5.

88 Girlanda P, Dattola R, Venuto C, Mangiapane R, Nicolosi C, Messina C. Local Steroid treatment in idiopathic carpal tunnel syndrome: short and long term efficacy. *J. Neurol.* 1993; **240**: 187–90.

89 Armstrong T, Devor W, Borschel L, Contreras R. Intracarpal steroid injection is safe and effective for short-term management of carpal tunnel syndrome. *Muscle Nerve* 2004; **29**: 82–8.

24

CHAPTER 24
Muscle disorders

Fiona Norwood, Michael R. Rose

Introduction

This chapter will evaluate the main management aspect for the following muscular disorders: Duchenne muscular dystrophy (DMD), Limb-girdle muscular dystrophies (LGMDs), Myasthenia gravis, Polymyositis.

Critical review of the evidence for each disorder

1. Duchenne muscular dystrophy

In a young boy with DMD, are there any effective drug treatments that are efficacious in halting deterioration or improving muscle strength? Might they have any harmful effects? At what age should treatment be started?

Background

The most common inherited muscle disorder, DMD, is also one of the most severe. Its incidence is 1 in 3500 liveborn males and thus it occurs in boys seen in general paediatric and paediatric neurology practice. Although mean survival has increased in the last couple of decades in particular, this is mainly due to improved general care and active management of respiratory insufficiency [1]. There has been much discussion over the past 40 years as to possible effective drug treatments and assessment of whether any may produce effective outcomes is clearly desirable. Administration of corticosteroids has been tried in previous decades but only recently subjected to full review.

Clinical scenario

Boys with DMD lose ambulation by 12 years of age. Wheelchair dependence increases the likelihood of complications such as scoliosis and ventilatory impairment. The aim of both drug and non-drug treatments is to prolong ambulation for as long as possible so as to delay the onset of these complications of which awareness and anticipation are essential. Physiotherapy techniques aim to prevent the development of fixed deformities such as limb contractures. For example, prevention or improvement of Achilles tendon contractures is an important factor in allowing walking stability to be maintained. If tendon contractures become excessively tight then surgical release may be indicated [2].

Evidence

Corticosteroid treatment has been the main drug modality used over the last few decades in an attempt to alter the natural history of the condition although the mechanism whereby it may produce stabilization or improvement in muscle strength has not been established. Despite the number of studies performed, evidence from just four randomized controlled studies was judged eligible for inclusion in the Cochrane Systematic Review [3–7]. This review had as its primary outcome measure the prolongation of ambulation but this was an outcome of only one study [3]. Therefore in the review secondary outcome measures of muscle strength and functional tests which were available from the other studies were also assessed. Three randomized controlled trials demonstrated improvements in muscle strength and function but for the relatively short period of 6 months [4,6,7] with the fourth study showing improvement for up to 2 years [3]. The studies reported data on a total of 161 patients treated with corticosteroids and compared with a total of 88 placebo patients. Most patients received prednisone ($n = 134$) with much smaller numbers treated with prednisolone ($n = 10$) and deflazacort ($n = 17$). The three studies of 6-month duration used prednisone or prednisolone given daily; deflazacort was used in an alternate-day regime at 2 mg/kg for the longer-time period of 2 years [3]. Prolongation of ambulation was reported by Angelini but Manzur et al. conclude that this conclusion was not supported by the statistical methods used. Secondary outcome measures of muscle strength assessments and tests of functional ability such as Gowers' time, timed walking tests and forced vital capacity were individually assessed from pooled data and all found to be better in the treated groups compared with placebo [4,6,7].

The Practice parameter produced by the American Academy of Neurology [8] also reviews relevant evidence for the treatment of DMD by corticosteroids. Seven class 1 trials were included [4,6,7,9–11], all showing improvement in various parameters including muscle strength, functional tests and lung function with minimum treatment durations of 6 months. Prednisone at three different daily doses (0.3, 0.75 or 1.5 mg/kg/day) was used and each was effective. 0.75 mg/kg/day produced an 11% net percentage increase in average strength score as well as improvement in timed functional tests. Alternate-day prednisone did not have the same effect when given at lower doses of 1.25 or 2.5 mg/kg but appears to be of possible benefit at doses of 5 mg/kg/day [11]. Deflazacort was used in two class 1 trials [3,12]. Mesa et al. used deflazacort at 1 mg/kg/day for 9 months whereas Angelini et al. used 2 mg/kg on alternate days for 2 years. Both groups showed sustained improvement in measured parameters.

Short-term adverse events from steroid treatment such as excessive weight gain and behavioural changes were found to be more common than placebo but deemed not severe. However there did appear to be a difference between deflazacort and prednisone in that only 6 months of treatment with the latter produced a statistically significant weight gain [4,6] whereas the longer 2-year treatment period with deflazacort did not [3]. Longer-term evaluation was not possible. Some of the weight gain may be from increased muscle mass as judged from 24-h urinary creatinine excretion [4]. Other potential side effects such as osteoporosis and dysglycaemia were not evaluated.

Summary

The dose of prednisone recommended in the conclusion of both reviews was 0.75 mg/kg/day. Side effects of treatment may necessitate dose reduction but even at the lower dose of 0.3 mg/kg/day improvement is seen. Deflazacort, if available, is recommended at a dose of 0.9 mg/kg/day [8]. There are no class 1 studies that examine the important question of the optimal age at which treatment should be started. The ideal duration of treatment is also unclear although class IV studies suggest continuation of improvement at 3 years [13].

2. Limb-girdle muscular dystrophies

Are there any effective interventions for these conditions and what is the evidence underlying their use?

Background

The LGMDs are all individually rare although for some conditions clear prevalence differences between different geographical populations are emerging. Although all the LGMDs are currently classified under one umbrella term, they are a heterogeneous group both in terms of their clinical features and molecular causation; they are classified together due to their general (but not exclusive) predilection for involvement of the proximal musculature. Establishing a precise molecular diagnosis may be a challenge and due to both this and to the uncommon nature of most of the LGMDs, randomized controlled trials of specific drug interventions are a distant prospect at present. The range of age of onset in the LGMDs is from childhood to late adult life. Despite this, general measures such as regular physiotherapy are applicable to the care of all these patients. Thus at present there is no clear unified molecular target for drug therapy and so clinical practice has emphasized the role of surveillance for, and timely intervention in, cardiac and respiratory complications. These can be treated with standard therapies.

Evidence

There is no RCT-based evidence to guide in the management of these collectively rare muscular dystrophies. However an expert panel has published useful guidelines [14]. Knowledge of the LGMD subtype may allow anticipation and timely intervention if respiratory and/or cardiac complications develop. Expert opinion currently recommends serial monitoring of respiratory function tests to be followed up by overnight oximetry if required. Provision of non-invasive ventilatory support has been shown to prolong life in conditions such as DMD and similar principles apply here. The frequency of monitoring may be modulated according to the expected prognosis associated with the particular LGMD subtype as some commonly involve the respiratory muscles whereas others rarely do so. For potential cardiac complications knowledge of the underlying diagnosis also guides onward referral for cardiac monitoring. Intervention in the development of cardiomyopathy and/or cardiac dysrhythmia may be needed.

3. Myasthenia gravis

1 *A 60-year-old man with acetylcholine receptor positive generalized myasthenia is referred to you. What should you use to treat him?*

2 *In a 20-year-old woman presenting with generalized and severe myasthenia gravis what is the evidence for and against thymectomy? At what stage of the disease should it be employed?*

Background

By far the most common neuromuscular junction disorder is acquired myasthenia gravis and this will be encountered in everyday clinical practice by the general neurologist. However, although the disorder is relatively common, each patient may present a unique set of circumstances with respect to possible therapeutic approaches. For example, consideration of age of onset, severity of disease, co-morbidities or a patient's wish to become pregnant may limit available drug and other options. We address two of many possible scenarios and the available evidence to guide treatment selection.

Corticosteroids

Oral corticosteroids are widely accepted as first line immunosuppressive treatment for autoimmune myasthenia gravis although there is surprisingly little definitive evidence of their efficacy compared with other treatments. Studies comparing corticosteroids with placebo are not possible due to ethical reasons. Evidence from randomized controlled trials was the subject of a Cochrane Review [15]. A variety of primary and secondary outcome measures were assessed in order to evaluate treatment efficacy in terms of clinical improvement, remission and adverse events. The authors found that treatment with prednisone did produce improvement in the short term compared with placebo but remarked on serious methodological flaws contained in all the studies. Two controlled studies comparing corticosteroids with placebo [16,17] are discussed. Both studies were of small numbers of patients, 13 for 2 years and 20 for 14 weeks, respectively. The 1998 study, which used intravenous methylprednisolone, produced the greater degree of strength enhancement with a relative rate of improvement of 7.2 times compared with the placebo group (Table 24.1). Zhang and Wu [21] examined different doses of corticosteroid in juvenile myasthenia and found that both were efficacious but that those receiving intravenous methylprednisolone improved more quickly and for longer.

Corticosteroids with azathioprine

Gajdos et al. compared corticosteroids with azathioprine [22] and found that similar percentages (72% and 74%, respectively) were in remission. Bromberg et al. also compared prednisone with azathioprine [19] over a year-long-study period; numbers were very small with only five patients in each group. The third randomized trial involving azathioprine is not discussed in the Cochrane Review but aimed to compare

prednisolone together with azathioprine against prednisolone alone [20]. This study demonstrated that a lower maintenance dose of prednisolone was required for those on combination treatment with azathioprine (Table 24.1).

Immunosuppressive treatments

Other immunosuppressive treatments have been tried. Cyclosporin treatment was examined by Tindall et al. and it was shown that patient strength measurements improved compared with placebo [23,24]. Cyclophosphamide induced remission compared with placebo in two further studies [25,26]. The latest agent to undergo close scrutiny is mycophenolate mofetil. The two studies conducted by Meriggioli et al. [27,28] were suggestive of improvement when compared with placebo but numbers were small. Tacrolimus at low dose has been studied in 19 patients with just under half showing improvement [29]. Overall, data from these studies is difficult to compare due to confounding factors such as whether or not the patient had undergone thymectomy and

Table 24.1 Corticosteroids and azathioprine for myasthenia gravis.

RCT	Intervention (dosage)	Outcome follow-up time	Results	
			n/N (%)	n/N (%)
			Corticosteroid	_Placebo_
Lindberg et al. [17]	_Corticosteroid_ MTPH 2 g intravenously on 2 consecutive days versus _Placebo_	Improvement in muscle after 2 weeks	8/10 (80%)	1/9 (11%)
Howard et al. [16]	_Corticosteroid_ Prednisone 100 mg on alternate days for 6 months, reduced by 10 mg every 2 weeks to 80 mg, then by 5 mg every 2 weeks to 20 mg if possible versus _placebo_	Improvement in muscle weakness at 6 months	3/6 (50%)	3/7 (43%)
			Corticosteroid	_AZTH_
MGCSG [18]*	_Corticosteroid_ Prednisone 1 mg/kg for 1 month, 0.5 mg/kg for 4 months, then 0.25 mg/kg p.o. daily versus _Azathioprine_ 3 mg/kg/day for 1 year then 2 mg/kg daily prednisone 1 mg/kg daily for 1 month	Number of patients Treatment failure within 5 years Remission or marked improvement	20 60%	21 24%
		after 1 year	72%	74%
		after 2 years	65%	76%
		after 3 years	67%	64%
Bromberg et al. [19]*	_Corticosteroid_ Prednisone 60 mg for 6 weeks versus _Azathioprine_ 50 mg	Improvement in muscle weakness, impairment and decrement after 1 year	4/5 (80%)	2/5 (40%)
			Corticosteroid	_Corticosteroids plus AZTH_
Palace et al. [20]	_Corticosteroids_ Prednisolone (1.5 mg/kg on alternate days) was tapered at remission to the minimal dose required to maintain remission plus placebo versus _Prednisolone plus azathioprine_ 2.5 mg/kg	Replaces and failures to remit over the 3 years	17/19 (89%)	9/15 (60%)

RCT: randomized controlled study. *unblind study.

so on. The evidence for the use of immunosuppressive agents in myasthenia gravis is currently receiving detailed evaluation and is the subject of a forthcoming Cochrane Review. The recent publication of consensus guidelines [30] reviews the results of published studies and recommends azathioprine together with corticosteroids, the aim of treatment being to progressively lower the steroid dose as the azathioprine becomes effective. This was a level A recommendation.

Thymectomy

The first step is to establish whether or not a thymoma is present. If it is then the decision as to whether to proceed to surgical removal is straightforward. Due to the potential of a thymoma to spread locally then excision is indicated. If necessary this should be followed by radiotherapy for those uncommon thymomas which are malignant.

In non-thymomatous patients the decision is less clear. Transsternal or transcervical thymectomy is a major procedure; perioperative risk may be increased by the concomitant use of corticosteroids or intravenous immunoglobulin, often used to increase a patient's respiratory and limb muscle strength before the operation. The aim of thymectomy in this group is to attain medication-free remission for as long a period as possible, or at least improvement in the underlying condition and reduction of medication. A review of thymectomy studies in non-thymomatous myasthenia gravis published as a Practice parameter for the American Academy of Neurology [31] appeared to demonstrate a definite benefit of the procedure although none of the trials reviewed was randomized controlled. Class II and III studies were evaluated and numerical adjustments were made in an attempt to reduce the impact of potential confounding factors. Twenty-eight articles ascertained from 1953 to 1998 were assessed; there was some overlap in the patient cohorts contained in these articles. All were designated class II studies as although patients either did or did not undergo thymectomy, none was assigned using a randomization procedure. Evaluation of the studies showed variation in patient type between cohorts (e.g. ocular myasthenia, presence or absence of thymic hyperplasia or not stated) as well as with study method (e.g. surgical technique, definition of remission criteria, duration of follow-up). Outcome assessments were not blinded. The outcome in most cohorts was consistent with the thymectomy patients showing a trend towards remission as judged by medication-freedom. The few exceptions to this were non-ideal studies in various respects, as the authors discuss. The issue of optimal timing of thymectomy was difficult to infer due to possible confounding factors such as prior treatments, gender differences and disease severity. Overall, adjusted median relative outcome rates showed a positive association between thymectomy and remission and improvement in myasthenia gravis. Consensus guidelines published recently concur with the above and recommend thymectomy for non-thymomatous patients as a level B recommendation [30].

Due to continuing uncertainties about the role of thymectomy, a multicentre randomized controlled trial has started recently and should eventually achieve the aim of allowing neurologists to assess the relative balance between benefits and risks of recommending surgery as well as the impact on subsequent medical treatments. For those patients with antibodies to muscle specific kinase (MuSK) the impact of thymectomy is unknown at present.

4. Polymyositis

Are there specific diagnostic criteria that I can apply to the diagnosis of myositis?
What is the best treatment for myositis?

Background

The precise incidence of myositis is hard to determine because of the lack of agreed diagnostic criteria and thus the lack of consistency in making the diagnosis. A number of diagnostic criteria for myositis have been proposed over the years but increasing knowledge of muscle diseases has widened the differential diagnosis that needs to be considered. Myositis is considered to be an acquired autoimmune inflammatory muscle disease that results in proximal muscle weakness; the so-called limb girdle distribution of weakness, a raised level of creatine kinase, abnormal electromyography and inflammation seen on muscle biopsy. It is generally considered to be responsive to anti-inflammatory or immunosuppressive suppressive treatment. Myositis may occur on isolation or in association with autoimmune lung disease, often with Jo-1 antibodies, and with other connective tissue diseases. Myositis can also be associated with overt or covert malignancy.

Clinical scenario

A 65-year-old lady is referred to your clinic by her GP. She was diagnosed as having myositis 3 months previously and has been treated with steroids which she continues to take as prednisolone 30 mg daily. However there has been no improvement in her symptoms and the patient has put on weight. The GP asks what should be done next.

Diagnosis

In the case scenario presented the first issue to resolve would be to confirm the diagnosis. You might want to look for specific diagnostic criteria for myositis to help you with the diagnosis. An attempted search for such criteria using MEDLINE will uncover many case reports and cases series and reviews of myositis but will not easily find agreed diagnostic criteria.

Probably the earliest quoted diagnostic criteria for myositis are those published by Bohan and Peters in 1975 [32]. The key elements of the criteria were that there should be weakness, a raised creatine kinase, EMG abnormalities supporting a diagnosis of myositis, evidence of inflammation on a muscle biopsy and exclusion of alternative muscle diseases.

The only distinguishing feature between polymyositis and dermatomyositis was that of a skin rash. The Bohan and Peters criteria however do not allow for the fact that the pathophysiology of polymyositis and dermatomyositis are different regardless of whether or not there is a skin rash. Polymyositis is a T-cell mediated disorder while dermatomyositis is a B-cell mediated disorder with activation of the complement cascade resulting in a vasculopathy. The Bohan and Peters criteria also do not allow the distinction between polymyositis and inclusion body myositis (IBM). IBM was first described in 1971 [33], with the first series published in 1989 [34] and therefore was not a recognized entity at the time of the Bohan and Peters criteria. It is now thought to be the commonest of the inflammatory myopathies. Advances in the diagnosis of hereditary muscular dystrophies has led to the appreciation that muscular dystrophies, such as LGMD type 2B with dysferlin deficiency, may have a late sub-acute consent with inflammation on muscle biopsy that mimics polymyositis. Although the Bohan and Peters criteria do require exclusion of other muscle diseases they could not have been specific about the exclusion of diseases such as IBM and dysferlinopathy which would require more detailed muscle biopsy analysis than would have been envisaged by Bohan and Peters. By contrast diagnostic criteria for IBM were agreed by an expert panel [35], have been endorsed by others [36] and seem uncontroversial.

More recent published diagnostic criteria for dermatomyositis or polymyositis that and tried to take account of latest advances in knowledge and muscle biopsy techniques will usually be by a few authors rather than by agreed multidisciplinary opinion [36–38]. As a result such diagnostic criteria will be the subject of dispute since polymyositis is a heterogeneous condition with different specialities having differing perspectives [39]. The neurologist will see polymyositis as part of a differential diagnosis of neuromuscular weakness, while the rheumatologist will see polymyositis more often in the context of muscle pain and with associated connective tissue disease.

In clinical practice it would therefore be important to review the diagnosis in our case scenario particularly with respect to the possibility of a revised diagnosis of IBM. In older people clinical experience shows this to be the commonest reason for the failure of a case of polymyositis to respond to treatment.

Treatment

If following diagnostic review the diagnosis is confirmed to be that of polymyositis then a review of the immunosuppressive or immuno-modulatory treatment would be appropriate. You might ask whether the dose of steroids is correct and whether an additional treatment is needed and if so which one. A search of the Cochrane Database of Systematic Reviews gives one relevant review of treatment of polymyositis [40,41]. However in this review by Choy et al. the emphasis is on the second line agents that are used to reduce if not replace the steroids for long-term immunotherapy. Such treatments are used in recognition of the fact that steroids while being good short-term immunosuppressive agents have side effects that preclude their long-term use. There is no evidence-based consensus on the dose or duration of treatment with steroids that would be appropriate in proven cases of polymyositis. However most clinicians would regard the 30 mg daily dose of prednisone being use in our clinical scenario as being a low dose and thus would advise an increased dose; perhaps as high as 1.5 mg/kg. If a second line agent is also being considered then the review by Choy et al. searched the Cochrane Neuromuscular Disease Group trials register for literature (searched February 2002 and updated November 2003) and MEDLINE (January 1966 to December 2002) identifying six qualifying trials. One of these trials was confined to dermatomyositis and is therefore not relevant to our scenario [42]. All the remaining trials used the Bohan and Peters diagnostic criteria [43–46]. Three were judged to be of high quality while two were open label with inadequate allocation concealment. The second line treatments assessed were plasma exchange, leukapheresis or sham apheresis with 12 treatments given over a 1-month period [43], 2 mg/kg/day azathioprine or placebo for 3 months in addition to 60 mg of prednisolone daily [47], prednisolone plus either low-dose methotrexate (15 mg weekly) or azathioprine (2.5 mg/kg daily) for 1 year [44], methotrexate 7.5 to 15 mg (mostly 10 mg) orally weekly or ciclosporin A 3.0 to 3.5 mg/kg/day for at least 6 months [45], oral methotrexate up to 25 mg weekly with azathioprine 150 mg daily for 6 months or intravenous methotrexate 500 mg/m^2 every 2 weeks for 12 treatments each with leucovorin rescue (50 mg/m^2 every 6 h for 4 doses) [46]. Thus only two of the relevant trials assessed immunosuppressive treatment against placebo. None of the trials gave statistically significant results in favour of any of the immunosuppressive treatments (Table 24.2). This is not to say that none of these treatments work but rather that the trials have not been adequately powered to show benefit. Since this systematic review fails to help answer our question we might try and seek guidance from less rigorous lines of evidence such as from non-randomized trials. Van de Vledkkert et al. conducted a MEDLINE and EMBASE search from 1966 to 2001 for French, German or English reports of treatment in dermatomyositis and polymyositis and found 92 eligible papers describing a total of 915 patients (92 of which were duplicated) in 74 single case reports and 18 case series. They assessed these reports using 10 standards that were thought important to allow any reader to recognize their own patient, copy the treatment and have some idea of the treatment effect. The conclusion was that the majority of the reports were of dubious quality and would not allow a useful systematic review [48]. Thus the decision as to what second line immunosuppressive treatment to use would have to be based upon expert opinion and personal preference.

Table 24.2 Second line treatments for polymyosites.

RCT	Intervention (dosage)	Outcome (follow-up time)	Active treatment Number of patients mean difference SD	Placebo Number of patients mean difference SD	WMD or relative risk (95% CI)	Comments
Bunch et al. [47]	Prednisolone 60 mg/day plus azathioprine (2 mg/kg/day) versus prednisolone plus placebo for 3 months.	Manual muscle testing after 3 months.	8 6.5 (23.5)	8 −1.1 (12.6)	5.40 (ns)	Azathioprine better
Dalakas et al. [42]	Intravenous immunoglobulin (2 g/kg/month) versus placebo for 3 months.	Manual muscle testing after 3 months.	8 8.50 (7.00)	7 −1.00 (2.40)	9.50 (4.33−14.67)	Intravenous immunoglobulin better
Miller et al. [43]	Plasma exchange or leukapheresis versus sham apheresis 12 treatments over a 1-month period.	Number of patients who improved after treatment.	6/26 (23%)	3/13 (23%)	1.00 (ns)	

ns: not statistically significant.

5. Facioscapulohumeral muscular dystrophy

Are there specific disease-modifying treatments or symptomatic treatments that could be used?

Background

Facioscapulohumeral muscular dystrophy (FSHD) is an autosomal dominant muscle disease with a characteristic pattern of muscle involvement as its name suggests. It is associated with contractions of the D4Z4 repeat in the subtelomere of chromosome 4q however the precise mechanism by which this results in the disease is unknown [49].

Clinical scenario

A 25-year-old man is referred to your clinic with a genetically proven diagnosis of FSHD. He wants to know if there is any treatment that could help him.

Evidence

Part of the difficulty of finding a suitable treatment for FSHD is that its precise pathogenesis is unknown and therefore disease specific approaches cannot be employed. Thus the search for potential treatments has been confined either to those treating aspects of the pathology or else generic muscle disease treatments. Occasional muscle biopsies from those with FSHD can show inflammatory cell infiltrates and so it is tempting to suggest steroid treatment. However this did not help in one open label study [50]. A Cochrane Systematic Review searched the Cochrane Neuromuscular Disease Group specialized register in August 2003, MEDLINE from January 1966 to August 2003 and EMBASE from January 1980 to August 2003 [51]. It identified one RCT which compared creatine supplementation with placebo finding a non-significant difference in favour of creatine [52]. One other RCT compared high- and low-dose albuterol (salbutamol) with placebo showing no significant difference in muscle strength at 1 year but some improvement in secondary measures such as lean body mass and handgrip [53]. A further RCT combining albuterol with exercise showed limited positive effects on muscle strength and volume but not of a sufficient degree as to justify its routine use [54].

Scapular winging can be a prominent and disabling feature of FSHD. The periscapular weakness results in inadequate scapular fixation such that the deltoid muscle which may be relatively preserved cannot elevate the arm. Thus scapular fixation may be a way to significantly improve shoulder elevation resulting in very worthwhile functional gains. A Cochrane Review which searched the literature up to March 2003 did not identify any RCTs for scapular fixation [55]. The review did highlight the potential benefits of the procedure but also the potential hazards which include post-operative pain, respiratory compromise due to splinting of the chest wall and failure of the fixation procedure. There was also a paucity of information regarding the long-term prognosis and benefit for this procedure.

References

1 Eagle M, Baudouin SV, Chandler C, Giddings DR, Bullock R, Bushby K. Survival in Duchenne muscular dystrophy: improvements in life expectancy since 1967 and the impact of home nocturnal ventilation. *Neuromuscl. Disord.* 2002; **12**(10): 926–9.

2 Sussman M. Duchenne muscular dystrophy. *J. Am. Acad. Orthop. Surg.* 2002; **10**(2): 138–51.

3 Angelini C, Pegoraro E, Turella E, Intino MT, Pini A, Costa C. Deflazacort in Duchenne dystrophy: study of long-term effect. *Muscle Nerve* 1994; **17**(4): 386–91.

4 Griggs RC, Moxley III RT, Mendell JR, Fenichel GM, Brooke M H, Pestronk A, Miller JP. Prednisone in Duchenne dystrophy. A randomized, controlled trial defining the time course and dose response. Clinical Investigation of Duchenne Dystrophy Group. *Arch. Neurol.* 1991; **48**(4): 383–8.

5 Manzur AY, Kuntzer T, Pike M, Swan A. Glucocorticoid corticosteroids for Duchenne muscular dystrophy. *Cochrane Database Syst. Rev.* 2004; 2: CD003725.

6 Mendell JR, Moxley RT, Griggs RC, Brooke MH, Fenichel GM, Miller JP, King W, Signore L, Pandya S, Florence J, Schierbecker J, Robison J, Kaiser K, Mandel S, Arkfen C, Gilder B. Randomised double blind six month trial of prednisone in Duchenne's muscular dystrophy. *N. Engl. J. Med.* 1989; **320**: 1592–7.

7 Rahman MM, Hannan MA, Mondol BA, Bhoumick NB, Haque A. Prednisolone in Duchenne muscular dystrophy. *Bangladesh Med. Res. Counc. Bull.* 2001; **27**(1): 38–42.

8 Moxley III RT, Ashwal S, Pandya S, Connolly A, Florence J, Mathews K, Baumbach L, McDonald C, Sussman M, Wade C. Practice parameter: corticosteroid treatment of Duchenne dystrophy: report of the Quality Standards Subcommittee of the American Academy of Neurology and the Practice Committee of the Child Neurology Society. *Neurology.* 2005; **64**(1): 13–20.

9 Backman E, Henriksson KG. Low-dose prednisolone treatment in Duchenne and Becker muscular dystrophy. *Neuromuscul. Disord.* 1995; **5**(3): 233–41.

10 Fenichel GM, Mendell JR, Moxley III RT, Griggs RC, Brooke MH, Miller JP, Pestronk A, Robison J, King W, Signore L. A comparison of daily and alternate-day prednisone therapy in the treatment of Duchenne muscular dystrophy. *Arch. Neurol.* 1991; **48**(6): 575–9.

11 Siegel IM, Miller JE, Ray RD. Failure of corticosteroid in the treatment of Duchenne (pseudo-hypertrophic) muscular dystrophy. Report of a clinically matched three year double-blind study. *IMJ. Ill. Med. J.* 1974; **145**(1): 32–3.

12 Mesa LE, Dubrovsky AL, Corderi J, Marco P, Flores D. Steroids in Duchenne muscular dystrophy–deflazacort trial. *Neuromuscul. Disord.* 1991; **1**(4): 261–6.

13 Fenichel GM, Florence JM, Pestronk A, Mendell J R, Moxley III RT, Griggs RC, Brooke MH, Miller JP, Robison J, King W.Long-term benefit from prednisone therapy in Duchenne muscular dystrophy. *Neurology* 1991; **41**(12): 1874–7.

14 Norwood F, de Visser M, Eymard B, Lochmuller H and Bushby K. Limb girdle muscular dystrophies. In: Hughes RAC, Brainin M & Gilhus NE, eds., *European Handbook of Neurological Management*, Blackwell Publishing, Oxford, 2006.

15 Schneider-Gold C, Gajdos P, Toyka KV, Hohlfeld RR. Corticosteroids for myasthenia gravis. *Cochrane Database Syst. Rev.* 2005; 2: CD002828.

16 Howard Jr FM, Duane DD, Lambert EH, Daube JR. Alternate-day prednisone: preliminary report of a double-blind controlled study. *Ann. NY Acad. Sci.* 1976; **274**: 596–607.

17 Lindberg C, Andersen O, Lefvert AK. Treatment of myasthenia gravis with methylprednisolone pulse: a double blind study. *Acta Neurol. Scand.* 1998; **97**(6): 370–373.

18 Myasthenia Gravis Clinical Study Group. A randomised clinical trial comparing prednisone and azathioprine in myasthenia gravis. Results of a second interim analysis. *Journal of Neurology, Neurosurgery and Psychiatry* 1993; **56**(11): 1157–63.

19 Bromberg MB, Wald JJ, Forshew DA, Feldman EL, Albers JW. Randomized trial of azathioprine or prednisone for initial immunosuppressive treatment of myasthenia gravis. *J. Neurol. Sci.* 1997; **150** (1): 59–62.

20 Palace J, Newsom-Davis J, Lecky B. A randomized double-blind trial of prednisolone alone or with azathioprine in myasthenia gravis. Myasthenia Gravis Study Group. *Neurology* 1998; **50**(6): 1778–83.

21 Zhang J, Wu H. Effectiveness of steroid treament in juvenile myasthenia. *Chinese J. Paediatr.* 1998; **36**: 612–14.

22 Myasthenia Gravis Study Group A randomised clinical trial comparing prednisone and azathioprine in myasthenia gravis. Results of the second interim analysis. Myasthenia Gravis Clinical Study Group. *J. Neurol. Neurosurg. Psychiatr.* 1993; **56**: 1157–63.

23 Tindall RS, Rollins JA, Phillips JT, Greenlee RG, Wells L, Belendiuk G. Preliminary results of a double-blind, randomized, placebo-controlled trial of cyclosporine in myasthenia gravis. *N. Engl. J. Med.* 1987; **316**(12): 719–24.

24. Tindall RS, Phillips JT, Rollins JA, Wells L, Hall K. A clinical therapeutic trial of cyclosporine in myasthenia gravis, *Ann. NY Acad. Sci.* 1993; **681**: 539–51.

25 De Feo LG, Schottlender J, Martelli NA, Molfino NA. Use of intravenous pulsed cyclophosphamide in severe, generalized myasthenia gravis. *Muscle Nerve.* 2002; **26**(1): 31–6.

26 Perez MC, Buot WL, Mercado-Danguilan C, Bagabaldo ZG, Renales LD. Stable remissions in myasthenia gravis. *Neurology* 1981; **31**(1): 32–7.

27 Meriggioli MN, Rowin J, Richman JG, Leurgans S., Mycophenolate mofetil for myasthenia gravis: a double-blind, placebo-controlled pilot study. *Ann. NY Acad. Sci.* 2003; **998**: 494–9.

28 Meriggioli MN, Ciafaloni E, Al Hayk KA, Rowin J, Tucker-Lipscomb B, Massey JM, Sanders DB. Mycophenolate mofetil for myasthenia gravis: an analysis of efficacy, safety, and tolerability. *Neurology* 2003; **61**(10): 1438–40.

29. Konishi T, Yoshiyama Y, Takamori M, Yagi K, Mukai E, Saida T. Clinical study of FK506 in patients with myasthenia gravis. *Muscle Nerve* 2003; **28**(5): 570–4.

30 Skeie GO, Apostolski S, Evoli A, Gilhus NE, Hart IK, Harms L, Hilton-Jones D, Melms A, Verschuuren J, Horge HW. Guidelines for the treatment of autoimmune neuromuscular transmission disorders. *Eur. J. Neurol.* 2006; **13**(7): 691–9.

31 Gronseth GS, Barohn RJ. Practice parameter: Thymectomy for autoimmune myasthenia gravis (an evidence-based review): Report of the Quality Standards Subcommittee of the American Academy of Neurology. *Neurology* 2000; **55**: 7–15.

32 Bohan A, Peter JB. Polymyositis and dermatomyositis (first of two parts). *N. Engl. J. Med.* 1975; **292**: 344–7.

33 Yunis EJ, Samaha FJ. Inclusion body myositis. *Lab. Invest.* 1971; **25**: 240–8.

34 Lotz BP, Engel AG, Nishino H, Stevens JC, Litchy WJ. Inclusion body myositis. Observations in 40 patients. *Brain* 1989; **112**: 727–47.

35 Griggs RC, Askanas V, DiMauro S, Engel AG, Karpati G, Mendell JR, Rowland LP. Inclusion body myositis and myopathies *Ann. Neurol.* 1995; **38**: 705–13.

36 Muller-Felber W, Pongratz D, Reimers C. 64th ENMC International Workshop: therapeutic approaches to dermatomyositis, polymyositis, and inclusion body myositis 29–31 January 1999, Naarden, The Netherlands. *Neuromuscul. Disord.* 2001; **11**(1): 88–92.

37 Dalakas MC. Polymyositis dermatomyositis and inclusion-body myositis. *N. Engl. J. Med.* 1991; **325**: 1487–98.

38 Dalakas MC, Hohlfeld R. Diagnostic criteria for polymyositis and dermatomyositis. *Lancet* 2003; **362**: 1763.

39 Miller FW, Rider LG, Plotz PH, Isenberg DA, Oddis CV., Diagnostic criteria for polymyositis and dermatomyositis. *Lancet* 2003; **362**: 1762–3.

40 Choy EH, Hoogendijk J, Lecky BR, Winer J. Immunosuppressant and immunomodulatory treatment for dermatomyositis and polymyositis. *Cochrane Database Syst. Rev.* 2005; **3**.

41 Rose MR, Griggs R, Dalakas M. Immunotherapy for inclusion body myositis (Protocol for a Cochrane Review). *The Cochrane Library*, 1999; 4, Update Software.

42 Dalakas MC, Illa I, Dambrosia JM, Soueidan SA, Stein DP, Otero C, Dinsmore ST, McCrosky S.,A controlled trial of high-dose intravenous immune globulin infusions as treatment for dermatomyositis. *N. Engl. J. Med.* 1993; **329**(27): 1993–2000.

43 Miller FW, Leitman SF, Cronin ME, Hicks JE, Leff RL, Wesley R, Fraser DD, Dalakas M, Plotz PH. Controlled trial of plasma exchange and leukapheresis in polymyositis and dermatomyositis. *N. Engl. J. Med.* 1992; **326**: 1380–4.

44 Miller J, Walsh Y, Saminaden S, Lecky BR.F, Winer JB. Randomised double blind controlled trial of methotrexate and steroids compared with azathioprine and steroids in the treatment of idiopathic inflammatory myopathy. *J. Neurol. Sci.* 2002; **199**(Suppl.): S53.

45 Vencovsky J, Jarosova K, Machacek S, Studynkova J, Kafkova J, Bartunkova J, Nemcova D, Charvat F. Cyclosporine A versus methotrexate in the treatment of polymyositis and dermatomyositis. *Scand. J Rheumatol.* 2000; **29**(2): 95–102.

46 Villalba L, Hicks JE, Adams EM, Sherman JB, Gourley MF, Leff RL, Thornton BC, Burgess SH, Plotz PH, Miller FW. Treatment of refractory myositis: a randomized crossover study of two new cytotoxic regimens. *Arthritis Rheum.* 1998; **41**(3): 392–9.

47 Bunch TW, Worthington JW, Combs JJ, Ilstrup DM, Engel AG. Azathioprine with prednisone for polymyositis. A controlled, clinical trial. *Ann. Intern. Med.* 1980; **92**(3): 365–9.

48 van de Vlekkert J, Tjin-A-Ton ML, Hoogendijk JE. Quality of myositis case reports open to improvement. *Arthritis Rheum.* 2004; **51**(1): 148–50.

49 Lemmers RJ, de Kievit P, Sandkuijl L, Padberg GW, van Ommen G. J, Frants RR, van der Maarel SM. Facioscapulohumeral muscular dystrophy is uniquely associated with one of the two variants of the 4q subtelomere. *Nat. Genet.* 2002; **32**(2): 235–6.

50 Tawil R, McDermott MP, Pandya S, King W, Kissel J, Mendell JR. A pilot trial of prednisone in facioscapulohumeral muscular dystrophy. FSH-DY Group. *Neurology* 1997; **48**: 46–9.

51 Rose MR, Tawil R. Drug treatment for facioscapulohumeral muscular dystrophy. *CochraneDatabaseSyst. Rev.* 2004; 2: CD002276.

52 Walter MC, Lochmuller H, Reilich P, Klopstock T, Huber R, Hartard M, Hennig M, Pongratz D, Muller-Felber W. Creatine monohydrate in muscular dystrophies: A double-blind, placebo-controlled clinical study. *Neurology* 2000; **54**(9): 1848–50.

53 Kissel JT, McDermott MP, Natarajan R, Mendell JR, Pandya S, King WM, Griggs RC, Tawil R. Pilot trial of albuterol in facioscapulohumeral muscular dystrophy. FSH-DY Group. *Neurology* 1998; **50**(5): 1402–6.

54 van der Kooi EL, Vogels OJ, van Asseldonk RJ, Lindeman E, Hendriks JC, Wohlgemuth M, van der Maarel SM, Padberg GW. Strength training and albuterol in facioscapulohumeral muscular dystrophy. *Neurology* 2004; **63**(4): 702–8.

55 Mummery CJ, Copeland SA, Rose MR. Scapular fixation in muscular dystrophy. *Cochrane Database Syst. Rev.* 2003; 3: CD003278.

Index

Note: Page numbers in italics refer to figures and tables.